MECHANISMS OF CELL-MEDIATED CYTOTOXICITY

ADVANCES IN EXPERIMENTAL MEDICINE AND BIOLOGY

Recent Volumes in this Series

Volume 137
THE RUMINANT IMMUNE SYSTEM
Edited by John E. Butler

Volume 138
HORMONES AND CANCER
Edited by Wendell W. Leavitt

Volume 139
TAURINE IN NUTRITION AND NEUROLOGY
Edited by Ryan Huxtable and Herminia Pasantes-Morales

Volume 140
COMPOSITION AND FUNCTION OF CELL MEMBRANES: Application to the Pathophysiology of Muscle Diseases
Edited by Stewart Wolf and Allen K. Murray

Volume 141
BIOCHEMISTRY AND FUNCTION OF PHAGOCYTES
Edited by F. Rossi and P. Patriarca

Volume 142
BIOCHEMISTRY AND BIOLOGY OF CORONAVIRUSES
Edited by V. ter Meulen, S. Siddell, and H. Wege

Volume 143
RELAXIN
Edited by Ralph R. Anderson

Volume 144
MUCUS IN HEALTH AND DISEASE II
Edited by Eric N. Chantler, James B. Elder, and Max Elstein

Volume 145
TERMINAL TRANSFERASE IN IMMUNOBIOLOGY AND LEUKEMIA
Edited by Umberto Bertazzoni and Fred J. Bollum

Volume 146
MECHANISMS OF CELL-MEDIATED CYTOTOXICITY
Edited by William R. Clark and Pierre Golstein

MECHANISMS OF CELL-MEDIATED CYTOTOXICITY

Edited by

William R. Clark
University of California
Los Angeles, California

and

Pierre Golstein
Centre d'Immunologie
INSERM-CNRS de Marseille-Luminy
Marseille, France

PLENUM PRESS • NEW YORK AND LONDON

Library of Congress Cataloging in Publication Data

International Workshop on Mechanisms in Cell-Mediated Cytotoxicity (1st: 1981: Carry-le-Rouet, France)
Mechanisms of cell-mediated cytotoxicity.

(Advances in experimental medicine and biology v. 146)
"Proceedings of the First International Workshop on Mechanisms in Cell-Mediated Cytotoxicity, held September 14-16, 1981, in Carry-le-Rouet, France"—T.p. verso.
Includes bibliographical references and index.
1. Cellular immunity—Congresses. 2. Cell-mediated lympholysis—Congresses. 3. Killer cells—Congresses. 4. Cell death—Congresses. I. Clark, William R., 1938- . II. Golstein, Pierre, 1939- III. Title. IV. Series. [DNLM: 1. Cytotoxicity, Immunologic—Congresses. W1 AD559 v. 146 / QW 568 I62 1981m]
QR185.5.I57 1982 616.07'9 82-5312

DOI 10.1007/978-1-4684-8959-0

Proceedings of the First International Workshop on Mechanisms in Cell-Mediated Cytotoxicity, held September 14–16, 1981, in Carry-le-Rouet, France

MyCopy version of the original edition 1982

A Division of Plenum Publishing Corporation
233 Spring Street, New York, N.Y. 10013

The following organizations provided financial support for this Workshop.

Centre National de la Recherche Scientifique (through a CNRS/NSF agreement)

Delegation Generale a la Recherche Scientifique et Technique

National Cancer Institute

Grand Island Biological Company

E. I. du Pont de Nemours and Company

Merck, Sharpe and Dome Research Laboratories

Pfizer, Inc.

The Upjohn Company

PREFACE

The First International Workshop on Mechanisms in Cell-Mediated Cytoxicity was held at Carry-le-Rouet, France, September 14-16, 1981. The Workshop brought together for the first time leading investigators in each of the principal areas of cell-mediated cytotoxicity, as well as experts in the area of complement-mediated cytoxicity. Formal research presentations were held to a minimum, the emphasis being on open discussion of current knowledge about mechanisms of cytoxicity in each of the systems under consideration. The major objectives of the Workshop were 1) to compare and integrate what is known about the mechanism(s) of cytoxicity in each system; 2) to determine whether, on the basis of information in hand, it seems likely that the mechanisms of cytotoxicity in the various systems are the same or are unique; and 3) to stimulate thinking about new approaches to elucidating the fundamental mechanisms by which certain cells are able to kill other cells.

This volume is intended as something more than a simple report or record of the Workshop. Various participants were asked to write either a review on a given topic, or a more detailed specific account of relevant current research. The mass of formal presentation in this volume thus far exceeds the amount of formal presentation that actually occurred. Each author has been encouraged to engage in a bit more speculation about possible mechanisms than might be appropriate for a standard research journal. Moreover, because most of the time in the various sessions was spent in open discussion we have tried to capture some of that flavor by appending portions of these discussions after papers, where appropriate. This may convey some impression of how at least some of us defend our present-day uncertainties.

Clearly a meeting of this scope could not have happened without the efforts and talents of a good many people. Gideon Berke helped formulate the original concept of a Workshop devoted exclusively to cell-mediated cytotoxicity. The Organizing Committee (G. Berke, M. Bevan, M. Hanna, P. Henkart, C. Henney, H.R. MacDonald, E. Martz) contributed valuable ideas about organization of the Workshop, potential participants, publication of the proceedings, etc. We would also like to express our appreciation to A.-M. Schmitt-Verhulst for her work with the local Organizing Committee, and to other participants who agreed to chair the various sessions not covered by members of the Organizing Committee (B. Bonavida, I.C.M. MacLennan, M. Mayer, P. Perlmann, E. Simpson). Their help and indeed that of the all participants contributed greatly to the success of the Workshop.

We hope that this book will provide not only a snapshot of the present state of the art, but an account of how a relatively small group of workers tries to tackle an apparently well-defined but difficult experimental problem. The aim of the book is to realize the first goal of the Workshop: to compare and integrate what is known about mechanisms of cytotoxicity. Whether the Workshop achieved its remaining two aims we leave to the reader of this volume to evaluate.

CONTENTS

SECTION I. LYSIS BY CYTOTOXIC T LYMPHOCYTES: MORPHOLOGICAL AND PHYSIOLOGICAL ASPECTS

SECTION III. THE USE OF ANTISERA, MONOCLONAL ANTIBODIES, AND CLONED EFFECTOR CELLS IN THE STUDY OF CELL-MEDIATED CYTOLYSIS

SECTION I. LYSIS BY CYTOTOXIC T LYMPHOCYTES: MORPHOLOGICAL AND PHYSIOLOGICAL ASPECTS

INTRODUCTION

T cell-mediated cytolysis has been thoroughly studied with respect to its morphological aspects, using a variety of techniques such as electron microscopy, microcinematography, fluorescence microscopy and interference contrast microscopy. In conjugates of effector and target cells there is, perhaps upon triggering by specific antigen recognition, a polarisation of the actin(not myosin) network in the effector cell towards the area of contact (Ryser and Vassali), and a localisation of the centriole in this region. There are strong movements in the contact zone (Ryser and Vassali) with effector-cell microfilament-containing projections "into" the target cell (Sanderson), with however no detectable rupture of the target cell plasma membrane. Target cell death manifests itself spectacularly as zeiosis, a way of dying that may be characteristic of lymphoid cell-mediated cytolysis (Sanderson). These observations have led to mechanical models for the lethal hit, the reorganisation of the actin network enabling a mechanical hit (Ryser and Vassali) perhaps via effector cell projections causing physical damage into the target cell (Sanderson). Studies with liposomes suggest the possibility that the disruption of the target cell sub-membranous matrix structure could lead to membrane destabilization and ultimately cell lysis (Mescher et al).

A mechanical model based on alterations of the biphysical properties of the target cell membrane itself, upon interactions with the effector cell membrane, has been developed (Berke and Clark, Clark and Berke). One aspect of it, namely the apparently necessary involvement of target cell MHC as target molecules, seemed to be supported by observations suggesting that in so-called "non-specific" lectin-mediated cytolysis the effector cell may see MHC molecules in conjunction with the lectin at the target cell surface (Berke and Clark). In particular, in a given system preincubation of target but not of effector cells in the presence of Concanavalin A led to lectin-mediated lysis. However, other situations were found; some cloned cytolytic T cells can mediate lectin-facilitated cytolysis if preincubated with Concanavalin A (Wall and Fitch), and evidence was given that lectin-mediated cytolysis may require that the lectin both bridges effector and target cells and activates the effector cells (Green). Peculiarities of the specificity of recognition by CTLs are described and discussed (Brondz et al).

Any hypothesis on the mechanism of T cell-mediated cytotoxicity that would relate it too exclusively to recognition may run the risk of not fully accounting for some post-recognition metabolic requirements and for polarity of cytolysis (briefly reviewed by Golstein). Especially the requirement for calcium is essential, and its site of action has been studied (Martz). Perhaps one way to reconcile the striking morphological observations supporting mechanical models and the post-recognition metabolic requirements is to consider a hybrid hypothesis: target cell death might result from the combined effect on the target cell membrane of a mechanical conjugation-induced fragilization and of effector cell-produced enzymes (Zagury).

MORPHOLOGICAL ASPECTS OF LYMPHOCYTE MEDIATED CYTOTOXICITY

Colin J. Sanderson

National Institute for Medical Research
The Ridgeway
Mill Hill, London NW7 1AA

INTRODUCTION

In this review I am going to discuss the contact-mediated killing of nucleated mammalian cells by cytotoxic T cells (Tc cells) and antibody-dependent K cells. I wish to suggest that the mechanism of killing by Tc cells and K cells is similar, although a different receptor-ligand interaction is involved in the two types of killing. Tc cells have a specific receptor which reacts with antigen on the target cell while K cells have an Fc receptor reacting with antibody on the surface of the target cell. Because of apparent similarities between NK cells and K cells it is possible that all three classes of lymphoid cell share the same mechanism of killing.

The lysis of cells by antibody and complement is relatively well characterized, and has often been proposed as a model for Tc cell killing. Thus, it has been suggested that the Tc cell may insert the final complement components or similar molecules into the target cell membrane, causing colloid osmotic lysis (1). However, because the morphological and biochemical changes in the target cell are not consistent with colloid osmotic lysis I suggest that the mechanisms of killing are different.

The most characteristic feature of cell death caused by cytotoxic lymphocytes is 'zeiosis.' This is a phenomenon in which blebbing of the membrane takes place, giving the impression that the cell is boiling (2), particularly when speeded up in time-lapse films. Although it is convenient to use this term to describe this stage of target cell death, it has also been used to describe other blebbing phenomena which may not be related to the changes occurring in lymphocyte-mediated cytotoxicity. For example, some types of cells show blebbing at mitosis. In the cell types that I have studied, mitotic blebbing is much less spectacular than that seen in lymphocyte-mediated cytotoxicity. It must also be remembered that zeiosis observed in time-lapse films depends very much on the time interval between frames, thus slow blebbing over several hours can be made to resemble fast blebbing lasting a few minutes, if different time intervals are used in filming. Zeiosis similar to that seen in lymphocyte-mediated cytotoxicity has been described in other types of cell death, and it will be suggested that an understanding of the mechanism of these types of cell death might lead to a better understanding of lymphocyte-mediated cytotoxicity.

LYSIS BY COMPLEMENT

Potassium is released more rapidly than macromolecules in complement mediated lysis (3), which was interpreted as colloid osmotic lysis. This was defined as the equilibration of ions between cell and medium, resulting in an increase in osmotic pressure in the cell caused by intracellular macromolecules and leadng to an influx of water. The cell membrane and its lesions were thought to become stretched as the cell swelled, permitting macromolecules to escape.

Fig. 1. Time-lapse sequences of the killing of P815 tumour cells (time shown in minutes). The fact that sequences B and C show similar timing is fortuitous.

(A) Lysis by antibody and complement. The two cells lyse at about the same rate. A progressive darkening under phase contrast can be seen in the frames at 13, 27 and 40 minutes. At 53 minutes cytoplasmic contents appear to burst out of the cell (this is only visible in the complete film). At about 60 minutes the cells swell suddenly and the remaining organelles can be seen in Brownian motion. Throughout the lytic process the cell membrane remains static.

(B) Phase-contrast film of Tc cell cytotoxocity. At time zero (an arbitrary time point in the film) two Tc cells (arrows) can be seen in contact wth a P815 tumour cell.

At 5 minutes the P815 cell is undergoing zeiosis, and two obvious blebs are visible opposite the Tc cells. At 10 minutes the cell has become quiescent. It retains phase contrast, indicating that significant loss of cytoplasmic contents has not occurred. The cell shows no membrane

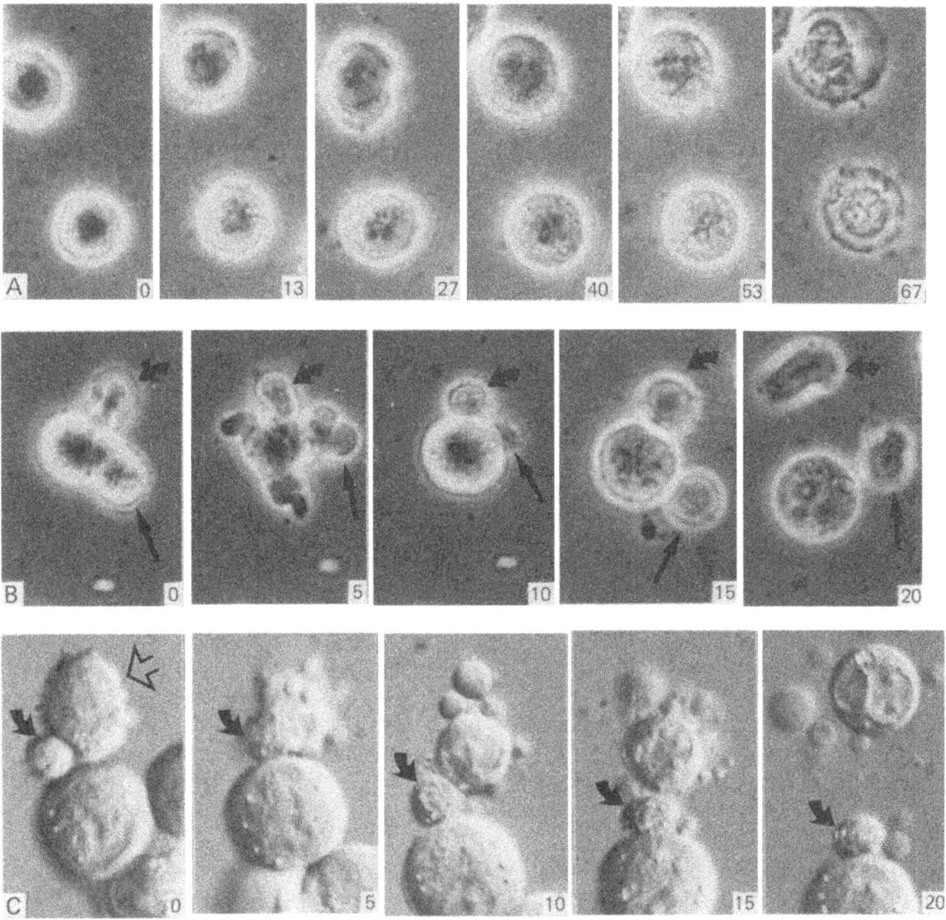

movement after zeiosis. By 15 minutes the cytoplasmic contents have burst out, and the cell swells. By 20 minutes the cell is a swollen ghost and the two T cells have detached and are migrating away.

(C) Nomarski optics of Tc cell cytotoxicity. At time zero (an arbitrary time point in the film) the Tc cell (curved arrow) can be seen in contact with two P815 tumour cells. One of these cells (broad arrow) is showing the very early signs of zeiosis. Small blebs are developing over the whole membrane. At 5 minutes the P815 cell is undergoing spectacular zeiosis. At 10 minutes some of the blebs can be seen to have broken away from the cell, and by 15 minutes there is massive bursting out of cell material. By 20 minutes the Tc cell has broken contact and the target cell is a swollen ghost. Cell debris is visible around the target cell. (From ref. 4)

Although the insertion of the complement components clearly leads to a leakage of cell contents (Lachmann, this volume), there remains some doubt that this definition of colloid osmotic lysis accurately describes the lytic process. For example, time-lapse films of mouse mastocytoma (P815) cells undergoing lysis by antibody and complement (Fig. 1A) show a gradual loss of refractile material (under phase contrast) followed by a burst of material from the cell. Cell swelling occurs after this burst. This and other experiments discussed more fully elsewhere (4) leave some doubt on the role of osmotic swelling in lysis by complement. It is clear, however, that zeiosis, which is characteristic of Tc cell killing does not occur in complement lysis. Neither with high concentrations of complement which leads to lysis within a few minutes, nor with limiting dilutions of complement when lysis occurs more slowly.

Tc CELL-MEDIATED CYTOTOXICITY

General Aspects

Despite earlier suggestions that colloid osmotic lysis was occurring in Tc cell killing (5-7), the first evidence that colloid osmotic lysis was not involved in Tc killing came from experiments in which the rate of release of different cytoplasmic markers was measured. Apart from rubidium (see below) small molecules and macromolecules are released at the same rate (4,8). This suggests that the lytic event is explosive, and not a result of small lesions.

The relationship between chromium release and the release of DNA provides further evidence against hypotheses involving colloid osmotic lysis. Russell et al (9) compared lysis by Tc cells, by antibody and complement, and hypotonic lysis. They demonstrated a clear difference between Tc cell killing and the other two mechanisms. Very little DNA was released by antibody and complement or by hypotonic lysis, whereas in Tc cell killing there was a progressive release of both cytoplasmic and nuclear contents. In an extension of this work Russell and Dobos (42), studied early changes in the nucleus. This was done by means of detergent to lyse the plasma membrane. Once nuclear disruption had begun in the lytic sequence, the detergent treatment would solubilize DNA. However, if the nucleus remained intact, DNA would not be released by the action of the detergent. Within minutes of Tc cell interaction, nuclear breakdown was detectable, whereas no such nuclear breakdown was detected in lysis by antibody and complement. In fact, in the latter case, the nucleus remained intact over an incubation period of one hour, by which time the release of cytoplasmic contents was complete. This suggests that Tc cell killing has a different mechanism from complement-mediated lysis.

A detailed study of the early stages of Tc cell interactions with target cells was carried out by Martz, who developed a detachment and dispersion procedure to define different stages in the process (10). He showed that once the cells were centrifuged to bring them into close apposition, contact (adherence) had a half-time of one minute. He defined the stage during which a viable effector cell was necessary as 'programming for lysis.' This had a half-time of 5 minutes, after which the target cells were irreversibly damaged; by contrast, lysis as measured by chromium release had a half-time of 100 minutes. Target cells could be rescued from lysis if the effector cells were detached within a few minutes of initial contact, thereby indicating that contact itself was not sufficient to cause lysis and clearly showing that contact and the lethal hit were separate events. The release of rubidium from target cells correlates with the timing of the lethal hit (11,12). Thus, the rapid rate of release of this marker compared to other cytoplasmic markers occurs because of undefined changes in ion fluxes at the time of the lethal hit. This cannot be used as evidence for osmotic lysis, as this would result in progressive release of all cell contents according to their molecular size. This does not happen (see above).

Another fascinating aspect of Tc cell killing is that it is unidirectional. Tc cells are susceptible to killing by other Tc cells. However, when two Tc cells interact killing proceeds only in the direction receptor to antigen (13). When two mutually cytotoxic Tc cells interact, only one is killed (14). Thus, although there is a receptor-antigen interaction in both directions, apparently the first to deliver a lethal hit survives the interaction.

Time-lapse Cinematography

Time-lapse cinematography (15) shows that target cell death follows a period of spectacular zeiosis (Fig. 1B, C). There is a wide variation in time between contact and zeiosis (from a few minutes to several hours). During this period of contact the target cell remains morphologically normal, retains normal membrane movement, and in several instances, target cells are observed to divide with the Tc cell in contact. This suggests that contact itself is not damaging to the target cell. In some cases, bubbles of cytoplasm could be seen bursting out of the cell during zeiosis. Cell swelling was a terminal event after the loss of cytoplasmic contents. This makes it unlikely that collod osmotic lysis was involved. In every case of target cell death the Tc cell remained in contact up to the time of zeiosis. The Tc cells detached at variable times after zeiosis, and often before the final swelling. In those cases where Tc cells detached without zeiosis occurring, the target cell did not die. When macrophages were used as targets, the cell cytoplasm retracted before zeiosis, indicating that changes were taking place in the cytoskeletal system at an earlier stage than zeiosis.

These studies showed that, like P815 tumour cells, some macrophages survived prolonged contact with a Tc cell and that the Tc cell remained in contact throughout zeiosis. The films gave the impression that the Tc cell was over the target cell nucleus just before the onset of zeiosis.

Films made at high magnification showed that four types of lytic event could be distinguished: (1) Zeiosis accompanied by loss of cytoplasmic contents, seen as dark spheres under phase-contrast which diffuse away into the medium. (2) Zeiosis in which blebs break away from the cell and remain intact (Fig. 1C). (3) Zeiosis followed by a period of quiescence before the cytoplasmic contents burst out of the cell (Fig. 1B). (4) Zeiosis followed by a quiescent period in which no contents were seen bursting out of the cell. Instead, the cell gradually darkened under phase contrast and finally swelled.

Time-lapse observations defined three stages in the lytic sequence; a variable interval between contact and the initiation of zeiosis, the phase of zeiosis, and the disintegration of the target cell. On the other hand, assay by chromium release experiments indicated that contact was followed in a few minutes by a lethal event, and then an effector cell independent step, before chromium was released. The reason for this apparent discrepancy became clear as a result of the following experiments in which the Tc cells were inactivated at different times by monoclonal IgM anti-Thyl and complement (4).

Anti-Thyl had no effect on the activity of the Tc cells, but addition of complement caused complete inactivation within two minutes. By allowing a short incubation in a tube at 37°C to allow lethal events to occur, followed by time-lapse filming, it was possible to show that the lethal event corresponded closely to the initiation of zeiosis (Fig. 2). Although Tc cells frequently remain in contact with the target cell during zeiosis, these observations indicated that zeiosis and eventual lysis continued after the inactivation of the Tc cell.

The timing of the lethal events depended on the frequency of the cell interactions (12). Thus, when one Tc cell interacts with one target cell, lethal events occurred over a period of at least 2 hours as was shown by time-lapse cinemaphotography (15). However, at high ratios of Tc cells to target cells the lethal events occurred within a few minutes, as was previously shown by (10). Hence, the timing of the lethal events depends very much on the frequency of cell interactions.

As a further complication to the lytic cycle it was shown that the continued presence of Tc cells after all the cells were lethally hit, increased markedly the rate of chromium release. This explains

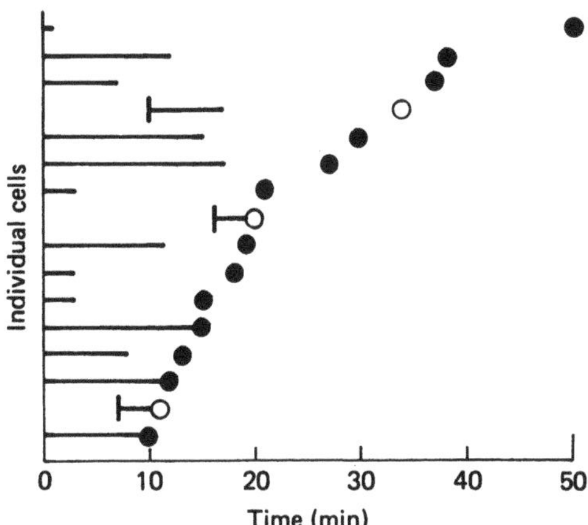

Fig. 2 Diagrammatic representation of the duration of zeiosis (horizontal bars) and the timing of the final swelling of the P815 target cells (circles). Effector cells (coated with IgM anti-Thy1) and target cells were centrifuged, and incubated at 37°C for 5 minutes to allow the lethal event to occur in a proportion of the targets. The effectors were then inactivated by adding complement, and the cells placed in a chamber for time-lapse filming. It can be seen that in each case zeiosis was visible from the beginning of the film. Three cells migrated into the field during filming and were in the phase of zeiosis. The time they entered the field is shown by a vertical bar, and the time of swelling with an open circle. This indicates that zeiosis follows very closely the lethal event, as no cells entered this phase after the beginning of filming. No cells that entered zeiosis recovered, and none of the other cells died. The cells shown represent about half the total cells in the field. (Adapted from ref. 12)

why chromium release requires three to four hours to reach plateau levels after inactivation of the Tc cells, but can reach maximum values within one hour with high ratios of Tc cells. The cell interactions in the lytic cycle are summarised in Fig. 3.

Electron Microscopy

The area of contact with target cells usually consists of microvilli on the Tc cell and point contacts (16), although in addition to point contacts wide areas of contact frequently develop (17,18). Grimm et al (18) described stretching and rupture of the target cell membrane near areas of broad contact and suggested these

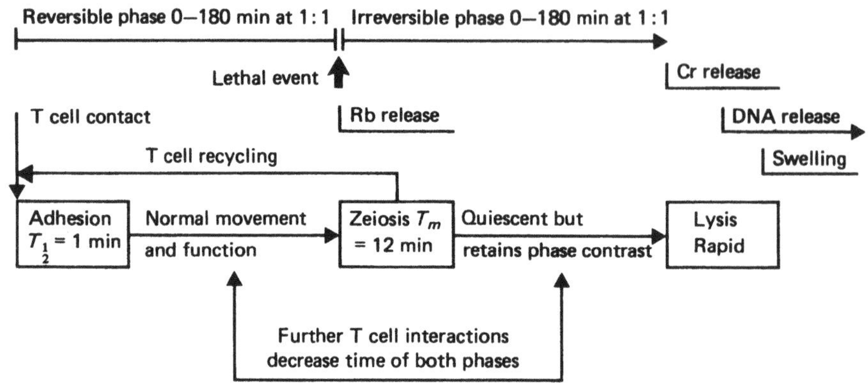

Fig. 3. Diagrammatic representation of the events taking place in the Tc cell lytic circle. The main feature of the cycle is that it consists of two phases of variable time. The reversible phase is the time before the lethal event, and if the Tc cell detaches or is inactivated, the target cell will survive. When a single Tc cell interacts with a single target cell, some lethal events occur within a few minutes, while others occur only after several hours. When multiple interactions are possible (in a cell pellet) all the lethal events can occur within a few minutes. Note that the lethal event causes rubidium release, zeiosis and nuclear damage (see text). Following the lethal event, there is a variable irreversible phase before the breakdown of the plasma membrane and loss of cytoplasmic contents (lysis). The Tc cell is not required after the lethal event, and can detach and recycle to other target cells; however, the continued presence of intact Tc cells during this phase does speed up the steps leading to lysis. The total effect of the variation between the length of these phases in different individual cells is to produce a release of cytoplasmic contents, which accumulate in the medium in approximately linear fashion. (From ref. 4)

Fig. 4. Examples of T cell and K cell projections into P815 target cells. Bars represent 1 µm.

(A) A T cell (T) projection pushed into a mitochondrion, which in turn is pushed back into the nucleus. The projection contains only microfilaments, and the tips is in close contact with the target cell membrane.

(B) A K cell (K) with projections into an antibody coated P815 cell. There is a zone of close contact (arrows) between the tip of the projection and the target cell membrane.

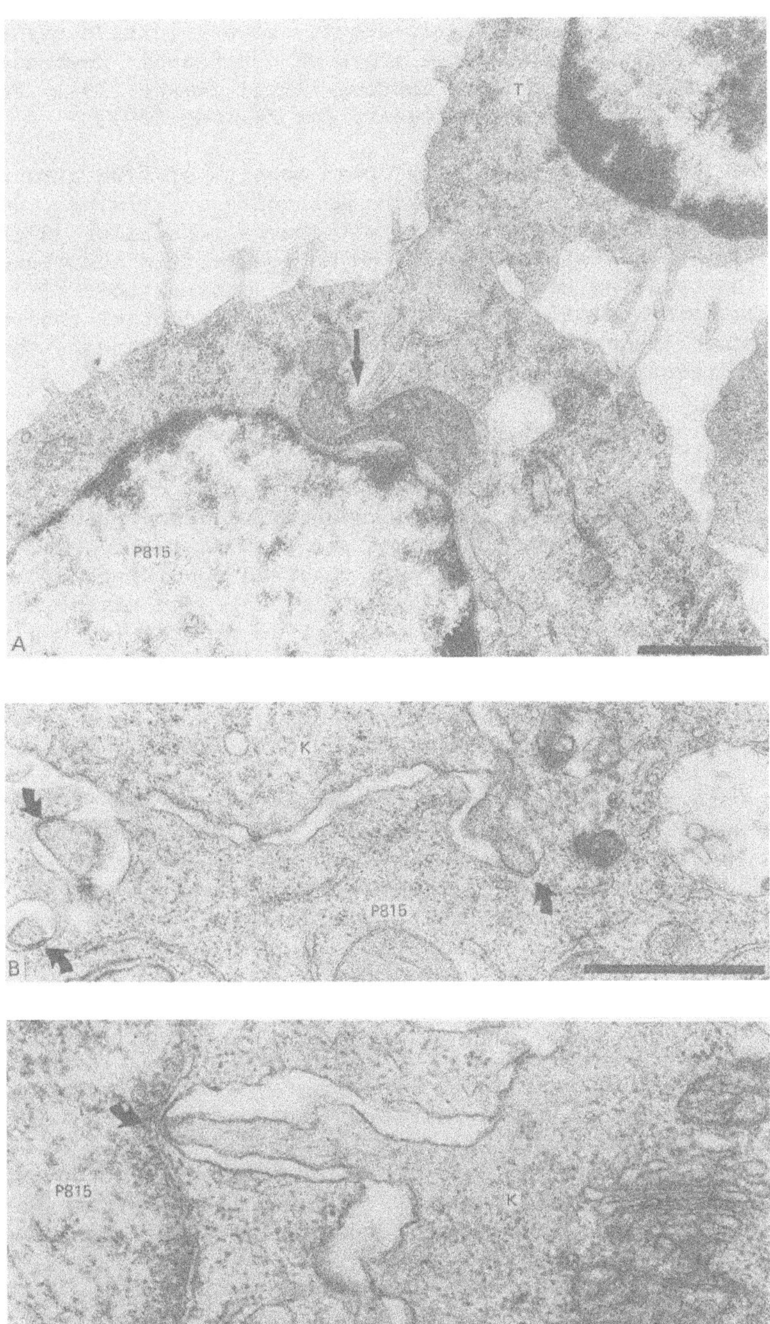

(C) A K cell (K) projection distorting the outline of a P815 nucleus. There is no suggestion of intracellular penetration. (A from ref. 28; B and C from ref. 40)

might represent the primary lytic event. However, these may represent fixation artifacts as large areas of cytoplasmic membrane can be cut away from cells without causing lethal damage (19). Furthermore, strong binding is not necessary for killing (20).

There is little agreement on other aspects of fine structure which might give some clue about the mechanism of killing. Some authors have described specialized structures resembling junctions (16,18,21), whereas others could find no specialized structures between the opposing membranes (17;22-24). Most authors find no convincing evidence of secretion at the zone of contact (16-18;24-26), although Bykovskaja et al. (27) described an organelle thought to be a secretory granule.

Several reports have noted projections from the effector cells pushing into the target cell (16,17;24-27). A study of material fixed at 37°C within 10 minutes of contact, under conditions giving very high rates of killing, provide a detailed description of these projections (28). It was noted that projections pushed into the target cell and, in some cases, were observed to distort organelles, including the nucleus, in their path (Fig. 4). The plasma membrane of both cells remained intact so that actual penetration was not involved. The projections contain microfilaments and other organelles, and an area of close contact between the two plasma membranes is usually seen at the tip of the projection. They are, therefore, different from passive interdigations, which contain ribosomes.

The fact that projections are relatively difficult to find in sections suggests that they form rapidly and disappear. This is reinforced by time-lapse films which show rapid movement of the Tc cell microvilli (unrelated to the area of contact with the target cell) and rapid movement of target cell organelles in the zone near the Tc

---

Fig. 5. Examples of zeiosis in P815 tumor cells in Tc cell (T) cytotoxicity. Bars represent 1 μm.

Note that in each case the P815 membrane is intact, and the organelles are normal. Slight mitochondrial swelling is also seen in controls, and may represent changes due to the culture conditions.

(A) Spectacular blebbing from a focus. The nucleus can be seen divided between different blebs. There is a mass of rod-like structures, which may be aggregates of microfilaments at the focus (an enlargement is shown in the original paper).

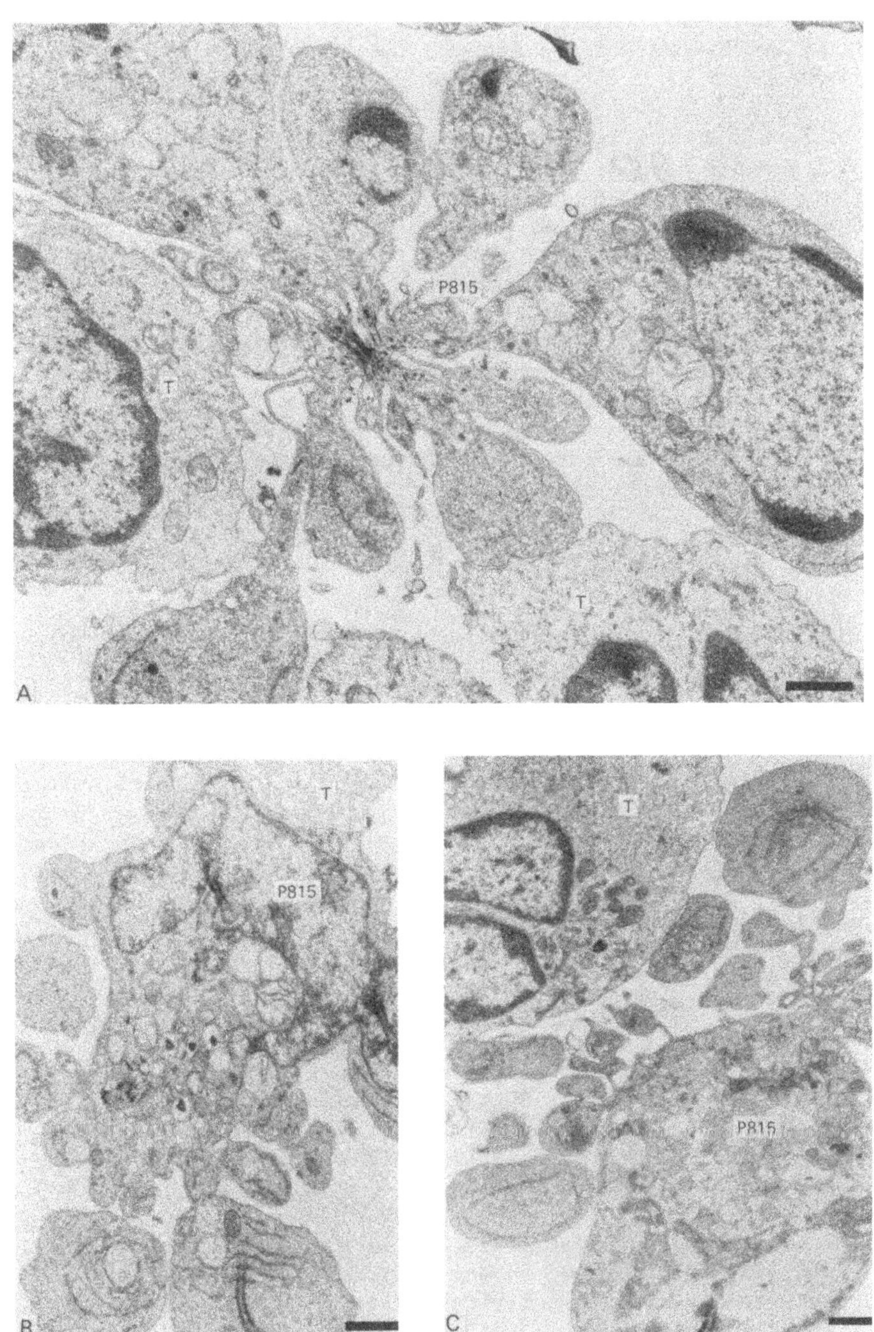

(B) Zeiosis showing the distortion of the nucleus. The blebs are away from the T cell.

(C) Zeiosis towards an effector cell. (From ref. 17)

cell. Furthermore, the fact that organelles in the target cell are distorted by the projections suggest they move rapidly and with some force.

Cells undergoing zeiosis (17) are clearly identifiable in electron micrographs because of the bizarre outline of the cell (Fig. 5). The cytoplasm forms blebs protruding from the cell. In some cases the whole cell may consist of blebs joining at a focus, in which dense rod-like structures are present, which may be aggregates of cytoskeletal filaments. The nucleus is usually distorted in shape and sometimes split into separate lobes in different blebs of the cell. It is noteworthy that no significant degenerative changes are observed. The plasma membrane and the nuclear envelope remain apparently intact, and the organelles remain morphologically normal. In some cases, which by analogy with time-lapse observations are assumed to be after the loss of cytoplasmic contents, the cells show vacuolation and loss of organelles.

K CELL-MEDIATED CYTOTOXICITY

General Aspects

The main problem in reviewing work on K cells is the considerable confusion in the literature concerning the type of effector cell being studied. Many authors discuss antibody dependent cell mediated cytotoxicity (ADCC) as though it is a single phenomenon. However, the number of effector cell types operating depends on the type of target cell. Chick red blood cells (CRBC) have been used widely as a target cell (29). Although susceptible to K cell activity, they are also highly susceptible to granulocyte and macrophage activity (30-33). Furthermore, normal mouse spleen (in contrast to rat spleen) has very low K cell activity (30,34). As reported by Holm (35), with human K cells, I have found no activity in defined rat K cell populations against mammalian red cells, whereas granulocytes and macrophages are highly active. Thus, studies in which unfractionated mouse spleen cells are tested against chick or mammalian red cells, are almost certainly concerned with phagocytic effector cells and not K cells. Similarly, work done with human peripheral blood effectors and antibody-coated mammalian cells may not be studying K cells.

The use of nucleated mammalian cells as target does not necessarily simplify the problem, as some of these are susceptible to granulocyte and macrophage activity. However, P815 tumour cells have low susceptibility to granulocyte killing (30) and even with susceptible tumour cell targets, granulocytes require much higher concentrations of antibody than K cells (36). Thus, systems involving P815 tumour cells as targets, and high dilutions of antibody that are optimal for K cell activity, are almost certainly only detecting K cells.

Kinetic analysis of the release of target cell contents from antibody-coated P815 cells showed that K cell contact was necessary, because centrifugation initiated chromium release immediately. In contrast to Tc cell killing of the same target cells (where chromium release is linear with time), K cells caused a rapid release over the first 15 minutes followed by a slower rate of release (34). This was not due to shedding of antibody. Resuspension of the cells followed by another centrifugation caused an additional burst of chromium release as new contacts were formed.

Time-Lapse Cinematography

Time-lapse films showed that K cells caused morphological changes in the target cells similar to those produced by Tc cells, except that the interval between contact and zeiosis was usually less than 15 minutes. This provided an explanation for the rapid rate of chromium over the first 15 minutes (38). As with Tc cells the K cell appeared to be over the target cell nucleus immediately before zeiosis. A single K cell could be observed to kill more than one target cell. However, the plateau usually found in the curve of chromium release after about 4 hours suggests that K cells become inactive over a period of a few hours (39).

Electron Microscopy

Examination of cells fixed at 37°C during the first 15 minutes of contact showed projections similar to those found in Tc cell killing (40). There was a zone of close contact at the tip (Fig. 4) and the projections contained only microfilaments. They were not randomly distributed over the K cell surface, but formed in the area of contact with the target cell. The projections could be seen to have distorted the outline of the nucleus of the target cell, but in no case was rupture of the target cell plasma membrane observed. Cells in zeiosis were observed, and resembled those seen in Tc cell killing.

Dourmashkin et al (41) reported ring-shaped membrane structures in a small proportion of dead cells. These were described as generally similar to 'lesions' seen on cells lysed by antibody and complement. They suggested that cell-mediated and complement lysis operate by similar mechanisms. However, the fact that these rings were seen after incubation periods of 4-10 hours, when K cell lysis occurs within 15 minutes, must raise the possibility that the rings are artifacts. Furthermore, the fact that K cell killing involves zeiosis, makes it possible that the rings result from the massive changes in the membrane during this stage, rather than the primary cause of death.

CONCLUSIONS

The primary cause of cell death in lymphocyte-mediated cytotoxicity remains unknown. There is little support for a role for secretory granules, so that it seems unlikely that a mechansim analogous to that of granulocytes, which release granule material onto the surface of the target object, is involved. The early changes in the nuclear envelope (42) indicate a mechanism of killing quite different from antibody and complement. Furthermore, the morphological changes are different from those seen in complement-mediated and hypotonic lysis, and so it seems unlikely that a membrane lesion is the primary cause of target cell death.

Lymphocyte-mediated killing involves a distinct and spectacular period of zeiosis (membrane blebbing). Zeiosis is an interesting and poorly understood phenomenon. It appears to have been overlooked for a long time in both time-lapse and electron microscope studies of lymphocyte killing. Zeiosis must result from massive changes in the cytoskeletal system, as similar blebbing is caused by agents that disrupt the cytoskeleton (43). Furthermore, zeiosis might provide a clue to the lethal event, as it represents a major difference between other forms of cell death such as complement lysis, hypotonic lysis and damage by light, which do not show zeiosis (Sanderson, unpublished). Time-lapse films of the killing of antibody-coated tumour cells by granulocytes indicated that cell death did not involve zeiosis, but resembled the changes seen in complement lysis (Sanderson and Lopez, unpublished). Death occurring in cultures of growing cells (natural cell death or mitotic death) also show zeiosis (15), but the events leading to death in these cells are unknown. Munro and Daniel (19) reported that manipulation of a micropipette in the nuclear region of a cell caused zeiosis followed by cell death. Little is known about other forms of cell death that involve zeiosis; however, it seems likely that internal changes in the cell rather than membrane damage are the primary lethal effect.

Lymphocyte projections might provide an explanation for target cell death. They appear to develop as a result of the receptor-ligand interaction when the effector cell makes contact with the target cell. Although there is no direct evidence to connect them with the mechanism of killing, there are a number of factors consistent with this. Time-lapse and electron microscopic observations show that the Tc cell produces considerable movement and distortion of target cell organelles, which might be enough to cause physical damage to sensitive structures in the cell. Alternatively, they may deliver a toxic substance close to a sensitive organelle, but in the absence of good evidence for a toxic substance, this seems unlikely at present. The concept of physical damage occurring inside the target cell, and caused by effector cell projections, is consistent with all the known facts about the mechanism of killing.

Firstly, zeiosis suggests some form of internal damage, rather than membrane damage, as discussed above. Secondly, the separation of contact from the lethal event as shown by Martz (10). Thirdly, lethal events appear to occur in a random fashion after contact, as shown by the variation in time between contact and zeiosis, and the sequential delivery of lethal events when a Tc cell interacts with several targets (44). Clearly, with high cell-cell interactions, the probability of a lethal event increases so that the total population is hit within a few minutes. Fourthly, the unidirectional nature of killing can be explained by proposing a role for projections in killing, as a cell delivering a lethal hit would not itself be damaged.

In summary, I would like to propose an hypothesis which links the receptors of the effector cell to its cytoskeletal system, so that occupation of the receptors would trigger the cytoskeletal system to push out projections. The projections (as distinct from interdigitations) appear to be unique, as similar projections have not been described in other biological systems. It seems hardly likely that such a mechanism would exist simply to maintain cellular contact, as the formation of broad areas of contact would serve the same purpose. In any event, strong binding is not necessary for killing to occur. This interaction between cell receptors and the cytoskeletal system preserves, at least in principle, the more primitive interaction of phagocytosis. Phagocytosis results from the occupation of a number of specialized membrane receptors (e.g., Fc receptors, but other recognition receptors preceded these), leading to the activation of the cytoskeletal system to produce pseudopodia for the engulfment of the target. It is proposed that K cells have evolved from phagocytic cells in such a way that activation of the cytoskeletal system by occupation of Fc receptors results in projections rather than pseudopodia, and that the projections are involved in killing. Tc cells have evolved specific receptors to deal with foreign antigens, especially the intracellular parasites (e.g., viruses), and to provide immunological specificity and memory. It is proposed that Tc cell receptors for antigen retain the interaction with the cytoskeletal system as the effector mechanism for killing. This proposed mechanism of killing, involving physical phenomena, overcomes the requirement for a well developed secretory system as in granulocytes and macrophages (which Tc cells do not have), and sidesteps the requirement for a membrane-bound toxin or enzyme (which has not been convincingly detected in Tc cells).

ACKNOWLEGEMENT

I wish to thank Dr. Audrey M. Glauert for providing the electron micrographs.

REFERENCES

1. Mayer, M.M. Mechanism of cytolysis by lymphocytes: a comparison with complement. J. Immunol. 119:1195-1203 (1977).
2. Price, Z.H. The micromorphology of zeiotic blebs in cultured human epithelial (HEp) cells. Exp. Cell. Res. 48:82-92 (1967).
3. Green, H., Barrow, P., and B. Goldberg. Effect of antibody and complement on permeability control in ascites tumor cells and erythrocytes. J. Exp. Med. 110:699-713 (1959).
4. Sanderson, C.J. The mechanism of lymphocyte-mediated cytotoxocity. Biol. Rev. 56:153-197 (1981b).
5. Henney, C.S. Studies on the mechanism of lymphocyte mediated cytolysis. II. The use of various target cell markers to study cytolytic events. J. Immunol. 110:73-84 (1973).
6. Ferluga, J., and A.C. Allison. Observations on the mechanism by which T lymphocytes exert cytotoxic effect. Nature 250: 673-675 (1974).
7. Martz, E. Burakoff, S.J., and B. Benacerraf. Interruption of the sequential release of small and large molecules from tumor cells by low temperature during cytolysis mediated by immune T cells or complement. Proc. Natl. Acad. Sci. 71:177-181 (1974).
8. Sanderson, C.J. The mechanism of T cell mediated cytotoxicity. I. the release of different cell components. Proc. Roy. Soc. Lond. B. 192:221-239 (1976a).
9. Russell, J.H., Masakowski, V.R., and C.B. Dobos. Mechanisms of immune lysis. I. Physiological distinction between target cell death mediated by cytotoxic T lymphocytes and antibody plus complement. J. Immunol. 124:1100-1105 (1980).
10. Martz, E. Mechanism of specific tumor cell lysis by alloimmune T lymphocytes: resolution and characterization of discrete steps in the cellular interation. Contemp. Top. Immunobiol. 7:301-361 (1977).
11. Martz, E. Early steps in specific tumor cell lysis by sensitized mouse T lymphocytes. II. Electrolyte permeability increase in the target cell embrane concomittant with programming for lysis. J. Immunol. 117:1023-1027 (1967).
12. Sanderson, C.J. The mechanism of T cell mediated cytotoxicity. VIII. Zeiosis corresponds to irreversible phase (programming for lysis) in steps leading to lysis. Immunology 42:201-206 (1981a).
13. Kuppers, R.C., and C.S. Henney. Studies on the mechanism of lymphocyte mediated cytolysis. IX. Relationships between antigen recognition and lytic expression in killer T cells. J. Immunol. 118:71-76 (1977).
14. Fishelson, Z. and G. Berke. T lymphocyte-mediated cytolysis: dissociation of the binding and lytic mechanism of the effector cell. J. Immunol. 120:1121 (1978).
15. Sanderson, C.J. The mechanism of T cell mediated cytotoxicity. II. Morphological studies of cell death by time-lapse micro-

cinematography. Proc. Roy. Soc. Lond. B. 192:241-255 (1976b).

16. Kalina, M., and G. Berke. Contact regions of cytotoxic T lymphocyte target cell conjugates. Cell. Immunol. 25:41-51 (1976).
17. Sanderson, C.J. and A.M. Glauert. The mechanism of T cell mediated cytotoxicity. V. Morphological studies by electron microscopy. Proc. Roy. Soc. Lond. B. 198:315-323 (1977).
18. Grimm, E., Price, Z., and B. Bonavida. Studies on the induction and expression of T cell mediated immunity. VIII. Effector target junctions and target cell membrane disruption during cytolysis. Cell. Immunol. 46:77-79 (1979a).
19. Munro, T.R., and M.R. Daniel. The effects of micro-operations on the morphology, survival, and lysosomes of Chinese hamster fibroblasts. Exp. Cell. Res. 38:483-494 (1965).
20. Shortman, K., and P. Golstein. Target cell recognition by cytolytic T cells: different requirements for the formation of strong conjugates or for proceeding to lysis. J. Immunol. 123:833-839 (1970).
21. Kalina, M., and H. Ginsburg. Ultrastructural aspects of the adherence to target cells of 'in vitro' differentiated lymphocytes. Proc. Soc. Exp. Biol. Med. 149:796-799 (1975).
22. Biberfeld, P., and Johansson, A. Contact areas of cytotoxic lymphocytes and target cells. Exp. Cell. Res. 94:79-87 (1975).
23. Liepins, A., Faanes, R.B., Lifter, J., Choi, Y.S., and E. De Harven. Ultrastructural changes during T lymphocyte mediated cytolysis. Cell. Immunol. 28:109-124 (1977).
24. Ryser, J.E., Sordat, B., Cerottini, J.-C., and K.T. Brunner. Mechanisms of target cell lysis of cytotoxic T lymphocytes. I. Characterization of specific lymphocyte target cell conjugates separated by velocity sedimentation. Eur. J. Immunol. 7:110-117 (1977).
25. Kalina, M., and N. Hollander. The effect of cytochalasin B on effector target cell interaction. Quantitative and ultrastructural study. Immunology 29:709-717 (1975).
26. Searle, R.F., and Flaks. A technique for liver transplantation in the inbred mouse. A fine structural study of allograft rejection. Transplantation 22:256-264 (1976).
27. Bykovsaja, S.N., Rytenko, A.N., Rauschenbach, M.O., and A.F. Bykovsky. ULtrastructural alteration of cytotoxic T lymphocytes following their interaction with target cells. Cell. Immunol. 40:175-185 (1978).
28. Sanderson, C.J., and Glauert, A.M. The mechanism of T cell mediated cytotoxicity. VI. T cell projections and their role in target cell killing. Immunology 36:119-129 (1979).
29. Perlmann, P., and G. Holm. Cytotoxic effects of lymphid cells in vitro. Adv. Immunol. 11:117-193 (1969).
30. Sanderson, C.J., Clark, I.A., and G.A. Taylor. Different effector cell types in antibody dependent cell mediated cytotoxicity. Nature 253:376-377 (1975).
31. Pollack, S.B., Nelson, K., and J.D. Grausz. Separation of

effector cells mediating antibody dependent cellular cytotoxicity (ADC) to erythrocyte targets from those mediating ADC to tumor targets. J. Immunol. 116:944-946 (1976).
32. Penfold, P.L., Green, A.H., and I.M. Roitt. Characteristics of the effector cells mediating cytotoxicity against antibody coated target cells. III. Ultrastructural studies. Clin. Exp. Immunol. 23:91-97 (1976).
33. Sanderson, C.J., and J.A. Thomas. A comparison of the cytotoxic activity of eosinophils and other cells by chromium release and time-lapse microcinematography. Immunology 34: 771-780 (1978).
34. Berger, A.E., and Amos, D.B. A comparison of antibody dependent cellular cytotoxicity (ADCC) mediated by murine and human lymphoid cell populations. Cell. Immunol. 33:377-290 (1977).
35. Holm, G. Lysis of antibody-treated human erythrocytes by human leukocytes and macrophages in tissue culture. Int. Arch. Allergy Appl. Immunol. 3:671-682 (1972).
36. Lopez, A.F., and C.J. Sanderson. Antibody dependent cell mediated cytotoxocity of nucleated mammalian cells by rat eosinophils and neutrophils. Int. Arch. Allergy Appl. Immunol. In press (1981).
37. Sanderson, C.J., and J.A. Thomas. The mechanism of K cell (antibody dependent) cell mediated cytotoxicity. I. The release of different cell components. Proc. Roy. Soc. Long. B. 197:407-415 (1977a).
38. Sanderson, C.J., and J.A. Thomas. The mechanism of K cell (antibody dependent) cell mediated cytotoxicity. II. Characteristics of the effector cell and mrophological changes in the target cell. Proc. Roy. Soc. Lond. B. 197:417-424 (1977b).
40. Glauert, A.M., and C.J. Sanderson. The mechanism of K cell (antibody-dependent) mediated cytotoxicity. III. The ultrastructure of K cell projections and their possible role in target cell killing. J. Cell. Sci. 35:355-366 (1979).
41. Dourmashkin, R.R., Deteix, P., Simone, C.B., and P. Henkart. Electron microscopic demnstration of lesions in target cells membranes associated with antibody-dependent cellular cytotoxocity. Clin. Exp. Immunol. 42:554-560 (1980).
42. Russell, J.H., and C.B. Dobos. Mechanisms of immune lysis. II. CTL induced nuclear disintegration of the targt begins within minutes of cell contact. J. Immunol. 124:1256-1261 (1980).
43. Godman, G.C., Miranda, A.G., Deitch, A.D., and Tanenbaum. Action of cytochalasin D on cells of established lines. III. Zeeiosis and movements of the cell surface. J. Cell. Biol. 64:644-667 (1975).
44. Zagury, D., Bernard, J., Jeannesson, P., Thierness, N., and J.-C. Cerottini. Studies on the mechanism of T cell mediated lysis at the single cell level. I. Kinetic analysis of lethal

hits and target cell lysis in multicellular conjugates. J. Immunol. 123:1604-1609 (1970).
45. Golstein, P., Foa, C., and I.C.M. MacLennan. Mechanism of T cell mediated cytolysis: the differential impact of cytochalasins at the recognition and lethal hit stages. Eur. J. Immunol. 8:302-309. (1978)

ROLE OF CELL MOTILITY IN THE ACTIVITY OF CYTOLYTIC T LYMPHOCYTES

J.-E. Ryser and P. Vassalli

Department of Pathology, Faculty of Medicine
University of Geneva
1211 Geneva 4, Switzerland

INTRODUCTION

The distinction between specific recognition and target cell (TC) lysis has been accepted as a useful concept in the analysis of cytolytic T lymphocyte (CTL)-mediated cytotoxicity. Recently, this process has been resolved by different methods into three steps: binding; "lethal hit"; and TC lysis; the first two of which require direct CTL-TC contact (1,2). As detailed in recent reviews (3-7), CTL-TC conjugates can be isolated physically before the lethal hit step (2,8-10), or binding and lethal hit can be separated on the basis of different cations requirements (11,12), and different susceptibilities to inhibition by low temperature (15°C) and drugs (3). These different sensitivities to temperature, extracellular cations and pharmacological compounds could mean that qualitatively different intracellular activities and/or membrane-associated phenomena operate in the binding and lethal hit steps.

Golstein (13) and Kuppers and Henney (14,15) made the important observation that lethal hit delivery has a polarity. Thus CTL of an irrelevant specificity can be used as TC and lysed specifically by effector CTL directed against them. Since, in this situation, binding has occurred between two cells endowed with cytotoxic ability, the lack of any demonstrable lesion to the effector CTL demonstrates the polarity of lethal hit, and appears to rule out models of the cytolytic process based on the production of diffusible cytotoxic molecules, or on the putative lethal effects of intimate membrane apposition.

The present contribution will attempt to connect the various aspects of CTL motility with the different steps of TC lysis by CTL, as they are defined functionally. Several aspects of the same topics have been discussed by Sanderson in a recent review (16). Cell motility can be explored either by direct observation of living cells, or deduced from modifications of the cell shape and cytoskeleton. One difficulty, however, is that the lethal hit, in contrast to binding and TC lysis, is defined in functional assays but cannot be readily and unambiguously detected in morphological studies (16, 17). Experiments performed with conjugates in conditions where lethal hit cannot occur allow, however, comparisons with CTL morphology and motility in conditions where TC lysis does eventually occur. The terms "permissive" and "non-permissive" will be used to describe experimental conditions in which the binding step is or is not followed by lethal hit, respectively.

The emphasis on cell motility during CTL activity will lead to the suggestion that CTL motility may play an essential role in CTL activity, a model which is easy to reconcile with the polarity of CTL function described above. As discussed in the last section, the polarization of CTL action and the localized motility of CTL in the area of binding with TC suggest that CTL motility might actually explain the functional link between specific recognition and the lethal hit event.

CTL TRANSLATIONAL MOVEMENTS BEFORE OR BETWEEN TC ENCOUNTERS

The motility of unbound CTL in culture chambers has been noted by different authors during the past 10 years (9,18-22). In a recent article, Chang et al. (20) reported that cell suspensions containing CTL comprise lymphocytes which, in the absence of TC, could be observed in culture chambers to change shape continuously and to move around. However, this experimental condition did not establish the CTL nature of the motile lymphocyte. Furthermore, a T lymphoma with lectin-mediated cytolytic capacity, corresponding presumably to CTL lines, was found to display "crawling" capacity which is not displayed by other T lymphomas (23). Rothstein et al. (24) used a different approach. To circumvent the need of a CTL marker, they separated T cell from the spleen of alloimmune mice and used the fraction of the cells which adhered to a layer of specific TC. CTL were then identified, on 10 hour timelapse microcinematographic films made under phase contrast microscopy, by their capacity to lyse TC. CTL were found to wander over the TC layer for prolonged periods of time and to lyse an average of 3 to 4 TC per hour, in agreement with conclusions based on functional demonstrations that CTL can be "recycled" (8,25). These observations indicate that unbound CTL display a high translational motility, this function being probably necessary to enter into contact with immobile TC. The prevention of in vitro cytotoxicity in the presence of cytochalasins (26,27), (drugs which interfere with cell motility), might thus simply reflect, in a first step at least, least, an inability of CTL to move and thus meet their TC. In the experiments of Chang et al, reported above, treating the cells with cytochalasin B or colchicine, or decreasing the temperature to 2025°C, suppressed crawling of the presumed CTL (20).

INITIAL CONTACT OF CTL WITH TC AND NON-SPECIFIC BY-STANDERS

Initial contact between CTL and TC can be observed in culture chambers where CTL and TC or irrelevant cells have been introduced separately (9,21,22,28). Encounters are not simply due to random collision since, when placed on a layer of adherent fibroblasts, immune but not normal T lymphocytes are found to crawl on a layer of fibroblasts (20). Similar crawling is observed whether the fibroblasts are specific TC or by-stander cells syngeneic to the immune T-cells. Thus, crawling can be interpreted as a specialized function which endows CTL with the capacity to actively explore the surface of other cells, and which eventually results in CTL-TC binding in the case of specific TC encounter. The nature of initial contact is not known. Since non-specific conjugates (see below) are relatively rare (2,10,29) in contrast to initial CTL contact with non-specific by-standers, it is possible that initial contact does not involve, as do conjugates, a mechanical bond strong enough to resist the shear forces of pipetting. Alternatively, the process of initial contact may not occur normally (and could be bypassed) in the technique of conjugate formation, by co-centrifugation of CTL-TC suspensions at room temperature. Initial contact with specific TC is not necessarily conducive to TC lysis. For example, in the experiments reported above (24), around half of the specific TC with which CTL made contact survived, even after prolonged CTL-TC contact (ca. 30 min.). Sanderson (9) also reported that close contact between CTL and specific TC in permissive conditions may dissociate spontaneously, with no apparent damage to the TC.

In summary, there is strong evidence that initial CTL-TC contact rests upon CTL movements allowing exploration of other cells' surface. This initial contact does not result in strong binding with by-stander syngeneic targets, and does not always result in lethal hit in the case of specific TC.

STRONG CTL-TC CONJUGATES IN "NON-PERMISSIVE" CONDITIONS

Since binding and lethal hit steps have been separated in functional studies, a description of the morphology and biological activity of CTL attached to specific TC in "non-permissive" conditions is needed in order to establish valid comparisons with additional structure and/or activity which may be related to lethal hit. Earlier studies relevant to CTL motility were generally performed only in "permissive" conditions (9,18,19,28). Because, in such conditions, CTL-mediated cytolysis is very rapid (30) and asynchroonous CTL and TC at all steps of the cytoytic process are present simultaneously, preventing a systematic study of each step separately. This difficulty can be avoided by the study of CTL-TC conjugates obtained in "nonpermissive" conditions. This can be achieved for example with lymphocytes purified from the peritoneal cavity of mice after rejection of an intraperitoneal graft of allogeneic tumor cells, which can be made to conjugate with TC by co-centrifugation at room temperature. In these conditions, conjugate formation occurs within a very short period of time, and the majority of CTL in conjugates can be demonstrated to be cytotoxic by different techniques (2,8,10,31); as already mentioned, "background" conjugates of these lymphocytes with nonspecific TC is low.

Light microscopic observations of conjugates either in suspension or on stained smears, shows an important heterogeneity in the tightness of attachment in different conjugates, and a predominance of conjugates made of one CTL and one TC (doublets). Distinctive structure are not seen in the binding areas (8,10). In contrast, both transmission and scanning electron microscopy have provided important information on the structure of the binding area. Several recent reports (10,21,28,32) agree that the surface of contact between CTL and TC corresponds to villous areas on both cells. Long microvillous projections from CTL and TC were found to interpenetrate with each other, giving the appearance of a tightly packed assembly of worm-like structures, and larger CTL projections extending deep into the TC cytoplasm were described (10). In other reports (21,28, 32), the binding area appears to have a looser general appearance, a discrepancy which is likely related to the heterogeneity of tightness of the conjugates. By transmission electron microscopy, microfilaments appear to be the major constituents of the CTL projections and to be contiguous to an area of well developed cytoplasmic microfilamentous network, devoid of organelles, which is the prominent feature of the CTL binding area (10, 32,33). No such structure is seen in the TC binding area.

The distribution of the contractile proteins actin and myosin has recently been explored in control CTL and CTL conjugated to TC (33). Fixed smears of cells and conjugates were prepared and stained by double immunofluorescence with anti-actin and antimyosin antibodies. In the majority of conjugated CTL, actin was detected as a brightly stained area near the binding area (Fig. 1), in contrast to control lymphocytes, which showed no polarization of actin in the CTL cytoplasm. Myosin, in contrast, showed no polarization in any CTL, including conjugated CTL with polarized actin. Although both antibodies stained CTL more brightly than TC, TC staining was sufficient to show that polarization of contractile proteins was not occurring in the TC.

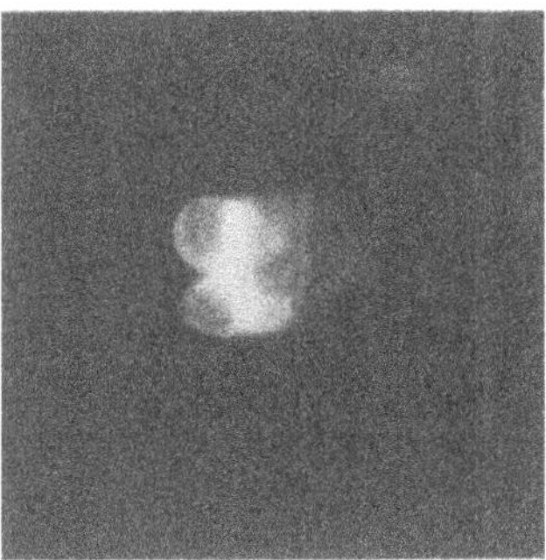

Fig. 1. Actin polarization in CTL. Actin stained by immunofluorescence is polarized in the binding area of two CTL, conjugated to the same P-815 TC.

Actin polarization was not observed in CTL displaying non-specific adherence with each other or with syngeneic TC. Failure to observe myosin polarization is considered a significant observation since myosin as well as actin polarization was readily detectable in B lymphocytes after capping of their surface Ig. Control experiments showed that, in the experimental conditions used, no lethal hit events were detectable (^{51}Cr release from labeled TC was identical to background ^{51}Cr release, when the conjugates were incubated with EDTA at 37°C), while TC lysis did occur when conjugates were incubated in permissive conditions. It was concluded that CTL conjugation in non-permissive conditions is accompanied by a striking modification of the CTL cytoskeleton in most conjugates, characterized by polarization of actin in the binding area, without polarization of myosin. (33).

THE CTL-TC BINDING AREA IN "PERMISSIVE" CONDITIONS"

CTL ultrastructure of the binding area in non-permissive and in permissive conditions has been directly compared in only a few studies. When comparisons were made (10), no morphological modifications of the CTL were reported following incubation at the permissive temperature. On the other hand, morphological studies restricted to permissive conditions were often interpreted to mean that a progression of CTL projections inside TC was related to the lethal hit event (18,19,21,34-36). Sanderson and Glauert (34,35) proposed that CTL projections, which developed after TC binding, penetrated into the TC, going in some cases as far as to form close apposition with the TC nuclear envelope.

Under phase contrast microscopy, observation in "permissive" conditions of living CTL bound to TC shows movements of the cells with respect to each other, which could precede the lethal hit (33). However, it must be pointed out that bright field, phase contrast and Nomarski optical microscopy cannot resolve great morphological detail in the binding area. For this reason, interference contrast microscopy, which allows observations wth a very narrow depth of field, has recently been used to obtain a more detailed picture of CTL motility in the binding area (33). Striking and rapid movements of the CTL membrane restricted to the binding area were observed, including back and forth formation and withdrawal of CTL projections against the TC surface.

Although these movements of the CTL membrane in the binding area preceded any drastic alterations in the morphology of TC, and might be considered as leading to or associated with the lethal hit, it must be pointed out, as already mentioned, that the correlation between the time of lethal hit and the first observation of TC damage is not established. As described by Sanderson (9,16), the main feature of CTL-bound TC incubated in permissive conditions is a phenomenon termed zeiosis, which occurs with no fixed time relation with CTL binding. It is characterized by a sudden and violent formation of cytoplasmic blebs on the surface of the TC, which immediately follows in some TC retraction to a spherical form. This spectacular event is not observed in complement-mediated lysis. It is followed by vacuolation, mitochondrial swelling and loss of cytoplasmic organelles. Elegant experiments by the same author (17) have recently provided evidence that TC zeiosis and lethal hit are closely related in time. However, in view of the rapidity with which both of these events occur, it cannot be formally excluded that zeiosis, like other morphologically detectable TC modifications, follows lethal hit after a short delay.

DISCUSSION AND CONCLUSION

From this review, it is apparent that high motility is a general property of CTL, already expressed before and during the initial contact of CTL with TC, and then during the period of CTL-TC firm binding. A detailed study of the binding step in this respect reveals an important characteristic: CTL bound to their TC are asymmetric, as shown by the polarization of microfilaments and actin in the binding area, which most likely corresponds to the localized high motility of the CTL in this area as detected by interference contrast microscopy. This CTL asymmetry does not exist before TC binding and, thus, must be triggered in some way during the process of conjugate formation.

Based on this asymmetry of CTL in conjugates, a new interpretation can be given to the observation by Golstein (13) and Kuppers and Henney (14,15) that TC killing is directional and apparently linked to TC recognition, as described above. In addition to their main function, which would be to ensure the specificity of CTL-mediated cytotoxicity, hypothetical specific CTL receptor(s) have been proposed to play the role of a mechanical bridge between CTL and TC. The structure of CTL attachment to TC, however, suggests that binding could be fully accounted for by the penetration into the cell body of TC, of CTL microvillosities and cytoplasmic projections rich in filamentous actin. Point and broad contacts described by most authors between CTL and TC membranes may or may not be required in this model of binding, which relies on the activity of CTL contractile actin molecules; it must be noted that, in any event, it is unlikely that these membrane contacts represent specific receptors (37). If this mechanism of binding is correct, it can be hypothesized that specific receptors, upon contact with TC surface, control the binding step by initiating a modification of the CTL actin network (e.g., a focal polymerization of actin), which would result in the establishment of the binding structure. In this way, specific structures would indirectly control the polarity of the lethal hit, which can be envisaged as a direct consequence of the polarity of the binding structure.

How the occupation of CTL specific receptor(s) by TC antigens could initiate this modification of CTL symmetry and motility remains conjectural. It has been shown recently that non-specific TC killing by CTL in lectin-mediated cytotoxicity cannot be used as evidence to minimize the role of CTL specific receptors (38). As discussed elsewhere (33), actin polarization in attached CTL is unlike that in B lymphocytes with capped surface Ig, which is accompanied by myosin polararization, and it differs from actin accumulation in fibroblasts ruffles, or in polymorphonuclear pseudopods during phagocytosis. This model is also distinct from others where CTL cytoskeleton was proposed to mobilize and/or expose membrane receptors, rather than to respond to a signal from membrane receptors. It may offer a more likely interpretation of the striking development of polymerized actin in the CTL binding area.

In addition to the model discussed above, which concerns the temporal and local relationship between recognition (localized signal to membrane receptors) and binding steps (focal actin polymerization leading to focal motility), is it possible that polarized CTL motility also plays a role in the lethal hit step? CTL motility has been proposed as instrumental in killing on the grounds of microcinematographic and ultrastructural studies of TC lysis. An hypothetical "mechanical" lethal hit might involve TC membrane disruption by tearing (21), pinching off (36) or shearing mechanisms (the latter mechanism has been considered as a possible cause of the TC initial lesion by analogy to the lysis of red blood cells subjected to shear forces in red cell rouleaux (39). The finding of high CTL motility localized to the binding area is in agreement with such a mechanical hypothesis (33).

A consequence of this extended model would be that binding and lethal hit steps are qualitatively similar, since they would both rely upon a special type of polarized CTL motility. One would thus expect some relationship between the binding activity and cytotoxic ability of a given CTL. It has indeed been reported by Glasebrook (40) that when CTL from different sources and of different cytolytic activities were compared, CTL with the higher cytolytic capacity were also found to show a higher avidity in TC binding (binding at lower temperature and/or more rapidly) and a higher recycling capacity. However, it has been shown that strong conjugate formation is not a strict requirement for CTL-mediated TC lysis (41) and a simple correlation between the frequencies of binders and of CTL among binders may not exist (42). It would be interesting to explore whether CTL with the lowest binding avidity and lower or slowest cytolytic capacity are also those with the lesser ability to polymerize actin and to display high motility in the contact area. Such a situation might result from an incomplete differentiation of the cells, containing less actin, or bearing less specific membrane receptors able to trigger focal actin polymerization.

Similarly, one major difficulty in assessing the validity of this type of model is that techniques used to distinguish between the steps of the cytotoxic process might be expected to influence, in the same way, the binding and lethal hit steps. There is, indeed, experimental evidence that this may well be the case. When a series of pharmacological inhibitors of the binding steps were tested for their effect on lethal hit, this last step was found to be inhibited, even when CTL and specific TC were maintained artificially in close physical contact (43). One interpretation of this observation was that the inhibition of lethal hit by the drugs was due to their capacity to relax the CTL-TC bond (43). It would be of interest to see if actin polarization had disappeared despite the maintenance of close physical contact, since this would be a requirement of the proposed "polarized motility" model. This type of analysis should be especially informative with known inhibitors of the cytoskeletal function, like cytochalasins. However, cytochalasin B, an inhibitor of actin polymerization (4) and other cellular biological functions was shown in certain experimental conditions to inhibit both binding and lethal hit steps (43,45) and to release bound CTL from their TC after the formation of doublets in nonpermissive conditions (43). Cytochalasins A and B have been reported to inhibit the binding but not the lethal hit step in other experimental conditions (3,45). Finally, some functional studies seem directly to contradict a model essentially based on cell motility acting at both steps, since they suggest that qualitative rather than quantitative differences exist between the binding and lethal steps. Thus, in addition to cytochalasins, the different effects of Ca^{++} and Mg^{++} (11,12,46) and of hyperthermia or diluted formaldehyde on binding and lethal hit might indicate fundamental differences between these two steps. It might be, however, that Ca^{++} entrance within the cells is part of the necessary signal for focal actin polymerization, while Mg^{++} might be required for more efficient contact between the CTL and TC membranes, without which the CTL cell motility would not be able to exert a strong effect on TC membrane.

In conclusion, the roles of CTL motility in CTL-TC interaction can be interpreted in at least two ways. There are indications that both binding and lethal hit steps following specific TC recognition by CTL might rely completely or largely on CTL motility. The finding that, in "permissive" conditions, the binding area is the site of rapid surface movements of the CTL supports this hypothesis (33) which is in line with previous similar models (21,35). Alternatively, CTL motility might be required until the lethal hit for the maintenance of tight binding, and the lethal hit event itself depending, however, on another CTL activities. On the basis of the striking asymmetrical changes of the CTL polymerized actin which rapidly follow TC recognition (33), it is proposed that a role of CTL motility which has not been appreciated until now could be to ensure both the mechanical bond between CTL and TC, and, consequently, the polarity of the lethal hit delivery.

ACKNOWLEDGEMENTS

The contributions of E. Rungger-Brandle and G. Gabbiano to the experimental work and discussions are gratefully acknowledged, as well as the expert technical assistance of M. Baumann and M.-C. Dubied. We also thank A. Tartakoff for reading this manuscrip.

REFERENCES

1. Martz, E., and B. Benacerraf. An effector-cell independent step in target cell lysis by sensitized mouse lymphocytes. J. Immunol. 111:1538 (1973).
2. Martz, E. Early steps in specific tumor cell lysis by sensitized mouse T-lymphocytes. I. Resolution and characterization. J. Immunol. 115:261 (1975).
3. Cerottini J.-C., and K.T. Brunner. Mechanisms of T and K cell-mediated cytolysis. In F. Loor and G.E. Roselants, B and T cells in immune recognition, p. 319, Wyley and Sons, Chichester, England (1977).
4. Golstein, P., and E.T. Smith. Mechanism of T-cell-mediated cytolysis: the lethal hit stage. Contemp. Top. Immunobiol. 7:273, Plenum Press, New York (1977).
5. Henney, C.S. T-cell-mediated cytolysis: an overview of some current issues. Contemp. Top. Immubiol. 7:245, Plenum Press, New York (1977).
6. Martz, E. Mechanism of specific tumor-cell lysis by alloimmune

T lymphocytes: resolution and characterization of discrete steps in the cellular interaction. Contemp. Top. Immunobiol. 7:301, Plenum Press, New York (1977).
7. Berke, G. Interaction of cytotoxic T lymphocytes and target cells. Prog. Allergy 27:69 (1980).
8. Zagury, D., Bernard, J., Thiernesse, N., Feldman, M., and G. Berke. Isolation and characterization of individual functionally reactive cytotoxic T lymphocytes: conjugation, killing and recycling at the single cell level. Eur. J. Immunol. 5:818 (1975).
9. Sanderson, C.S. The mechanisms of T cell mediated cytotoxicity. II. Morphological studies on cell death by time-lapse microcinematography. Proc. Roy. Soc. Lond., Ser. B 192:241 (1976).
10. Ryser, J.-E., Sordat, B., Cerottini, J.-C., and K.T. Brunner. Mechanism of target lysis by cytotoxic T lymphocytes. I. Characterization of specific lymphocyte-target cell conjugates separated by velocity sedimentation. Eur. J. Immunol. 7:110 (1977).
11. Golstein, P., and E.T. Smith. The lethal hit stage of mouse T and non-T cell mediated cytolysis: differences in cation requirements and characterization of an analytical "cation pulse" method. Eur. J. Immunol. 6:81 (1976).
12. Plaut, M., Bubbers, J.E., and C.S. Henney. Studies on the mechanism of lymphocyte-mediated cytolysis. VII. Two stages in the T cell-mediated lytic cycle with distinct cation requirements. J. Immunol. 116:150 (1976).
13. Golstein, P. Sensitivity of cytotoxic T cells to T cell-mediated cytotoxicity. Nature 252:81 (1974).
14. Kuppers, R.C., and C.S. henney. Evidence for direct linkage between antigen recognition and lytic expression in effector T cells. J. Exp. Med. 143:684 (1976).
15. Kuppers, R.C. and C.S. Henney. Studies on the mechanism of lymphocyte-mediated cytolysis. IX. Relationships between antigen recognition and lytic expression in killer T cells. J. Immunol. 118:71 (1977).
16. Sanderson, C.J. The mechanism of lymphocyte-mediated cytotoxicity. Biol. Rev. 56:153 (1981).
17. Sanderson, C.J. The mechanism of T cell mediated cytotoxicity. VIII. Zeiosis corresponds to irreversible phase (programming for lysis) in steps leading to lysis. Immunology 42:201 (1981).
18. Koren, H.S., Ax, W., and E. Freund-Moelbert. Morphological observations on the contact-induced lyis of target cells. Eur. J. Immunol. 3:32 (1973).
19. Matter, A. Microcinematographic and electron microscopic analysis of target cell lysis induced by cytotoxic T lymphocytes. Immunology 36:179 (1979).
20. Chang, T.W., Celis, E., Eisen, H.N., and F. Salomon. Crawling movements of lymphocytes on and beneath fibroblasts in culture.

Proc. Natl. Acad. Sci. USA 76:2917 (1979).
21. Grimm, E., Price, Z., and B. Bonavida. Studies on the induction and expression of T cell-mediated immunity. VIII. Effector-target junctions and target cell membrane disruption during cytolysis. Cell. Immunol. 46:77 (1979).
22. Matter, A., and P. Vassalli. Ultrastructure and fuctional study of cytotoxic T lymphocytes. In G. Raspe, Advances in the biosciences 12, p. 57, Pergamon Press, Vieweg (1973).
23. Chang, T.W., and H.N. Eisen. Lymphomas with cytotoxic activity. nature 280:406 (1979).
24. Rothstein, T.L., Mage, M., Jones, G., and L.L. McHugh. Cytotoxic T lymphocyte sequential killing of immobilized allogenic tumor target cells measured by time-lapse microcinematography. J. Immunol. 121:1652 (1978).
25. Berke, G., Sullivan, K.A., Amos, D.B. Tumor immunity in vitro: destruction of a mouse ascites tumor through a cycling pathway. Science 177:433 (1972).
26. Cerottini, J.-C., and K.T. Brunner. Reversible inhibition of lymphocyte-mediated cytotoxicity by cytochalasin B. Nature (New Biol.) 237:272 (1972).
27. Plaut, M., Lichtenstein, L.M., and C.S. Henney. Studies on the mechanism of lympocyte-mediated cytolysis. III. The role of microfilaments and microtubules. J. Immunol. 110:771 (1973).
28. Liepins, A., Foanes, R.B., Lifter, J., Choi, Y.S., and E. de Harven. Ultrastructural changes during T-lymphocyte-mediated cytolysis. Cell. Immunol. 28:109 (1977).
29. Berke, G., Gabison, D., and M. Feldman. The frequency of effector cells in populations containing cytotoxic T lymphocytes. Eur. J. Immunol. 5:813 (1975).
30. MacDonald, H.R. Early detection of potentially lethal events in T cell mediated cytolysis. Eur. J. Immunol. 5:251 (1975).
31. Grimm, E.A., and B. Bonavida. Studies on the induction and expression of T-cell mediated immunity. VI. Heterogeneity of lytic efficiency exhibited by isolated cytotoxic T lymphocytes prepared from hghly enriched populations of effector-target conjugates. J. Immunol. 119:1041 (1977).
32. Kalina, M., and G. Berke. Contact regions of cytotoxic T lymphocyte-target cell conjugates. Cell. Immunol. 25:41 (1976).
33. Ryser, J.-E., Rungger-Brandle, E., Chaponnier, C., Gabbiani, G., and P. Vassalli. The area of attachment of cytotoxic T lymphocytes to their target cells shows high motility and polarization of actin, but not myosin. J. Immunol. (in press) (1982)
34. Sanderson, C.J., and A.M. Glauert. The mechanism of T cell mediated cytotoxicity. V. Morphological studies by electron microscopy. Proc. Roy. Soc. Lond., Ser. B. 198:315 (1977).
35. Sanderson, C.J., and A.M. Glauert. The mechanism of T cell mediated cytotoxicity. VI. T-cell projections and their role

in target cell killing. Immunology 36:119 (1979).
36. Barber, T.A., and B.J. Alter. Ultrastructure of effector-target cell interaction in secondary cell-mediated lympholysis. Scand. J. Immunol. 7:57 (1978).
37. Biberfeld, P., and A. Johansson. Contact areas of cytotoxic lymphocytes and target cells. An electron microscopic study. Exp. Cell Res. 94:79 (1975).
38. Berke, G., Hu, V., McVey, E., and W.R. Clark. T lymphocyte-mediated cytolysis. I. A common mechanism for target recognition in specific and lectin-dependent cytolysis. J. Immunol. 127:776 (1981).
39. Seeman, P. Ultrastructure of membrane lesions in immune lysis, osmotic lysis and drug-induced lysis. Fed. Proc. 33:216 (1974).
40. Glasebrook, A.L. Conjugate formation by primary and secondary populations of mruine immune T lymphocytes. J. Immunol. 121:1870 (1978).
41. Shortman, K., and P. Golstein. Target cell recognition by cytolytic T cells: Different requirements for the formation of strong conjugates or for proceeding to lysis. J. Immunol. 123:833 (1979).
42. Grimm, E., and B. Bonavida. Mechanism of cell-mediated cytotoxocity at the single cell level. I. Estimation of cytotoxic T lymphocyte frequency and relative lytic efficiency. J. Immunol. 123:2861 (1979).
43. Gately, M.K., Wechter,, W.J., and E. Martz. Early steps in specific tumor cell lysis by sensitized mouse T lymphocytes. IV. Inhibition of programming for lysis by pharmacological agents. J. Immunol. 125:783 (1980).
44. Fox, J.E.B., and D.R. Phillips. Inhibition of actin polymerization in blood platelets by cytochalasins. Nature 292:650 (1981).
45. Golstein, P., Foa, C., and I.C.M. McLennan. Mechanism of T cell mediated cytolysis: the differential impact of cytochalasins at the recognition and lethal hit stages. Eur. J. Immunol. 8:302 (1978).
46. Martz, E. Immune T lymphocyte to tumor cell adherion. Magnesium sufficient, calcium insufficient. J. Cell. Biol. 84:584 (1980).
47. Berke, G., Fishelson, Z., and B. Schick. Hyperthermia and formaldehyde can dissociate the binding and killing activities of cytolytic T lymphocytes. Transplant. Proc. 11:804 (1979).

DISCUSSION

W. Clark

In your films, was it clear that the localization of actin was in the CTL and not in the target cell, or was it in both?

J.-E. Ryser

It was absolutely clear. Actin is detectable in the targets, but there are lesser amounts, and it's clear from the picture that it's only CTL actin which is polarized, TC actin remaining in a diffuse pattern.

C. Henney

Were these studies done using a cloned CTL line?

J.-E. Ryser

We used PEL cells immunized *in vivo*.

C. Henney

If you use lymphocytes as targets, then does the actin still not move to the points of contact? Is it only at the effector level that that happens?

J.-E. Ryser

This experiment wasn't done.

C. Henney

Can you get myosin to cap under any condition in effector T cells?

J.-E. Ryser

No. Well, we didn't see any capping of myosin, but the same technique can be used to show myosin capping in B cells.

M. Mescher

In your experiments, did you see any killer bound to two different targets, and if so, what did the actin look like in that case?

J.-E. Ryser

I can't answer for sure to that, because conjugates were made in lymphocyte excess.

W. Clark

That's a good point, since it's thought the CTLs can only kill one target at a time.

G. Berke

We have made a similar study related to tubulin accumulation (Geiger, Rosen and Berke, 1981, submitted). By forming conjugates, fixing and staining them with an antitubulin antibody we have been able to show the localization of the centriole of the effector, but not of the target, exquisitely at the contact site, which corresponds to the finding of accumulation of actin. We cannot offer any immediate interpretation of that fact, but it may be related to the great deal of membrane activity and to other structures that are localized at that site.

P. Henkart

What I see here does not really strike me as something I would call extensive interdigitation. I would just like to clarify to what extent there is agreement between your studies and those of others.

J.-E. Ryser

I think there is full agreement. But interference contrast microscopy, unlike electron microscopy (Eur. J. Immunol. 1977, 7:110), doesn't allow to see all interdigitations between the cells. This technique has the advantage that details of the binding can be studied between living cells, but the drawback is that you only see the portion of the cell which is in close contact with the glass substrate. So, you don't see the center of the binding structure, you just see its periphery.

E. Martz

It seems that many groups are in agreement that these kinds of extensive motile interdigitations occur during killing conjugation. As has been mentioned, cytochalasin A does not appear to block the completion of the lethal hit and we have done quite a bit of work with cytochalasin B, and we would agree that cytochalasin B acts very strongly on probably the strengthening of the adhesion, but does not prevent the completion of the lethal hit. So, I think the experiment that needs to be done is to observe these interdigitations, perhaps in the film situation or videotape, while taking the conjugates through stages and applying one of the cytochalasins in such a way that one can decide whether the interdigitations are necessary for the lethal hit. Not sufficient, but necessary. They may be unnecessary, i.e., you may be able to prevent that kind of motile interdigitation and penetration and still see completion of the lethal hit, because it has been shown by several groups, that you can complete the lethal hit in the presence of cytochalasin.

G. Berke

If one wants to know whether a reagent affects conjugation, which may be the sole reason why it prevents killing, one could explore the possibility that conjugates seen under the light microscope are disturbed (poor interdigitation, for example) when examined under the electron microscope (Transplant. Proc. 1981, 13:1073). Another approach is to use fluorescently-labeled killer cells and non-labeled target cells and videotape the interaction under the fluorescent light microscope at 37°C, using a light intensifier (Berke and Schlessinger, unpublished). With this technique we could see finger-like structures penetrating the target cell back and forth. We estimate that about 20% of the entire surface area of the killer is involved. If you consider how much energy and movement is required to interject those finger-like structures you can get an idea of how easy it can be to disturb conjugation.

M. Mescher

Gideon, do you see those extensive interdigitations under conditions which don't allow lysis to occur? In the absence of calcium, in other words?

G. Berke

To some extent, it is a quantitative thing.

M. Mescher

You mean the number of interdigitations or are you talking about the depth of penetration, or points of contact?

G. Berke

No, I'm talking about the extent of interdigitation.

A. Allison

Gideon, if you use cytochalasin A, do you block these interdigitations?

G. Berke

There is a substantial reduction and also the kinetics of formation is slower (Rosen et al., Transpl. Proc. 1981, 13:1073). In addition, cytochalasin A at higher (>0.2 μg/ml) concentrations totally eliminates.

A. Allison

It seems an appealing interpretation that microfilaments are actually involved in these interdigitations.

G. Berke

I think it's an almost inevitable conclusion.

E. Martz

Gideon, have these interdigitations been observed in lectin-dependent, non-specific T cells?

G. Berke

Yes, these interdigitations are indistinguishable in specific or lectin-dependent cytolysis.

B. Bonavida

We have done some studies of effector-CTL conjugates by electron microscopy a few years ago and we have also seen those interdigitations (Cellular Immunology, 1979, 46:77). Do you see them when you have binding with target cells in a system in which lysis does not take place?

W. Clark

You get pretty good conjugate formation at room temperature, but not lysis, and there it's clear that the extent of interdigitation is qualitatively different than at 37°C.

S. Ladisch

I just would like to take that question one step further and ask whether those interdigitations might exist between cells that are not cytotoxic at all.

G. Berke

We don't have firm evidence whether they're absolutely positively playing a role in the cytolytic process. We do see them associated with it, but we can't say more than that.

M. Hanna

Josh Fidler has been able to select *in vitro* lymphocyte resistant B16 melanoma lines. These are almost totally resistant to sensitized lymphocytes. The electron microscopic analysis of the conjugates shows many fewer sensitized lymphocytes approaching or surrounding these B16 cells, and a total absence of interdigitations. The cells may approach, and we have seen lymphocytes pairing to form rosettes around these lymphocyte-resistant B16 cells, but no interdigitation. It's interesting that there seems to be a uniform separation between the lymphocytes and the target cells.

P. Golstein

We may be faced with the conclusion that interdigitations might be necessary for kill, but the whole problem is, are they sufficient?

CYTOLYTIC T LYMPHOCYTE RECOGNITION OF SUBCELLULAR ANTIGEN

Matthew F. Mescher, Steven P. Balk, Steven J. Burakoff and Steven H. Herrmann

Department of Pathology and the Sidney Farber Cancer Institute, Harvard Medical School
Boston, Massachusetts 02115

INTRODUCTION

Specific antigen recognition is required to stimulate generation of a cytolytic T lymphocyte (CTL[1]) response and to allow the resulting effector CTLs to bind and lyse the target cells. Reliable assays allow in vitro assessment of stimulation of a primary and secondary response and of the effector-target interaction. The antigens required to trigger generation of a response are the same as those required to allow binding and lysis by the effector CTL.

The antigens recognized by murine CTLs are cell surface proteins present on allogeneic, virus-infected or chemically-modified cells or tumor cells. In each case, recognition involves the Class I Major Histocompatibility Antigens (H-2 antigens) present on the stimulating and target cells (1). The H-2 antigens are transmembrane glycoproteins having the bulk of the protein exposed on the cell surface (Fig. 1, ref. 2). CTL specific for syngeneic targets recognize both the H-2 antigens and the foreign protein on the target cell: the viral, chemically-modified or tumor-specific protein. CTL specific for allogeneic targets may recognize only the foreign H-2 present on the target, although it has been suggested that this may also involve joint recognition of H-2 and other surface proteins (3).

---

[1]Abbreviations: CTL, cytolytic T lymphocytes; pCTL, primed precursor CTL, T_HF, T cell helper factor; LPS, lipopolysaccharide.

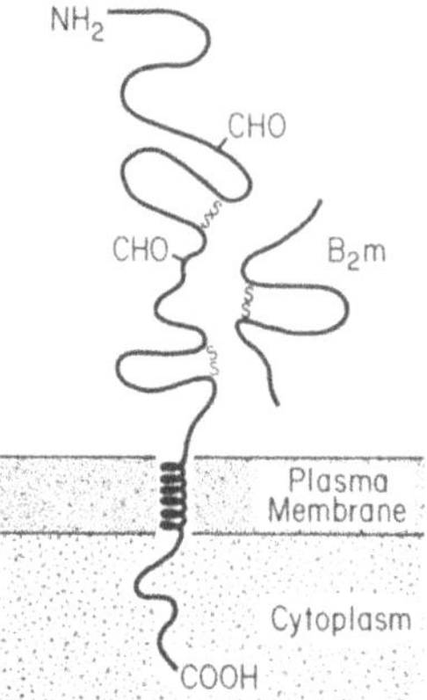

Fig. 1 Schematic diagram of a Class I murine MHC antigen in the plasma membrane. CHO: carbohydrate units.

Although genetic and immunological approaches have allowed definition of most of the relevant antigens, the recognition process is poorly understood at the molecular level, as is the mechanism by which CTL lyse the target cell. This is due in part to the complex milieu of the stimulating and target antigens - the surface of live, intact cells. For this reason considerable effort has been made to measure CTL recognition using subcellular antigen preparations. This approach has begun to provide better definition of the requirements for recognition and holds promise for providing a means of studying the lytic mechanism. The use of artificial membranes (liposomes) has contributed greatly to understanding the mechanism of complement-mediated lysis (4). Artificial antigen-containing membranes which could be lysed by CTL would similarily provide an invaluable means of studying the molecular mechanisms involved in the lytic agent.

Early work with subcellular antigen preparations demonstrated that particulate fractions from allogeneic cells would stimulate generation of a secondary CTL response (5-8) but would not effectively block the CTL-target interaction (8,9). The stimulating activity was immunologically specific (5-8), was localized to the plasma membrane (8) and could be blocked by anti-H-2 antisera specific for the antigens on the membranes (10). It thus appeared that recognition of antigen on the isolated membranes mimicked, at least in some respects, recognition of cell bound antigen. We have continued, over the past several years, to pursue this approach to the study of CTL recognition. Efforts to examine recognition during stimulation of a response, done largely in collaboration with Dr. Steven Burakoff and his co-workers (Sidney Farber Cancer Research Institute, Harvard Medical School) have thus far been most successful and are briefly reviewed here. Attempts to measure subcellular antigen recognition at the effector CTL stage have been less successful. These efforts have, however, revealed novel features of the CTL-target interaction and suggested possible explanations for the difficulties of measuring subcellular antigen recognition. Furthermore, the findings suggest new approaches to attempting to use artificial membranes to study lysis by CTL and these are discussed.

STIMULATION OF A CTL RESPONSE

It was found that plasma membranes could be solubilized with detergent and reconstituted (by dialysis to remove the detergent) in a form which retained activity for stimulation of a secondary allogeneic CTL response (11,12). This made it possible to manipulate the composition of the stimulating antigen preparation by adding or removing proteins before reconstitution. Thus, it could be demonstrated that reconstituted membranes containing both H-2 and viral proteins would stimulate a Sendai virus-specific response (13). Effective stimulation occurred only if both the H-2 and viral proteins were present in the same lipid bilayer. Similar results have been obtained by others in studying stimulation of responses to other viruses (14,15) and to syngeneic tumor (16). It was also shown that purified human histocompatibility antigens HLA-A, B and C, incorporated into unilamellar liposomes would stimulate generation of a xenogeneic (mouse anti-human) CTL response (17). More recently it has become possible to purify H-2 antigens on a relatively large scale using monoclonal antibody affinity columns (18,19). The purified H-2 antigens in liposomes will stimulate an allogeneic response (20) and Hale et al. (21) have shown that liposomes containing purified H-2 and viral proteins will stimulate a virus-specific response.

While the studies described above have demonstrated the ability of artificial membranes of defined composition to stimulate generation of secondary CTL responses, the nature of the assay placed severe limitations on studying recognition by the primed, precursor CTL (pCTL). Assays were done by mixing liposomes and primed responder cells, placing them in culture and assaying CTL activity on the appropriate targets five days later. It was not known when antigen recognition occurred during the five days nor if the liposomes were in the same form at the time of recognition as when they were added. Thus, for example, meaningful results regarding the effect of lipid composition of the membrane or antigen density could not be obtained because of the possibility that these parameters had changed (lipid exchange, proteolysis, etc.) by the time interaction with the pCTL occurred.

It was also becoming apparent, from work being done in a number of laboratories, that helper T cells could augment CTL responses.

Thus, the magnitude of the CTL response might be determined by the effectiveness of pCTL antigen recognition or, alternatively, by the level of helper cell activity in the cultures. Recent results, obtained in collaboration with Dr. Steven Burakoff and his coworkers, have demonstrated that generation of a secondary allogeneic CTL response to H-2 containing lipsomes is dependent on T helper cell activity (22). Use of liposomes and helper factor (T_HF) has made it possible to separate pCTL-antigen recognition from delivery of help and study each signal separately (23). Furthermore, the pCTL-antigen interaction can be limited to short times, thus allowing meaningful results to be obtained regarding parameters which affect this recognition.

Liposomes provide unique advantages in studying the requirements for generation of a CTL response. The liposomes can be mixed with cells for varying periods of time and subsequently removed by differential centrifugation. Furthermore, including radioactively labeled antigen makes it possible to monitor the effectiveness of antigen separation from the cells and to monitor the fate of the antigen in culture. These properties of H-2 containing liposomes together with techniques for separating subpopulations of spleen cells have mde it possible to study the requirements for generation of a secondary allogeneic CTL response. As previously proposed by others (24-28), the response requires two different signals, both involving T cell recognition of alloantigen (ref. 23 and Fig. 2).

Signal 1 delivery occurs via specific recognition of the alloantigen by Ly 1^-2^+ primed precursor CTL. Pulsing cells with liposomes under different conditions, followed by removal of the antigen, has demonstrated that exposure of the cells to the liposomes for two hours at 4°C is sufficient to trigger a maximum response when the cells are subsequently placed in culture at 37°C and signal 2 provided at the optimum time (23 and Hermann and Mescher, unpublished). No adherent cell requirement could be demonstrated for this recognition event, suggesting that the pCTL recognize native antigen. Furthermore, non-primed cells which have been pulsed with liposomes and washed fail to stimulate a significant response when mixed with primed cells. This result suggests that the pCTL may directly interact with the H-2 antigen on the liposome and not with antigen bound to the surface of other cells in the culture. Following interaction with alloantigen, pCTL require 12 to 24 hours in culture to become maximally responsive to signal 2, suggesting that alloantigen recognition triggers synthesis and/or expression of receptors for signal 2. The pCTL differentiate to effector CTL only if signal 2 is available following antigen recognition.

Signal 2 is provided by T cell helper factor. Production of this factor also requires alloantigen recognition and recognition in this case is dependent on adherent cells (23,29,30). Evidence indicates that antigen is taken up by the adherent cells, 'processed' and presented to $Ly1^{+}2^{-}$ T helper cells. Effective recognition by the T helper cells appears to require both processed alloantigen and Ia antigen on the adherent cells. Only Ia bearing adherent cells are effective in antigen presentation and anti-Ia antisera (and anti-Ia monoclonal antibodies) block presentation. Antigen recognition triggers T helper cells to produce a soluble factor(s), probably IL2, thus providing signal to the pCTL. Signal 2 can also be provided by factors prepared from culture supernatants of conconavalin A stimulated rat lymphocytes or phytohemagglutinin stimulated human lymphocytes (T_HF). Primed spleen cells depleted of $Ly1^{+}2^{-}$ T cells and adherent cells are able to make a CTL response if pulsed with H-2 containing liposomes and T_HF is added 12 to 24 hours later. The response remains strictly dependent on alloantigen; addition of T_HF alone gives no response.

The results described above have clarified the events occurring during generation of a CTL response. They have also provided methodology which allows study of parameters affecting pCTL recognition of alloantigen. Thus, responder cells can be pulsed with liposomes of varying size, antigen density, lipid composition, etc., and subsequently provided with an optimum amount of T_HF. The magnitude of the resulting CTL response is then a measure of the effectiveness of recognition of the H-2 by the pCTL.

It was previously shown that the composition of the H-2 containing liposomes affects the efficiency of stimulation of a CTL response (20,31). Stimulation occurs at a lower antigen dose if liposomes are prepared in the presence of a detergent-insoluble fraction isolation from plasma membranes than if the liposomes are prepared using just lipid and H-2. The detergent insoluble membrane fraction appears to consist of a group of proteins which form a skeletal structure on the inner membrane surface (32). Extraction of purified plasma membranes with non-ionic detergents removes most of the lipid and protein but the matrix remains insoluble and is in the form of closed structures. When isolated matrix is mixed with H-2 and lipid in deoxycholate and liposomes are then formed by dialysis it appears that the lipid reforms a bilayer on the matrix and the H-2 antigens become incorporated on their surface. Such liposomes are larger and more irregular in shape than liposomes prepared using just lipid and H-2. When liposomes prepared from matrix, H-2 and lipid were compared to those prepared from just lipid and H-2, they were found to be 3 to 6 fold more efficient in stimulating a response. Those experiments were done by mixing liposomes with responder cells, culturing the cells for 5 days and measuring the response. Thus, the greater efficiency of matrix-containing liposomes could have resulted from more effective recognition by CTL, greater stimulation of helper factor production (e.g., by more effective adherent cell uptake), or both.

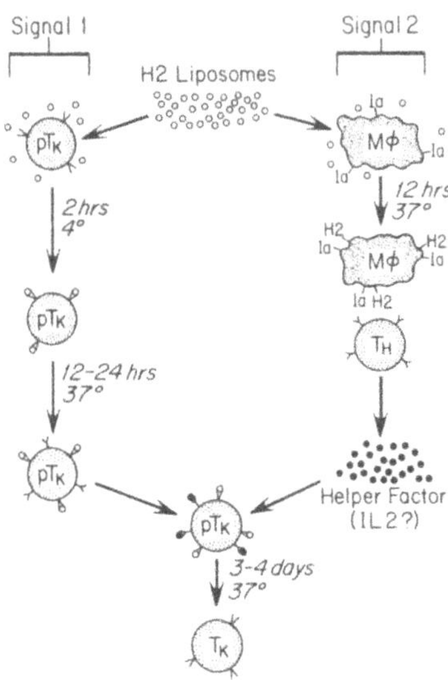

Fig. 2 Two signals are required for stimulation of a secondary allogeneic CTL response by H-$2K^k$ in liposomes. See text for discussion. (pT_K, primed precursor: MØ, adherent cell: T_H, T-helper cell).

More recently, we have compared the two types of liposomes in assays similar to that shown in Fig. 2 (23). Responder cells were pulsed with varying doses of one or the other type of liposome, washed to remove antigen and placed in culture. T_HF was then added 24 hours later to provide optimum signal 2, thus insuring that the magnitude of the response would be determined by pCTL interaction with H-2. It was again found that matrix-containing liposomes were 3-5 fold more effective than liposomes lacking the matrix. Thus, it appears that the structure of the liposome affects the efficiency of pCTL recognition of H-2.

The greater efficiency of the matrix-containing liposomes might result from an interaction between the transmembrane H-2 protein and a component of the matrix which affects the manner in which the H-2 is arrayed on the liposome surface. Alternatively, the matrix-containing liposomes may allow for a greater number of receptor-antigen interactions in a localized area on the cell surface due to their larger size and irregular shape. A requirement for highly multivalent interaction is suggested by the observations that the soluble papain cleavage product of H-2 will not stimulate a response despite the fact that it retains serological activity (5). Furthermore, removal of detergent from intact H-2 in the absence of lipid, a procedure which probably yields small protein aggregates, results in antigen which will stimulate only a marginal response even at doses 50 to 100 times greater than those required for stimulation by H-2 containing liposomes (Stallcup, Burakoff, and Mescher, unpublished).

Using the approach decribed above, it will now be possible to examine the basis for more effective recognition of H-2 on matrix-containing liposomes and to determine what other parameters (e.g., lipid fluidity, H-2 modifications, antigen density, etc.) might affect pCTL recognition. It seems not unreasonable to expect that factors which influence pCTL recognition may also affect the CTL-target cell interaction.

THE CTL-TARGET CELL INTERACTION

Purified membranes or liposomes bearing the appropriate H-2 antigens, as demonstrated by their ability to specifically stimulate a CTL response, might also be expected to block lysis of targets of CTL. Despite considerable effort in this and other laboratories (8,9,33,34), it has proven very difficult, thus far, to use this approach as a realiable and reproducible means of assessing CTL recognition of subcellular antigen. These difficulties could arise due to a failure of the CTL to recognize subcellular antigen or, alternatively, due to inability of subcellular antigen to compete with intact target cells in the assays used.

Several features of the standard assay used to measure CTL-target cell interaction result in suboptimal conditions for attempting to block the interaction with membranes. CTL and targets are allowed to settle or are pelleted by centrifugation under conditions where membrane vesicles remain in suspension. Thus, the effective cell concentration is greatly increased and the cells are removed from exposure to the majority of the membrane. The CTL and targets are then allowed to interact for a relatively long period, usually four hours. During this time an individual CTL probably lyses several target cells. Lysis of a target cell involves binding by the CTL to form a conjugate and subsequent programming for lysis and lysis of the target (35). Membranes would be expected to interfere only with the binding event, not with programming and lysis of an already bound target. Unless binding of the target by the CTL were the rate limiting step in the assay, membranes might significantly affect the rate of CTL-target interaction without affecting the chromium release measured at the end of four hours.

For these reasons, an assay was developed which eliminates these potential problems (33). It was found that effective allogeneic CTL-target interaction occurred when the cells were mixed and kept in uniform suspension on a rotating shaker. This was true for tumor cell and lipopolysaccharide (LPS) blast targets but not for normal spleen cell targets. Furthermore, it was possible to develop an assay which measured the rate and extent of functional conjugate formation in suspension, independent of the lytic events. This was done by taking advantage of the observations that conjugate formation occurs in the absence of calcium but programming for lysis does not (35). Chromium release from targets bound by CTL in the absence of calcium can then be measured under conditions where formation of new conjugates cannot occur by shifting the cells to medium containing calcium and dextran. The calcium allows programming and lysis to occur while the viscous dextran prevents new conjugates from forming.

Using this assay, it was possible to measure the rate and extent of conjugate formation in suspension (33). It was found that the CTL-target interaction had the properties of an equilibrium binding process. Conjugate formation proceeded at a rapid initial rate but the number of conjugates plateaued within one to two hours. It could be shown that free CTL and target cells were present at this time despite the fact that no increase in the total number of conjugates was occurring: the plateau level of conjugates was dependent on the target cell concentration in suspension. Data obtained at several different target cell concentrations could be analyzed by Scatchard analysis to yield a value for the apparent affinity of the CTL for the target cell.

An equilibrium binding between CTL and targets implies a finite rate at which the conjugates fall apart. This reversal could be measured by allowing conjugates to form, diluting the cells to lower the target cell concentration and measuring the number of functional conjugates remaining following further incubation in suspension for several hours. It was found that reversal occurred more rapidly when conjugates were formed using spleen cell targets than when tumor cell targets were used. In fact, the slow rate of reversal with tumor targets was difficult to measure due to the problem of spontaneous chromium release from the targets during the course of the necessarily long incubations.

While spontaneous reversal was difficult to measure, it was found that addition of unlabeled target cells after dilution of the conjugates resulted in a rapid decrease in the number of labeled targets present in functional conjugates (36,37). This occurred only if the unlabeled target cells were of the appropriate H-2 haplotype. When the same experiment was done using unlabeled targets to form the initial conjugates and labeled targets were then added following dilution, it was found that functional conjugate formation occurred with the labeled targets. These results are most easily interpreted as indicating that a CTL having a bound target cell can interact with a second target and release the first, i.e., it appears to be an exchange process. It should be emphasized that the assay employed in these experiments measures 'functional' conjugates, i.e., CTL-target binding that leads to chromium release. It is possible that a CTL having a bound target may bind a second target and lyse only that second target without releasing the first. The failure to observe significant numbers of multiple conjugates (i.e., lymphocytes having two or more targets bound) when these cells are examined under the microscope suggests that this is not the case. However, rigorous quantitative data to demonstrate this has not yet been obtained.

The results obtained using the assay to measure conjugate formation in suspension indicate that the CTL-target interaction is an equilibrium binding process. Furthermore, it appears that a CTL can release a bound target upon interaction with a second target cell. These proposed interactions are summarized in Fig. 3. Recent data has provided further support for the view that CTL-target interaction is an equilibrium binding process (Balk and Mescher, manuscript in preparation). Treatment of preformed conjugates with anti-H-2 antiserum specific for the target cell H-2 results in reversal of the conjugates. Similarly, treatment with anti Lyt 2 antiserum, specific for the CTL, results in rapid reversal. In this case, quantitative conjuate counting has demonstrated that the target is released from the CTL upon reversal with antibody. Treatment of conjugates with antibodies directed at other CTL surface proteins (Thy 1 and H-2) does not cause reversal.

The approaches described above have provided novel ways to attempt to measure CTL recognition of membranes bearing the appropriate alloantigens. Thus, membranes can be examined for an effect on the initial rate of conjugate formation, an effect on the equilibrium level of binding or the ability to cause reversal of preformed conjugates. Numerous attempts to demonstrate such specific effects at membrane concentrations of up to 1-2 mg/ml have been unsuccessful (33,36,37). Consideration of the apparent CTL affinity for different types of target cells, however, suggests that these negative results may be due to ineffective competition of membranes with intact target cells and not due to an inability of the CTL to recognize and interact with subcellular antigen.

Allogeneic CTL appear to have a much higher apparent affinity for tumor cells and LPS blast targets than for spleen cell targets. This is suggested by the observation that conjugate formation with tumor cell and LPS blast targets an occur in suspension while it only occurs with spleen cell targets when cell contact is increased

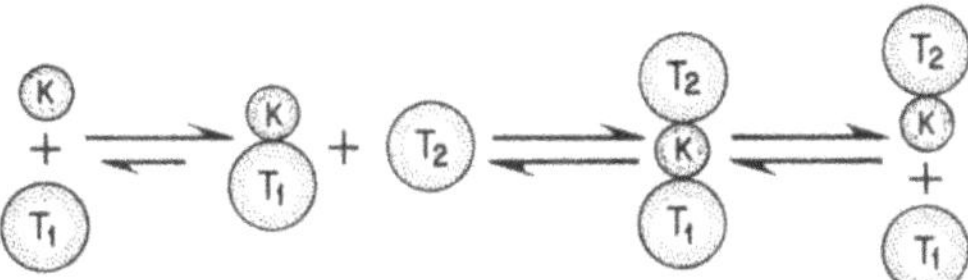

Fig. 3 The CTL-target cell interaction has the properties of an equilibrium binding process. See text for discussion.

by allowing cells to settle or pelleting them together by centrifugation (33). Furthermore spontaneous reversal of CTL-spleen cell conjugates occurs rapidly if the conjugates are formed by pelleting and then suspended (37). In contrast, as described above, reversal of conjugates made from tumor cell targets is very slow. The most striking demonstration of the difference in apparent affinity is provided by experiments done to examine exchange between preformed conjugates and added unlabeled targets (37). Conjugates made from spleen cell targets readily exchange upon addition of unlabeled tumor targets and to a lesser degree upon addition of unlabeled spleen cell targets. In contrast, conjugates made fom tumor cell targets exchange upon addition of cold tumor cells but are not significantly affected by addition of spleen cell targets. Thus, this experiment provides an example of ineffective competition of one target with another despite the fact that the spleen cell can clearly be recognized and lysed by the CTL under appropriate conditions.

Tumor cells and normal spleen cells clearly have a large number of differences which might contribute to their interaction with CTL. Tumor specific antigens do not appear to be one of these. The experiments described above were done using allogeneic CTL populations obtained by in vitro secondary stimulation of cells from previously primed mice. CTL obtained by secondary stimulation with either irradiated tumor cells or spleen cells showed the same relative preference for tumor versus spleen cell targets. A difference in H-2 antigen density on the surface also appears unlikely to account for the differences in apparent CTL affinity. P815, the tumor target used in most of the above experiments, appears to have about the same surface density of $H-2^d$ as $H-2^d$ spleen cells (19).

One obvious difference between tumor and LPS blast targets in comparison to spleen cells is their larger size. The results described in the previous section suggest that the extent of multivalency may affect pCTL triggering by liposomes. A more extensive area of surface interaction between the tumor target and CTL may similarly account for the apparently higher affinity of this interaction. If so, it would not be surprising that membranes fail to compete with intact target cells since the membranes are in the form of small vesicles, only up to about 1 micron in diameter (8).

These considerations suggested that attachment of the membranes to a large surface might allow effective competition and blocking of the CTL-target interaction. Therefore, polycationic beads with a diameter of 75-150 microns were coated with membrane vesicles and tested for blocking (Balk and Mescher, manuscript in preparation). Membranes bind to the beads via the positive charge on the bead surface. Membrane-coated beads were found to block allogeneic CTL-target cell interaction. Numerous experiments examining beads coated with membranes bearing different H-2 haplotypes and using CTL populations of several specificities have shown that there is a reproducible and specific component to the blocking. Very significant non-specific blocking is also seen in these experiments, probably due to residual positive charge on the surface of the coated beads. These results are consistent with the possibility that the area of surface interaction, and thus the extent of multivalency, plays a critical role in determining the effectiveness of CTL-antigen binding. The possibility cannot be ruled out, however, that the positive charge on the bead surface helps to stabilize the CTL-membrane interaction. Varying the size and charge density of the beads should make it possible to investigate the relative importance of these parameters. It should also be possible to begin to examine CTL recognition of purified antigen by using beads coated with H-2 containing liposomes.

CONCLUSIONS

Results obtained in studies of stimulation of a CTL response and blocking of effector-target interactions with subcellular antigen have suggested that a highly multivalent interaction may be critical for effective CTL (or pCTL) binding of the antigen. This may prove to be an important consideration in attempting to design antigen bearing liposomes capable of being lysed by CTL. Thus small, unilamellar vesicles prepared from lipid and H-2 are unlikely to act as targets. Large liposomes may be more effective but methods for preparing such vesicles under conditions which allow incorporation of non-denatured protein antigens are limited.

Hollander et al. (38) have reported successful specific lysis of liposomes by allogeneic CTL. The liposomes were prepared in the presence of protein extracted from human eye muscle preparations. The resulting liposomes were large, up to 1 micron in diameter. Difficulty was encountered in attempting to reproducibly obtain liposome preparations capable of acting as targets. Examination of effective and ineffective preparations suggested that the liposomes were good targets only if they were large and irregular in shape (39).

The detergent insoluble plasma membrane matrix may provide a means of preparing reproducibly large vesicles bearing H-2 antigen on their surface. In the experiments described in a previous section it was found that liposomes formed in the presence of matrix isolated from membrane vesicles effectively stimulated generation of a CTL response (20). Although larger than vesicles prepared using just lipid and H-2, the matrix containing liposomes were still relatively small, up to 0.3 microns in diameter; probably too small to act as effective targets. Their size is limited by the size of the matrix structure which can be isolated from plasma membrane preparations.

We have recently found that detergent treatment of enucleated cytoplasts removes most of the membrane lipid and protein and the cytoplasmic proteins (Herrmann and Mescher, unpublished). The structures remaining following extraction have the appearance of empty bags of the same size as the cytoplasts and consist of the membrane matrix. Preliminary experiments suggest that mixing these structures with H-2 and lipid in deoxycholate and dialyzing to remove detergent results in very large vesicles having H-2 incorporated. These vesicle preparations appear to be more effective in stimulating a CTL response than liposomes prepared using matrix derived from membrane vesicles. If conditions can be found which allow preparation of such vesicles which will retain trapped markers, they may provide effective CTL targets useful for studying both recognition and the lytic mechanism.

It should be pointed out that a lytic mechanism involving, for example, poisoning of the target cells' ability to pump ions would not allow lysis of liposomes. Only a lytic mechanism which acts directly on the membrane (e.g., by changing its permeability properties or destabilizing its structure, see below) would be expected to be effective with liposomes. However, liposomes which are effectively recognized by CTL and trigger the lytic mechanism might prove useful even if they are not lysed. For example, they could provide a means of examining possible transfer of CTL components to the target.

It is interesting to speculate that the plasma membrane matrix might be involved in lysis by CTL. This matrix appears to form a membrane skeleton over the entire inner face of the plasma membrane (32, Herrmann and Mescher, manuscript in preparation). This is indicated by the fact that Triton X-100 extraction of intact cells (tumor cells or lymphocytes) under appropriate conditions yields 'ghosts' consisting of an intact nucleus surrounded by a structure with a bag-like appearance. The extraction procedure removes most (>95%) of the cell surface and cytoplasmic proteins. The bag-like structure appears to consist of the plasma membrane matrix. If this matrix plays a structural role in stabilizing the surface membrane, as appears likely, then disruption of the matrix structure by the CTL could lead to membrane destabilization and ultimately cell lysis. Matrix-containing liposomes which could be used as targets for CTL attack would provide a means of investigating this possibility.

REFERENCES

(1) Klein, J. 1979. The major histocompatibility complex of the mouse. Science 203:516.
(2) Nathenson, S.G., Uehara, H., and Ewenstein, B.M. 1981. Primary structural analysis of the transplantation antigens

of the murine H-2 major histocompatibility complex. Ann. Rev. Biochem. 50:1025.
(3) Matzinger, P., and Bevan, M.J. 1977. Hypothesis. Why do so many lymphocytes respond to major histocompatibility antigens. Cell. Immunol. 29:1.
(4) Kinsky, S.C., and Nicolotti, R.A. 1977. Immunological properties of model membranes. Ann. Rev. Biochem. 46:49.
(5) Engers, H.D., Thomas, K., Cerottini, J.C., and Brunner, K.T. 1975. Generation of cytotoxic T cells in vitro. V. Response of normal and immune spleen cells to subcellular alloantigen. J. Immunol. 115:356.
(6) Wagner, H., Hess, M., Feldmann, M., and Rollinghoff, M. 1976. Secondary cytotoxic allograft responses in vitro. III. The immunogenicity of allogeneic membrane fragments. Transplantation 21:282.
(7) Häyry, P., and Anderson, L.C. 1976. Generation of T memory cells in one-way mixed lymphocyte culture. IV. Primary and secondary responses to soluble and insoluble membrane preparations and to ultraviolet light inactivated stimulator cells. Scand. J. Immunol. 5:391.
(8) Lemonnier, F., Mescher, M.F., Sherman, L., and Burakoff, S. 1978. The induction of cytolytic T lymphocytes with purified plasma membranes. J. Immunol. 120:1114.
(9) Todd, R.F., Stulting, R.D., and Amos, D.B. 1975. Lymphocyte-mediated cytolysis of allogeneic tumor cells in vitro. I. Search for target antigens in subcellular fractions. Cell. Immunol. 18:304.
(10) Lemmonier, F., Burakoff, S., Mescher, M., Dorf, M., and Benacerraf, B. 1978. Inhibition of the induction of cytolytic T lymphocytes with alloantisera directed aginst H-2K and H-2D gene products. J. Immunol. 120:1717.
(11) Mescher, M., Sherman, L., and Burakoff, S. 1978. The induction of secondary cytolytic T lymphocytes by solubilized membrane proteins. J. Exp. Med. 147:946.
(12) Fast, L.D, and Fan, D.P. 1978. Dissociated and reconstituted subcellular alloantigen capable of stimulating mouse cytotoxic T lymphocytes in vitro. J. Immunol. 120:1092.
(13) Finberg, R., Mescher, M., and Bufakoff, S.J. 1978. The induction of virus-specific cytotoxic T lymphocytes with solubilized viral and membrane proteins. J. Exp. Med. 148:1620.
(14) Loh, D., Ross, A.H., Hale, A.H., Baltimore, D., and Eisen, H.N. 1979. Synthetic phospholipid vesicles containing a purified viral antigen and cell membrane proteins stimulate the development of cytotoxic T lymphocytes. J. Exp. Med. 150:1067.
(15) Ciavarra, R.P., Kang, C.Y., and Forman, J. 1980. Vesicular stomatitis antigens recognized by cytotoxic cells: analysis with defective intefering particles and reconstituted membrane vesicles. J. Immunol. 125:336.

(16) Alaba, O., and Law, L.W. 1980. Specific induction of syngeneic cytotoxic T lymphocytes by solubilized tumor antigen: fractionation of the specific R-MuLV-induced leukemia antigen. J. Immunol. 125:414.
(17) Engelhard, V.H., Strominger, J.L., Mescher, M., and Burakoff, S. 1978. Induction of secondary cytotoxic T lymphocytes by purified HLA-A and HLA-B antigens reconstituted into phospholipid vesicles. Proc. Natl. Acad. Sci. USA 75:5688.
(18) Herrmann, S.H., and Mescher, M.F. 1979. Purification of the H-2K^k molecule of the murine major histocompatibility complex. J. Biol. Chem. 254:8713.
(19) Stallcup, K.C., Springer, T.A., and Mescher, M.F. 1981. Characterization of an anti-H-2 monoclonal antibody and its use in large scale antigen purification. J. Immunol. 127:923.
(20) Herrmann, S.H., and Mescher, M.F. 1981. Secondary cytolytic T lymphocyte stimulation by purified H-2K^k in liposomes. Proc. Natl. Acad. Sci. USA 78:2488.
(21) Hale, A.H., Ruebush, M.J., and Harris, D.T. 1980. Elicitation of anti-viral cytotoxic T lymphocytes with purified viral and H-2 antigens. J. Immunol. 125:428.
(22) Weinberger, O., Herrmann, S.H., Mescher, M.F., Benacerraf, B., and Burakoff, S.J. 1981. Cellular interactions in the generation of cytotoxic T lymphocyte responses. Analysis of the helper T cell pathway. Eur. J. Immunol. 11:1105.
(23) Herrmann, S.H., Weinberger, O., Burakoff, S.J., and Mescher, M.F. 1981. Analysis of the two-signal requirement for precursor CTL activation using H-2K^k in liposomes. Manuscript submitted.
(24) Lalande, M.E., McCutcheon, M.J., and Miller, R.G. 1980. Quantitative studies on the precursors of cytotoxic lymphocytes. VI. Second signal requirements of specifically activated precursors isolated 12 hours after stimulation. J. Exp. Med. 151:12.
(25) Teh, H.-S., and Teh, S.-J. 1980. Direct evidence for a two-signal mechanism of cytotoxic T-lymphocyte activation. Nature 285:163.
(26) Symington, F.W., and Teh, H.-S. 1980. A two-signal mechanism for the induction of cytotoxic T lymphocytes. Scand. J. Immunol. 12:1.
(27) Bach, F.H., Bach, M.L., and Sondel, P.M. 1976. Differential function of major histocompatibility complex antigens in T lymphocyte activation. Nature 259:273.
(28) Lafferty, K.L., and Woolnough, J. 1977. The origin and mechanism of the allograft reaction. Immunol. Rev. 35:231.
(29) Weinberger, O., Herrmann, S.H., Mescher, M.F., Benacerraf, B., and Burakoff, S.J. 1980. Cellular interactions in the generation of cytolytic T lymphocyte responses. Role of Ia positive splenic adherent cells in the presentation of H-2 antigen. Proc. Natl. Acad. Sci. USA 77:6091.
(30) Weinberger, O., Hermann, S.H., Mescher, M.F., Benacerraf, B.,

and Burakoff, S.J. 1981. Antigen presenting cell function in the induction of helper T cells for cytolytic T lymphocyte responses. Proc. Natl. Acad. Sci. USA 78:1796.

(31) Herrmann, S.H., and Mescher, M.F. 1981. Lymphocyte recognition of H-2 antigen in liposomes. J. Supramol. Struct. and Cellular Biochem., in press.

(32) Mescher, M.F., Jose, M.J.L., and Balk, S.P. 1981. Actin-containing matrix associated with the plasma membrane of murine tumor and lymphoid cells. Nature 289:139.

(33) Balk, S.P., Walker, J., and Mescher, M.F. 1981. Kinetics of cytolytic T lymphocyte binding to target cells in suspension. J. Immunol. 126:2177.

(34) Linna, T.J., Engers, H.D., Cerottini, J.-C., and Brunner, K.T. 1978. Inhibition of cytolytic T lymphocyte activity with subcellular alloantigen preparations and with unlabeled allogeneic target cells. J. Immunol. 120:1544.

(35) Martz, E. 1977. Mechanism of specific tumor cell lysis by alloimmune T lymphocytes: resolution and characterization of discrete steps in the cellular interaction. Contemp. Top. Immunobiol. 7:301.

(36) Balk, S.P., and Mescher, M.F. 1981. Specific reversal of cytolytic T cell-target cell functional binding is induced by free target cells. J. Immunol. 127:51.

(37) Balk, S.P., and Mescher, M.F. 1981. Specific reversal of cytolytic T lymphocyte-target cell interaction. J. Supramol. Struct. and Cellular Biochem., in press.

(38) Hollander, N., Mehdi, S.Q., Weissman, I.L., McConnnell, H.M., and Kriss, J.P. 1979. Allogeneic cytolysis of reconstituted membrane vesicles. Proc. Natl. Acad. Sci. USA 76:4042.

(39) Mehdi, S.Q., Lewis, J.T., Copeland, B.R., and McConnell, H.M. 1980. Freeze-fracture of reconstituted model membranes used as targets for cell-mediated cytotoxicity. Biochim. Biophys. Acta. 600:590.

T LYMPHOCYTE-MEDIATED CYTOLYSIS - A COMPREHENSIVE THEORY
I. THE MECHANISM OF CTL-MEDIATED CYTOLYSIS

Gideon Berke[1] and William R. Clark[2]

[1]Department of Cell Biology
Weizmann Institute of Science
Rehovot, Israel

[2]Department of Biology and the
Molecular Biology Institute
University of California
Los Angeles, California 90024

INTRODUCTION

The mechanism(s) by which cytotoxic T lymphocyte (CTL) cause lethal and irreversible damage to target cells (TC) has been the subject of considerable research during the past 10-15 years. A number of mechanisms have been proposed, examined, and either have been disproved or have generally not been pursued for lack of convincing experimental evidence in their support. These have included involvement of CTL-associated complement-like components (1,2); direct transfer of molecules, from the CTL to the TC membrane or cytoplasm, that eventually result in death of the target cell (3,4); localized extracellular secretion by the CTL, upon specific contact with the TC, of cytotoxic molecules (5,6); tangential shearing of the TC membrane as a result of CTL-TC conjugation (7); distortion of TC membrane potential (8); and implication of the CTL membrane as a generalized cytotoxic agent (9). These and other proposed mechanisms have been extensively reviewed (see ref. 10-13). Despite a great deal of imaginative experimentation in pursuit of these various hypotheses, none of them has attracted widespread support as a principle mechanism of CTL-mediated cytolysis.

Substantial information has been gathered concerning the phyiological requirements for direct, antigen-specific CTL-mediated lysis, and indeed these studies have contributed important general insights into the permissive environmental conditions under which the lytic mechanism will function. As a result of these studies the events associated with cytolysis have been grouped into three principal stages: binding of the CTL to the TC; programming of the TC for lysis; and target cell dissolution (for reviews see ref. 10-13). This division has led to a general consensus that binding and lysis involve distinct molecular mechanisms. Although such studies certainly do support the notion that TC binding and delivery to the TC of the lethal hit are distinct steps in the lytic process, they by no means demand, or in fact even imply, the involvement of molecularly distinct entities of the CTL in the binding and lytic steps. Indeed, the failure, after a search of a dozen years or more, to isolate a CTL component with either specific or nonspecific cytolytic activity, or to obtain convincing evidence for the existance of a lytic apparatus in the CTL membrane separate and distinct from the CTL receptor(s) for TC binding, might in itself occasion reconsideration of the basic premises upon which such a search was founded.

A re-evaluation of the existing literature regarding the mechanism of CTL-mediated lysis, plus additional recent data (14,15) has led us to suggest (16) that CTL are not equipped with a cytolytic apparatus, distinct from the binding entity, that is activated upon binding to the TC. We propose here a model for CTL-mediated lysis in which target cell destruction follows as a direct consequence of CTL-TC binding, through interaction of CTL receptors with TC MHC components, provided that permissive environmental conditions for the lytic phase of the reaction are met.

THE MODEL

Briefly stated, our proposal is as follows. The binding of TC MHC antigens, which are transmembrane glycoproteins, by CTL surface receptors, the molecular nature of which are unknown, occurs across a fairly extensive portion of the two dimensional surface of the CTL and TC surfaces. We postulate that this interaction in and of itself leads to alterations in the biophysical properties of the TC membrane that ultimately lead to TC destruction.

Our underlying assumption is that the integrity of the plasma membrane as a permeability barrier depends on appropriate interactions of the constituent lipids with each other and with integral membrane proteins, particularly transmembrane proteins. Membrane lipids and proteins coexist in the lowest feasible energy state; interference with their freedom to interact properly creates an unstable interface between them, and the potential, around transmembrane proteins, for ion leakage and loss of the permeability barrier function of the membrane. We propose that the physical restriction, rearrangement, or conformational distortion of the MHC proteins in the plane of the TC plasma membrane, by the imposition of what is in effect a two dimensional crosslinking grid consisting of the CTL surface and its embedded MHC receptors, creates instabilities at the target cell MHC protein-bilayer lipid interface that lead to increased membrane permeability. We do not consider MHC proteins as unique in this respect; we suppose that such disturbances would occur were any transmembrane proteins similarly restricted or distorted. Conformational distortions in the hydrophobic regions of the MHC proteins may or may not involve the exposure of hydrophilic residues, but in any case will lead to molecular mismatching at the protein-lipid interface, which in turn leads to increased membrane permeability followed ultimately by TC dissolution.

LIPID-PROTEIN INTERACTIONS AND PERMEABILITY IN MODEL MEMBRANE SYSTEMS

Increased membrane permeability as a result of destabilization of membrane structure is well documented in model membrane systems. There are a number of ways in which structural instabilities leading to permeability alterations can be generated, involving both lipid-lipid and lipid-protein interactions. DeGier et al. (17) reported that simply increasing the frequency of cis-unsaturated fatty acids in synthetic vesicles made them more permeable to glycerol and erythritol. This was correlated with increasing lipid disorder, due to poor molecular packing of the acyl chains. Conceivably, changes in biological membranes that increase local concentrations of phospholipids containing unsaturated fatty acids (i.e., in protein annular lipids) might lead to alterations in permeability. Numerous investigators have shown that cholesterol is very important in reducing permeability in liposomes (18-21). Structural alterations imposed on membranes that cause local exclusions of cholesterol, or interfere with its interaction with other membrane molecules (lipid or protein), could also increase membrane permeability.

Increased permeability to ions and other small molecules has been observed in artificial membranes in the region of the phase transition temperature (22). This permeability can be influenced by overall membrane lipid composition (23,24) and by membrane proteins (25). Marsh et al (26) observed that the uptake of Tempocholine into lipid vesicles composed of mixed function phospholipids is highly correlated with lateral phase separations and the existence of gel-liquid boundaries. They felt, as did Papahadjopoulos et al (27), that this arose because of areas of molecular mismatch occurring at the interface between the phases. A similar conclusion was reached by Blok et al (28) concerning water permeability at the transition temperature in liposomes. Nagle and Scott, on the other hand, felt that the permeability increase was more likely due to local fluctuations in headgroup density which could create transient openings in the headgroup region, through which ions pass into the hydrocarbon region (29).

The existence of such instabilities in biological membranes, leading to permeability changes, has yet to be demonstrated and indeed would be difficult to test for directly. Nevertheless, the generation of instabilities in lipid-lipid interactions, for example by sequestration of lipid molecules in ordered arrays around integral membrane proteins (annular lipids), could conceivably lead to the equivalent of local phase separations (or head-group density fluctuations), postulated as causes of leakiness in synthetic membrane systems. For example, glycophorin, when incorporated into synthetic lipid vesicles, causes a dramatic increase in membrane permeability. Van Zoelen et al. (30) showed that each molecule of glycophorin incorporated into synthetic phospholipid bilayers caused the ordering of up to 80-100 surrounding phospholipid molecules. They postulated that this created discontinuities at the ordered/disordered lipid interface, leading to the observed increase in membrane permeability.

Inappropriate interactions of membrane proteins with surrounding bilayer lipids has also been shown in other systems to lead to increased membrane permeability. Kimmelberg and Papahadjopoulos (31) reported that the incorporation of lysozyme, cytochrome c or poly-L-lysine increased the permeability of lipid vesicles to Na^+. The effects of the proteins on permeability depended very much on the lipid composition of the vesicle, and was postulated to be due to poor molecular matching at the protein-lipid interface. Cytochrome A and gramicidin were shown in a separate study to increase synthetic phospholipid membrane permeability, most likely through a deformation of contact lipids (32). Similar observations were made with cytochrome b_5 (33). Such increases in permeability are not always offset by the presence of cholesterol in the phospholipid bilayer (34).

One of the more interesting and perhaps relevant systems studied is the reconstitution of the passive Ca^{++} transport ATPase of sacroplasmic reticulum (35,36). When this protein is incorporated into lipid vesicles, the passive diffusion of Ca^{++} is increased many-fold, as is the permeability to other ions. The magnitude of the effect depends on the fatty acid composition of the vesicle, and increases with temperature. One suggested explanation of this effect, both in vivo and in phospholipid vesicles, is that leakage may be a result of improper molecular packing at the protein-lipid interface. Metcalfe and Warren (37), on the other hand, in a very thorough study of the interaction of the reconstituted ATPase with surrounding phospholipids, concluded that the site of leakage was at the boundary between the ordered annular lipids of the ATPase and the disordered bulk vesicle lipds, as described above for glycophorin.

The point we wish to emphasize, based on the above and other similar studies, is that target cell destruction as a result of membrane leakage may not require participation of a discrete CTL membrane-disrupting apparatus. Each MHC protein exists in dynamic equilibrium with surrounding lipids, through interactions between neighboring lipid molecules and transmembrane amino acid residues. This interaction is highly specific; distortion of the MHC protein molecule, resulting in altered secondary or tertiary structure, will alter interactions with surrounding lipids. Since normal, resting lipid-protein interactions are presumably the most favorable energetically, it is highly likely that any disturbance of these interactions will result in a less stable state of the membrane. Increased membrane permeability (lysis) may thus be understood simply in terms of disruption of normal molecular interactions in the target cell membrane, resulting from the binding process alone.

DISCUSSION

A minimum requirement of any theory is that it be consistent with all observations of the phenomenon it attempts to explain. The present theory is clearly consistent with many observations concerning CTL killing: the requirement for a viable effector cell; the effects of known chemical inhibitors; the requirement for direct cell contact; target cell specificity; etc. We thus discuss here only those observations that might be viewed as possibly inconsistent with the model we are proposing. We then extend discussion of our model (see accompanying paper) in an attempt to understand CMC in the context of other, non-lytic T cell functions, and we provide corollary hypotheses that we feel may unify all T cell-partner cell interactions at the membrane level.

Failure of Soluble Ligands to Cause Target Cell Death

The objection could immediately be raised that MHC proteins can, at appropriate concentrations, be bound, crosslinked and structurally altered by ligands such as antibodies or lectins, and this does not lead to cell lysis.[1] There are, however, various reasons why such binding and crosslinking might not lead to irreversible changes in membrane permeability. Binding by ligands may not lead to conformational alterations of the MHC proteins of the type, or to the extent imposed by, the CTL. Most ligands are bivalent and probably never more than tetravalent with respect to cell surface antigens, and may not impose sufficient structural restraints or alterations to lead to interfacial instability. Moreover, even though some degree of structural instability may be imposed by cross-

[1]It should be noted that those lectins binding to MHC proteins <u>are</u> toxic to cells at high concentrations.

linking with ligands, this might not necessarily lead to cell lysis because the crosslinked proteins are able to redistribute into energetically more favorable microclusters or patches, which can then be capped and shed or endocytosed. In fact, conformational distortions of integral membrane proteins induced by ligands, and subsequent thermodynamically driven redistributions, may be a hitherto unsuspected driving force behind patch formation. On the other hand, the enforced maintenance on the target cell surface (or more appropriately, in the plane of the target cell membrane) of MHC proteins in thermodynamically unfavorable configurations, across broad areas of contact with the multivalent CTL as suggested in our model, may lead to longer term molecular instability at the protein-lipid interface, which in turn could cause increased membrane permeability. At some critical point after collapse of the permeability barrier the target cell will be irreversibly damaged and proceed to dissolution.

Nonspecific Lysis by CTL as an Argument for Distinct Binding and Lytic mechanisms

Perhaps a more serious challenge to the notion of a single CTL entity mediating both binding and lysis has come from the study of non-specific lytic systems such as lectin-dependent cell-mediated cytotoxicity (LDCC). In the single entity model we are proposing, lysis ordinarily occurs as a direct consequence of, and is thus dependent upon, binding of the CTL receptor to TC MHC antigens. In the traditional view of LDCC, CTL receptor-TC MHC interactions are bypassed; the CTL and target cell are brought together by the multivalent lectin, which binds to sugar residues on the surface of each cell, and lysis is thought to ensue through activation and/or engagement of a lytic entity or apparatus unrelated to the CTL MHC receptor (38-40). If this view were true, our model would clearly be invalid as an explanation of LDCC in particular, and would be seriously challenged as an explanation of CTL killing generally. We have recently re-examined the role of lectin (Concanavalin A) in LDCC (15,16). We found that in Con A-mediated LDCC, the primary role of lectin is <u>not</u> in the bridging or binding of CTL and TC. Rather, the lectin acts primarily at the TC surface, modifying it in such a way as to make it recognizable by the CTL, through a receptor unrelated to the CTL lectin binding site. More importantly, we have shown that TC MHC antigens are required for Con A-mediated LDCC to take place, implying that the CTL receptor involved is recognizing MHC antigens. It has also been found that only those lectins binding to MHC proteins are able to mediate LDCC (G. Berke and D. Rosen, in preparation; A. Kimura, personal communication). A definite though considerably lower degree of LDCC has been observed against TC expressing very low or perhaps no MHC antigens on their surface (17,41,42). This may be mediated by related surface molecules mapping outside of the classical MHC region, or by other transmembrane structures currently being defined (Moscowitz and Berke, in preparation).

Experiments examining the interaction of CTL with TC that are themselves CTL provide a strong argument in favor of the identity of the binding and lytic mechanism in CTLs. For example, when A anti-B and B anti-C CTL are cocultured, only the B anti-C partner is killed (41,42). Yet B anti-C is as fully potent a CTL as A anti-B, and is clearly equally proximal to A anti-B as a potential TC. Obviously, intimate proximity of CTL and TC is in itself no guarantee that the lytic function can be expressed. These results argue that at the very least the CTL receptor must be occupied in order for lysis to occur, and strongly suggest that a free and independent lytic apparatus, capable of functioning independently of the binding receptor, does not exist. Identical results were obtained in our LDCC experiments. When CTL from a common source were split in half, and only one half pre-treated with Con A, upon subsequent coincubation only the Con A pre-treated partner was lysed, even though in this case the functional CTL and TC were otherwise absolutely identical (16). Again, the physical proximity of both partners was identical; if a lytic apparatus distinct from the CTL receptor were operating, lysis should have been symmetrical.

These findings have a number of important implications. First, they reconcile the apparent discrepancy between direct CTL killing and so-called non-specific CTL lysis (at least as exemplified by Con A-mediated LDCC), in that both can now be viewed as involving TC MHC antigens. Second, lytic systems such as LDCC may no longer be cited as *a priori* major arguments for the physical separateness of CTL recognition and killing functions. Finally, these results are fully consistent with our proposal that participation of TC MHC antigens (and possibly other transmembrane proteins) is obligatory for CTL-mediated lytic processes.

Apparent Dissociation of Binding and Lysis by Hyperthermic or Formaldehyde Treatment of CTL

Another serious challenge to the concept of a single mechanism for TC binding and TC lysis as proposed here is posed by recent data from one of our own laboratories. The lytic activity of CTL in direct, specific reactions with TC is abolished following brief exposure to hyperthermia (43°C) or mild formaldehyde treatment, whereas the ability to bind to TC is considerably less diminished (43). At firt glance, this would seem to provide clear evidence for the existence of distinct binding and lytic entities. A closer analysis of the system, however, showed that only those treatments that were just barely sufficient to abolish cytolysis (10 minutes at 43°; 0.2% HCHO for 30 minutes at 0°C) left the binding function relatively intact. Extended treatment by either method also abolished binding (43). Moreover, ultrastructural analysis of CTL-TC conjugates formed using CTL treated under conditions just sufficient to abolish lysis showed that the number and integrity of the conjugates was in fact compromised. The extent of interdigitation of heat-treated CTL and TC was noticeably reduced, suggesting that the conjugates may be considerably weaker than normal, with not enough receptor-determinant contacts to cause cytolysis. Furthermore, although heat-treated CTL could not induce ^{51}Cr release from labeled TC, a marked reduction in TC ATP content was observed, indicating some degree of TC damage (45). We feel these results point out that simple CTL-TC contact in and of itself is not necessarily sufficient for cytolysis to occur, but rather a certain threshold level of interaction of CTL and TC membranes is required to inflict a lethal degree of damage to the TC. The threshold level of membrane interdigitation required to form a specific conjugate may simply be lower than the level required for lysis. This conclusion would also seem to be supported by the effects of temperature on binding and cytolysis. The binding of CTL and tumor TC is optimal at about 23°, whereas lysis does not begin to be significant until about 30°, reaching a maximum at 37-40° (46). We would suggest that the membrane interactions that take place at 23° are sufficient for conjugate formation to occur, but not for inflicting irreversible TC damage. There could be several possible mechanisms for this. Higher temperatures may be necessary for more extensive interdigitation of CTL and TC membranes, or for permitting engagement of a greater number of CTL receptors and TC MHC proteins per unit area of membrane. The greater translational mobility of membrane proteins at higher temperature could facilitate a larger number of correct receptor-determinant interactions. Moreover, thermodynamic instabilities leading to leakage at boundaries or interfaces, created by TC MHC binding, would clearly increase with temperature.

CONCLUSION

In addition to providing a new approach to understanding the mechanism of cell-mediated cytotoxicity, our model also suggests a new interpretation of the physiological role of class I MHC proteins. Current views of the role of these proteins include self-recognition, T cell ontogeny, cell-cell communication, and "immune surveillance," among others. In particular, the need to perceive viral or tumor antigens in association with or in the context of "self" antigens has been postulated as a principal function for MHC proteins. But why, in the essentially closed system of "self," is there a need to perceive viral or tumor antigens in the context of self antigens? Self as opposed to what? Self restriction, on a purely recognition level, makes no biological sense.

Our model for the mechanism of cell-mediated cytotoxicity suggests a more fundamental role for at least class I MHC proteins. We propose that the _primary raison d'etre_ for these proteins is to provide an absolute guarantee that every cell in the body can be destroyed if it becomes virally or neoplastically transformed. These ubiquitously distributed, transmembrane proteins provide a potential channel through which the delicate osmotic balance necessary for cell viability can be lethally disrupted. The system for CTL-self MHC interaction was most likely selected precisely on this basis, and can be guaranteed to work in every situation. It cannot be left to chance that a CTL would be able to deliver a lethal blow to an infected cell through the viral components associated with the cell membrane. If this were true, viruses would rapidly evolve and be selected to escape any such mechanism, and the host species would be faced with the problem of continually modifying its own defense mechanisms.

Each cell thus has built into it a means for its own destruction, under those conditions that lead to lethal interactions with CTL. The possible nature of these conditions, and how they relate to non-lethal T cell interactions, are addressed in the accompanying paper.

REFERENCES

1. Canty, T.C., and J.R. Wunderlich. Quantitative in vitro assay of cytotoxic celular immunity. J. Natl. Cancer Inst. 45:761 (1970).
2. Henney, C.S., and M.M. Mayer. Specific cytolytic activity of lymphocytes: Effect of antibodies against complement components C_2, C_3 and C_5. Cell. Immunol. 2:702 (1971).
3. Selin, D., Wallach, D.F.H., and H. Fischer. Intercellular communication in cell-mediated cytotoxicity. Fluorescein transfer between $H\text{-}2^d$ target cells and $H\text{-}2^b$ lymphocytes in vitro. Eur. J. Immunol. 1:453 (1971).
4. Sanderson, C.J., Hall, P.J., and J.A. Tomas. The mechanism of T cell mediated cytotoxicity. IV. Studies on communicating junctions between cells in contact. Proc. R. Soc. Long. B 196:73 (1977).
5. Granger, G.A., and W.P. Kolb. Lymphocyte in vitro cytotoxicity: Mechanism of immune and non-immune small lymphocyte mediated target L cell destruction. J. Immunol. 101:111 (1977).
6. Berke, G., Sullivan, K.A., and D.B. Amos. Rejection of ascites tumor allografts. I. Isolation, characterization and in vitro reactivity of peritoneal lymphoid effector cells from BALB/c mice immune to EL4 leukosis. J. Exp. Med. 135:1334 (1972).
7. Seeman, P. Ultrastructure of membrane lesions in immune lysis, osmotic lysis and drug induced lysis. Fed. Proc. 33:2116 (1974).
8. Berke, G., and D.B. Amos. Mechanisms of lymphocyte-mediated cytolysis. The LMC cycle and its role in transplantation immunity. Transplant. Rev. 17:71 (1973).

9. Ferluga, J., and A.C. Allison. Cytotoxicity of isolated plasma membranes from lymph node cells. Nature, Lond. 255:708 (1975).
10. Berke, G. Interaction of cytotoxic T lymphocytes and target cells. prog. in Allergy 27:69 (1980).
11. Golstein, P., and E.T. Smith. Mechanism of T cell-mediated cytolysis: The lethal hit stage. Contemp. Top. Immunobiol. 7:273 (1977).
12. Henney, C.S. T-cell-mediated cytolysis: An overview of some current issues. Contemp. Top. Immunobiol. 7:245 (1977).
13. Martz, E. Mechanisms of specific tumor cell lysis by allo-immune T-lymphocytes: Resolution and characterization of discrete steps in the cellular interaction. Contemp. Top. Immunobiol. 7:301 (1977).
14. Berke, G., Hu, V., McVey, E., and W.R. Clark. T lymphocyte-mediated cytolysis. I. A common mechanisms for target recognition in specific and lectin-dependent cytolysis. J. Immunol. 127:776 (1981).
15. Berke, G., McVey, E., Hu, V., and W.R. Clark. T lymphocyte-mediated cytolysis. II. Role of target cell MHC antigens in recognition and lysis. J. Immunol. 127:782 (1981).
16. Berke, G., and W.R. Clark. How do cytotoxic T lymphocytes lyse target cells? Fourteenth Internat. Leuc. Cult. Conf. - Heidelberg. In "Mechanism of Lymphocyte Activation (Elsevier/North Holland), in press (1981).
17. DeGier, J., Vandersloot, J.G., and L.L.M. van Deenen. Lipid composition and permeability of liposomes. Biochem. Biophy. Acta 150:666 (1968).
18. Nakamura, T., Nishikawa, M., Inoue, K., Nojima, S., Akiyama, T., and U. Sankawa. Phosphatidylcholine lipsomes containing cholesterol analogs with side chains of varying lengths. Chem. Phys. Lipids 26:101 (1980).
19. Gallucci, E., Micelli, E., and C. Lippe. Effectof cholesterol on the non-electrolyte permeability of planar lecithin membranes. Nature 255:722 (1975).
20. Cooper, R.A. Influence of increased membrane cholesterol on membrane fluidity and cell function in human red blood cells. J. Supramolec. Struct. 8:413 (1978).
21. Papahadjopoulos, D., and J.C. Watkins. Phospholipid model membranes. II. Permeability properties of hydrated liquid crystals. Biochem. Biophys. Acta 135:639 (1967).
22. Antonov, V., Petrov, V., Molnar, A., Predvoditelev, and A. Ivanov. The appearance of single ion channels in unmodified lipid bilayer membranes at the phase transition temperature. Nature 285:585 (1980).
23. Blok, M.C., Van de Neut-Kok, E.C., van Deenen, L., and J. De Gier. The effect of chain length and lipid phase transitions on the selective permeability peroperties of liposomes. Biochem. Biophys. Acta 406:187 (1975).
24. van Deenen, L., DeGier, J., and R. Demel. Relations between lipid composition and permeability of membranes. Biochem. Soc.

Symp. 35:377 (1972).
25. Blok, M.C., van Deenen, L., DeGier, J., Opdenkamp, J., and A. Verkleij. Some aspects of lipid phase transition on membrane permeability and lipid-protein association. In "Biochemistry of Membrane Transport. Edited by G. Sewenya and E. Carafoli, Springer-Verlag, Berlin., pp. 38-46 (1977).
26. Marsh, D., Watts, A., and P.F. Knowles. Evidence for phase boundary lipid. Permeability of tempo-choline into dimyristoyl phosphatidylcholine vesicles at the phase transition. Biochem. 15:3570 (1976).
27. Papahadjopoulos, D., Jacobson, K., Nir, S., and T. Isac. Phase transitions in phosphoipid vesicles. fluorescence polarization and permeability measurements concerning the effect of temperature and cholesterol. Biochem. Biophys. Acta 311:330 (1973).
28. Blok, M.C., van Deenen, L.L.M., and J. DeGier. Effect of the gel to liquid crystalline phase transition on the osmotic behaviour of phosphatidylcholine liposomes. Biochem. Biophys. Acta 433:1 (1976).
29. Nagle, J.F., and H.L. Scott, Jr. Lateral compressibility of lipid mono- and bilayers. Theory of membrane permeability. Biochem. Biophys. Acta 513:236 (1978).
30. Van Zoelen, E., Van Dijck, P., De Kruijff, Verkleij, A., and L. van Deenen. Effect of glycophorin incorporation on the physico-chemical properties of phospholipid bilayers. Biochem. Biophys. Acta 514:9 (1978).
31. Kimelberg, H.K., and D. Papahadjopoulos. Interactions of Basic Proteins with Phospholipid Membranes. Binding and Changes in the Sodium Permeability of Phosphatidylserine Vesicles. J. Biol. Chem. 246:1142-1148 (1971).
32. Papahadjopoulos, D., Moscarello, M., Eylar, E., and T. Isac. Effects of Proteins on the Thermotropic Phase Transitions of Phospholipid Membranes. Biochem. Biophys. Acta 401:317- (1976).
33. Holloway, P., and J. Katz. Effect of Cytochrome b_5 on the Size, Density and Permeability of Phosphatidylcholine Vesicles. J. Biol. Chem. 250:9002- (1975).
34. Papahadjopoulos, D., Vail, W., and M. Moscarello. Interaction of a Purified Hydrophobic Protein from Myelin with Phospholipid Membranes: Studies on Ultrastructure, Phase Transition and Permeability. J. Membr. Biol. 22:143- (1975).
35. DeBoland, A.R., Jilka, R.L., and A.N. Martonosi. Passive Ca^{++} Permeability of Phospholipid Vesicles and Sarcoplasmic Reticulum Membranes. J. Biol. Chem. 250:7501-7510 (1975).
36. Jilka, R.L., Martonosi, A.N., and T.W. Tillack. Effect of Purified [Mg^{++} Ca^{++}]-Activated ATPase of Sarcoplasmic Reticulum Upon the Passive Ca^{++} Permeability and Ultrastructure of Phospholipid Vesicles. J. Biol. Chem. 250:7511-7524 (1975).
37. Metcalfe, J., and E. Warren. Lipid-Protein Interactions in a Reconstituted Calcium Pump. In "International Cell Biology" (R.B. Brinkley and K.R. Porter, editors), Rockefeller Univer-

sity Press, pp. 15-23 (1977).
38. Bevan, M.J., and M. Cohn. Cytotoxic effects of antigen- and mitogen-induced T cells on various targets. J. Immunol. 114: 559 (1975).
39. Bonavida, B., and T.P. Bradley. Studies on the induction and expression of T cell-mediated immunity. V. Lectin-induced non-specific cell-mediated cytotoxicity by alloimmune lymphocytes. Transplantation 41:94 (1976).
40. Green, W.R., Ballas, Z.K., and C.S. Henney. Studies on the mechanism of lymphocyte-mediated cytolysis. XI. The role of lectin in lectin-dependent cell-mediated cytotoxicity. J. Immunol. 121:1566 (1978).
41. Golstein, P. Sensitivity of cytotoxic T cells to T cell mediated cytotoxicity. Nature 252:81 (1974).
42. Kuppers, R.C., and C.S. Henney. Evidence for direct linkage between antigen recognition and lytic expression in effector T cells. J. Exp. Med. 143:684 (1976).
43. Berke, G., Fishelson, Z., and B. Schick. Hyperthermia and formaldehyde can dissociate the binding and killing activities of cytolytic T lymphocytes. Transplant. Proc. 11:804 (1979).
44. Rosen, D., Fishelson, Z., and G. Berke. The role of CTL projections in Tc lysis. Transpl. Proc. 13:1073 (1981).
45. Fishelson, Z., and G. Berke. In preparation (1981).
46. Berke, G., and G. Gabison. Energy requirements for the binding and lytic steps of T lymphocyte mediated cytolysis of leukemic cells in vitro. Eur. J. Immunol. 5:671 (1975).

(See Discussion after next paper.)

T LYMPHOCYTE-MEDIATED CYTOLYSIS - A COMPREHENSIVE THEORY

II. LYTIC vs. NONLYTIC INTERACTIONS OF T LYMPHOCYTES

William R. Clark[1] and Gideon Berke[2]

[1]Department of Biology and the
Molecular Biology Institute
University of California
Los Angeles, California 90024

[2]Department of Cell Biology
Weizmann Institute of Science
Rehovot, Israel

In the model for CTL-mediated lysis presented in the preceding paper, we postulated that the binding of CTL to target cells through interaction of an array of MHC-specific T cell receptors with a corresponding array of TC MHC antigens is sufficient, under permissive environmental conditions, to cause TC destruction. However, a variety of other T cell subsets interact with target or partner cells in an MHC-restricted fashion, implying the existence of MHC-specific receptors on these T cells as well. In the mouse, T cells displaying Ly 1 antiens but not Ly 2,3 antigens recognize I region associated (Ia) antigens, and serve as amplifying cells in the differentiation of B cells to plasma cells, and in the activation of pre-CTL to mature, functional CTL. Cells with reduced levels of Ly 1 and high levels of Ly 2,3 serve effector functions as CTL and as suppressors of Ly 1 amplifier cells. Ly 2,3 CTL bear receptors for K/D antigens, whereas Ly 2,3 suppressor cells have receptors for determinants coded for by genes in the I-J subregions. Ly 1 T cells do not normally function as CTL; whether Ly 2,3 suppressor T cells utilize a cytotoxic mechanism in their function is uncertain.

Since all T cell functional subsets ultimately derive from the same cell lineage, and mature under similar selective pressures with respect to development of a repertoire of cell surface antigen receptors, it is not unreasonable to assume that they are potentially capable of similar MHC receptor-mediated interactions with partner cells. Both Ly 1 T helper (T_h) cells and Ly 2,3 CTL have the potential to interact with MHC-coded proteins on other cells, and according to our model this should result in lysis of the non-T partner cell. Why then do only Ly 2,3 CTL appear to be able to cause lethal and irreversible damage to the cells with which they interact? Any model for the mechanism of CMC should at least attempt to come to grips with this problem.

One rather simple solution might be that Ly 1 T cells recognize I region-associated (Ia) antigens, whereas Ly 2,3 CTL are specific for antigens coded for by the K/D region. The distortion of Ia antigens via T cell surface receptors specific for Ia could be postulated not to lead to cytolysis. However, it has been shown that CTL specific for Ia antigens can be generated (1). Thus, Ia antigens _can_ serve as target antigens for cytolytic damage. In the accompanying paper we predicted that _any_ transmembrane protein could serve as an active participant in the lytic process, and Ia antigens are transmembrane in nature. Why then are Ly 1 amplifier cells not normally cytotoxic for their partner cells?

We believe the answer lies in the way each of these T cell types interacts with its partner cell in the execution of its specific function. Ly 1 helper T cells appear to interact almost exclusively with antigen-presenting cells (APC), which may be macrophages or dendritic cells. APC present antigen to pre-T_h cells in asociation with APC membrane-bound Ia molecules (self Ia in the normal course of events). Pre-T_h cells capable of recognizing APC Ia antigen(s) plus the foreign antigen are triggered to mature to T_h cells. This antigen presenting function can also be carried out by soluble factors derived from antigen-pulsed APC cultures (2), potentially eliminating the need for cell-cell contact at this stage. Upon continued or subsequent exposure to antigen (on an APC displaying the same Ia allotype as the original stimulating APC, or in association with the corresponding APC factor) the mature T_h cell can aid in the maturation of the B cell response to the same antigen. This amplifying effect can _also_ be mediated by secretion of a soluble factor that can be picked up by an APC and presented to an appropriate B cell (3), again obviating a requirement for direct cell-cell contact between activated T_h cell and either the APC or the B cell. These latter factors appear to contain receptor components for the antigen involved (4), but as yet have not been shown definitely to contain elements of the T cell receptor for MHC. The mediation of T_h cell-partner cell interactions by soluble factors at both interfaces of the reaction of T_h cells with other cell types would certainly offer one means for partner cells to avoid T cell-inflicted lytic damage. Of course, the fact that T_h interactions with partner cells _can_ be mediated by soluble factors in experimental systems in vitro does not mean that they necessarily do so in vivo. Nevertheless, we feel that the very existence of such factors, and the apparent ease of their release from the surfaces of T_h cells, may provide an important clue to the fundamental difference between the interactions of these cells and CTL with target cells.

We assume that the driving force behind the evolution of the CTL system is the need to eliminate virally transformed syngeneic (self) cells, and possibly neoplastic cells (which may be a subset of or related to the former). In the syngeneic CTL system, which is the system any model must primarily account for, the T cell is responding to antigen in the context of a class I MHC protein. As far as we know at present, then, this system is in fact high analogous to the T_h system, with the important difference that CTL-TC interactions are lethal. As just noted, in T_h-AFC interaction the non-MHC antigenic component is associated with the cell surface as an extrinsic entity, probably readily detachable. In syngeneic CMC systems, on the other hand, the non-MHC antigen (on a sensitizing cell or a TC) would be very tightly associated with the presenting cell surface. Viral antigens, for example, are associated with viral glycoproteins which themselves are integral membrane components and thus not at all readily detachable from the cell surface. We suggest that the nature of the interaction of the T cell MHC receptor with partner cell MHC determinants is in fact probably the same for both T_h and CTL, the crucial difference being that in the case of CTL-TC reactions this interaction is stabilized by the interaction of the T cell with the additional foreign, surface-stable determinants, whereas in the case of T_h-presenting cell interactions it is not. Thus the interaction of CTL receptors with self MHC proteins, which clearly must under normal circumstances be of low avidity, is not rendered stable and lethal. Whether the interaction of the T cell with the foreign determinant occurs through a single receptor recognizing both MHC and foreign antigen, or through separate receptors recognizing MHC and foreign antigen (see below), is unclear but also unimportant. It is the stable and continuous interaction of MHC related receptors on the CTL, and transmembrane proteins on the TC, that leads to TC death.

THE RELATIONSHIP BETWEEN SYNGENEIC AND ALLOGENEIC CYTOTOXICITY

How can this point of view be extended to allogeneic reactions? It is our view that syngeneic and allogeneic CMC reactions mediated by Ly 2,3 cells must be an expression of the same mechanism, not only in a general sense but in the finest detail. What then are the homologs of self MHC antigen and of the membrane-integral foreign antigenic determinant vis-a-vis allogeneic CTL-TC interactions? We believe there are two equally attractive approaches to this problem.

Janeway *et al* have proposed that T cells in general have two classes of receptors, one of which is positively selected on the basis of low affinity for self-MHC products (5,6). They postulate that a portion of such receptors will, by analogy with heteroclitic antibody, have a high affinity for any given allogeneic MHC product. Whereas under normal (syngeneic) conditions, this T cell receptor would not be engaged in a sufficiently avid way to activate the T cell, the occupation of a postulated second receptor for nominal antigen would stabilize T cell-partner interaction and permit expression of T cell function.

Matzinger and Bevan (7,8) make perhaps the most eloquent case for a single T cell receptor recognizing MHC products in association with nominal antigen, perhaps through uniquely generated neoantigens. In the case of virally infected self, the T cell would be recognizing some "interaction antigen" composed of self MHC and viral protein. In the case of alloreactivity, it is assumed that the responding T cell recognizes an interaction antigen generated by the association of the allogeneic MHC product with some other normally occurring cell-surface protein.

Both of these models, as applied to allogeneic CMC reactions, deal with the problem of recognition, not with the nature of the actual lytic mechanism itself. Both absolutely account for and require target cell MHC proteins in the interaction of CTL and target cells. Thus, from our point of view, the possibility of an involvement of target cell MHC proteins in post-binding stages of the lytic reaction sequence is assured in both cases.

WHY DON'T PRE-CTL KILL PARTNER (STIMULATING) CELLS?

One final aspect of CTL killing may deserve comment. Since only antigen-specific subsets of pre-CTL are selected in response to stimulating antigen, we must conclude that the same set of receptors recognizing both MHC and "other" determinants, is present on the pre-CTL. Yet pre-CTL are not cytotoxic. Why? There may be a number of reasons for this. The cells may not have enough surface membrane to form adequate (lethal) intercellular contacts with TC; the surface density of receptors may be too low to allow sufficiently avid interactions with TC to lead to lysis. We do not know the answer. However, as we pointed out some years ago (8), the development of cytotoxicity in allogeneic reactions may not in fact represent the generation of a cytotoxic function *per se*, but rather the development of the ability to bind properly to target cells.

REFERENCES

(1) Dennert, G., S. Weiss and J. Warner. T cells may express multiple activities: allohelp, cytolysis and DTH are expressed by a cloned CTL line. Proc. Natl. Acad. Sci. USA 78:4540 (1981).
(2) Erb, P., M. Feldmann and N. Hogg. Role of macrophage in the generation of T helper cells. IV. Nature of genetically related factor derived from macrophages incubated with soluble antigen. Eur. J. Immunol. 6:365 (1977).
(3) Munro, A., M. Taussig and J. Archer. I-region products and cell interactions. In, Ir genes and Ia antigens. Ed. by H.O. McDevitt, Academic Press, New York, p. 487 (1978).
(4) Mozes, E. Some properties and functions of antigen specific T cell factors. In, I genes and Ia antigens. Ed. by H.O. McDevitt, Academic Press, New York, p. 475 (1978).
(5) Matzinger, P., and M. Bevan. Why do so many lymphocytes espond to major histocompatibility antigens? Cell. Immunol. 29:1 (1977).
(6) Matzinger, P. A one receptor view of T cell behavior. Nature 292:497 (1981).
(7) Janeway, C., H. Wigzell and H. Binz. Hypothesis: Two different V_H gene products make up T cell receptors. Scand. J. Immunol. 5:993 (1976).
(8) Janeway, C., et al. T cell receptor idiotypes. Scand. J. Immunol. 12:83 (1980).
(9) Kimura, A.K., and W.R. Clark. Functional characteristics of T cell receptors during sensitization against histocompatibility antigens in vitro. Cell. Immunol. 12:127-139 (1974).

DISCUSSION

I. MacLennan

I think your message is quite clear, that MHC is being recognized in lectin-mediated cytolysis by cells generated in CTL reactions. You didn't positively show us that CTL was doing this. You presumably have data on that.

G. Berke

I think most if not all authors would agree that the cells involved in lectin-mediated killing are similar if not identical, or perform identically, to cells that are operational in specific CTL-mediated killing. In spite of that, as you noticed, I was careful not to refer to our killer cells as CTL. I called them effector cells although I believe they are CTL. With CTL clones or hybridomas, this could now be checked more directly.

P. Perlmann

Could it be that the lectins, regardless of whether they sit on a target cell or on an effector cell, activate those lymphocytes which are susceptible to activation and this may then in an indirect way trigger cytolytic effector cells? This could also be the case when you have hybridomas or cell lines.

G. Berke

I think you are absolutely right in suggesting that there is a possibility that the effect is indirect. But the point is, that we think that MHC is the key element in the process, regardless at which step it is involved.

M. Mayer

I want to question the philosophy of your argument. The fact is that the cytolytic system does work, albeit less efficiently, with the H-2-less targets. What that says to me, is that the basic mechanism does not require H-2. By analogy, in the complement area, it is accepted that the membrane attack requires complement proteins 5, 6, 7, 8 and 9. I can show you experiments in which C3 will potentiate that action as much as 2,000-fold, not just twice, but 2,000-fold, and yet C3 is not required. It just improves the efficiency.

M. Nabholz

One type of evidence on which your hypothesis is based is the effect of the pretreatment of the killers or the targets with a lectin. But the fate of the lectin, on the killer cells or on the target cells, may be very different. The lectin may, for instance, disappear more quickly from the effector cells. The lentil lectin works when you treat either killers or targets, and I would like to know how you explain that.

G. Berke

Whether the lectin is sort of 'misbehaving' on killers and 'behaving' on targets has been treated fairly adequately by utilizing targets which themselves are killers (J. Immunol. 1982, 127:776). In that case we cannot argue that there is any difference between killers and targets.

M. Nabholz

Except that the populations are always heterogeneous. They are not 100% killer cells.

G. Berke

Of course, Marcus, of course they are not. That's the best we could do. As to the lentil lectin, it behaves differently from Con A, probably because it has a lower affinity for H-2 antigens than Con A (Berke, Rosen and Moscovitch, 1981, submitted).

F. Fitch

We have two sets of data, one obtained with a cloned L3 line, which Andy Glasebrook developed and derived in my lab, and T18, which is a B10 anti-TNP B10 clone which Kathy Wall developed in the laboratory. In general, we find results similar to Gideon's, but with some differences. If one pretreats the targets one gets similar levels of lysis, and with T18 if one pretreats the effector cells, one does not really get much lysis. L3, on the other hand, does give some lysis and I guess the question is, is the cup half full or the cup half empty? Also, there are differences with different target cells. EL4 shows the effect best with L3 whereas B10 blasts would give about as good killing with pretreatment of the effectors and the targets. So it would appear that at least with some effectors and with some targets, pretreatment of the target cells with lectin gives better lectin-mediated lysis than pretreatment of the effector cells, although with some effector cells apparently the reverse can be true (see paper in this volume).

I. MacLennan

K and T cell mediated cytolysis have so many metabolic similarities and in K cell kill you can probably not demonstrate MHC independence.

W. Clark

Two points I can make quickly about that. One is that, in searching the literature and looking at experiments, I'm not entirely convinced that MHC proteins could not have been involved in ADCC. The second point is, that we would generalize our hypothesis to the possibility that any trans-membrane protein could potentially serve as a channel. Such that if the antibody were directed toward another trans-membrane protein, distortion of that might lead to lysis.

P. Perlmann

ADCC experiments can be performed with measles virus-infected target cells but lacking MHC antigens. When ADCC is induced by monoclonal antibodies against viral components the results are the same, regardless of the pesence or absence of MHC antigens. So at least in this system, I see no implication of MHC in ADCC.

W. Clark

Viral coat proteins are in many instances integral membrane proteins and again distortion of them could provide a channel.

M. Mayer

I think what you propose, Bill, is an extremely valuable concept because it leads to certain predictions that can be experimentally tested. The type of interface channel that you are suggesting involving an integral membrane protein, in the first place, would be a small channel and, in the second place, would be a fluctuating channel. And both properties can be measured, so that if the channel size were measured and if the time fluctuations were measured, one could ascertain whether this type of channel is operative, because the other kind of channel that we have studied, made of inserted hydrophobic peptides, can be quite large. It doesn't have to be large, but it may be large so that if you were to find in cell-mediated lysis that the channel size is indeed large, that would argue against your concept. Furthermore, if you were to find that the sizes of the channels do not fluctuate much with time, that also would argue against it. Conversely, if you were to find otherwise, it would argue for it. I think this is experimentally ascertainable.

E. Simpson

If recognition were, in fact, enough, since all T cells are H-2 restricted and T helper cells see antigen X in the context of self Ia, you would expect that T helper cells would kill. As far as I know, there is no evidence that this is so.

W. Clark

But there is no evidence that it is not so. We don't know what happens to the antigen-presenting cell... I'm not arguing that there is kill, Liz, but I don't think experiments have been done offhand to test whether the antigen-presenting cell is killed.

Valerie Hu

As I understand it, the mechanism that you're proposing for the transduction of the lytic signal is microclustering of the H-2 components in the target membrane. Do you want to clarify this?

G. Berke

I think one should not confuse between what we have proposed the lectin is doing to the target to make it recognizable and our ideas as to how the lytic signal is conveyed. I don't think that it's imperative that there is clustering of H-2 so that the lytic signal is conveyed.

Valerie Hu

My first point would be that lectins may facilitate lysis by increasing the avidity of the killer cell receptor for target antigens. The other point I have is addressed to Dr. Mayer's point, that is one could test such a model by assuming that this would give rise to fluctuating channels. This may not be necessarily so, if there is a rearrangement of proteins in the membrane forming some sort of a stable cross-link grid.

B. Bonavida

I think so far we have been discussing the role of MHC products on the target cells, as a mechanism for explaining lysis in ADCC. What I would like to propose is that the lectin activates the CTL to mediate LDCC. There is some circumstantial evidence to support this notion. First, most lectins that mediate LDCC have been shown to be T cell mitogens. Non-T cell mitogens would not induce any LDCC (Transplantation, 1976, 24:94). Second, PNA and soybean agglutinin bind very poorly to effector cells; if the latter are treated with neuraminidase, those lectins become T-cell mitogens and also can mediate LDCC (unpublished).

G. Berke

I would like to comment on our ODCC studies (J. Immunol. 1981, 127: 782). In ODCC, oxidation either by periodate or by neuraminidase followed by galactose-oxidase, renders target cells susceptible to killing by any CTL, regardless of its specificity. We have found that only oxidation of the target cells renders them susceptible to killing; doing the same thing to the killer cells produces very little killing. Interestingly, the inhibition by alloantisera is also seen in ODCC.

P. Perlmann

This is also a mitogenic system. In our hands, if we pretreat human lymphocytes, we get a perfect cytolytic reaction.

B. Bonavida

We have done hundreds of experiments, showing that CTL modified by either periodate or NA/GO mediate non-specific cytotoxicity. Preliminary findings have been presented (Fed. Proc. 1981, 40:1147; manuscript in preparation).

F. Fitch

We have cloned T helper cell lines that react with Mls determinants. They will not mediate LDCC. LDCC, in our hands, thus appears to be mediated by CTL only.

STUDIES ON THE MECHANISM OF LECTIN-DEPENDENT T CELL-MEDIATED CYTOLYSIS: USE OF LENS CULINARIS HEMAGGLUTININ A TO DEFINE THE ROLE OF LECTIN

William R. Green

Program in Basic Immunology
Fred Hutchinson Cancer Research Center
Seattle, Washington 98104

INTRODUCTION

Alloimmune cytotoxic T cell populations demonstrate exquisite immunologic specificity, killing only target cells which display alloantigens related to those used for immunization (1,2). It was noted some time ago, however, that in the presence of the plant lectins concanavalin A (Con A) and phythohemagglutinin such specificity is not maintained; rather a variety of target cells, including those syngeneic to the effector cell source, are lysed (3-5).

In initial attempts at explaining this phenomenon of lectin-dependent cell-mediated cytoxocity (LDCC), it was hypothesized that the lectin served merely as a "bridge" or "glue", bringing the cytotoxic cell into close approximation with its target (4). This explanation reinforced the concept, then prevalent, that the effector T cell was an inherently lytic cell whose antigen receptor, although conferring specificity, simply served to bridge the effector cell to its appropriate target. In this way the roles of antigen receptors and lectins were viewed analogously.

This appealing interpretation was seriously questioned by the finding that the antigen-receptor sites of effector T cells do not serve merely a simple bridging function in lytic expression (6,7). Kuppers and Henney observed that when two cytotoxic lymphocyte populations were mixed under circumstances in which antigen recognition occurred in only one direction (e.g., a anti-d killer cells mixed with d cells of anti-b specificity), then effector cell inactivation occurred only in the direction of antigen recognition (6,7). Hence, simple proximity to a cytotoxic T cell did not, in itself, lead to cytolysis. Occupation of the effector cell's antigen receptor was necessary before lytic activity was demonstrable. Antigen recognition, then seemed intimately associated with lytic expression, a clear demonstration that cytolysis is more than a simple collision between effector and target cells.

This conclusion was confirmed and extended with effector cell populations containing a high percentage of killer T cells and employing conjugate formation (microscopically observed cell clusters) as an index of cell-cell interaction (8). When studied at the population level, incubation of two effector cell sources directed against each other's alloantigens led to conjugate formation and to lysis of both sets of effector cells. In all cases, however, when individual conjugates were followed microscopically, lysis occurred only in one direction. These results suggested that the bidirectional lysis observed at the level of the whole population reflected the accumulation of many random lytic events each of which was unidirectional. These results suggested that when two killer cells interacted with each other, under conditions in which mutual recognition could occur, only one cell (perhaps the one whose receptors had the greatest affinity for antigen) was "triggered"; the other effector cell did not express its lytic attack and served as the target for attack. Occupation of the T cell receptor by antigen was thus viewed as necessary to "activate" the cytotoxic effector cell to engage the metabolic machinery associated with lysis.

In keeping with these findings, subsequent studies on LDCC by Green et al (9) and Parker and Martz (10) strongly suggested that, analogous to the T cell receptor's function in specific lysis, lectin also was required to do more than just bridge the effector cell to the target cell. This conclusion was based on the following findings:

1. Only T cell mitogens supported lectin-dependent cytolysis; agglutinating nonmitogenic agents were ineffective whether or not B cell mitogens were present (9).
2. For many lectins, including at least some that mediate LDCC, conditions could be defined under which stable adhesions formed between target and effector cells that were "non-lethal", i.e., did not result in lysis (10).
3. T effector cell populations "activated" by T cell mitogen did not lyse target cells when cell-cell bridging was intentionally precluded (9).

Thus, consistent with the mechanistic similarities (in terms of susceptibility to inhibition by various drugs) between lectin-dependent and direct T cell-mediated cytolysis (11), it appeared that lectin, like the antigen receptor, performed the dual role of bridging effector to target cells and of activating the cytotoxic machinery of the effector cell.

Recently, this view that lectin performs a dual role of bridging and activation has been questioned. An intriguing alternative hypothesis has been advanced by Berke et al in which the sole function of lectin in LDCC is to modify and/or redistribute target cell H-2 antigens in such a way that these altered H-2 products can then be recognized in a cross-reactive but specific manner by the effector cell's antigen receptors (12,13). Thus, this model argues that lectin per se neither binds effector and target cell nor activates the effector cell. Rather, it is argued that specific T cell lysis and LDCC are not only analogous, but identical, in that in both cases the cytotoxic T cell receptor is required to bind specifically to antigen on the target cell. The basis for this hypothesis stems largely from the observation, previously made by several investigators, that while Con A pretreated effector cells do not mediate appreciable levels of non-specific lysis of untreated target cells, Con A pretreated target cells are quite susceptible to lysis (9,14, 15). It is this finding that has been interpreted as the evidence that lectin (Con A) acts exclusively on the target cell, not the effector cell.

In view of this provocative new model for LDCC, the present communication is intended first to reexamine and extend the findings that led to the previous hypothesis that the function of lectin in LDCC is the dual one of bridging effector and target cells and activating the effector cells. To do this, a lectin very similar to Con A in terms of carbohydrate specificity, _Lens culinaris_ hemagglutinin A (LcH-A), is uniquely employed. Secondly, LcH-A is further used in conjunction with Con A to argue forcibly that lectins, including Con A, do not act exclusively on target cells in mediating LDCC.

RESULTS

Evidence Against the "Glue" Hypothesis

The contention that lectin does not mediate LDCC by merely bringing the cytotoxic T cell into close contact with a target cell is substantiated by the data summarized in Table I. As mentioned above, LDCC is not mediated by several reagents capable of bridging including both allogeneic and xenogeneic antiserum, wheat germ agglutinin (WGA), and soybean agglutinin (SBA), the latter an efficient agglutinin providing the cells are first treated with neuraminidase. These results are consistent with the previous observation by Bonavida and Bradley that poly-L-lysine, another nonmitogenic agglutinin, failed to support lectin-dependent lysis (14).

In spite of these findings, the "glue" hypothesis has been invoked to account for the lack of success in obtaining continuously growing hybrid lines exhibiting cytotoxic activity. In a recent study in which murine cell hybrids were obtained by fusion of thy-

TABLE I. Comparison of the agglutinating and mitogenic properties of various agents with their ability to support LDCC[a]

Lectin/Antiserum	Agglutination	Mitogenesis[b]	LDCC[c]
Con A	+++	+++(T)	++
LcH-A	+++	+++(T)	+++
PHA-L	+++	++(T)	++
LPS	-	++(B)	-[d]
WGM	-	++(B)	-[d]
WGA	++	-	-
SBA	-	-	-
SBA + neuraminidase[e]	+++	±(ND)	-
CBA anti-EL4 serum	+++	-	-
Rabbit anti-EL4 serum	+++	-	-

[a]Various lectins and antisera (range 0 to 200 μg/ml lectin and 1:4 to 1:256 antisera) were concurrently assessed for their ability to cause: agglutination of alloimmune C57BL/6 spleen cells and of EL4 cells, increased ^{3}H-TdR incorporation in alloimmune spleen cell populations, cytolysis of EL4 cells in the presence of alloimmune (C57BL/6 anti-P815) effector cells and scored using a relative scale based on the concentration of agent required to yield 50% agglutination, the extent of proliferation (stimulation index), or the level of LDCC, respectively. (Adapted from Green, W.R., Z.K. Ballas, and C.S. Henney, J. Immunol. 121:1566. With permission. Copyright 1978, Williams and Wilkins, Baltimore, MD).

[b]The responding lymphocyte population in parentheses was determined by both positive and negative selection of the T cell compartment. T cells were removed by treating spleen cells with an anti-Thy 1.2 antiserum in the presence of complement. T cells were conserved by passage through a nylon wool column. In the case of PHA-L this was not determined empirically, but this classification has been widely reported. (N.D., not determined.)

[c]The lectin-dependent cytolytic activity of C57BL/6 spleen cells obtained 10 to 14 days after immunization with 10^{7} P815 cells was measured by using a microcytotoxicity assay employing ^{51}Cr-labeled syngeneic EL4 target cells and an effector to target cell ratio of 100:1, essentially as described previously (9). Lectin-dependent specific cytolysis was defined as follows:

moma cells with "allo-activated" T cells, of 16 hybrid lines formed, no effector cell function was observed (16). This lack of killing activity was attributed to the possibility that the agent used to promote fusion acted like a lectin in causing non-specific lysis of the partner thymoma cell whenever a killer cell was about to be fused to it. Thus, it has been speculated that such hybridoma cytotoxic lines would be very difficult to isolate. To test this possibility, polyethylene glycol (PEG), the agent most commonly used to fuse cells during hybridoma formation, was tested for its ability to mediate LDCC. As shown in Table II, over a wide concentration range, PEG was unable to support the lysis of syngeneic EL4 target cells by alloimmune cytotoxic T cells. Unfortunately, PEG could not be tested at the concentrations often employed in cell fusion because at levels of 100 mg/ml or higher, there was an interference with the specific T cell lysis of P815 target cells. Even so, these data provided no support for the suggestion that fusion agents can mediate non-specific cell-mediated lysis. Although cell fusion and lectin-dependent cytotoxicity both clearly involve cell-cell interaction, the agents which induce the two events appear to be quite distinctive. Furthermore, fusion-derived hybrid cytotoxic T cell lines have recently been obtained by both Nabholz and co-workers (17) and Kaufman and co-workers (18).

<u>The Utility of Lens culinaris Hemagglutinin (LcH-A) to Mediate LDCC</u>

As schematically depicted in Table I, LcH-A was routinely found to support higher levels of LDCC than the more commonly employed lectins, concanavalin A (Con A) and the leucoagglutinin of phytohemagglutinin (PHA-L). Con A and PHA-L usually supported similar levels of lysis. It was thus important to determine whether LcH-A was perhaps allowing effector cells of other than T cell origin to lyse syngeneic target cells. Positive and negative enrichment experiments employing nylon wool column fractionation and conventional anti-Thy 1.2 and complement treatments, respectively, confirmed that LcH-A-mediated LDCC by alloimmune spleen cells was exclusively performed by cytotoxic T cells (data not shown), as is the case for

---

$$\%\ \text{specific lysis} = \frac{\begin{matrix}{}^{51}\text{Cr release}\\ \text{with immune}\\ \text{cells + lectin}\end{matrix} - \begin{matrix}{}^{51}\text{Cr release}\\ \text{with normal}\\ \text{cells + lectin}\end{matrix}}{\begin{matrix}{}^{51}\text{Cr released after three}\\ \text{cycles of freeze-thaw}\end{matrix}} \times 100\%$$

[d]These levels were not increased when reagents with the ability to agglutinate a majority of the cells (either WGA or rabbit-anti-EL4 serum) were added together with LPS or WGM.

[e]SBA was added to cells which had been pretreated with 10-100 units/ml of neuraminidase.

TABLE II. Inability of the fusion agent PEG to mediate LDCC of EL4 target cells[a]

Agent/Lectin Added to Assay	% Specific Lysis of:	
	P815	EL4
None	24.3	1.3
2.5 μg/ml LcH-A	ND.	21.7
1 μg/ml PEG	25.3	0.2
10	26.5	0.6
100	25.1	0
1 mg/ml	24.0	-0.6
10	21.3	-0.7
100	-1.2	2.4

[a]Effector cells and cytolytic assays were performed as in Table I. Percent specific lysis of P815 target cells was calculated using the same formula as in the legend to Table I except that lectin was not present.

both Con A and PHA-L. Because of this finding, it was of interest to determine the relationship of the cytotoxic T cells killing in the presence of LcH-A to those doing so in the presence of Con A or PHA-L. Did these lectins functionally define distinct or overlapping populations of CTL?

To approach this question, experiments were conducted in which the lysis of syngeneic EL4 target cells by alloimmune effector cells was conducted in the presence of various concentrations of each lectin alone, or in the presence of all permutations of concentrations of LcH-A and Con A or LcH-A and PHA. If separate populations of CTL were defined by these lectins, then the amount of lysis occurring in the presence of two lectins might approach the sum of that occurring in the presence of each individual lectin. As shown in Table III, however, the amounts of lysis approached additivity only when one or both lectins were present in suboptimal concentrations. At optimal or supra-optimal concentrations, the level of lysis was always equal to, or less than, the level observed in the presence of LcH-A alone. Although this finding was not unexpected in the case of LcH-A and Con A, because of their similar carbohydrate specificities, it was also found for LcH-A and PHA-L. In a second experiment in which the relationship of Con A and PHA-L was also examined, a similar lack of additivity was observed for this combination as well. Thus, it appeared that while these lectins

TABLE III. Relationship of killer cells mediating LDCC of EL4 target cells by LcH-A, Con A and PHA-L[a]

	% Specific Lysis in Presence of:					
	LcH-A (μg/ml)					
	0	0.5	1.0	2.5	5	10
Con A (μg/ml)						
0	0.5%	16	33	36	33	24
0.5	2	19	32	41	35	26
1	8	22	30	39	34	26
2.5	21	25	30	35	30	23
5	23	24	25	26	24	17
10	18	18	15	17	14	11
PHA-L (μg/ml)						
0.5	6	27	33	44	37	26
1	11	29	35	41	38	25
2.5	23	35	32	38	35	23
5	24	30	36	37	33	17
10	21	29	29	32	25	14

[a]The lysis of EL4 target cells by sungeneic C57BL/6 spleen cells from mice previously immunized with P815 tumor cells was measured at an E/T ratio of 100:1 as in Table I.

might not define identical populations of CTL, these populations were largely overlapping. Those CTL responsive to LcH-A might constitute a larger population of CTL, or alternatively, LcH-A might define the same population but be more efficient, perhaps by allowing a faster recycling time.

LcH-A was also examined for its ability to support LDCC following pretreatment of either effector or target cells. As mentioned above, Con A has the peculiar property of allowing non-specific lysis when target, but not effector, cells are pretreated, and this observation has been used to suggest that lectin acts exclusively on the target cell in LDCC (12,13). Previously, my co-workers and I had reported that effector cells pretreated with LcH-A exhibited as much lytic activity as was observed when LcH-A was merely added to untreated effector and target cells (9). In the experiments published, however, excess lectin not bound to the effector cells was not washed out but was present when effector and target cells were combined. Hence, the possibility existed that it was this free lectin that actually mediated lysis by binding to target cells. In the experiment of Table IV in which care was taken to remove excess lectin, it can be seen that LcH-A pretreated CTL did cause optimal levels of LDCC. LcH-A pretreated target cells, on the other hand, were less susceptible than untreated target cells to LcH-A mediated LDCC. Furthermore, even these lower levels of lysis following target cell pretreatment required higher concentrations of LcH-A on a per cell basis than those used to pretreat effector cells. Thus, there is no evidence that LcH-A acts exclusively on target cells in supporting LDCC. In contrast, the ability of LcH-A to mediate lysis following either effector of target cell pretreatment appeared to make it especially suitable for further study of the role of lectin in LDCC.

Activation in the Absence of Bridging is Insufficient for LDCC to Occur

In a previous section evidence was provided which argued that lectin bridging of a cytotoxic T cell to a syngeneic target cell was insufficient for LDCC to occur, thus implying that a function of effector cell activation was also required to be performed by lectin. Because there were no non-agglutinating T cell mitogens to test, these data did not exclude the possibility that lectin was only required to activate the effector cell. To address this possibility, effector cells were pretreated with LcH-A and the cytolytic assay was conducted in the presence of its specific sugar, α methylmannoside (αMM) to preclude bridging (9). The problem with this approach was that αMM might have removed the lectin from the effector cell surface and thus reversed the state of activation.

An alternative method avoided these problems associated with the use of αMM by instead employing anti-lectin antiserum to preclude or diminish bridging of target and effector cells (9). As shown in a more extensive version of this type of experiment (Table V), target cells pretreated with Con A were susceptible to LDCC by syngeneic effector cells as previously described. Subsequent pretreatment with anti-Con A antiserum completely inhibited this lysis. This protocol thus served to occupy those cell surface structures capable of being bound by both Con A and LcH-A, since their carbohydrate specificities were so similar. Because the anti-Con A serum

TABLE IV. The effect of LcH-A pretreatment of effector versus target cells of lectin-dependent lysis[a]

Pretreatment Conditions			
Effector Cells	Target Cells	Lectin Added to Assay	% Specific Lysis of EL4
Untreated	Untreated	None	0
		1 μg/ml LcH-A	30.2
		2.5	46.6
		5	49.0
		10	37.6
		20	17.3
2.5 μg/ml LcH-A	Untreated	None	31.2
5.0 μg/ml			42.5
10.0 μg/ml			44.7
20.0 μg/ml			43.2
40.0 μg/ml			39.7
Untreated	2.5 μg/ml LcH-A	None	1.7
	5.0 μg/ml		4.0
	10.0 μg/ml		10.9
	20.0 μg/ml		15.9
	40.0 μg/ml		21.3

[a]Alloimmune (C57BL/6 anti-P815) effector or EL4 target cells were preincubated at 10^7 cells ml with various concentrations of LcH-A for 30 minutes at 37°C. The cells were then washed three times with medium containing 10% FCS. Normal C57BL/6 spleen cells were employed in all cases, including pretreatments, as a control to calculate lysis as described in the legend to Table I.

TABLE V. The effectof anti-Con A antiserum on the susceptibility of Con A-pretreated EL4 target cells to LDCC[a]

Target Cell Pretreatment		% Specific Lysis of EL4		
Lectin	Antiserum	no added lectin	presence of LcH-A[b]	presence of PHA-L[c]
None	None	-0.2	35.8	25.8
5 μg/ml Con A	None	19.9	N.D.	N.D.
	Anti-Con A	-0.3	37.9	30.5
10 μg/ml Con A	None	34.3	N.D.	N.D.
	Anti-Con A	3.2	33.8	22.2
20 μg/ml Con A	None	34.4	N.D.	N.D.
	Anti-Con A	0.5	19.5	21.1

[a]Lectin pretreatment was performed as described in the legend to Table IV but with Con A. In this experiment, the lectin pretreated target cells were further incubated (30 minutes, room temperature) with 1 ml of rabbit anti-Con A serum. After centrifugation and removal of the supernatant, the cells were resuspended for use in cytotoxic assays. Adapted in part from Green, W.R., Z.K. Ballas, and C.S. Henney, J. Immunol. 121:1566. With permission. Copyright 1978. Williams and Wilkins, Baltimore, MD.

[b]5 μg/ml LcH-A final concentration.

[c]5 μg/ml PHA-L final concentration.

does not bind LcH-A (data not shown), however, LcH-A could be delivered relatively exclusively and normally to effector cells for activation purposes under conditions where bridging to target cells was diminished. It was observed that when a high concentration of Con A was used to approach a saturation of target cell LcH-A binding sites, a significant inhibition of the ability of LcH-A to mediate lysis occurred. Such pretreatment of target cells had only a slight effect, however, on the extent of lysis caused by PHA-L, which exhibits a different sugar specificity. The inhibitory effect was therefore specific and not due to gross steric effects. These results were taken as evidence that effector cell activation in the absence of lectin bridging to target cells is not sufficient for LDCC to occur.

The possibility exists, of course, that "activation" did not occur in these experiments, perhaps because effector cells require interaction with cell-bound mitogen in order to express their cytotoxic potential. Although this explanation cannot be excluded, it seems unlikely to be the case because the lectin-dependent T killer cells undoubtedly encountered LcH-A bound to other cells within the effector cell population. These findings, taken together with those showing bridging per se to be insufficient, are thus consistent with a dual role of activation and bridging for lectin in LDCC.

The Bridging Function of Lectin in Cytolysis Cannot Be Served by a Non-mitogenic Agglutinin

Although two functions thus appeared to be required of lectin, it was not clear whether both had to be performed by the T cell mitogen. It was possible that a non-mitogenic agglutinin could fulfill the bridging requirement when the T cell mitogen was only functioning to activate. To address this possibility, anti-lectin antibody was again employed to compromise bridging by cell bound T cell mitogen (Table VI). In this case, however, alloimmune effector cells were pretreated with LcH-A. Subsequent pretreatment with a specific anti-LcH-A serum completely abrogated lysis, presumably by inhibiting bridge formation. Addition of the non-mitogenic agglutinins WGA or rabbit anti-EL4 serum to promote cell-cell contact, however, did not restore lysis. These results were interpreted as favoring the hypothesis that the T cell mitogen itself must also supply the bridging function.

An alternative explanation would be that the interaction of anti-LcH-A antibody with effector cell bound LcH-A inhibited activation of the effector cell. To avoid this possibility, specific antigen, rather than lectin, was used to activate the alloimmune effector cells. Thus, unlabeled P815 target cells were added to mixtures of C57BL/6 anti-P815 effector cells and ^{51}Cr-labeled EL4 target cells, and the "bystander lysis" of the syngeneic EL4 target cells was examined in the presence of WGA or anti-EL4 antiserum (Table VII). Although these non-mitogenic agglutinins had only a small effect on the lysis of the specific target cell (P815), they did not support non-specific lysis of the syngeneic target cell (EL4). This lack of lysis occurred even though the effector cells were activated by the process of lysing their specific target cells and should have been bridged to syngeneic target cells by the presence of the agglutinating reagents. This data was taken as further evidence that a given lectin must perform both the activating and bridging roles for LDCC to occur. Furthermore, this data suggests that the sites on the T cell surface through which activation is effected, and those which result in bridging to the target cell, appear to be closely linked. Evidence to support this contention has also been obtained with directly cytotoxic T cell populations. When two populations of effector cells (A anti-B and B anti-D) were

TABLE VI. Inability of non-mitogenic agglutinins to subserve the bridging role of lectin in LDCC[a]

Effector Cell Pretreatment		% Specific Lysis of EL4		
Lectin	Antiserum	no added lectin	presence of WGA[b]	presence of anti-EL4[c]
5 μg/ml LcH-A	None	20.3	N.D.	N.D.
	Anti-LcH-A	0.6	1.0	-1.2
10 μg/ml LcH-A	None	19.5	N.D.	N.D.
	Anti-LcH-A	2.0	1.0	2.9
20 μg/ml LcH-A	None	17.1	N.D.	N.D.
	Anti-LcH-A	0.8	0.6	2.2

[a]Effector cells were of C57BL/6 anti-P815 origin and the E/T ratio was 100:1.

[b]Highest value observed with 10 or 100 μg/ml WGA as final concentration.

[c]Highest value observed with 1:8 or 1:16 dilution as final concentration.

coincubated, only effector cells of the B type were lysed. Effector cells of type A were not lysed even when cells of the D phenotype were added, in order to "trigger" the other effector cell population (17,19).

Evidence That Lectins, Including Con A, Are Required to Interact With Both Target and Effector Cells

The data to this point, obtained largely by using LcH-A, support the hypothesis that in mediating LDCC, lectin performs the dual roles of effector cell activation and bridging of effector and target cells. An alternative model that lectin per se acts exclusively on target cells to modify their H-2 for antigen specific recognition and does not activate or bridge is largely based on the inability of Con A pretreated effector cells to mediate LDCC. Certainly, this model cannot be a general one for LDCC because higher levels of lysis occur when effector cells, not target cells are pretreated with LcH-A (Table IV). Similarly, PHA has also been shown to support LDCC following pretreatment of effector or target cells, although the extent to which excess PHA was removed was unclear in these pretreatment studies (14). Nonetheless, the possi-

TABLE VII. Inability of non-mitogenic agglutinins to mediate "bystander lysis" of syngeneic target cells[a]

Target Cells[b] ^{51}Cr-labeled	unlabeled	Lectin/Antiserum added	% Specific Lysis
P815	None	None	33.9
		50 μg/ml WGA[c]	28.4
		1:64 Anti-EL4[d]	24.8
EL4	None	None	0.4
		50 μg/ml WGA[c]	0.1
		1:64 Anti-EL4[d]	-0.7
P815	EL4	None	33.4
		50 μg/ml WGA[c]	24.3
		1:64 Anti-EL4[d]	22.5
EL4	P815	None	0.2
		50 μg/ml WGA[c]	0.5
		1:64 Anti-EL4[d]	-0.8

[a]Effector cells were C57BL/6 spleen cells from mice previously immunized with 10^7 P815 tumor cells.

[b]$2x10^4$ ^{51}Cr-labeled $\pm$ $2x10^4$ unlabeled target cells were used.

[c]5, 10, 20 and 100 μg/ml final concentrations of WGA were also tested and were unable to support lysis of EL4 target cells.

[d]1:16 and 1:32 dilutions of anti-EL4 antiserum also tested did not support lysis of EL4 and were somewhat more inhibitory to the lysis of P815 target cells.

bility remained that in the particular case of Con A-mediated LDCC, lectin does act exclusively on target cells.

To approach this question, advantage was taken again of the similar binding specificities, but different properties with respect to LDCC, of Con A and LcH-A in the experiment of Table VIII. The possibility that Con A per se was required to bridge effector and target cells was investigated by mixing Con A-pretreated target cells, which are very susceptible to lysis by untreated effector cells, with lectin pretreated effector cells. If Con A pretreated target cells are lysed by untreated effector cells without target cell-bound Con A bridging effector and target cells, then the extent of lysis should be unchanged whether the effector cells are pretreated with lectin or not, provided that the pretreated effector cells are actively lytic. Although this latter criterion cannot be unambiguously met with Con A pretreated effector cells, it is fully met with LcH-A pretreated effector cells, which vigorously lyse untreated target cells.

Overall, the data shown in Table VIII show that as the concentration of Con A used to pretreat target cells or that of LcH-A used to pretreat effector cells increased, the amount of lysis declined when both partners were pretreated. This was particularly true at the higher concentrations of lectin where saturation of binding sites was approached and competition between effector cell-bound LcH-A and target cell-bound Con A for bridge formation would be maximized. For example, combining target cells pretreated with 20 µg/ml Con A, which were lysed 52% by untreated effector cells, and effector cells pretreated with 40 µg/ml LcH-A, which lysed untreated target cells at the 54% level, led to only 21% lysis. This level was substantially less than would have been predicted if Con A was only required to interact with target cells and not promote bridging. For any particular preparation of LcH-A-pretreated target cells or Con A-pretreated effector cells, the amount of lysis progressively declined as the concentration of lectin used to pretreat either effector cells or target cells, respectively, was increased. Although Con A-pretreated cells lysed untreated target cells very sluggishly, a similar trend was generally observed. Moreover, the use of LcH-A pretreated target cells yielded results which were qualitatively very comparable to those depicted with Con A-pretreated target cells (data not shown).

Taken together, these results argue forcibly against a model of LDCC in which lectin in general, or Con A in particular, does not bind the effector and target cell together but only antigenically modifies the target cell. Certainly, lectins do modify the target cell surface to which they bind, but these data show that conditions must also be such that lectin is allowed to bridge effector and target cells if LDCC is to occur. Thus, the results presented here coupled with those just cited collectively support the previously advanced hypothesis that lectin performs the dual functions of bridging effector and target cells and activating the effector cell.

The discrepancy between Con A and LcH-A in their ability to support LDCC following effector cell pretreatment remains a puzzle. One notable difference between the two lectins -- their valence, Con A being tetravelent and LcH-A divalent-- is an appealing possibility but does not seem to provide the answer. Succinylated-Con A (S-Con A), which is divalent, did not behave like LcH-A in pretreatment experiments. While S-Con A was only modestly able to mediate LDCC, compared to Con A, when added to untreated cells, it was even less effective in supporting lysis, if at all, upon pretreatment of effector or target cells (Table IX).

TABLE VIII. The effect of Con A pretreatment of target cells on their susceptibility to LcH-A pretreated effector cells[a]

Effector Cell Pre-treatment	Lectin Added to Assay	% Specific Lysis of				
		EL4	5μg/ml Con A-EL4	10μg/ml Con A-EL4	20μg/ml Con A-EL4	40μg/ml Con A-EL4
Untreated	None	-1	23	39	52	35
	5 μg/ml LcH-A	53				
	10	29				
	20	16				
	40	10				
	5 μg/ml Con A	35				
	10	23				
	20	14				
	40	7				
5 μg/ml LcH-A	None	89	45	45	36	25
10		72	40	34	29	23
20		65	33	24	27	19
40		54	25	23	21	15
5 μg/ml Con A	None	2	8	20	23	22
10		6	5	7	11	9
20		10	5	6	5	4
40		6	3	2	0	0

[a]Lectin and antiserum pretreatment of effector and/or target cells was perfomed as described in the legends to Tables V and VI using the appropriate anti-lectin antiserum.

TABLE IX. Ability of succinylated-Con A to mediate LDCC[a]

Pretreatment Conditions		Lectin Added to Assay	% Specific Lysis of EL4
Target Cells	Effector Cells		
Untreated	Untreated	5 μg/ml Con A	24.5[b]
		2.5 μg/ml SCA[c]	4.8
		5	7.5
		10	12.1
		20	13.7
		40	14.7
2.5 μg/ml SCA[c]	Untreated	None	1.7
5			3.4
10			2.2
20			3.2
40			5.3
Untreated	2.5 μg/ml s-Con A		0.4
	5		1.4
	10		1.4
	20		3.0
	40		2.1

[a]Pretreatments were performed as described in the legend to Table IV.

[b]The highest amount of lysis observed over the range of 2.5-40 μg/ml Con A.

[c]Succinylated Con A

DISCUSSION

The results presented in this paper favor the view that in order to mediate lectin-dependent cell-mediated cytolysis, a lectin must be a T cell mitogen and must both bridge the effector to the target cell as well as activate the cytotoxic "machinery" of the effector cell. The evidence supporting this hypothesis can be summarized as follows:

1. Bridging alone is insufficient for lysis to occur; non-mitogenic agglutinating agents do not mediate LDCC (Table I).
2. B cell mitogens in the presence or absence of non-mitogenic agglutinating agents do not mediate LDCC (Table I); only T cell mitogens allow LDCC to occur, consistent with a requirement for cytotoxic T cell activation.
3. Imposing conditions under which activation of effector cells should have occurred but bridging of these effector cells to target cells was discouraged, resulted in an inhibition of lysis (Table V) suggesting that activation, though necessary, is not sufficient for LDCC to occur.
4. Non-mitogenic agglutinins are not able to subserve the bridging role of the T cell mitogen in LDCC (Table VI and VII) implying that the T cell mitogen per se must perform both the activating and bridging functions.

Much of this evidence was obtained by the use of LcH-A in a lectin-dependent lytic system. LcH-A appeared to be particularly suited for defining the role of lectin in LDCC because it consistently supported higher levels of lysis than either Con A or PHA-L (Table I) and yet appeared to define the same or a somewhat larger population of cytotoxic T cells than did the other two lectins (Table III). Furthermore, and unlike Con A, LcH-A was able to cause LDCC following lectin pretreatment of either effector or target cells. The ability of LcH-A to mediate higher levels of LDCC when effector, rather than target cells, were pretreated argues strongly against the general hypothesis of Berke et al. (12,13) that the role of lectin in LDCC is only to modify target cell H-2 and does not act on effector cells either to activate them or bridge them to target cells. Moreover, the results of experiments presented here utilizing Con A pretreated target cells and LcH-A pretreated effector cells are not consistent with this kind of role for lectin even for Con A (Table VIII). Thus, the competitive inhibition of lysis obtained by combining these pretreated partner cells suggests that in the case of Con A pretreated cells, as well, Con A is required to bind the effetor cell to the target cell.

Three other findings are difficult to reconcile with the model of Berke et al. First, and most incisive of these, is the observation made by Todd on trypsin-treated effector T cells (20). While trypsin treatment appeared to have abrogated T cell receptor function as evidenced by the inability of the treated cells to lyse their specific target cells or to bind to appropriate allogeneic monolayers, substantial lectin-dependent killing activity remained. These results are thus inconsistent with a model of LDCC which is based on specific recognition by the T cell receptor. The second finding that bears upon this new model for LDCC, made by Kuppers et al. (21), is that with some target cells, at least., partial papain stripping of target cell H-2 results in a much more severe inhibition of specific cytolysis than LDCC. For a sub-line of the L5178 tumor, only 14% inhibition of LDCC was noted following papain treatment compared to 63% inhibition of specific allogeneic cytolysis. This observation also suggests that recognition by the T cell receptor may not be required in LDCC. Finally, Ballas et al (22) have reported that Con A-coupled Sepharose 4B beads are able to mediate levels of LDCC as high as those caused by soluble Con A. It is somewhat difficult conceptually to envision the ability of Con A in very large insoluble form to modify and/or redistribute target cell H-2 molecules.

A striking observation noted by Berke et al. seems to more readily explain the inability of Con A-pretreated effector cells to exhibit their lytic potential. These investigators found that Con A-pretreated effector cells were unable to form conjugates with untreated target cells (12). Since cell-cell contact is the first prerequisite for cell-mediated lysis to occur, this is a very satisfying explanation. Further experimentation is obviously needed to confirm this observation and to thus determine whether the "Con A effect" has any significance for our understanding of lectin-dependent and, by inference, specific cell-mediated cytolysis. Perhaps the recent availability of homogeneous cloned cytotoxic T cell lines will allow us to more precisly define the roles of lectin and the antigen receptor in T cell-mediated lysis.

REFERENCES

1. Brunner, K.T., and J.C. Cerottini. Cell-mediated cytotoxicity, allograft rejection and tumor immunity. Adv. Immunol. 18:67 (1974)
2. Wagner, H.S., S.W. Harris, and M. Feldman. Cell-mediated immune response _in vitro_. II. The role of thymus and thymus-derived lymphocytes. Cell. Immunol. 4:39. (1972)
3. Moller, E. Contact-induced cytotoxicity by lymphoid cells containing foreign isoantigens. Science 147:873. (1964)
4. Forman J., and G. Moller. Generation of cytotoxic lymphocytes in mixed lymphocyte reactions. I. Specificity of the effector cells. J. Exp. Med. 138:672. (1973)
5. Bevan M.H., and M. Cohn. Cytotoxic effects of antigen and mitogen-induced T cells on various targets. J. Immunol. 114:559. (1975)
6. Kuppers, R.C., and C.S. Henney. Evidence for direct linkage between antigen recognition and lytic expression in effector T cells. J. Exp. Med. 143:684. (1976)
7. Kuppers, R.C., and C.S. Henney. Studies on the mechanism of lymphocyte-mediated cytolysis. IX. Relationships between antigen recognition and lytic expression in killer T cells. J. Immunol. 118:71. (1977)
8. Fishelson, Z., and G. Berke. T lymphocyte-mediated cytolysis:

Dissociation of the binding and lytic mechanisms of the effector cell. J. Immunol. 120:1121. (1978)

9. Greeen, W.R., Z.K. Ballas,, and C.S. Henney. Studies on the mechanism of lymphocyte-medited cytolysis. XI. The role of lectin in lectin-dependent cell-mediated cytotoxicity. J. Immunol. 121:1566. (1978)
10. Parker, W.L., and E. Martz. Lectin-induced nonlethal adhesions between cytolytic T lymphocytes and antigenically unrecognizable tumor cells and nonspecific "triggering" of cytolysis. J. Immunol. 125:25. (1980)
11. Gately, M.K., and E. Martz. Comparative studies on the mechanisms of nonspecific, Con A-dependent cytolysis and specific T cell-mediated cytolysis. J. Immunol. 119:1711. (1977)
12. Berke G., V. Hu, E. McVey, and W.R. Clark. T lymphocyte-mediated cytolysis. I. A common mechanism for target recognition in specific and lectin-dependent cytolysis. J. Immunol. 127:776. (1981)
13. Berke, G., E. McVey, V. Hu, and W.R. Clark. T lymphocyte-mediated cytolysis. II. Role of target cell histocompatibility antigens in recognition and lysis. J. Immunol. 127:782. (1981)
14. Bonavida, B., and T.P. Bradley. Studies on the induction and expression of T cell-mediated immunity. V. Lectin-induced nonspecific cell-mediated cytotoxicity by alloimmune lymphocytes. Transplantation 21:94. (1976)
15. Rubens, R.P., and C.S. Henney. Studies on the mechanism of lymphocyte-mediated cytolysis. VIII. The use of Con A to delineate a distinctive killer T cell subpopulation. J. Immunol. 118:180. (1977)
16. Kohler, G., I. Lefkovits, B. Elliott, and A. Coutinho. Derivation of hybrids between a thymoma line and spleen cells activated in a mixed leukocyte reaction. Eur. J. Immunol. 7:758. (1977)
17. Nabholz, M., M. Cianfriglia, O. Acuto, A. Conzelman, W. Haas, H.V. Bohmer, H.R. MacDonald, and J.P. Johnson. Cytolytically active murine T cell hybrids. Nature 287:437. (1980)
18. Kaufmann, Y., G. Berke, and Z. Eshhar. Cytotoxic T lymphocyte hybridomas that mediate specific tumor-cell lysis _in vitro_. Proc. Natl. Acad. Sci. 78:2502. (1981)
19. Gensheimer G.G., and J.R. Neefe. Cell-mediated lympholysis: A receptor-associated lytic mechanism. Cell. Immunol. 36:54. (1978)
20. Todd, R. Functional characterization of membrane components of cytotoxic peritoneal exudate T lympocytes. II. Trypsin sensitivity of the killer cell receptor. Transplantation 20:314. (1975)
21. Kuppers, R.C., Z.K. Ballas, W.R. Green, and C.S. Henney. Quantitative appraisal of H-2 products in T cell-mediated lysis by allogeneic and syngeneic effector cells. J. Immunol. 127:500. (1981)

22. Ballas, Z.K., W.R. Green, and C.S. Henney. Studies on the mechanism of T cell-mediated lysis. XIII. Lectin-dependent T cell-mediated cytotoxicity is supported by Con A-coupled Sepharose beads. Cell. Immunol. 59:411. (1981)

EFFECTS OF CONCANAVALIN A PRETREATMENT ON CLONED CYTOLYTIC T CELLS

Katherine A. Wall and Frank W. Fitch

Department of Pathology
University of Chicago
Chicago, Illinois 60637

Concanavalin A (Con A) and some other lectins have been shown to facilitate lysis of antigenically irrelevant target cells by otherwise specific cytolytic T cells (CTL). The mechanism of the nonspecific recognition in such lectin-facilitated cytolysis is not yet understood; however, simple bridging is apparently not sufficient since some lectins may agglutinate cells and yet not cause target cell lysis (1).

Recent observations made with polyclonal effector cells suggested that the target cell is the critical site of Con A action (2). Target cells preincubated with Con A were lysed as effectively by cytolytic T cells in the absence of additional Con A, as when Con A was present throughout the assay. Effector cells preincubated with Con A produced lysis subsequently only when additional Con A was present during the assay.

We have analyzed the effects produced by preincubation of target or effector cells with Con A on the lytic activity of several cloned cytolytic T cells. We find that the pattern of lysis observed is dependent on the cloned CTL used, and the results differ from those previously described. Some cloned CTL can mediate lectin-facilitated cytolysis if preincubated with Con A.

MATERIALS AND METHODS

CTL Clones

Four cloned cytolytic T cells were studied. L3 and B18 clones were derived from secondary C57BL/6 anti-DBA/2 mixed leukocyte culture (MLC) and specifically lysed H-$2D^d$ and H-$2K^d$ bearing target cells, respectively (3). T18 and T38 clones were derived from a primary C57BL/10 (B10) anti-TNP-B10 MLC and specifically lysed TNP-modified cells bearing H-$2D^b$ antigen and H-$2D^{b,d,s}$ antigen, respectively (unpublished observations). None of the clones alone lysed the syngeneic target cells used. The specificity of lysis is shown for these lines in Table I.

The conditions for deriving and maintaining alloreactive cytolytic T cell clones have been previously described (3). Briefly, clones were maintained by weekly transfer of 1.6×10^4 cells into Linbro 24 cluster wells containing 6×10^6 irradiated (1200R) stimulator cells in 1.5 ml Dulbecco's minimal essential medium (DMEM, Gibco) supplemented with 2% fetal calf serum, 5×10^{-5} M 2-mercaptoethanol, 10mM morpholinopropanesulfonic acid (MOPS), penicillin/streptomycin and containing 33% of a supernatant from mixed lymphocyte cultures of Con A-stimulated rat spleen cells (3). B18 and L3 cells were passaged on DBA spleen cells; T18 and T38 were passaged on a mixture of 3×10^6 each unmodified and TNP-modified B10 spleen cells. These cells were modified by incubation in 10 mM trinitrobenzenesulfonate (TNP, Eastman, 1x recrytallized) in Dulbecco's phosphate buffered saline (DPBS), pH 7.4, for 10 minutes at 37°C. The culture medium for the TNP-reactive clones contained 10% fetal calf serum, 10 mM N-2-hydroxyethylpiperazine-N'-2-ethanesulfonic acid (HEPES), 0.03% glutamine, and 2-mecaptoethanol, antibiotics, and supernatants as above.

Target Cells

Con A stimulated spleen cells were prepared as described (3). EL-4 and AKR-A are tumor cells of C57BL/6 and AKR origin, respectively. TNP-modified target cells were prepared as described above. Cells were labeled with 0.2 mCi sodium ^{51}Cr-chromate for 1.5 h before assay.

TABLE I. SPECIFICITY OF CTL CLONES

	% Specific Lysis of ^{51}Cr-T (E/T = 10:1)[a]			
Clone	B10	TNP-B10	DBA/2	TNP-DBA/2
T18	0	100	0	5
T38	0	62	0	64
L3	-	0	92	-
B18	0	-	90	-

[a]Target cells were Con A stimulated spleen cells, modified as described in the text. Lysis is the average of duplicate samples and is corrected for spontaneous release. (-) indicates not tested.

Cytolytic Assay

For Con A pretreatment, effector cells or ^{51}Cr-target cells at 2×10^5/ml were incubated in 20 μg/ml Con A (Pharmacia Fine Chemicals) at 37°C for 30 minutes. Cells were washed twice with medium before assay. Five thousand ^{51}Cr-target cells and 7.5×10^4 effector cells were mixed in microtiter wells in 200 μl DMEM containing 5% agamma horse serum, 1% MOPS. In some cases, Con A was added to give a final concentration of 20 μg/ml. The plates were centrifuged for 1 minute at 600 rpm and incubated at 37°C for 90 minutes. Fifty μl 0.04M (ethylenedinitrilo)tetraacetic acid (EDTA) was added to each well and incubation was continued for an additional 90 minutes. The plates were centrifuged for 5 minutes at 1500 rpm and 100 μl supernatant was removed for determination of ^{51}Cr release. Results are reported for a single effector:target cell ratio (E/T) for ease of presentation; however, full curves with varying E/T ratios gave the same pattern of results for each clone. Maximal release (100%) was determined from a frozen and thawed sample of target cells.

TABLE II. CONDITIONS FOR CONCANAVALIN A DEPENDENT LYSIS BY L3 CTL

^{51}Cr	Incubation	Percentage ^{51}Cr Release[b] (E/T=10:1) with Concanavalin A at:			
Target	Time (min)[a]	0 μg/ml	10 μg/ml	20 μg/ml	30 μg/ml
B10	60	0	14	17	16
AKR-A	30	-	14	26	-
	60	-	29	-	-
	90	-	37	52	-
	120	-	40	-	-
	180	2	41	-	-
P815	0	0	-	-	-
	30	88	-	-	-
	180	108	105	-	-

[a] Effector and ^{51}Cr-target cells were mixed, centrifuged at 600 rpm for 1 minute, and incubated at 37°C for the indicated time. EDTA was added to 10mM and the cells were incubated at 37°C for an additional period to equal 180 minutes total incubation time.

[b] The average of duplicate samples, corrected for spontaneous release: AKR-A, 5%; B10, 22%; P815, 7%.

(-) Indicates not tested.

RESULTS

Effect of Con A Pretreatment on Lectin-Facilitated Lysis by L3 and T18 Cells

Preliminary dose response studies established that maximal lysis of target cells was observed when the Con A concentration was 20 μg/ml (Table II). The extent of lectin-facilitated lysis increased with incubation time and reached near maximal levels at 90 minutes (Table II). This time was chosen for all subsequent assays, with an additional 90 minutes after addition of EDTA to allow ^{51}Cr release. A similar time course was observed for T18 on AKR-A and P815 target cells (data not shown).

Both L3 and T18 lysed B10 and EL-4 target cells only in the presence of Con A (Table III). Similar extent of lysis was observed with both CTL clones when the target cells were pretreated with Con A and the assay was performed in the absence of additional Con A. However, when only the effector cells were pretreated with Con A, the two clones showed different patterns of lysis. B10 target cells

TABLE III. CONCANAVALIN A-PRETREATED CTL CLONES VARY IN EFFICIENTY OF LECTIN-DEPENDENT KILLING

Effector	Cell Pretreated with Con A[a]	Con A Present (20 μg/ml)	% ^{51}Cr Release by Target (E/T = 15:1)[b] B10	EL-4
L3	-	-	0	2
(B6 anti-DBA)	-	+	20	62
	B10,EL-4	-	17	40
	L3	-	15	18
	L3	+	21	56
T18	-	-	0	2
(B10 anti-TNP-B10)	-	+	14	56
	B10,EL-4	-	10	67
	T18	-	1	3
	T18	+	12	40

[a] Effector cells or ^{51}Cr-target cells at 2×10^5/ml were incubated in 20 μg/ml Con A for 30 minutes. Cells were washed twice with medium before assay.

[b] 5×10^3 ^{51}Cr-target cells and 7.5×10^4 effector cells were assayed as described in Materials and Methods. Spontaneous release: B10, 22%; EL-4, 4%. These values were unaffected by Con A treatment.

were lysed as effectively by pretreated L3 cells as by L3 when Con A was present during the assay; EL-4 target cells were lysed less efficiently by pretreated L3 cells than by L3 in the presence of Con A. Pretreated T18 cells gave background levels of lysis on both target cells. The viability of both L3 and T18 pretreated effector cells was demonstrated by their lytic activity in the presence of Con A.

Lectin-Facilitated Lysis by B18 and T38 Clones

One known difference between the L3 and T18 clones is that L3 is an alloreactive cell, whereas T18 recognizes syngeneic H-2, in combination with TNP. To ask whether the differences observed in response to Con A pretreatment would correlate with H-2 antigenic specificity, we analyzed one additional alloreactive clone, B18, and one additional syngeneic H-2 restricted clone, T38. Table IV shows that B18 gave a pattern similar to that of L3; Con A pretreated B18 was almost as effective against EL-4 target cells as was B18 in the presence of Con A. However, in contrast to the results with T18, Con A pretreated T38 also lysed EL-4 target cells, although the extent of lysis was somewhat less than that observed with B18. Therefore, three out of four clones tested gave substantial lysis of untreated target cells when only the CTL were pretreated with Con A.

TABLE IV. LECTIN-DEPENDENT KILLING BY B18 AND T38 CTL

Effector	Cell Pretreated with Con A[a]	Con A Present (20 μg/ml)	% ^{51}Cr Release by EL-4 (E/T = 15:1)
B18	-	-	2
(B6 anti-DBA)	-	+	88
	EL-4	-	66
	B18	-	54
	B18	+	78
T38	-	-	4
(B10 anti-TNP-B10)	-	+	72
	EL-4	-	108
	T38	-	31
	T38	+	65

[a] See Table III. Spontaneous release: EL-4, 14%; Con A-EL-4, 17%.

Con A-Pretreated CTL as Effector and Target Cells

One possible explanation for the differences observed between the L3 and T18 clones could be a difference in the amount of Con A bound per cell. We asked whether both CTL clones could serve as effective targets for Con A-facilitated lysis.

Equal levels of lysis of ^{51}Cr-L3 target cells by L3 effector cells were achieved with Con A present during the assay and with Con A pretreated target cells (Table V). Con A pretreated L3 effector cells on untreated ^{51}Cr-L3 gave a similar extent of lysis, in agreement with our previous results.

Analogous experiments with T18 as effector and target cell confirmed that Con A pretreated effector cells did not lyse ^{51}Cr-T18 or ^{51}Cr-L3 cells. However, Con A pretreated ^{51}Cr-T18 and ^{51}Cr-L3 target cells were lysed by untreated T18 cells. Con A pretreated ^{51}Cr-T18 cells were also lysed by untreated L3 effector cells. These results indicate that T18 cells are capable of binding sufficient Con A to be effective target cells for lectin-facilitated lysis. Varying the concentration of Con A used for pretreatment of T18 effector cells did not change the levels of lectin-facilitated lysis (Table VI). The inhibition of lytic activity in the presence of Con A with increasing concentration during pretreatment could be similar to the inhibition observed with high concentrations of Con A present during the assay (4).

TABLE V. CONCANAVALIN A-PRETREATED CTL CLONES CAN SERVE AS BOTH TARGET AND EFFECTOR CELLS IN LECTIN-DEPENDENT KILLING

Effector	Cell Pretreated with with Con A[a]	Con A Present (20 μg/ml)	% Specific Lysis of ^{51}Cr-T (E/T = 15:1)[a] L3	T18
L3	-	-	3	-
(B6 anti-DBA)	-	+	35	-
	^{51}Cr-L3,-T18	-	31	52
	L3	-	21	-
T18	-	-	-	2
(B10 anti-TNP-B10)	-	+	-	30
	^{51}Cr-L3,T18	-	23	31
	T18	-	7	4

[a] See Table III. Spontaneous release: L3, 17%; Con A-L3, 21%; T18, 7%; Con A-T18, 29%.

TABLE VI. EFFECT OF CONCANAVALIN A PRETREATMENT ON T18 CTL LYSIS OF ^{51}Cr-EL-4

Pretreatment with[a] Con A (μg/ml)	% ^{51}Cr-Release by EL-4 (E/T = 5:1) with Con A present During Assay at	
	0 μg/ml	20 μg/ml
0	2	19
20	1	6
40	2	8
80	4	8

[a] T18 effector cells were incubated with Con A for 30 minutes at 37°C and were washed twice before assay.
[b] Corrected for spontaneous release by EL-4: 8%.

CONCLUSIONS

The extent of lysis observed with Con A pretreated effector cells relative to the lysis obtained in the presence of Con A was dependent on both the effector cell and target cell studied. Lysis of untreated B18 and L3 target cells by Con A pretreated L3 CTL was similar to that observed in the presence of Con A. Lysis of EL-4 target cells by pretreated L3, B18, and T38 cloned CTL was also substantial. However, with one CTL clone, T18, Con A pretreatment of the effector cells gave background levels of lysis on all target cells tested. Therefore, a majority of the CTL studied required effector cell pretreatment only for lectin-facilitated lysis. The reason for the lack of lytic activity by Con A pretreated T18 is as yet unclear, since this CTL clone is capable of lysing target cells when Con A is present.

The results indicate that the sensitization of a cell by Con A to serve as a target cell for lectin-facilitated lysis is apparently different from that which allows the cell to act as an effector cell, as has been previously suggested (1,5). Pretreatment with Con A was sufficient to allow T18 cells to serve as target cells but not as effector cells. This comparison has the difficulty that the numbers of pretreated CTL differ depending on whether they are effector or target cells; up to 15 fold more pretreated CTL are present when the CTL is used as the effector cell than as the target cell. This is necessary because very low levels were measured in the short term assay with E/T equal to 1. If Con A treated effector cells preferentially lysed other effector cells rather than the target cells, then low levels of ^{51}Cr-release would result. However, all pretreated CTL would be expected to show similar reductions in target cell lysis.

Variations in lytic activity after pretreatment might also be due to lysis or aggregation during Con A treatment. The spontaneous ^{51}Cr-rlease of CTL target cells and verification by cell counting showed that CTL autolysis was only slightly increased during Con A treatment. Treatment at 4°C should reduce this problem. The use of succinyl Con A, which facilitates lysis but caused less aggregation, would reduce problems with inaccurate E/T ratios caused by aggregation.

The response to Con A pretreatment observed with the T18 clone is similar to that observed previously (2) with Con A stimulated spleen cells and alloimmune peritoneal exudate cells (PEC). The CTL clones studied here are all MLC-derived cells. Comparisons between cytolytic PEC and CTL derived from MLC have shown other differences, for example, the failure of anti-Lyt-2 antibodies to inhibit the cytolytic activity of PEC (6). It has been suggested that this difference could be due to differences between MLC cells and PEC in avidity for target cell antigens. The lytic activity of the four MLC clones studied here is similar. However, it is difficult to estimate the effect of the avidity of a cell for its specific antigen on lectin-facilitated lysis, because the nature of the target antigen is unclear.

ACKNOWLEGMENTS

This research was supported by USPHS Grants AI-04197 and CA-19226. Katherine Wall is the recipient of USPHS Fellowship 1F32-AI-06253. The authors gratefully acknowledge the technical assistance of Yukio Hamada, LaVerne Decker, and Daisy Freeman. We also acknowledge the assistance of Frances Mills in the preparation of the manuscript.

REFERENCES

1. Bonavida, B., and T.P. Bradley. Studies on the induction and expression of T cell-mediated immunity. V. Lectin-induced nonspecific cell-mediated cytotoxicity by alloimmune lymphocytes. Transplantation 21:94 (1976).
2. Berke, G., V. Hu, E. McVey, and W.R. Clark. T lymphocyte-mediated cytolysis. I. A common mechanism for target recognition in specific and lectin-dependent cytolysis. J. Immunol. 127:776 (1981).
3. Glasebrook, A.L., and F.W. Fitch. Alloreactive cloned T cell lines. I. Interactions between cloned amplifier and cytolytic T cell lines. J. Exp. Med. 158:876 (1980).
4. Tartof, D. Inhibition of cytotoxic T lymphocytes with concanavalin A. Cell. Immunol. 50:48 (1980).
5. Green, W.R., Z.K. Ballas, and C.S. Henney. Studies on the

mechanism of lymphocyte-mediated cytolysis. XI. The role of lectin in lectin-dependent cell-mediated cytotoxicity. J. Immunol. 121:1566 (1978).

6. MacDonald, H.R., N. Thiernesse, and J.-C. Cerottini. Inhibition of T-cell mediated cytolysis by monoclonal antibodies directed against Lyt-2: heterogeneity of inhibition at the clonal level. J. Immunol. 126:1671 (1981).

SEQUENTIAL ANALYSIS OF T CELL-MEDIATED CYTOLYSIS: A BRIEF REMINDER OF SOME POSSIBLY INFORMATIVE MARKERS AT THE RECOGNITION AND LETHAL HIT STAGES

Pierre Golstein

Centre d'Immunologie INSERM-CNRS de Marseille-Luminy
Case 906 - 13288 Marseille cedex 9 - France

The mechanism of T cell-mediated cytolysis can be considered as a "metabolic" pathway leading to a specialized functional effect, much like the pathways in microorganisms leading to the processing of a given metabolite. The comparison is useful mostly in the sense that it suggests a multi-step process. The latter may be studied genetically.

It can also be physiologically dissected. Several groups (reviewed in 1-4) have attempted such a physiological, step-by-step analysis of the cytolysis pathway. A few years ago, a division of the cytolytic process into three stages was proposed (5): a "recognition" stage was followed by a "lethal hit" stage, leading to a "target cell distintegration" stage. Perhaps an important question now is to define how much the lethal hit is distinct from recognition, and in particular whether effector cell surface molecules are uniquely involved in delivering the lethal hit. This communication aims (a) at underlining the practical difficulties of this sort of analysis, and (b) at recalling some of the results thus obtained, with selected, possibly informative metabolic markers (i.e., required metabolites or inhibitory agents).

IT CAN BE EXPERIMENTALLY DIFFICULT TO ASSIGN THE EFFECT OF A GIVEN AGENT TO RECOGNITION OR LETHAL HIT

The standard methods used (culture conditions, media, generation of cytolytic cells by mixed leucocyte culture, origin of the target cells and the 4 h ^{51}Cr-release cytolysis test) have all been described in detail (6-8). Two more specialized approaches were necessary for a sequential analysis of the mechanism of T cell-mediated cytolysis, namely a "Ca^{++} pulse" method (6) and conjugate formation (8-10), either in isolation, or in combination. Other methods have been used (see for instance ref. 3), which could be discussed similarly.

Ca^{++} pulse

The Ca^{++} pulse approach was based on the realization that the Ca^{++} requirement for T cell-mediated cytolysis (11-15) was localized at the lethal hit stage (2,6). In practice (2,6), the sequential addition to effector and ^{51}Cr-labeled target cell mixtures in EGTA-containing medium of Ca^{++} 40 min. after the beginning of incubation and EDTA 20 min. after Ca^{++} allowed dissection of the cytolytic process very schematically into the recognition stage before addition of Ca^{++}, the lethal hit stage between addition of Ca^{++} and addition of EDTA and the killer cell-independent target cell disintegration stage after addition of EDTA. On this experimental backbone, a given agent (e.g., a metabolic inhibitor) could be added either initially, or 10 min. before addition of Ca^{++}, or just after addition of EDTA. Total incubation time was 4 h.

When studying in this manner the effect of a given cytolysis-inhibiting agent, three situations were encountered:

(a) No inhibitor added post-pulse blocked cytolysis (2,3). This argued in favor of a simple (osmotic?) process operating at the target cell disintegration stage. The only exception is the inhibition reported using RAT* antiserum (6).

(b) One drug, namely cytochalasin A, did not inhibit cytolysis when added prepulse at given concentrations. At the same concentrations, this drug inhibited cytolysis when added initially. This showed that cytochalasin A affected preferentially recognition rather than lethal hit (7).

These first two situations were directly conclusive because they were characterized by an absence of inhibition of cytolysis when an agent was added at a given step.

(c) Apart from these two situations, the general case is inhibition of cytolysis when a given agent is added either initially or "pre-pulse." This was observed for many metabolic inhibitors (2,3) and was also found recently with cytolysis-inhibiting mAb (this volume). The question then is whether they inhibit recognition or lethal hit or both. This cannot be solved using Ca^{++} pulse methodology alone.

Conjugate formation

The formation of microscopically observable "conjugates" between effector cells and target cells was proposed to investigate the recognition stage of cytolysis (9,10).

This approach was very useful in particular to obtain a quantitative estimate of the proportion of antigen-specific cells in a population (9,10). However, when used to investigate mechanisms it suffers from at least one drawback. The visualization of conjugates requires the resuspension of the cell mixtures, which subjects potential conjugates to significant shearing forces. The formation and persistance of stable conjugates seems linked to (a) specific recognition, comparable to what happens when cells are maintained in a pellet, plus (b) non-specific strengthening binding forces, necessary to resist shear (8,17). Many agents which block conjugate formation may act on the latter rather than on specific recognition per se.

Because of this, again the absence of inhibition of conjugates would be more telling than inhibition, when testing a given agent. In fact, by investigating inhibition of either conjugate formation (8) or its equivalent specific adsorption on cell monolayers (2), we never encountered any agent that inhibited lethal hit without inhibiting conjguate formation. A detailed study strongly suggested that some agents were affecting the non-specific strengthening binding necessary for obtaining conjugates, rather than specific recognition as such (8). Similarly, Mg^{++} appeared to be necessary for this binding rather than for recognition in itself (8).

Combinatin of Ca^{++} pulse and conjugates

In the general case when an agent inhibits cytolysis in a Ca^{++} pulse experiment both initially and prepulse"

1. It is usually not possible to ascertain whether specific recognition as such is affected, because of the drawback of the conjugate approach mentioned above.

2. It is sometimes possible to show that lethal hit is affected. A prepulse inhibition of cytolysis could be due, either to a "downstream" block of lethal hit, or to an "upstream" reversal of recognition. Gross reversal of recognition was ruled out for the drugs azide, DMSO, phenol, cytochalasin B and theophylline (which did not reverse specific adsorption on monolayers (2) and for the B35-27.9 mAb (which did not reverse preformed conjugates (18). This strongly suggested that these agents affected lethal hit.

FIVE AGENTS WHICH MAY GIVE SOME INFORMATION ON LETHAL HIT

From the studies mentioned above, it was clear that five agents could provide some information on the mechanism of lethal hit, and perhaps contribute to distinguish it from recognition.

Ca^{++}

The Ca^{++} requirement is unique to lethal hit. Ca^{++} seems not required anywhere else in the cytolytic process, nor is it required for the formation of conjugates (even for the non-specific strengthening binding, which is Mg^{++} dependent). In fact, in the Ca^{++} pulse method the Ca^{++} requirement defines the lethal hit stage. There are very few published data on the site of this Ca^{++} requirement (e.g., whether intra or extra-cellular, whether acting on effector or target cells) which thus may or may not be an indication for a stimulus-secretion pathway as part of the cytolytic process (but see E. Martz, this volume).

Cytochalasin A

Cytochalasin A at certain concentrations inhibited cytolysis in a Ca^{++} pulse set-up when added initially but not prepulse (7). This showed that cytochalasin A inhibited recognition but not lethal hit. Similar conclusions were reached by Thorn and Henney (19). Most interestingly, the same concentrations of cytochalasin A which did not inhibit lethal hit were disruptive for microfilaments, which suggested that these may not be involved in lethal hit (7). Thus, the redistribution of the microfilamental network observed in "Conjugated" effector cells, mentioned elsewhere in this volume, may not be relevant to the mechanism of lethal hit.

Glucose

At least using certain effector cell populations, provision of glucose in the extracellular fluid is necessary for cytolysis (20, 21). Sequencing experiments showed that the glucose requirement (or the inhibition by deoxyglucose) occurred after the cytochalasin A-sensitive step (21). Glucose may then be required for lethal hit, which would be consistent with the inhibition of lethal hit by cytochalasin B, a drug which unlike cytochalasin A affects not only microfilaments but also cell permeability to glucose (7). However, it was been suggested (22) that glucose was necessary at recognition, on the basis of inhibition of conjugate formation by deoxyglucose (8,22) which we would argue may reflect glucose requirement for strengthening forces rather than for specific recognition *per se* (8). Interestingly, glucose is required for a reason probably other than just energy provision (21) or glycosylations (23).

Cytolysis-inhibiting mAb (18,24,25)

Protease inhibitors

Some protease inhibitors depress the cytolytic activity of T lymphocytes. This is the case in particular for N -tosyl-L-lysyl-chloromethyl-ketone (TLCK) which affects the effector cells in a slowly reversible manner, probably at the lethal hit stage (26). This is one of a series of observations suggesting the participation of trypsin-like or other enzymes in the cytolytic process (see also Zagury, this volume). How distant the site of action of these enzymes is from the actual cytolytic mechanism is not known.

CONCLUSION

Clearly the determination of a sequence of events on the cytolytic pathway, using either Ca^{++} pulse or conjugate formation or both, can be sometimes experimentally difficult. It was however possible to individualize five characteristics of the lethal hit stage.

(a) The requirement for Ca^{++}.

(b) The possible requirement for glucose.

(c) The probably absence of involvement of microfilaments.

(d) The question of effector cell surface molecules, detected with mAb.

(e) The possible involvement of trypsin-like or other enzymes.

Also, the fact that several inhibitors (each of which most probably act on a different metabolic step) were able to inhibit lethal hit can be taken as an argument for metabolic complexity of the lethal hit stage (2). Finally, whatever the mechanism of lethal hit is, it has to be somehow polarized from the effector to the target cell, since the potentially susceptible (27) effector cell is spared when it kills. All these points should be taken into consideration when discussing possible mechanisms for lethal hit.

ACKNOWLEDGEMENTS

Our research quoted here was done with the expert technical assistance of M.-F. Luciani and with the support of CNRS, INSERM and DGRST.

REFERENCES

1. Henney, C.S. T-cell-mediated cytolysis: an overview of some current issues. Contemp. Top. Immunobiol. 7:245 (1977).
2. Golstein, P., and E.T. Smith. Mechanism of T-cell-mediated cytolysis: the lethal hit stage. Contemp. Top. Immunobiol. 7:273 (1977).
3. Martz, E. Mechanism of specific tumor-cell lysis by alloimmune lymphocytes: resolution and characterization of discrete steps in the cellular interaction. Contemp. Top. Immunobiol. 7:301 (1977).
4. Berke, G. Interaction of cytotoxic T lymphocytes and target cells. Progress in Allergy. 27:69 (1979).
5. Wagner, H., and M. Rollinghoff. T cell-mediated cytotoxicity: Discrimination between antigen recognition, lethal hit and cytolysis phase. Eur. J. Immunol. 4:745 (1974).
6. Golstein, P., and E.T. Smith. The lethal hit stage of mouse T and non-T cell-mediated cytolysis: differences in cation requirements and characterization of an analytical "cation pulse" method. Eur. J. Immunol. 6:31 (1976).
7. Golstein, P., Foa, C., and I.C.M. MacLennan. Mechanism of T cell-mediated cytolysis: the differential impact of cytochalasins at the recognition and lethal hit stages. Eur. J. Immunol. 8:302 (1978).
8. Shortman, K., and P. Golstein. Target cell recognition by cytolytic T cells: different requirements for the formation of strong conjugates or for proceeding to lysis. J. Immunol. 123:833 (1979).
9. Berke, G., Gabison, D., and M. Feldman. The frequency of effector cells i populations containing cytotoxic T lymphocytes. Eur. J. Immunol. 5:813 (1975).
10. Martz, E. Early steps in specific tumor cell lysis by sensitized mouse T lymphocytes. I. Resolution and characterization. J. Immunol. 115:261 (1975).
11. Mauel, J., Rudolf, H., Chapuis, B., and K.T. Brunner. Studies of allograft immunity i mice. II. Mechanism of target cell inactivation in vitro by sensitized lymphocytes. Immunology 18:517 (1970).
12. Henney, C.S., and J.E. Bubbers. Studies on the mechanism of lymphocyte-mediated cytolysis. I. The role of divalent cations in cytolysis by T lymphocytes. J. Immunol. 110:63 (1973).
13. Dickmeiss, E. Comparative study of antibody-dependent and direct lymphocyte-mediated cytotoxicity in vitro after alloimmunisation in the human. II. Chemical inhibitors. Scand. J. Immunol. 3:817 (1974).
14. Golstein, P., and C. Fewtrell. Functional fractionation of human cytotoxic cells using differences in their cation requirements. Nature (London) 255:491 (1975).
15. Plaut, M., Bubbers, J.E., and C.S. Henney. Studies on the mechanism of lymphocyte-mediated cytolysis. VII. Two stages

in the T cell mediated lytic cycle with distinct cation requirements. J. Immunol. 116:150 (1976).

16. Hiserodt, J.C., and B. Bonavida. Studies on the induction and expression of T cell-mediated immunity. XI. Inhibition of the "lethal hit" in T cell-mediated cytotoxicity by heterologous rat antiserum made against alloimmune cytotoxic T lymphocytes. J. Immunol. 126:256 (1981).
17. MacLennan I.C.M., and P. Golstein. Recognition by cytolytic T and K cells: identification in both systems of a divalent-cation-independent, cytochalasin A-sensitive step. J. Immunol. 121:2542 (1978).
18. Hayot, B., Pierres, M., and P. Golstein. Mechanism of T cell-mediated cytolysis: an investigation of cells and stages affected by cytolysis-inhibiting monoclonal antibodies. This volume.
19. Thorn, R.M., and C.S. Henney. Enumeration of specific cytotoxic T cells. Nature (London) 262:75 (1976).
20. MacDonald, H.R. Energy metabolism and T cell-mediated cytolysis. II. Selective inhibition of cytolysis by 2-deoxy-D-glucose. J. Exp. Med. 146:710 (1977).
21. MacLennan, I.C.M., and P. Golstein. Requirements for hexose, unrelated to energy provision, in T cell-mediated cytolysis at the lethal hit stage. J. Exp. Med. 147:1551 (1978).
22. MacDonald, H.R., and J.C. Cerottini. Inhibition of T cell-mediated cytolysis by 2-deoxy-D-glucose (2-DG): differential effect of 2-DG on effector cells isolated early or late after allo-antigenic stimulation in vitro. J. Immunol. 122:1067 (1979).
23. MacDonald, H.R., and J.C. Cerottini. Inhibition of T cell-mediated cytolysis by 2-deoxy D. glucose: dissociation of the inhibitory effect from glycoprotein synthesis. Eur. J. Immunol. 9:466 (1979).
24. Pierres, M., Goridis, C., and P. Golstein. Inhibition of murine T cell-mediated cytolysis and T cell proliferation by a rat monoclonal antibody immunoprecipitating two lymphoid cell surface polypeptides of 94,000 and 180,000 molecular weight. Eur. J. Immunol, in press.
25. Golstein, P., Pierres, M., Schmitt-Verhulst A.M., Luciani, M.F., Buferne, M., Eshhar, Z., and Y. Kaufmann. Functional relationships of lymphocyte membrane structures probed with cytolysis and/or proliferation-inhibiting H35-27.9 and H35-89.9 monoclonal antibodies. This volume.
26. Chang, T.W., and H.N. Eisen. Effects of Nα-tosyl-L-lysyl-chloromethylketone on the activity of cytotoxic T lymphocytes. J. Immunol. 124:1028 (1980).
27. Golstein, P. Sensitivity of cytotoxic T cells to T cell-mediated cytotoxicity. Nature 252:81 (1974).

DISCUSSION

R. Herberman

How are you separating the recognition stage into two substages?

P. Golstein

Together in particular with I.C.M. Mac Lennan and Ken Shortman, we showed that cytochalasin A affected recognition (Eur. J. Immun. 1978 - 8 : 302) before any divalent cation-dependent step of T kill (J. Immunol. 1978-121:2542). It followed that the cytochalasin A-sensitive step preceded any possible magnesium requirement for recognition. It was then shown that, while conjugate formation or absorption on a monolayer was magnesium dependent, recognition between cells packed in a pellet was not or far less magnesium dependent (J. Immunol. 1979-123:833). We think 'recognition' includes two stages; one which is magnesium independent, and one which is magnesium-dependent, required only to establish the strong binding forces necessary for conjugate formation or maintenance.

W. Clark

Most of us define conjugates as something resisting three strokes, five strokes, seven strokes of a Pasteur pipette and how that relates to the quality of the bond required for lysis is really not clear. It's something we always have to keep in mind in talking about conjugates and the relationship to cytotoxicity.

R. Herberman

How do you think microfilaments could be required for recognition?

P. Golstein

One possibility is that microfilaments are necessary for a flattening of the killer cell on the target cell, to increase the area of contact. Microfilaments may also be necessary to establish and maintain the killer cell 'digitations' described by others.

THE ROLE OF CALCIUM IN THE LETHAL HIT OF T LYMPHOCYTE-MEDIATED CYTOLYSIS

Eric Martz[b], Wendy L. Parker[c], Maurice K. Gately[d], and Constantine D. Tsoukas[e]

[b]Department of Microbiology, University of Massachusetts Amherst, MA 01003

[c]Department of Microbiology, University of Massachusetts Medical Center, Worcester, MA 01605

[d]Surgical Neurology Branch, National Institute of Neurological and Communicative Disorders and Stroke, National Institutes of Health, Bethesda, MD 20205

[e]Department of Clinical Research, Scripps Clinic and Research Foundation, 10666 N. Torrey Pines Road, La Jolla, CA 92037

INTRODUCTION

The cytolytic T lymphocyte (CTL)[1] inflicts lethal damage within minutes after contact with a specific antigen-bearing target cell. The mechanism of this damage remains a mystery. Elsewhere in this volume (1), we have reviewed progress during the past decade towards understanding the mechanism of CTL-mediated killing.

The CTL-target interaction has been resolved into three separately-assayable stages: recognition-adhesion (probably two steps but not yet operationally resolved); the lethal hit (also termed programming for lysis); and killer cell-dependent lysis (2-4,

[1]Abbreviations used in this paper:

cAMP, cyclic adenosine monophosphate; CTL, cytolytic T lymphocyte; EGTA, ethylene glycol-bis-(β-aminoethyl ether)-N,N'-tetraacetic acid, a chelator with specificity for calcium over magnesium; WGA, wheat germ agglutinin.

reviewed in 5). Recognition-adhesion is very rapid (one to several minutes), and the lethal hit is typically completed within 2-20 minutes after contact. Subsequent (killer cell independent) lysis is a slower and apparently passive process, requiring 0.5-4 hr.

Each stage has been characterized in some detail (5-8) but the mechanism of the lethal hit remains an enigma. It is generally supposed that the primary attack is on the target cell membrane, producing an ionophoretic lesion (hole) which secondarily leads to colloid osmotic lysis. Thus, the lytic mechanism is thought to resemble that of the complement system on a functional level, but probably does not employ complement components _per se_.

UNIQUE IMPORTANCE OF CALCIUM IN REGULATING THE LETHAL HIT

One approach towards elucidating the mechanism of the lethal hit has been to search for pharmacologic inhibitors which act selectively on this stage. (Early pharmacological work has been reviewed and tabulated in 5.) That is, such inhibitors should have no effect on recognition-adhesion or on killer cell-independent lysis.

Contrary to this goal, these studies have shown that nearly all inhibitors of CTL-mediated killing inhibit the formation of shear-resistant adhesions, i.e., the recognition-adhesion step. Included in this category are: EDTA, cytochalasins, inhibitors of energy metabolism (e.g., azide, 2-deoxyglucose), local anaesthetics (e.g., lidocaine, benzyl alcohol), dibutyryl cyclic AMP, dimethyl sulfoxide, trypan blue, heparin Rosenthal's inhibitor (6), colchicine (9), proteases, concanavalin A (as a CTL pretreatment, 10), and monoclonal antibodies to Lyt-2,3 and LFA-1 (reviewed in 1). (See also 11 and 5 for data on most of the inhibitors in this list.)

There appears to be only one clearcut exception to this pattern: removal of Ca^{++} from the assay medium (in the presence of ample Mg^{++}) greatly inhibits the lethal hit without impairing adhesion formation (4,5,12-14).

In a detailed quantitative study (14), we found that Ca^{++} was not only unnecessary, but also insufficient to support adhesion formation.[2] The most convincing experiments utilized EGTA, which reduces the free Ca^{++} concentration 1000-fold below that in "calcium-free" medium. In the presence of a physiological concentration of Mg^{++} (2-4 mM), Ca^{++} (1 mM) vs. EGTA (0.1-10 mM in Ca^{++}-free medium) had no effect on the rate of adhesion formation, its shear-resist-

[2] Ca^{++} did augment the adhesion-supporting ability of suboptimal Mg^{++}; this effect of Ca^{++} was later shown to be distinct from that of Ca^{++} in the lethal hit, and unnecessary for killing (22).

ance, temperature dependence, or sensitivity to cytochalasin B (14).

Thus, the extracellular Ca^{++} concentration is unique in strongly regulating the lethal hit without affecting the recognition-adhesion step.

INHIBITION OF THE LETHAL HIT BY DRUGS

Although no drug has been shown selectively to inhibit the lethal hit without inhibiting adhesion formation, it appears that many inhibitory drugs do act on the lethal hit as well as on adhesion, at least in an operational sense. The demonstration of a "direct" effect on the lethal hit is complicated by the fact that many drugs not only inhibit adhesion formation, but also greatly weaken or detach adhesions formed before drug addition. EDTA (2,5, 8,15), cytochalasins (8,16), 2-deoxyglucose (8), and dimethylsulfoxide (16) have been shown to weaken and/or detach CTL-target adhesions. Since efficient lethal hit delivery appears dependent upon intimate adhesive contact ,the fact that post-adhesion of these and other drugs inhibits killing clearly falls short of demonstrating that the drugs act directly on the lethal hit.

Gately (16) got around this problem by using concanavalin A to strengthen specific CTL-target adhesions. Such con A-strengened adhesions were no longer detachable by EDTA (unless accompanied with 100 mM α-methyl-mannoside) or any of ten other inhibitory drugs tested. However, all eleven agents remained able to inhibit the lethal hit in the presence of the con A-strengthened adhesions. Thus, these inhibitors appear to act on the lethal hit as well as on adhesion, although their action on the lethal hit might involve the same sort of disruption of membrane function which would normally lead to detachment.

FAILURE TO RESOLVE STEPS WITHIN THE LETHAL HIT

Having found this evidence consistent with the hypothesis that some drugs inhibit the lethal hit "directly", we wondered if the inhibited step(s) could be resolved from each other or from the calcium or temperature-dependent step(s). To answer this question, we used an inhibitor sequencing approach (cf. earlier experiments by Henney, 17). The rationale for these experiments is explained in Fig. 1.

The experiments were designed to resolve two temporally and mechanistically distinct steps within the lethal hit (programming for lysis) process. Not all inhibitors are suitable for such experiments, since both a profound inhibition and a rapid and complete reversal of inhibition following drug dilution are required. How-

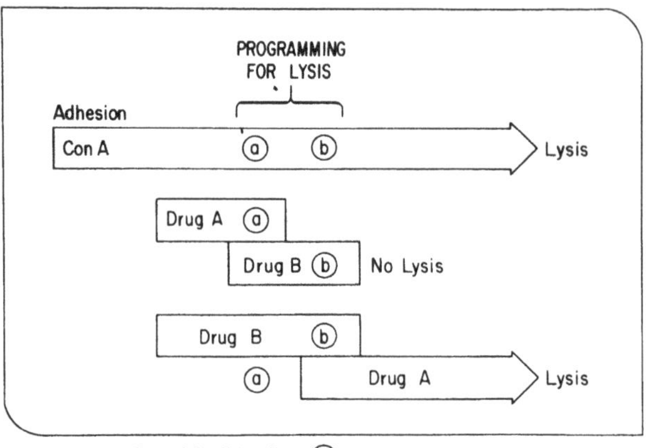

Fig. 1. Principle of drug sequencing experiments. The assumption is made that programming for lysis (the lethal hit) comprises at least two mechanistically and temporarily distinct steps, "a" and "b", and that two inhibitory drugs ("A" and "B") are available, each of which acts on only one of these steps. Irreversible adhesions (strengthened by con A) are allowed to form before addition of one of the inhibitory drugs. (Adhesion formation was conducted for 5 minutes in EGTA to prevent programming for lysis during this interval. The first drug was then allowed to equilibrate 5 minutes before free Ca^{++} was restored to 1 mM.) After 10 minutes to allow possible completion of step "a", the second drug is added (and allowed to equilibrate for 5-10 minutes in the presence of the first drug) followed by dilution of the first drug to a subinhibitory concentration (while maintaining the second drug at the inhibitory level). The rate of ^{51}Cr release is monitored during continued incubation at 37°C. Further details are in Gately, Wechter, and Martz (16), on which this figure is based.

ever, four drugs met these criteria in addition to EGTA and low temperature. Unfortunately, neither sequence of any pair of inhibitors permitted lysis. The pairs tested are summarized in Fig. 2. This result could mean that all inhibitors act at the same single step, or that some of them act at multiple steps. In any case, this approach failed to resolve the calcium-dependent step from any other putative step within the lethal hit (programming for lysis).

By relaxing the restriction that both steps be within the lethal hit, it was possible to show that the protocol employed was capable of demonstrating a sequence of steps. When the adhesion-strengthening con A was omitted, the sequence cytochalasin B-EGTA

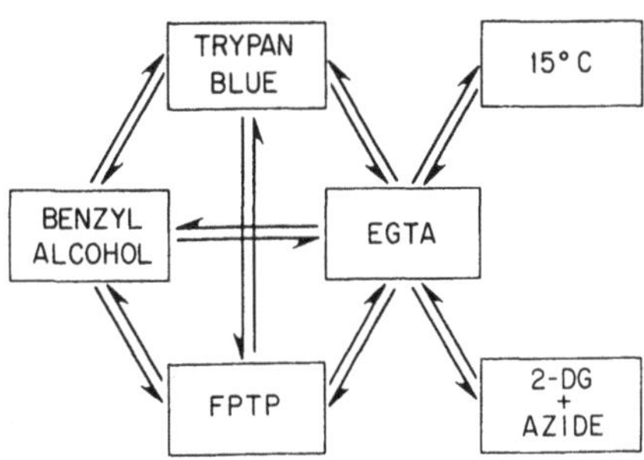

Fig. 2. Pairs of inhibitors tested in an attempt to resolve the calcium-dependent step from other possible step(s) within the lethal hit delivery process (programming for lysis). The experimental design is explained in Figure 1. For all pairs tested, neither sequence permitted lysis. Thus, the Ca^{++}-dependent step was not resolved from the temperature-dependent step or the drug inhibitable steps within programming for lysis. EGTA is a calcium-specific chelator which blocks the calcium-dependent step; 2-DG is 2-deoxyglucose; FPTP is a fluoro-compound shown to inhibit CTL-mediated killing by Barbara E. Loughman and associates at the Upjohn Co. This Figure is based on data in Gately, Wechter, and Martz (16).

gave 12% lysis, while the reverse gave 43% lysis (for additional details and controls, see Fig. 3 in 16). This demonstration that cytochalasin B blocks a step earlier than EGTA within the whole cytolytic process is in accord with other data showing that cytochalasin B blocks adhesion formation (reviewed in 5), but inhibits the lethal hit only slightly (16).

The failure to find a sequence of drug-inhibitable steps within the lethal hit delivery process contrasts with the results of similar protocols in other systems, which demonstrate a clear sequence of inhibitable steps in the mast cell secretory response (18,19), the terminal stages of complement-mediated lysis (20), and in the immunoglobulin capping response of B lymphocytes (21).

AGONIST SELECTIVITY SEQUENCE OF ALKALINE EARTH CATIONS

We found that Sr^{++} can replace Ca^{++} in supporting CTL-mediated killing (22). The optimal concentration of Sr^{++} is about 10-fold higher than than of Ca^{++}, and can support an equally high rate of killing. Neither Mg^{++} nor Ba^{++} could substitute for Ca^{++}. Thus, the order of efficacy (selectivity sequence) of alkaline earth metal ions in supporting the lethal hit is $Ca^{++} > Sr^{++} > Ba^{++}$ > or Mg^{++} (22).

This selectivity sequence is by no means universal in biological or chemical systems. It is compatible with only one of thirty experimentally observed sequences reviewed by Diamond and Wright (23). The most commonly observed sequences are seven predicted on theoretical grounds by Sherry (23), none of which agrees with the sequence observed in CTL-mediated killing. Nevertheless, the same sequence has been observed with some frequency in two types of phenomena: stimulus-secretion coupling and binding of divalent cations by calcium-stabilized or -activated extracellular enzymes. Examples are documented in Table I.

INHIBITION BY MANGANESE AND OTHER CALCIUM ANTAGONISTS

It may also be noted in Table I that many Ca^{++}-dependent biological processes are antagonized by Mn^{++}. On the other hand, Mn^{++} typically substitutes effectively for Mg^{++} in Mg^{++}-dependent processes (reviewed in 14). In accord with these patterns, we found that Mn^{++} will substitute for Mg^{++} in supporting adhesion formation (14), but blocks the lethal hit in a manner consistent with it acting on the Ca^{++}-dependent site (24). The inhibition by Mn^{++} was competitive with Ca^{++} but not Mg^{++}. The step inhibited by Mn^{++} could not be resolved from the Ca^{++}-dependent step by inhibitor sequencing experiments such as those described in Fig. 1 (24).

Thus, Mn^{++} represents only the second example ("Ca^{++}-free" medium or EGTA being the first) of an inhibitor of CTL-mediated killing which acts selectively on the lethal hit. Unfortunately, it has not led to new insights, since it appears to function in the same way and at the same site as EGTA.

DOES CALCIUM ACT INSIDE THE CTL?

Three sites where calcium might act in the lethal hit are listed in Table II. We shall now consider each in turn.

Similarity Between CTLs and Mast Cells

For many years, a remarkable similarity has been evident between secretory responses and lethal hit delivery by CTLs (17). The list of drugs and doses which inhibit mast cell secretion is virtually identical to that for inhibition of CTL-mediated killing (5,17,25). As already emphasized (Table I), both require Ca^{++}, have about the same optimal Ca^{++} concentration, and have nearly identical alkaline earth selectivities (22,24). Intracytoplasmic Ca^{++} is believed to serve as a stimulus-secretion coupler (second messenger) in secretory responses (26). Ca^{++} may move to the cytoplasm either (a) from outside the cell via some natural ionophore in the plasma membrane, or (b) from intracellular stores, such as mitochondria or other

TABLE I. Divalent Cation Selectivity Sequences and Antagonists: Comparison Among Various Biological Systems

Test System	Agonist Selectivity Sequence	Antagonists#
Lethal hit in CTL-mediated killing	Ca > Sr > Mg or Ba	Mn, La, Co, Ni
Stimulus-secretion coupling: Mast cells; acetylcholine from neuromuscular junctions and sympathetic ganglia; oxytocin from neurohypophysis	Ca > Sr > Mg (effect of Ba varies)	Mn, La
Muscle contractility: rat serum	Ca > Sr > Mg or Ba	Mn
Calcium activated or stabilized enzymes: Staph. aureus nuclease, bovine pancreatic DNAse, B. subtilis α-amylase* or neutral proteinase, α-chymotrypsinogen*	Ca > Sr > Mg $\geq$ Ba	Mn
Phase separation of phosphatidyl serine from phosphatidyl choline in lipid bilayer	Ca > Ba > Sr > Mg	

* Ba not tested.

Tested in some but not all systems listed.

References and additional details will be found in 22 and 24.

organelles. Agents which are known or believed to block transmembrane fluxes of Ca^{++} block both mast cell secretion and CTL-mediated killing (27): Mn^{++} and La^{+++} (24,28), ruthenium red (24,2873), and verapamil (24,29).

TABLE II. Hypothetical Sites for the Role of Calcium in the Lethal Hit of CTL-Mediated Cytolysis

Site	Role	Tentative Conclusion (and Basis)
Inside the CTL	Second Messenger to Trigger Lethal Hit Delivery	Unlikely (Failure of A23187 to Trigger)
Inside the Target Cell	Ca^{++} Accumulation Sufficient to Kill Target Cell	Unlikely (Mast Cell Targets Don't Secrete)
At Cell Surface(s)	Calcium Stabilized or Activated Enzyme?	Likely

It should be noted that ultrastructural studies of CTL (30-32) have not revealed the numerous prominent membrane-lined granules or vesicles seen in secretory cells. Nevertheless, it is clearly possible that the role of calcium in the lethal hit is similar to its role in secretory systems.

Evidence for a Triggering Step Prior to the Lethal Hit

It is not obvious, however, that a triggering step exists for the lethal hit of CTLs. It is possible that the lytic mechanism is constantly deployed in a fully-active state on the CTL surface, and thus that extensive adhesive contact with a potential target is sufficient for killing. The antigen specificity of killing would then reside solely in the recognition-adhesion step; that is, the only function of the antigen-specific receptors would be to create extensive adhesive contact.

We tested this hypothesis by looking for lectins which might induce adhesions between CTLs and (antigenically nonspecific) target cells, yet fail to induce killing. Such nonlethal adhesions were obtained under certain conditions with wheat germ allutinin (WGA, 33). The CTL remained functional, since addition of Con A converted the nonlethal adhesions into lethal ones. We were able to rule out several trivial explanations for the nonlethality of the WGA-induced adhesions, including lack of persistence, inadequate contact (centrifugation at 37°C did not induce lethality), or inhibition of killing by WGA. We believe that this demonstration of persistent, nonlethal CTL-target adhesions provides the best evidence yet offered against the hypothesis that CTL-target adhesion is sufficient for killing, and suggests a requirement for a triggering event to initiate lethal hit delivery. A requirement for triggering by the antigen receptors is also supported by elegant unidirectional recognition experiments involving two CTL populations (Kuppers and Henney, 34).

Failure to Trigger the Lethal Hit with Calcium Ionophore A23187

In mast cell secretion, one of the major pieces of evidence supporting a triggering role for Ca^{++} is the ability to trigger secretion with the calcium ionophore, A23187 (26). A23187, a hydrophobic compound of 523 M_r extracted from Streptomyces chartreusensis, carries complexed divalent cations across lipid membranes. It greatly accelerates passive transmembrane fluxes of Ca^{++} and Mg^{++} but not Na^+ or K^+ (35). Cells typically maintain exceedingly low free Ca^{++} activities in the cytoplasm (36,37), two to four orders of magnitude below the 1 mM typical of plasma or culture medium. Thus, the addition of A23187 greatly accelerates passive Ca^{++} influx, raising the calcium activity in the cytoplasm.

Preliminary experiments in which CTLs and specific or non-specific targets were incubated in various concentrations of Ca^{++} and A23187 showed no triggering effects (Parker and Martz, unpublished; cf. 11). However, it seemed possible that A23187 might induce a very brief lethal hit response, which would be detected only when a potential target cell was already in suitable contact with the CTL prior to the application of the ionophore.

For this reason, the WGA-induced nonlethal adhesion system seemed an ideal one in which to test the possibility of lethal hit triggering by A23187. Such experiments were carried out as shown in Fig. 3. No killing was induced by A23187.

While this experiment gave negative results, we were able to rule out certain potential reasons for failure which had not been considered in previous similar attempts (11,38). First, we had already shown that under our conditions, the adhesions induced by WGA were strong and persistent, and that the adhering CTL remained functional, since killing of the attached targets could be induced by con A (27, 33). Adhesion persistence, the failure of A23187 to detach the adhesions, and the failure of A23187 to inactivate the CTLs were all verified by the ability of con A to induce killing after addition of A23187 to the dispersed clumps of cells as shown in Fig. 3.

Second, it was important to verify that mast cell secretion could be triggered by the A23187 in the same medium employed for the CTL experiments. Mg^{++} is a competitive antagonist of A23187-induced calcium influx, and serum albumin binds A23187 avidly (27). Thus, the serum concentration and Mg^{++}/Ca^{++} ratio employed , among other possibilities, can make the difference between a positive or negative result with A23187. The ability of A23187 to trigger mast cell secretion in the same media in the same experiment is verified in Fig. 3.

Finally, it was important to test the entire range of A23187 concentrations, from a level ineffective on mast cells up to the toxic level. Since we limited toxicity by employing a 30-min A23187 pulse terminated by dilution in albumin, we were able to test a 30-fold range of concentrations effective on mast cells (Fig. 4).

The inability to trigger CTL-mediated killing is consistent with the hypothesis that intracytoplasmic Ca^{++} does not trigger lethal hit delivery. However, it is important to interpret these negative results with caution. It is possible, for example, that A23187 triggers lethal hit delivery, but that the triggering is localized, not globally distributed over the entire CTL. If the regions of CTL-target adhesion were relativly inaccessible to A23187, killing would not be induced. There is, indeed, some additional evidence consistent with local as distinct from global CTL triggering (27, 39).

Does A23187 "Bypass" Inhibition by Calcium Flux Blockers?

Inhibition of IgE or antigen-induced mast cell secretion by cyclic-AMP (cAMP), quercetin, D600 (a verapamil derivitive), and ruthenium red (but not by other inhibitors, e.g. azide) can be an-

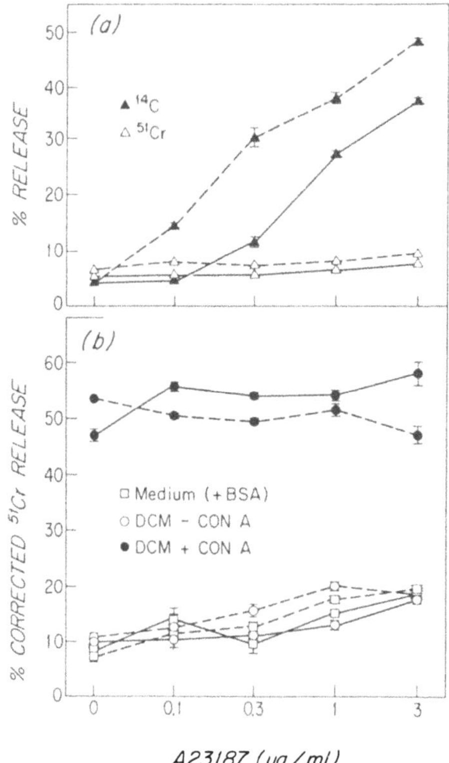

tagonized by A23187 (reviewed in 29). It has been proposed that this antagonism results when the direct Ca^{++} influx produced by A23187 bypasses the need for the normal Ca^{++} gating mechanism (26, 40, 41). It follows that the bypassable inhibitors must limit secretion solely by impairing physiological calcium gating. That is, were they to inhibit other cellular functions essential for secretion, A23187 would fail to bypass such inhibition. This hypothesis gains credence from the fact that D600, verapamil, and ruthenium red are well-known blockers of calcium transport in various systems (reviewed in 27, 29).

Fig. 3. Failure of A23187 to trigger CTL-mediated killing (taken from Parker, 27).

Panel (b) shows the CTL portion of the experiment. Alloimmune ($H-2^d$ anti-$H-2^b$) CTL were agglutinated nonlethally to P815 ($H-2^d$) with WGA (33). A23187 was added for 30 minutes at 37°C. Cells were then dispersed in dextran-containing medium (DCM) $\pm$ 10μg/ml Con A, or diluted in 0.5% albumin in medium and held on ice 15 minutes (albumin has a high avidity for A23187 in the cold, 59). ^{51}Cr release was measured after an additional 3.5 hr at 37°C.

Dextran dispersion was required in order that all killing induced by con A be dependent on the CTL-target adhesions previously produced with WGA (33). No killing is seen in DCM + con A when the WGA agglutination step is omitted.

Two Mg^{++} concentrations were tried, 1.8 mM (solid lines) and 0.45 mM (broken lines). Ca^{++} was 1.2 mM.

Lysis in DCM + con A shows that CTL were agglutinated to targets by the WGA step and that A23187 neither detached these WGA-induced adhesions nor inactivated the adhering CTL. Failure to lyse in medium shows that A23187, unlike Con A, did not trigger concentrations. (At 10 μg/ml, A23187 induced chromium release from the P815 in the absence of CTL. 1 μg/ml A23187 equals 1.9 μM.)

Panel (a) shows the control using rat mast cells. Mast cells were incubated for 2 minutes with A23187, and isotope release was measured. The mast cells had been doubly labeled with ^{14}C-serotonin and ^{51}Cr. A23187-induced release of ^{14}C without ^{51}Cr shows that non-lytic exocytotic secretion was induced (29,55). The same two Mg^{++} concentrations were employed as in Panel (b).

For both panels, the medium employed during A23187 treatment was Liebowitz-15 plus 10 mM HEPES buffer pH 7.3 and 2% fetal calf serum. Additional details are in 27.

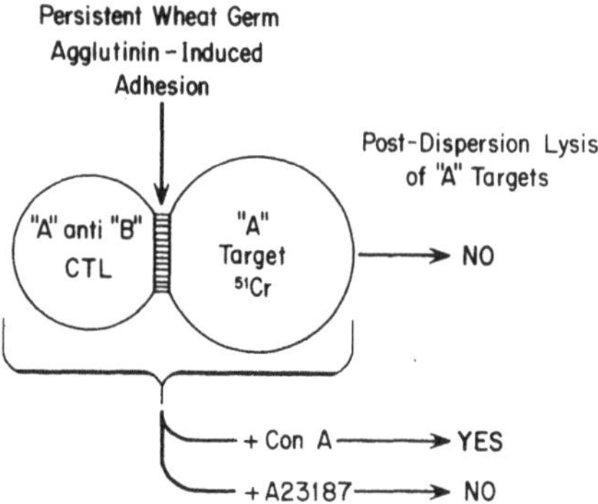

Fig. 4. A23187 does not trigger lethal hit delivery across WGA-induced CTL-target adhesions. Schematic representation of result in Fig. 3.

We thought it might be possible in certain cases to bypass inhibition of CTL-mediated killing with A23187. Such an experiment would seem worthwhile if it would argue that calcium influx is important in triggering the lethal hit. We were able to show that ruthenium red, verapamil, and quercetin inhibit CTL-mediated killing when added after the formation of con A-strengthened adhesions (27), and therefore that they inhibit the lethal hit.

First, however, it seemed important to verify the bypass phenomenon in the mast cell system. We were surprised to find that upon closer scrutiny, the "bypass" interpretation of the results in the mast cell did not seem well founded (29).

Using $^{45}Ca^{++}$, Foreman and coworkers (42) have directly demonstrated that dibutyryl-cAMP (db-cAMP) inhibits calcium influx in antigen-triggered mast cells, and that A23187 can restore the calcium influx. However, we found not only that db-cAMP was an inconsistent inhibitor of IgE-induced secretion, but also that it consistently augmented (by up to 100%) A23187-induced mast cell secretion (29). This would appear to represent an action of cAMP above and beyond its inhibitory effect on calcium gating, making the bypass hypothesis overly simplistic in the case of cAMP.

Our studies with quercetin (29) suggested that what had previously been taken for A23187-induced bypass secretion (43) was likely a lytic release of histamine resulting from A23187 toxicity.

Verapamil (the parent compound for D600) had not been studied in the mast cell previouly. We found that verapamil was equally effective at inhibiting IgE-induced or A23187-induced mast cell secretion, providing no basis for a bypass hypothesis.

We found that ruthenium inhibition of αIgE-induced mast cell secretion could be antagonized by A23187 in a classic "bypass" type phenomenon. Unfortunately, it seems likely that this can be accounted for by a direct stoichiometric complexing between A23187 and ruthenium red, which would remove the latter from its inhibitory site on the cell, regardless of whether that site is the Ca^{++} gate (29). A similar explanation is difficult to rule out for other "bypassable" inhibitors.

In summary, we found that in the mast cell system, the A23187 "bypass" hypothesis is either too simplistic or cannot be substantiated for the inhibitors studied. We therefore did not search for similar phenomena in the CTL system.

DOES CALCIUM ACT INSIDE THE TARGET CELL?

Ca^{++} is a Cytotoxin

Let us now consider the second hypothesis listed in Table II. We have already alluded to the belief that all mammalian cells maintain a very low free Ca^{++} concentration in the cytoplasm, and that transient increases in cytoplasmic Ca^{++} are used to regulate diverse functions, including cytoskeletal movements and secretion. Clearly, a massive influx of Ca^{++} will derange many functions, and may be sufficient to kill cells.

This excess Ca^{++} toxicity hypothesis is supported by the widespread observation that A23187 is a potent cytocidal agent, its toxicity being strictly dependent upon the availability of Ca^{++} outside the cell. This has been for diverse target cells including thymocytes and lymphocytes (44, 45, and Martz, unpublished), muscle (46), rat basophilic leukemia cells (47), pancreatic acinar cells (48), erythrocytes (49), and rat mast cells and various tumor cells (Martz, unpublished). Ca^{++}-"free" medium (typically contaminated with up to 50 μM calcium) affords considerable but incomplete protection against A23187-induced lysis. EGTA, the calcium-specific chelator, provides complete protection. In our hands, rat splenocytes and mast cells give half-maximal ^{51}Cr-release in 1 hr at about 2 μM A23187 (1.2 mM calcium, 1.8 mM magnesium, 1% fetal calf serum). Yet in EGTA little or no ^{51}Cr-release is induced in these cells by 200 μM A23187 (Martz, unpublished). These results indicate that excess calcium influx is sufficient to kill diverse cells.

Evidence Against Ca^{++} Being a Common Final Mediator for Diverse Cytolysins.

Schanne, Kane and Farber (50) showed that a diverse list of cytolysins were remarkably calcium-dependent in their ability to kill normal rat liver cells within a few hours. In addition to A23187, the list included amphotericin B (a polyene channel-forming ionophore), lysolecithin, mellitin (a detergent-like peptide from bee venom), phalloidin (an actin-binding mushroom toxin), alkylating mutagens, and particles of silica or asbestos.

We subsequently studied many of these agents on mouse P815 (mastocytoma) cells and normal mouse splenocytes. These two targets were picked because they differ 30-fold in their sensitivity to A23187-induced cytolysis (half maximal at 60 and 2 μM respectively for 1 hr in 1.2 mM Ca^{++}, 1.8 mM Mg^{++}, 1% fetal calf serum; Martz, unpublished).

We picked a dose of each cytolysin which gave only partial lysis (typically 20-40%) in short-term incubation (0.5-2 hr), so it would be sensitive to inhibition by low calcium. The lysis of neither cell type was sensitive to calcium for amphotericin B or mellitin. Similar results were obtained for lysolecithin (tested only on P815) and silica (in serum-free medium, tested only on splenocytes). In addition to these agents which had been studied by Schanne, Kane and Farber (50), we also studied peroxide, polylysine, and wheat germ agglutinin. Little or no effect of calcium was seen (Martz, unpublished).

Evidently, the importance of Ca^{++} as a final common mediator of cell death in rat hepatocytes does not extend to mouse ascites tumor cells or lymphocytes[3]. While calcium influx appears sufficient to kill all of these cells (based on results with A23187), calcium influx does not appear to play a crucial role in cytolysis by other agents.

Evidence Against Ca^{++} Being the Primary Cytolysin in CTL-Mediated Killing: Use of Mast Cells as Targets.

It remained worthy of consideration that CTLs might kill target cells by admitting a lethal influx of Ca^{++}. In order to test this possibility, we studied the responses of mast cells to CTL-mediated killing[4] (51). We reasoned that if Ca^{++} influx into the target cell is the primary effect of attact by CTLs, the mast cell targets should display secretory degranulation before lysing.

[3]Most of our results were based on ^{51}Cr release in Ca^{++} + 1% fetal calf serum with or without EGTA, while Schanne, Kane and Farber used trypan blue in serum-free medium + calcium. However, using trypan blue, we found the same results. Also, amphotericin B- and mellitin-induced lysis of splenocytes remained calcium-independent in serum-free medium, and when calcium-"free" medium was used instead of Ca^{++} + EGTA.

[4]Tsoukas, C.D., Wechter, W.J., and E. Martz. Manuscript in preparation.

For this study, we developed a technique of double isotopic labeling of the mast cell population with ^{14}C-serotonin and ^{51}Cr. We used rat mast cells because they can readily be purified (52), whereas mouse mast cells cannot. Serotonin release has been shown to correlate well with histamine release (53, 54), and ^{51}Cr release has also been used for mast cells (55). The release of these markers from doubly labelled cells has not previously been studied, but reflects an independent compartment, as expected. Release of > 90% of ^{14}C with < 10% of ^{51}Cr can obtained with any potent secretagogue (48/80, polymyxin B, A23187), release of ^{51}Cr without ^{14}C can also be obtained (see below and Fig. 5). Together, these markers provide a sensitive (5000 cells/test) assay for secretion with a built-in control for lysis which may well see wider use in the future (for details, see 29).

A23187 is well known as a mast cell secretagogue; as discussed above, it is also a lysin. We have tested A23187 from the minimal secretory dose (0.2 μM) up to the maximal dose giving calcium-dependent lysis (200 μM); at all doses, secretion clearly precedes

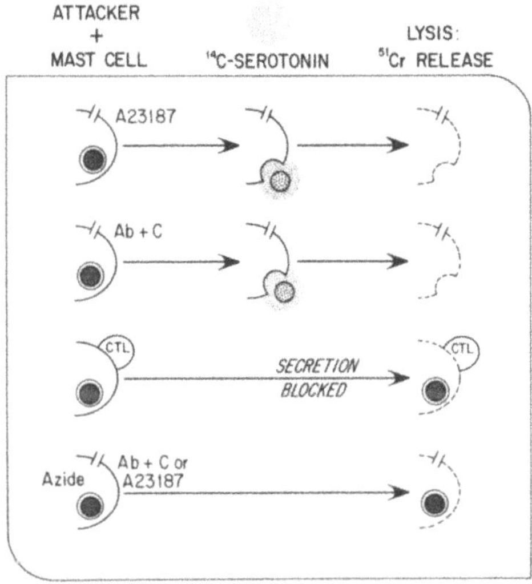

Fig. 5. Evidence against Ca^{++} poisoning as the mechanism of CTL-mediated killing: mast cells do not secrete prelytically when attacked by CTLs. The mast cell is represented schematically as having a single secretory granule. A23187 produces prelytic secretion at all doses (first line); the secretion is energy dependent (last line, 60,61). Antibody + complement (Ab + C) induces a similarly energy-dependent, prelytic secretion (second and last lines, 55). CTL lyse mast cells without inducing prelytic secretion, and indeed block secretory responsiveness shortly before lysis[4] (third line, 51). For details, see text.

lysis[4]. Moreover, pretreatment of mast cells with subsecretagogic doses of A23187 for 30 min does not render them unable to respond to a subsequent secretagogic dose of A23187[4]. Thus, if CTL attack allows Ca^{++} to enter a mast cell target at a rate sufficient to lyse it within one hour, prelytic secretion would be expected.

Mouse anti-rat killer cells were prepared by priming mice *in vivo* with rat lymphoma cells, and later restimulating primed splenocytes *in vitro* with the same rat lymphoma (56). The killers were shown to be Thy-1^+ and Lyt-2^+ (56), and antigen specific for BN rat mast cells over Lewis rat mast cells[4], hence CTL.

Rat mast cells were specifically killed by the mouse CTL, releasing 50% of their ^{51}Cr in 1 hr at a lymphocyte/target cell ratio around 20 to 50. ^{14}C-serotonin was released an hour or more *after* ^{51}Cr; that is, prelytic secretion was *not* observed during CTL-meiated killing.

In order to test whether the mast cell targets were capable of secretion 48/80 or A23187 (both potent secretagogues producing maximal secretion in less than 2 min) were added at various times to mast cells under attack by CTLs. The mast cells were able to secrete in response to 48/80 or A23187 for 10 min, then gradually lost the ability to respond (50% loss at 25 min). The loss of secretory ability prededed ^{51}Cr release by about 10 min, and did not occur when non-immune lymphocytes were substituted for CTL. Increasing the doses of secretagogues (to compensate for binding by cell debris) did not restore secretion.

These results exclude the simplest hypothesis, that calcium influx is the sole primary effect of the CTL on the target cell, since prelytic secretion would be expected according to this hypothesis. The results do not exclude the possibility that the CTL produces early calcium influx into the target cell simutaneously with other effects (such as depletion of ATP) which block secretion. Indeed, we have described above how the CTL is able to block secretory ability shortly before lysis of mast cell targets.

Ko and Lagunoff (55) studied the lysis of mast cells by antibody and complement. ^{51}Cr was accompanied by histamine release[5],

---

[5]Ko and Lagunoff (55) utilized a rabit anti-rat mast cell antiserum and rabbit complement. Under their conditions, antiserum-coated mast cells produced little or no histamine release in the presence of C6-deficient rabbit serum. Therefore, the histamine release observed in the presence of normal rabit serum could be attributed neither to an anti-IgE or anti-IgE-receptor effect of the antibody on the mast cells, nor to release of anaphylatoxin during complement fixation. Thus, in their study, the release of histamine required the production of lytic complement lesions.

as many had observed previously. However, they made the remarkable observation that the (presumably prelytic) release of histamine could be blocked by inhibitors of ATP production (dinitrophenol, antimycin A, or KCN), without inhibiting ^{51}Cr release. Under these conditions, their electron micrographs showed that "cell lysis occurred but most of the mast cell granules remained intact" (55). These results are consistent with the hypothesis that calcium entering via the lytic complement lesions (known to be equivalent to pores up to 50 Å in diameter, 57, 58) triggers energy-dependent, exocytotic prelytic histamine release.

This interpretation is summarized, together with the CTL and A23187 results, in Figure 5.

We draw two conclusions from these experiments. First, it is unlikely that CTL-mediated killing is brought about primarily by the introduction of a calcium-selective ionophore into the target membrane. While calcium influx into the target cell may contribute to its demise, it seems unlikely that calcium influx is the early programming-for-lysis event primarily responsible for target cell death. Second, it appears that the primary lesion produced by the CTL differs functionally (and therefore structurally) from that produced by complement. A "pore" permeable to sodium and potassium but not to divalent cations might, for example, be employed by the CTL.

WHERE DOES CALCIUM ACT?

As indicated in Table II, we presently favor the hypothesis that the calcium requirement in CTL-mediated killing resides outside the plasma membranes of the CTL-target cell conjugate, and that Ca^{++} probably acts as a stabilizing or activating factor for some essential protein(s). At present, however, the evidence is far from conclusive, and we look forward to future experimentation.

SUMMARY

Ca^{++} is necessary for the lethal hit in CTL-mediated killing. Despite studies of many inhibitory drugs, Ca^{++} is the only agent presently known which regulates the lethal hit selectively, that is, without affecting the preceding recognition-adhesion step. For this reason, Ca^{++} provides a uniquely important tool for exploring the mechanism of the lethal hit.

The selectivity sequence with which the alkaline earths support the lethal hit (Ca > Sr > Mg = Ba = 0) is consistent with a secretory process or with a calcium activated/stabilized extracellular enzyme. There is also a strong parallel between the actions of inhibitory drugs on mast cell secretion and CTL-mediated killing.

In mast cells, the calcium ionophore A23187 can antagonize inhibition of secretion by cyclic AMP and calcium flux blockers, and this has been regarded as A23187-induced "bypass" of blockade of the normal calcium gating mechanism. Thinking that the bypass phenomenon might be attempted in the CTL system, we repeated the mast cell experiments, but upon close scrutiny concluded that the "bypass" hypothesis cannot be substantiated in the mast cell system.

A23187 triggers mast cell secretion, but has been unable to trigger the lethal hit in CTLs despite extensive trials. It therefore seems unlikely that calcium influx into the cytoplasm of the CTL serves as a triggering signal for the lethal hit.

Alternatively, calcium influx into the cytoplasm of the target cell might be responsible for target cell death. Excessive calcium influx appears sufficient to kill a wide variety of cell types, based on the calcium-dependent toxicity of A23187. Contrary to a recent report, however, we found that the toxicity of unrelated chemical lysins (amphotericin B, mellitin, lysolecithin, silica, etc.) was not calcium dependent, at least for mouse lymphocytes and tumor cells, and thus that Ca^{++} is not a common final mediator for these lysins.

Nevertheless, CTLs might kill by admitting excess Ca^{++} into the target cell. To test this possibility, we used normal mast cells as specific targets for CTL-mediated killing. We reasoned that early calcium influx into the target cell would induce secretion of the mast cell mediators. However prelytic secretion was not seen during CTL-mediated killing of mast cells. In contrast, Ko and Lagunoff have reported an energy-dependent prelytic secretion during killing of mast cells by antibody and complement. We conclude that it is unlikely that the CTL uses calcium influx to poison the target cell, and that the primary lesion produced by the CTL differs from that produced by complement.

Since we have obtained evidence against an intracytoplasmic role for Ca^{++} in either the CTL or the target cell, we favor an extracellular site of action for calcium in the lethal hit of CTL-mediated killing.

ACKNOWLEDGEMENT

Supported by NIH grants CA-14723, CA-09141, AI-00458, AI-18003, and by postdoctoral fellowships from the Helen Hay Whitney Foundation (M.K.G.) and the Runyon-Winchell Fund (C.D.T.).

REFERENCES

1. Martz, E., Davignon, D., Jurzinger, K., and T.A. Springer. The molecular bsis for cytolytic T lymphocyte function: analysis with blocking monoclonal antibodies. This volume (1982).
2. Martz, E. Early steps in specific tumor cell lysis by sensitized mouse T-lymphocytes. I. Resolution and characterization. J. Immunol. 115:261-267 (1975).
3. Wagner, H., and M. Rollinghoff. T cell-mediated cytotoxicity: Discrimination between antigen recognition, lethal hit and cytolysis phase. Eur. J. Immunol. 4:745-750 (1974).
4. Golstein, P., and E.T. Smith. The lethal hit stage of mouse T and non-T cell-mediated cytolysis. Differences in cation requirements and characterization of an analytical "cation pulse" method. Eur. J. Immunol. 6:31-37 (1976).
5. Martz, E. Mechanism of specific tumor cell lysis by alloimmune T-lymphocytes: Resolution and characterization of discrete steps in the cellular interaction. Contemp. Top. Immunobiol. 7:301-361 (1977).
6. Berke, G. Interaction of cytotoxic T lymphocytes and target cells. Progress in Allergy 27:69-133 (1980).
7. MacLennan, I.C.M., and P. Golstein. Recognition by cytolytic T and K cells: Identification in both systems of a divalent-cation-independent, cytochalasin A-sensitive step. J. Immunol. 121:2542-2546 (1978).
8. Shortman, K., and P. Golstein. Target cell recognition by cytolytic T cells: Different requirements for the formation of strong conjugates or for proceeding to lysis. J. Immunol. 123:833-839 (1979).
9. Barber, T.A., and B.J. alter. Ultrastructures of effector-target cell interaction in secondary cell-mediated lympholysis. Scand. J. Immunol. 7:57-66 (1978).
10. Berke, G., McVey, E., Hu, V., and W.R. Clark. T lymphocyte-mediated cytolysis. I. A common mechanism for target recognition in specific and lectin-dependent cytolysis. J. Immunol. 127:776-781 (1981).
11. Golstein, P., and E.T. Smith. Mechanism of T cell-mediated cytolysis: The lethal hit stage. Contemp. Top. Immunol. 7:273-300 (1977).
12. Gately, M.K., and E. Martz. Comparative studies on the mechanisms of nonspecific, Con A-dependent cytolysis and specific T cell-mediated cytolysis. J. Immunol. 119:1711-1722 (1977).
13. Plaut, M., Bubbers, J.E., and C.S. Henney. Studies on the mechanism of lymphocyte-mediated cytolysis. VII. Two stages in the T cell-mediated lytic cycle with distinct cation requirements. J. Immunol. 116:150-155 (1976).
14. Martz, E. Immune lymphocyte to tumor cell adhesion: magnesium sufficient, calcium insufficient. J. Cell Biol. 84:584-598 (1980).

15. Stulting, R.D., and G. Berke. Nature of lymphocyte-tumor interaction. A general method for cellular immunoabsorption. J. Exp. Med. 137:932-942 (1973).
16. Gately, M.K., Wechter, W.J., and E. Martz. Early steps in specific tumor cell lysis by sensitized mouse T lymphocytes. IV. Inhibition of programming for lysis by pharmacologic agents. J. Immunol. 125:783-92 (1980).
17. Henney, C.S. On the mechanism of T-cell mediated cytolysis. Transplant. Rev. 17:37-70 (1973).
18. Kaliner, M., and K.F. Austen. A sequence of biochemical events in the antigen-induced release of chemical mediators from sensitized human lung tissue. J. Exp. Med. 138:1077-1094 (1973).
19. Ranadive N.S., and C.G. Cochrane. Mechanism of histamine release from mast cells by cationic protein (band 2) from neutrophil lysosomes. J. Immunol. 106:506 (1971).
20. Boyle, M.D.P., Langone, J.J., and T. Borsos. Studies on the terminal stages of immune hemolysis. IV. Effect of metal salts. J. Immunol. 122:1209-1213 (1979).
21. Young-Karlan, B.R., and R.F. Ashman. Order of events leading to surface immunoglobin capping: analysis of a transmembrane signal. J. Immunol. 127:1177-1181 (1981).
22. Gately, M.K., and E. Martz. Early steps in specific tumor cell lysis by sensitized mouse T lymphocytes. III. Resolution of two distinct roles for calcium in the cytolytic process. J. Immunol. 122:482-489 (1979).
23. Diamond, J.M., and E.M. Wright. Biological membranes: The physical basis of ion and nonelectroltyte selectivity. Ann. Rev. Physiol. 31:581-646 (1969).
24. Gately, M.K., and E. Martz. Early steps in specific tumor cell lysis by sensitized mouse T lymphocytes. V. Evidence that manganese inhibits a calcium-dependent step in programming for lysis. Cellular Immunol., in press (1981).
25. Becker, E.L., and P.M. Henson. In vitro studies of immunologically induced secretion of mediators from cells and related phenomena. Adv. Immunol. 17:93-193 (1973).
26. Foreman, J.C., Garland, L.G., and J.L. Mongar. The role of calcium in secretory processes: model studies in mast cells. Symp. Soc. Exp. Biol. 30:193-218 (1976).
27. Parker, W.L. Studies on the mechanism of T cell-mediated cytolysis. Ph.D. Thesis, Harvard University, Cambridge, Mass., 191 pages (1980).
28. Foreman, J.C., and J.L. Mongar. The action of lanthanum and manganese on anaphylactic histamine secretion. Brit. J. Pharmacol. 48:527-537 (1973).
29. Parker, W.L., and E. Martz. Calcium ionophore A23187 as a secretagogue for rat mast cells: Does it bypass inhibition by calcium flux blockers? Submitted for publication (1981).
30. Matter, A. The differentiation pathway of T lymphocytes. Evidence for two differentiated cell types. J. Exp. Med. 140:566-577 (1974).

31. Grimm, E., Price, Z., and B. Bonavida. Studies on the induction and expression T cell-mediated immunity. VIII. Effector-target junctions and target cell membrane disruption during cytolysis. Cellular Immunol. 46:77-99 (1979).
32. Sanderson, C.J., and A.M. Glauert. The mechanism of T-cell mediated cytotoxicity. VI. T-cell projections and their eole in target cell killing. Immunololgy 36:119-129 (1979).
33. Parker, W.L., and E. Martz. Lectin-induced nonlethal adhesions between cytolytic T lymphocytes and aitngenically unrecognizable tumor cells, and nonspecific "triggering" of cytolysis. J. Immunol. 124:25-35 (1980).
34. Kuppers, R.C., and C.S. Henney. Studies on the mechanism of lymphocyte-mediated cytolysis. IX. Relationships between antigen recognition and lytic expession in killer T cells. J. Immunol. 118:71-76 (1977).
35. Truter, M.R. Chemistry of the calcium ionophores. In "Calcium in biological systems," C.J. Duncan, Ed., Cambridge University Press, Cambridge, pp. 19-40 (1976).
36. Wasserman, R.H. Calcium transport by selected animal cells and tissues. In "Metabolic Pathways, Vol. 6, Metabolic Transport," L.E. Hoken, Ed., Academic Press, pp. 351-384 (1972).
37. Blaustein, M.P. The interrelationship between sodium and calcium fluxes across cell membranes. Rev. Physiol. Biochem. Pharmacol. 70:33-82 (1974).
38. Green, W.R., Ballas, Z.K., and C.S. Henney. Studies on the mechanism of lymphocyte-mediated cytolysis. XI. The role of lectin in lectin-dependent cell-mediated cytotoxicity. J. Immunol. 121:1566 (1978).
39. Wei, W.-Z., and R.R. Lindquist. Alloimmune cytolytic T lymphocyte activity: Triggering and expression of killing mechanisms in cytolytic T lymphocytes. J. Immunol. 126:513-516 (1981).
40. Kazimierczak, W., and B. Diamant. Mechanisms of histamine release in anaphylactic and anaphylactoid reactions. Prog. Allergy 24:295-365 (1978).
41. Lichtenstein, L.M. The mechanism of basophil histamine release induced by antigen and by the calcium ionophore A23187. J. Immunol. 114:1692-1699 (1975).
42. Foreman, J.C., Hallett, M.B., and J.L. Mongar. The relationship between histamine secretion and ^{45}calcium uptake by mast cells. J. Physiol. 271:193-214 (1977).
43. Fewtrell, C.M.S., and B.D. Gomperts. Quercetin: A novel inhibitor of Ca^{2+} influx and exocytosis in rat peritoneal mast cells. Biochim. Biophys. Acta 469:52-60 (1977).
44. Kaiser, N., and I.S. Edelman. Calcium dependence of ionophore A23187-induced lymphocyte cytotoxicity. Cancer Res. 38:3599-3603 (1978).
45. Kaiser, N., and I.S. Edelman. Further studies on the role of calcium in glucocorticoid-induced lymphocytolysis. Endocrinology 103:936-942 (1978).
46. Publicover, S.J., Duncan, C.J., and J.L. Smith. The use of

A23187 to demonstrate the role of intracellular calcium in causing ultrastructural damage in mammalian muscle. J. Neuropath. Exp. Neuro. 37:544-557 (1978).

47. Siraganian, R.P., Kulczycki, A., Jr., Mendoza, G., and H. Metzger. Ionophore A23187 induced histamine release from rat mast cells and rat basophil leukemia (RBL-1) cells. J. Immunol. 115:1599-1606 (1975).

48. Chandler, D.E., and J.A. Williams. Intracellular uptake and alpha-amylase and lactate dehydrogenase releasing actions of the divalent cation ionophore A23187 in dissociated pancreatic acinar cells. J. Membrane Biol. 32:201-230 (1977).

49. MacDermott, R,P., and B.S. Nash. Cellular cytotoxicity induced by calcium ionophore A23187. In "Regulatory mechanisms in lymphocyte activation, 11th Leucocyte Culture Conference," Academic Press, New York, pp. 671-673 (1977).

50. Schanne, F.A.X., Kane, A.B., Young, E.E., and J.L. Farber. Calcium dependence of toxic cell death: A final common pathway. Science 206:700-702 (1979).

51. Martz, E., Tsoukas, C.D., and W.J. Wechter. Evidence against Ca^{++} poisoning by killer cells: Mast cells killed by T lymphocytes do not secrete prelytically. J. Supramol. Struct. Suppl. 3:311 (Abstract 818)(1979).

52. Cooper, P.H., and D.R. Stanworth. Isolation of rat peritoneal mast cells in high yield and purity. Methods in Cell Biol. 14: 365-378 (1977).

53. Morrison, D.C., Roser, J.F., Henson, P.M., and C.G. Cochrane. Activation of rat mast cells by low molecular weight stimuli. J. Immunol. 112:573-582 (1974).

54. Bloom, G.D., Diamant, B., Hagermark, O., and M. Ritzen. The effects of adenosine-5'-triphosphate (ATP) on structure and amine content of rat peritoneal mast cells. Exp. Cell Res. 62:61-75 (1970).

55. Ko, L., and D. Lagunoff. Depletion of mast cell ATP inhibits complement-dependent cytotoxic histamine release. Exp. Cell Res. 100:313-321 (1976).

56. Davignon, D., Martz, E., Reynolds, T., Kurzinger, K., and T.A. Springer. Lymphocyte function-associated antigen one (LFA-1): a surface antigen distinct from Lyt-2/3 that participates in T lymphocyte-mediated killing. Proc. Natl. Acad. Sci. USA 78:4535-4539 (1981).

57. Simone, C.B., Henkart, P. Permeability changes induced in erythrocyte thost targets by antibody-dependent cytotoxic effector cells: Evidence for membrane pores. J. Immunol. 124:954-963 (1980).

58. Giavedoni, E., Yu, B., Chow, M., and A.P. Dalmasso. The functional size of the primary complement lesion in resealed erythrocyte membrane ghosts. J. Immunol. 122:240 (1979).

59. Sarkadi, B., Szasz, I., and G. Gardos. The use of ionophores of rapid loading of human red cells with radioactive cations for cation-pump studies. J. Membrane Biol. 26:357-370 (1976).

60. Foreman, J.C., Mongar, J.L., and B.D. Gomperts. Calcium ionophores and movement of calcium ions following the physiological stimulus to a secretory process. Nature 245:249-252 (1973).
61. Diamant, B., and S.A. Patkar. Stimulation and inhibition of histamine release from isolated rat mast cells. Dual effects of the ionophore A23187. Int. Archs. Allergy Appl. Immun. 49: 183-207 & Proc. Natl. Acad. Sci. USA (1975).

DISCUSSION

A. Allison

The possibility that calcium-activated enzymes participate in cytolysis seems intriguing, and I wonder whether anyone has made serious attempts to look at it. The first group of enzymes to be considered would be phospholipases. Both neutral phospholipase A2, which hydrolyses phosphatidylethanolamine and phosphatidylcholine, and phospholipase C, which hydrolyses phosphatidylinositol, are calcium-dependent (Biochem. J. 1981, 197:523). A second possibility is calcium---activated neutral membrane proteases, which appear to be involved in cell fusion (Biochem. J. 1980, 192:829). The membrane perturbations involved in cell fusion may be analogous to those occurring in target cells during cytolysis.

R. Goldfarb

In this regard, it is interesting that the ionophore A 23187 can induce phospholipase A2 activity in red blood cell membranes. In addition, neutral serine proteases, such as trypsin and alphathrombin can also activate phospholipase A2. Therefore, the link that Tony suggests may be real.

E. Martz

We think of calcium acting on a protein, although there are other possibilities and notably phospholipases directly binding calcium in the membrane. The question that I tried to discuss is, where that calcium-dependent target is, and I would still say that I tend to favor the idea that it's outside the cell. Whether it's a phospholipase, protease or whatever, as far as I know there is no good evidence on that.

R. Goldfarb

It's certainly possible that some of these enzymes can function in a cell surface externally associated form, and therefore there may be no controversy there.

M. Mayer

It's well known that calcium produces a reorientation of membrane lipids by changing the angle of the head group. This, I think, may have something to do with what you're talking about, Eric. Calcium does alter the bilayer by changing the angular orientation of the phospholipid molecules. It is also well known that Ca^{++} binds to anionic head groups on phospholipid bilayers, which decreases membrane fluidity and triggers phase separations. (Shlatz, L. and Marinetti, G.A. 1972. BBA, 290:70. Gordon, L.M., Sauerheber, R.D., Esgate, J.A. 1978. J. Supra. Mol. Struct. 9:299. Trauble, H., and Eibl, H. 1974. Proc. Natl. Acad. Sci. USA, 71:214.)

I. MacLennan

I think the reason why we talk about calcium-dependence of the lethal hit stage is simply because of the existence of EDTA. If EDTA had a higher affinity for magnesium than calcium, then we would call it the magnesium-dependent lethal hit stage, because there is a magnesium requirement for full expression of cytolytic capacity. Also, in the presence of magnesium, you can get some kill without calcium. However, in terms of lytic units it is reduced by more or less an order of magnitude (Immunology. 1980. 39:109). The other thing is that there is a requirement for other types of cations and you require really quite high concentrations of potassium in order to get killing. I was surprised to hear that an energy requirement was being claimed on the basis of azide inhibition, because most leukocytes, probably preferentially, use glycolysis and not the cytochrome system to get energy and certainly bypass cytochrome blocks. I think that simply means that you're getting a non-energy block by azide (J. Biol. Chem. 1959, 234:1355).

E. Martz

I think the only azide I mentioned is in the mast cell. There it has been shown by others (Int. Artch. allergy 1975, 69:155) that the ATP ATP turnover is very rapid and that azide alone will cause a very rapid decay in a couple of minutes of the ATP pool. You are absolutely right about T cells for which it has been shown that both 2-deoxyglucose and azide are required to get a good block (J. Exp. Med. 1977. 146:698).

I. Maclennan

Your slide indicated that magnesium did not have much role in cytolysis. Is not cytolysis relatively inefficient in the absence of magnesium plus calcium?

E. Martz

No, I didn't mean to give the impression that magnesium isn't involved. I simply wasn't discussing that point. I tend to feel as you do that magnesium is crucial in the normal lytic pathway to establish a strong adhesion, probably more, as Pierre has said, in the strengthening of the adhesion than in the actual recognition event. It's very difficult to get evidence as to whether magnesium is required in a direct sense for the lethal hit for technical reasons, but it may well be required there as well. So I don't mean to say that magnesium is not important. I think it's very important in early events and may also be in later events. It's just not testable.

DIRECT ANALYSIS OF INDIVIDUAL KILLER T CELLS: SUSCEPTIBILITY OF TARGET CELLS TO LYSIS AND SECRETION OF HYDROLYTIC ENZYMES BY CTL

D. Zagury

Laboratoire de Physiologie cellulaire
Université Pierre et Marie Curie
4, place Jussieu
Paris Cedex 05, France

and

Laboratoire de Cytologie
Institut Jean-Godinot
51100 Reims, France

INTRODUCTION

T cell mediated lysis has been extensively studied using the standard chromium release test (1) which measures semi-quantitatively the activity of cytotoxic T lyphocyte (CTL) suspensions from _in vivo_ (2, 3) and _in vitro_ (4) experimental systems. As reviewed by Berke (5) and more recently by Henney (6, 7), biological conditions required for T cell mediated cytotoxicity (T CMC) were well defined and the lytic process was dissected into three succesive stages: A) Binding, which is dependent upon the specific recognition by effector cells (E) of sensitizing antigens carried by targets (T). E-T cell contact is a necessary step for target lysis. B) Lethal hit during which stage a lesion occurs on the target cell. This process is at once "the most interesting and most enigmatic," (7) since we do not know yet the nature of the "hit." One hypothesis indeed proposed that target cell destruction is caused by a soluble mediator secreted by the killer lymphocytes (8). C) Cytolysis which does not require the continuous presence of the effector cell. The target cell undergoes a series of membrane permeability alterations leading to cell destruction (5-7).

As mentioned, the lethal hit is a concept not yet well understood and numerous questions are still unanswered concerning the mechanism of T CMC. Our knowledge is indeed limited by the use of the total effector cell suspension in the T CMC analysis. This heterogeneous cellular material excludes direct morphological and biochemical investigations of killer cells (7). These limitations can, however, be overcome in part by a direct approach of the functionally homogeneous killer cell subpopulation isolated by micromanipulation from the mass effector cell suspension (9-11).

RESULTS AND DISCUSSION

Direct Study Of The Isolated Killer Cell Population

As diagrammed in Fig. 1, killer cell subpopulations were isolated from the effector T cell suspensions of in vivo and in vitro T CMC systems. Effector cells from in vivo systems were lymphoid cell suspension collected from lymphoid organs (spleen; lymph nodes) or fluids (peritoneal exudates; blood) of immunized organisms sensitized against allogeneic or virus-modified syngeneic cells (2-3). T lymphocyte suspensions were purified after passage through a nylon wool column (12). Effector cells from in vitro systems were responder cells stimulated by sensitizing cells (4).

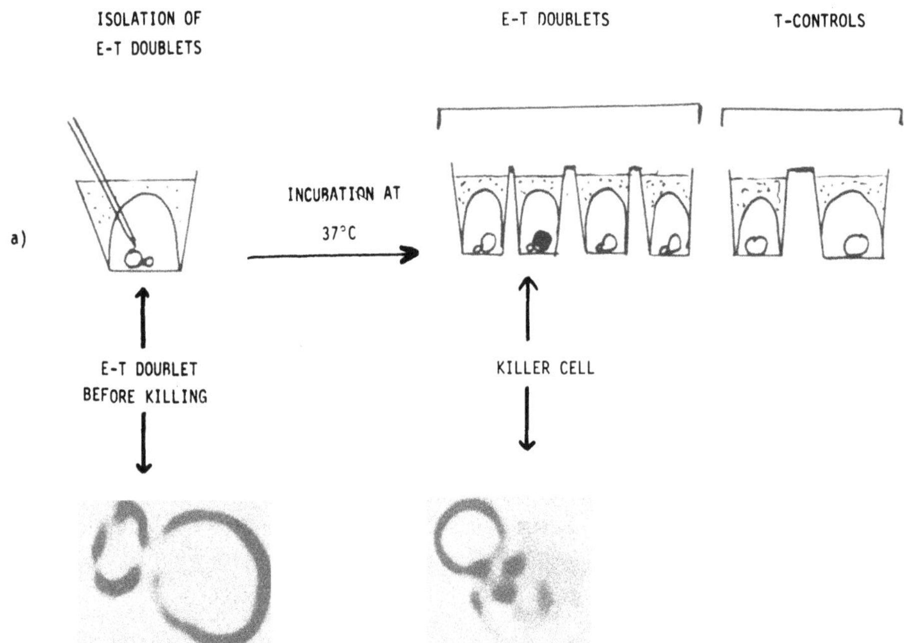

Fig. 1 a) Diagrammatic representation of the CTL identification.
b) E-T doublets before (left) and after (right) target lysis.

E-T doublets formed either by direct microassociation (10,11) or after conjugation (9) were first individually isolated at the bottom of a culture microwell at room temperature (Fig. 1a) and subsequently incubated at 37°C. In the microassociation technique (10-11), effectors cells were collected at random and put into contact with a target cell forming E-T doublets. At the beginning of the 37°C incubation, some E-T doublets dissociated, while others formed stable binding. This procedure had the advantage to investigate the lytic function of all the effector cells. In conjugation (9), E-T doublets named conjugates were formed by centrifugation and resuspension at room temperature of mixed effector and target cell suspension. These conjugates which were individually isolated usually formed stable binding during the subsequent incubation at 37°C. Investigation of the lytic function was, however, limited in the conjugation procedure to the selected subpopulaton of effectors which formed conjugates.

After the 37°C incubation of the E-T doublets, killer cells were identified by the lysis of their associated target which was appreciated by the loss of cell refringency (Fig. 1b).

Identified killer cells were enumerated, isolated and collected separately. This functionally homogeneous cell subpopulation was available for further morphological (9,13), cytochemical (14,15) or physiological (15) investigations and for long-term clone culture (16,17). Such investigations performed on pure killer T cells provided new information concerning the mechanism of the T CMC, as discussed below.

E-T Binding And Conjugation

Direct killing assays performed on E-T doublets coming from microassociation or conjugation provided the following results:

a) As reported previously (5-7), E-T cell contact (binding) is necessary for target lysis to occur. When E and T were not bound at the beginning of 37°C incubation, no target lysis was subsequently observed.

b) After E-T binding only a percentage of bound effectors lysed the associated target (Table 1). This result demonstrated that 1) an effector killer can lyse a target without the cooperation of any accessory cell and 2) binding even though necessary is not sufficient for lysis to occur.

c) As indicated in Table 1, enumeration of killer cells (column 3) showed that within the total effector cell suspensions the number of killers is higher than provided by the killer conjugates. Also, a number of non-conjugated effectors exhibited killing activity when bound to a target by microassociation.

Table I : ENUMERATION OF CTL BY SINGLE CELL ASSAY

Immunization	Day of immunization	Conjugation		Microassociation		Number of CTL per 100 effector cells	
		lymphocytes bound	Proportion of CTL	lymphocytes bound	Proportion of CTL	Conjugation	Microassociation
In vivo[3]	9	34	44[c]	100	32	15	32
	10	32	62	100	35	26	35
	11	40	55	100	25	22	25
In vitro[b]	5	21	14	100	9	3	9
	6	17	41	10	12	7	12

[a]Peritoneal exudate lymphoid populations obtained after i.p. inoculation of BALB/c (H-2^d) mice with 10^8 EL-4 (H-2^b) tumor cells.

[b]MLC populations obtained from cultures of DBA/2 (H-2^d) spleen cells and irradiated (200 rads) C56B11/6 (H-2^b) spleen cells.

[c]Each value repesents the mean of 3 experiments in which 150 lymphocyte-EL-4 tumor doublets were scored for CTL.

d) Not all effectors from E-T conjugates exhibited killing activity, as shown in Table 1 (column 1).

e) Multiple effector target binding occured. After conjugation, multiple effector cells conjugated to one target were not observed while multiple target cells (2-4) conjugated to one effector are often seen. Moreover, when one associated a fresh effector cell to a previously bound target, the second effector dissociated. These observations provide evidence that membrane changes existed in the target cell after binding to an effector.

Rapid Delivery Of Lethal Hit And Lytic Cycle

a) Even though target lysis usually was observed between 0.5 to 3 hours of incubation at 37°C after binding to the effector cell, the lethal hit apparently occured within the first ten minutes of incubation. The rapid occurrence of the lethal hit was directly demonstrated when E-T doublets were dissociated by EDTA after a variable lag period of a 37°C incubation (19).

b) Experiments performed with total effector cell suspensions suggested that a killer cell could lyse more than one target cell, proceeding through lytic cycles (20). Multiple-target hits by one killer can be directly demonstrated either by experiments in which effector cells were conjugated with 2, 3 or 4 targets (19) or by recycling which already lysed one target and reassociated to a fresh target. Since in all these instances target hits were given sequentially (19), the CTL lytic cycle concept was confirmed.

Evidence For a Localized Exocytosis Of Hydrolases by CTL

Presence of lysosomes and lysosomal enzymes. In E-T conjugates isolated after different times of incubation at 37°C and treated for electron microscopy, effector killer cells presented lysosomal granules, localized around the Golgi region and near target junction (9, 21). Histochemical reactions of the killer conjugates showed acid phosphatase activity in lysosomal granules and also at the level of the target junction (Fig. 2)(14). Enzyme activity was not found at the target junction in non-killer effector conjugates. These results suggested that killer cells secrete hydrolases at the level of the target junction which could account for a target cell lesion. This hypothesis is also supported by the following observations.

Biological requirements for effector cell to lyse targets

These requirements are those necessary for other secretory processes, such as zymogen secretion by pancreatic acinic cells, insulin secretion of Langerhans islets, histamine containing granules by mast cells, or hydrolytic enzymes by polymorphonuclear cells (2).

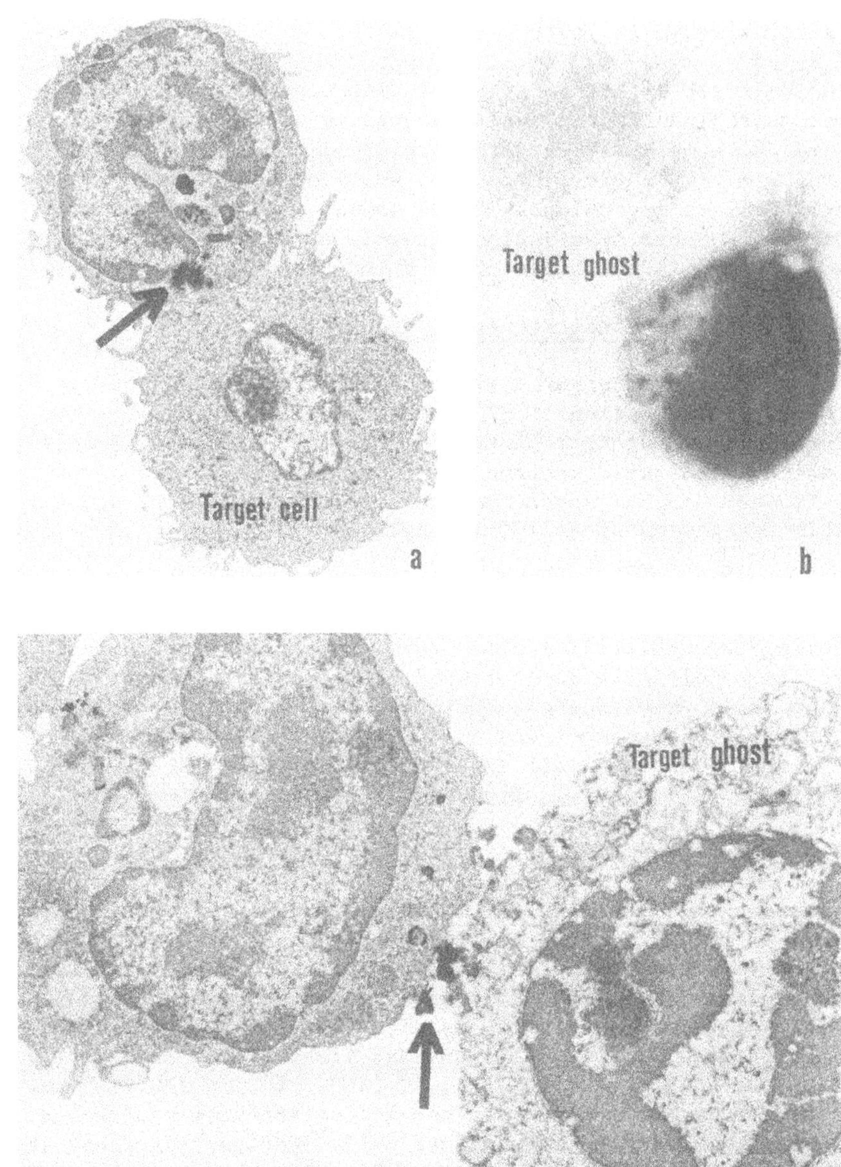

Fig. 2 a) Electron microscopy of CTL-T conjugates treated for detection of acid phosphatase enzymes (Gomori reaction). Note the presence of acid phosphatase in the lysosomes [↗].
b) Killer CTL after May Grunwald-Giemsa stain. Note the number of lysosomal-like granules and, near the CTL, target cell debris.

These conditions, as defined for killer cells by studies using total cell suspensions, are: presence of divalent ions, integrity of the cellular microskeleton, energengy dependency, and low level of cAMP (5-7,23).

Freeze fracture electron microscopy observations

On a study on E-T conjugates by freeze fracture (13), Nicolas and Zagury described at the E-T junctions along the killer cell membrane the presence of open vesicles, the size of which corresponds to lysosomal granules. In addition, the authors observed amorphous material at the target junction of CTLs which could represent hydrolytic enzymes.

Lysis of targets bound to effectors in presence of Phospholipase A2

In recent experiments performed on isolated E-T conjugates and free targets, phospholipase (hog pancreatic phospholipase A2 from Boehringer 600 U/mg) was added to the medium. As shown in Table 2, the addition of phopholipase did not lyse free target cells. However, targets bound in E-T conjugates were lysed to a much higher extent when phospholipase A2 was present in the medium.

Cell Lysis

a) The target lytic process was directly studied on EL4 target cells conjugated to peritoneal exudate T lymphocytes collected from BALB/c mouse immunized against allogeneic EL4 cells (9). Before lysis the conjugated targets were refringent, showing a well-defined contour and no apparent nucleus by phase contrast microscopy. The earliest cell modification observed was an ill-defined contour; it was followed successively by a loss of cell refringency, appearance of the nucleus, swelling of the cytoplasm, and, later on, cytoplasmic disintegration. These progressive modifications reflect ionic and/or osmotic membrane permeability disorders.

b) Target cytolysis has been also investigated by microcinematography (24). Through the film one can observe directly lysis of targets in isolated E-T conjugates. Such observations confirm the phenomenon of zeiosis which is related to disturbance of osmotic and/or ionic permeability states between intracellular and extracellular compartments.

---

c) Electron microscopy of CTL-T conjugates treated for detection of acid phosphatase enzymes (Gomori reaction). Note the presence of acid phosphatase at the target junction [↗].

TABLE II : EFFECT OF PHOSPHOLIPASE TREATMENT ON TARGET CELL LYSIS.

EXPERIMENTS	MLC RESPONDERS (a)	TARGET (b)	PHOSPHOLIPASE TREATMENT(c)	% OF TARGET LYSIS
I	+	Conjugated	+	33
	-	Free	+	0
	+	Conjugated	-	12
	-	Free	-	6
II	+	Conjugated	+	39
	-	Free	+	6
	+	Conjugated	-	10
	-	Free	-	0
III	+	Conjugated	+	23
	-	Free	+	0
	+	Conjugated	-	3
	-	Free	-	0
IV	+	Conjugated	+	25
	-	Free	+	3
	+	Conjugated	-	6
	-	Free	-	0
V	+	Conjugated	+	33
	-	Free	+	0
	+	Conjugated	-	18
	-	Free	-	6

[a]Effector cells[a] were responder cells originated from normal human peripheral blood lymphocytes stimulated in vitro by irradiated (5000 rads) allogenic Epstein-Barr virus transformed B cells.
[b]Target cells were the sensitizing B^{EBV+} cells.
[c]Phospholipase treatment was administered on E-T conjugated for 15'. E-T conjugates or free targets in experimental samples were incubated at 37°C first in a RPMI medium containing 500µg/ml of Hog pancreatic Phospholipase A2 (Boehringer) (600U/mg) and 1% FCS. After 15' the phopholipase medium was replaced by RPMI containing 10% FCS. Control samples were incubated in the same conditions without phospholipase. 100µg/ml of phospholipase A2 was toxic and 100µg/ml was not active in these experimental conditions.
[d]Killer enumeration test (9) was performed on effector-target conjugates isolated after centrifugation and resuspension of mixed responder and target cell suspension 2-4 days after a secondary boost. Each sample was constituted of 40 ± 10 conjugates and an equal number of free target cells were tested. Experiments lasted 3-5 hours.

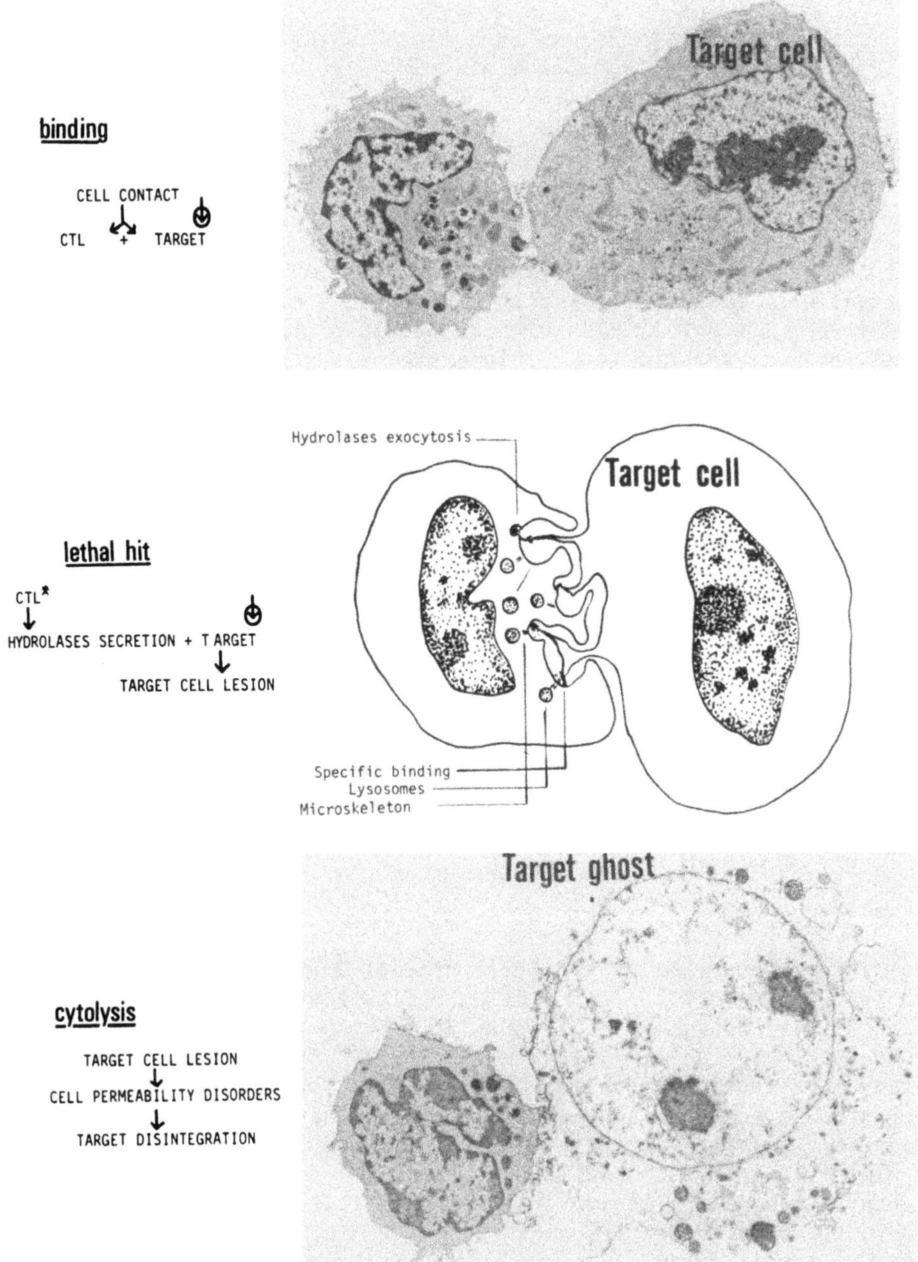

Fig. 3 Illustrative scheme of the different CMC stages. CTL* = activated killer cell; T = susceptible target.

Interpretative T CMC Scheme Extracted From Direct Study of Killer Cell Subpopulations

Direct studies performed on isolated CTL have enabled us to analyze three successive stages of T-CMC, as follows (Fig. 3):

Binding

It is determined by effector cell recognition of sensitizing antigens carried by specific targets. Section III demonstrated that the binding necessary to initiate T-CMC is not restricted to conjugation. Additional binding can occur in mixed effector target cell through random Brownian motion or, at the single cell level, by microassociation. This explains why killer cells were observed in both conjugate and non-conjugate effector populations.

Binding allows cell to cell contact. In addition, it should promote modifications of bound effector and target cells preparing each for the lethal hit. Concerning the killer cell partner, activation of membrane receptor by target cell antigens might well trigger the effector functions (7). Binding also modifies target cells either by local alterations of transmembrane electrical potential, as hypothesized by Berke (5), or, more simply, if one considers histocompatibility antigen displacements, by molecular reorganization of the cell surface. Such a membrane reorganization would explain 1) the inability of the bound target cell to accept a second effector cell and 2) the lytic action of phospholipases exhibited on bound targets and not on free ones.
Membrane modifications of the target cells may render the target cell susceptible for the lethal hit.

Lethal hit

This major stage of the lytic process lasts only a few minutes and is performed by a single killer cell without the help of accessory cells. The killer cell "hits" its bound target causing an irreversible lesion resulting in cytolysis. Of the suggestions offered by classical studies to account for the lethal lesion, secretion of a factor by the killer cell (8) appears to be confirmed by direct investigation of the killer cell subpopulation. Secretion of hydrolytic enzymes localized at the CTL-T junction would indeed account for a lethal lesion on the susceptible target. In this event, two questions are posed:

1) Which hydrolytic enzyme(s) would be concerned in the lethal hit? Even though no decisive experimental evidence is yet available

it seems likely that phopholipases are involved for the following reasons: a) the molecular permeability changes of the target cell with the external compartment during the lytic process results from ionic and/or osmotic alternations. This suggests that the initial lesion is at the level of the lipid bilayer cell membrane; b) the nature of the membrane permeability changes and inhibition of these changes by solutions of high osmotic pressure parallel remarkably the mechanism of complement induced cytotoxicity, which is determined by action of a hole on the lipid bilayer membrane (25); c) interferon which activates phospholipiases (26) increases T-CMC (27) as well as other cellular (28) and molecular (29) mediated cytotoxicity processes (29); prostaglandins E and cAMP which are inhibitors of phopholipase (26) inhibit also CMC (6, 7); d) moreover, phospholipase treated targets bound to effector cells are lysed to a much higher extent than the untreated ones (Table 2). Also, enzymes from killer cells which would hydrolyze target membrane (glyco)proteins could induce activation of endogenous phospholipase anbd thus generate a hole in the lipid bilayer.

2) Why hydrolytic enzymes secreted at the E-T cell junction determine a lesion on the target and not on the effector cell? A tentative explanation is that hydrolytic enzymes act only upon susceptible cell membranes, such as those of the modified bound targets.

Cytolysis

This terminal stage, which is the consequence of target cell lesion performed during the lethal hit, does not require the continuous presence of killer cells. It consists of a series of membrane permeability changes resulting in the demise of the target cell and lasts usually 0.5-3 hours according to the type of target cell and experimental conditions.

CONCLUSION

T-CMC, which affects elimination of foreign allogeneic or transformed syngeneic cells, represents a specialized immune process, requiring differentiation of specific CTL from precursor cells. Other immune and non-immune defense mechanisms (27,28) exist to eliminate undesirable cells. Recent studies performed on NK cells (30) and on interferon mediated cytotoxicity (29), together with the results presented here, suggest that a basic target lesion - an alteration of the membrane permeability, as found in T-CMC - should account for the different lytic processes. Membrane alterations could be, however, performed differently according to the lytic system, either by transmembrane channel due to insertion of hydrophobic peptides, as demonstrated for complement dependent cytotoxicity (25) or through hydrolytic enzyme(s) action as described for polymorph (22) or T lymphocyte (31) mediated cytotoxicity.

SUMMARY

Direct identification, enumeration and biological characterization of cytolytic T lymphocytes (CTL) complementing the chromium release test has allowed us to propose a mechanism for T-cell mediated cytotoxicity (T-CMC). One CTL without accessory cells is able to lyse a specific target. Binding which allows cell contact (E-T doublets), should activate effector CTLs and render target cells susceptible to lysis. Secretion of hydrolytic enzymes localized at the CTL-target junction accounts for the lethal hit given by CTLs to susceptible targets. This hypothesis that the resulting cell lesion is identified with an alteration of the lipid bilayer membrane has been confirmed by single killer cell study. Furthermore, we have proposed that phospholipase enzymes are involved in the membrane alterations, since susceptible targets bound to effector cells (conjugates) were lysed in a much higher yield in the presence of phospholipase. Membrane cell lesion determined by hydrolytic enzyme (phospholipase) could represent a basic general mechanism for other cellular or molecular mediated processes.

ACKNOWLEDGMENTS

We are grateful to Doctor Doris-Ann Morgan for her contribution and skilled advice.

This work was supported by grants from INSERM, DRET and DGRST, and by help from the Ligue Nationale Francaise contre le Cancer, ADRC (Villejuif), and La Fondation pour la Recherche Medicale.

REFERENCES

(1) Brunner, K.T., Cerottini, J.C., and Chapuis, B., 1968. Quantitative assay of the lytic action of immune lymphoid cells on chromium-labeled allogenic targets in vitro; inhibition by isoantibody a,d by drugs. Immunology, 14, p. 181.

(2) Brunner, K.T., Mauel, J., Rudolf, H., and Chapuis, B., 1970. Studies of allograft immunity in mice. I.- Induction, development and in vitro assay of cellular immunity. Immunology, 18, p. 501.

(3) Berke, G., Sullivan, K.A., and Amos, D.B., 1972. Rejection of ascites tumor allograft. I. - Isolation, characterization and in vitro reactivity of peritoneal lymphoid effector cells from BALB/c mice immune to EL_4 leukosis. J. Exp. Med., 135, p. 1334.
(4) Hayry, P. and Defendi, V., 1970. Mixed lymphocyte cultures produced by effector cells; model in vitro for allograft rejection. Science, 168, p. 133.
(5) Berke, G. and Amos, D.B., 1973. Mechanism of lymphocyte-mediated cytolysis; the LMC cycle and its role in transplantation immunity. Transplant. Rev., 17, p. 71.
(6) Henney, Ch.S., 1977. T cell-mediated cytolysis: an overview of some current issues. Contemporary Topics in Immuno-Biology, ed. O. Stutman, Plenum Press, New York - London.
(7) Henney, Ch. S., 1980. The mechanism of T-cell mediated lysis. Immunology Today, 1, p. 36.
(8) Granger, G.A. and Kolb, W.P., 1968. Lymphocyte in vitro cytotoxicity. Mechanisms of immune and non-immune small lymphocyte mediated target destruction. J. Immunol., 101, p. 111.
(9) Zagury, D., Bernard, J., Thiernesse, N., Feldman, M., and Berke, G., 1975. Isolation and characterization of individual functional reactive cytotoxic-T-lymphocytes conjugation, killing and recycling at the single cell level. Eur. J. Immunol., 5, p. 818.
(10) Zagury, M., Fouchard, M., & Petit, 1979. Cytolyse à médiation cellulaire dépendante d'une immunisation contre des antigènes cellulaires; identification et numération des cellules cytotoxiques. C.R. Acad. Sci., Paris, série D, 288, p. 1243.
(11) Zagury, D., Fouchard, M., Morgan, D.A., and Cerottini, J.C., 1980. Enumeration of T effector cells mediating direct and/or lectin dependant lysis. Immunology Letters, 1:335.
(12) Berke, G., Sullivan, K.A., and Amos, D.B., 1972. Rejection of ascite tumor allografts. I. - Isolation, characterization and in vitro reactivity of PEL from BALB/c mice immune to EL_4 leukosis. J. Exp. Med., 135, p. 1334.
(13) Nicolas, G., and Zagury, D., 1980. Etude par cryofracture de la zone de contact entre cellule cytolytique et cellule cible. Biol. cell., 3, p. 231.
(14) Thiernesse, N., David A., Bernard J., Jeannesson, P., and Zagury, D., 1977. Activité phosphatasique acide de la cellule T cytolytique au cours du processus de cytolyse. C.R. Acad. Sci., Paris, 285, p.713.
(15) Jeannesson, P., Bernard, J., Thiernesse, N., Cerottini, J.C., Brochier, J., and Zagury, D., 1978. Isolation and characterization of single killer K cells from human peripheral blood. In "Human leukocyte differentiation: its application to cancer." INSERM, Symposium n°8, B. Serrou and C. Rosenfeld, Elsevier, North-Holland Medical Press.

(16) Zagury, D., D.A. Morgan, and Fouchard, M., 1980. Evidence for cytotoxic functions in well-defined human T cell clones. Biomedicine, 33, p. 272.
(17) Zagury, D., Morgan D.A., and Fouchard, M., 1981. Production of well-defined human T lymphocyte clones. I. - Monoclonal culture and functional cytotoxicity maturation. J. Immunol. Methods, 43, p. 67.
(18) Golstein, P., Svedmyr, E.A.J., and Wigzell, H., 1971. Cells mediating specific in vitro cytotoxicity. I. - Detection of receptor-bearing lymphocytes. J. Exp. Med., 134, p. 1385.
(19) Zagury, D., Bernard, J., Jeannesson, P., Thiernesse, N., and Cerottini, J.C., 1979. Studies on the mechanism of T cell-mediated lysis at the single effector cell level. I. - Kinetic analyses of lethal hits and target cell lysis in multicellular conjugates. J. Immunol., 123, p. 1604.
(20) Martz, E., 1975. Early steps in specific tumor cell lysis by sensitized T lymphocytes. I. - Resolution and characterization. J. Imunol., 115, p. 261.
(21) Bykovskaja, S.N., Rytenko, A.N., Renschenbach, M.O., and Bykovsky, A.F., 1978. Ultrastructural alteration of cytolytic T lymphocytes. II. - Morphogenesis of secretory granules and intracellular vacuoles. Cell. Immunol., 40, p. 175.
(22) Weissmann, G., Goldstein, I., Hoffstein, S., Chauvet, G., and Robineaux, R., 1975. Yin/Yang modulation of lysosomal enzyme release from polymorphonuclear leucocytes by cyclic nucleotides. In Part IV "Role of Inflammatory cells in the Destruction of Synovid Tissues." Annals N.Y. Acad. of Sciences, 222, 253 and 750.
(23) Henney, Ch. S., and Lichtenstein, L.M., 1971. The role of cyclic AMP in the cytolytic activity of lymphocytes. J. Immunol., 107, p. 610
(24) Zagury, D., Bernard, J., Thiernesse, N., and Benoist, H., 1976. "Killer cells in action."
(25) Mayer, M.M., 1977. Mechanisms of cytolysis by lymphocytes: a) a comparison with complement. J. Immunol., 119, p. 1195.
(26) Wallach, D., and Revel, M., 1979. Hormonal protection of interferon-treated cells against double-stranded RNA induced cytolysis. FEBS Letters, 101, p. 364.
(27) Lindahl, P., Leary, P., and Gresser, I., 1972. Enhancement by Interferon of the specific cytotoxicity of sensitized lymphocytes. Proc. Natl. Acad. Sci., 60, p. 721.
(28) Trinchieri, G., Santoli, D., and Koprowski, H., 1978. Spontaneous CMC in Humans: Role of Interferon and Immunoglobulins. J. Immunol., 120, p. 1849.
(29) Stewart, W.E. II, DeClerco, E., and DeSomer, P., 1973. Specificity of Interferon induced enhancement of cytotoxicity for double stranded RNA induced cytolysis. J. General Virology, 18, p. 237.

(30) Carpen, O., Virtanen, I., and Saksela, E., 1980. The cytotoxicity activity of human NK cells requires an intact secretóry apparatus. Cell. Immunol. (in press).

(31) David, A., Bernard, J., Thiernesse, N., Nicolas, G., Cerottini, J.C., and Zagury, D., 1979. Le processus d'exocytose lysosomale localisée est-il responsable de l'action cytolytique des lymphocytes T tueurs? C.R. Acad. Sci., Paris, 288, p. 441.

DISCUSSION

P. Lachmann

Investigations of T cell cytotoxicity might benefit from the experience of complement workers who spent a lot of effort looking at phospholipase as a lytic mediator with negative results. Does Dr. Zagury use 10% fetal calf serum in his experiments?

D. Zagury

No, we used phospholipase in 1% fetal serum for 15 minutes, then we remove phospholipase and then we add 10% fetal serum without phospholipase.

P. Lachmann

I wonder how much lysolecithin is generated from the lechithin in the fetal calf serum by the phospholipase? Do you have evidence that the phospholipase is acting on the membrane phospholipids rather than those in solution, and that it is not a lytic agent generated in solution which damages the membrane?

D. Zagury

This is still a possibility; our experiments are very preliminary.

P. Golstein

Actually, it may not matter too much, because whatever the toxic agent at play here, perhaps the interesting point is that when the target cells are conjugated they are more susceptible to it.

P. Lachmann

I do not doubt that when a membrane is perturbed in any of a number of ways it becomes more susceptible to phospholipase A2. Complement lysis of liposomes does give rise to small amounts of phospholipid breakdown products. But it has been shown (Lachmann et al., Immunology, 1973, 24:135) that they are not the cause of the lysis.

G. Berke

The comment by Zagury may be of great importance since involvement of phospholipase in cell-mediated killng was suggested (Frye and Friou, Nature 1975, 258:333) on the basis of inhibition by Rosenthal's inhibitor, a lecithin analog. In CTL-mediated lysis, this has been shown to be due to inhibition of conjugate formation rather than to inhibition of phospholipase activity (Prog. Allergy 1981, 27:69). However, as Zagury pointed out, target cells appear to become susceptible to phospholipase activity upon interaction with killer cells. This is reminiscent of an exciting finding that Van Dienen published some years ago: in snake venom, phospholipase activity is enhanced by an additional (basic) protein. Only upon pretreatment of cells with that venom component are they rendered susceptible to the phospholipase activity.

R. Herberman

As I recall from that paper by Frye and Friou (Nature 1975, 258:333), it wasn't clearly related to CTL. I wonder if you could clarify whether Rosenthal's inhibitor will inhibit CTL action.

G. Berke

In the Tucson Leucocyte Culture Conference (in "Regulatory Mechanisms in Lymphocyte Activation," Acad. Press, New York, 1977, p. 809), we reported on the effects of Rosenthal's inhibitor on CTL mediated killing showing quite conclusively that it was blocking CTL mediated killing because it was preventing conjugate formation.

M. Mayer

I want to get back to Gideon Berke's comment on the phospholipase. It is true that you can influence the attack of exogenous phospholipase with co-factor to improve accessibility of the membrane phospholipids to the exogenous phospholipase. I think much of this is really irrelavant because it's well known that one can hydrolyze a very high proportion of membrane phospholipid, as much as 50-60% and sometimes more, without destroying the bilayer. As long as the lysophosphatide fatty acid products stay in the bilayer, the integrity is preserved. So this notion that you can destroy a cell with phospholipase is not necessarily true.

There is a very interesting paper by Jain (Nature 284:486, 1980) from the University of Delaware on that. He used erythrocytes that had been 80% hydrolyzed and remained intact, until he pulled out the fatty acid with a high concentration of albumin outside and then the orientation was disturbed. The way Jain interpreted that was very simple. He said that even though you have cleaved off the fatty acid, the fatty acid molecules remained in more or less the same orientation within the bilayer, which remained intact.

P. Lachmann

As Manfred says, phospholipase A2 doesn't attack most membranes in the absence of a "priming" agent. This priming agent is commonly lysolecithin itself produced by phospholipase action on exogenous lecithin. In cobra venom there are basic proteins which, as Manfred says, insert into the membrane and allow phospholipase access to membrane phospholipid. Low concentrations of polylysine can be used for the same purpose.

D. Zagury

In our experiments with phospholipases, among free effectors, free targets, conjugated effectors and conjugated targets, only the latter were lysed. This means that the target cells are rendered susceptible through the association with the effectors.

A. Allison

The most interesting phospholipases are those in the plasma membrane which are activated when a cell is triggered to perform a particular function. An example is activation of calcium-dependent phospholipase A2 in the membranes of macrophages which releases arachidonic acid, which is then used in the cyclo-oxygenase and lipoxygenase pathways (Biochem. J. 1981, 197:523). In this way phospholipase activation could have a series of metabolic consequences.

M. Mayer

The question of sequence has to be kept in mind. The cytotoxic action of lymphotoxin, which we studied, produces a calcium influx. A group of Japanese investigators subsequently showed that this is actually preceded by phospholipase activation, not followed. One would have thought that lymphotoxin produces a calcium pulse and then endogenous phospholipase gets activated. They say that phospholipase activation precedes the calcium influx. The second comment that I would make is in relation to secretion and the cytotoxic event. I think it is much more reasonable to regard these as independent but parallel events, not necessarily sequential, which fit in with Eric's results, and not to make the assumption that is so widely made that they are, indeed, sequential.

R. Goldfarb

In collaboration with Ron Herberman and Tom Hoffman, we have demonstrated that Rosenthal's inhibitor can block human natural killer cell activity and that exogenously added phospholipase A2 can augment the activity of killing.

Valerie Hu

I had a question to people talking about the possible involvement of phospholipases. Are they thinking about the phospholipases being activated in the target or the killer cell?

G. Berke

We have made direct measurements to investigate this question by using P^{32} labeled target cells, exposing them to killer cells, extracting their phospholipids and analyzing them. The rationale was that if the phospholipase A2 were involved in disintegration of target cell phospholipids, then we should see an accumulation of lysolecithin. The results were conclusively that this was not the case.

Valerie Hu

Yes, but there could be a phospholipase activated in the killer cell that would be cleaving the target cells, or alternatively the killer cell could induce phospholipase action in the target cell. That's what I was asking.

W. Clark

I suppose most of us naively are thinking of phospholipase in the killer cell.

R. Goldfarb

I'm intrigued by the possibility that, at least in some killer cell populations, endogenous protease, which is produced, might then activate a latent phospholipase. Both enzymes would be in the killer cells.

E. Martz

An important observation was made by John Hiserodt (J. Immunol. 123: 332) of a plausible candidate for a cell-free mediator for T cell mediated lysis. In addition to being cell-free it was T cell dependent, antigen-specific and lysed the standard kinds of target cells that are used, such as P815 and EL4, and it has a short half-life *in vitro*. After that came out, we made some attempts to repeat it but I don't think we spent enough time at it to give it fair trial, although we did not obtain any evidence of a confirmatory nature. I would like to know if anyone else feels that they have given a fair amount of effort to trying to repeat that observation.

B. Bonavida

I don't want to speak for John Hiserodt or the experiments that he's published with Dr. Granger. Actually we have started to carry out this sort of experiment and came up with a soluble cytotoxin mediator from NK effector cells, with selective cytotoxicity for NK targets. It still may be that the cytotoxic material doesn't have to be antigen-specific although it may be derived from antigen-specific CTL. We have not pursued the CTL antigen-specific factor and became interested in the natural killer system.

E. Martz

It would seem we can state that no one here knows of any other laboratory which has made a serious effort to repeat these experiments.

THE DIFFERENCES IN RECEPTOR CROSS REACTIVITY AND CLONAL STRUCTURE BETWEEN CYTOTOXIC T LYMPHOCYTES, SPECIFIC SUPPRESSOR T CELLS AND MEMORY T CELLS IMMUNE TO ANTIGENS OF THE H-2 COMPLEX

B.D. Brondz, I.F. Abronina, Z.K. Blandova, A.V. Karaulov, A.A. Pimenov

Laboratory of Tumour Immunochemistry and Diagnosis, Cancer Research Centre
Kashirskoye Shaussae 6, Moscow 115478, USSR

INTRODUCTION

Study of the T lymphocyte clonal structure is complicated by striking inhomogeneity of T cells responding to the same antigen. T cells are shown to perform various functions; killer, suppressor, helper, delayed hypersensitivity reactions. The relevant T cell subsets appear not to be identical as to the structure of their antigen-binding receptors (1). Moreover, effector T cell receptor contact with an antigen, in addition to providing antigenic recognition, simultaneously promotes triggering of the specific T cell function, particularly the killer activity of cytotoxic T lymphocytes (CTL)(2,3). As other T cell subsets responding to the same H-2 antigen are unable to lyse target cells (TC), it remains unclear in what way the specific T cell function is due to peculiarities of the determinant recognizable by the relevant receptors. In other words, what is the property of the determinant, recognition of which leads to activation of the CTL function.

CTL induced by differences in the whole H-2 complex bear receptors to the products of one H-2 region only, either K or D (4,5). Moreover, CTL directed to a single K/D antigen and shown to respond selectively to a single CTL-determinant, either to the private H-2 specificity or to the adjacent serologically silent determinant (6,7), also proved to be inhomogeneous displaying a cross lysis of third-party TC (8-10). This cross-reactivity has been shown to be due to the capacity of the particular CTL cross-reactive (CR) fractions to adhere to the relevant extraneous TC monolayers, bearing either mutant (11,12), or third-party H-2 haplotypes (13). The same cross absorption was found to be a feature of the anti-H-2 specific suppressor T cells (SSTC), whose particular CR fractions were shown to be capable of adhering to the relevant third-party TC (14).

At the same time, a non-identity could be demonstrated between determinants of tumor antigens recognized by anti-tumor syngeneic CTL and SSTC (15,16). Besides, determinants of hapten- or virus-modified syngeneic TC seemed also to be non-identical, when they are recognized by secondary CTL or their precursors (memory cells, MC) devoid of cytotoxic activity (17).

In the present report, the nature of cross-reactivity of CTL, SSTC and MC receptors was examined in the H-2 system using the technique of CR subset isolation by elution of the lymphocytes adherent to TC monolayers of different origin (18).

ABBREVIATIONS

SSTC, specific suppressor T cells; CTL, cytotoxic T lymphocytes; MC, memory cells; TC, target cells; CR, cross reactive; MLR, mixed lymphocyte reaction; CI, cytotoxic index; II, inhibition index; SD, serologically defined.

MATERIALS AND METHODS

Mice of H-2 congenic strains C57BL/10Sn, abbreviated B10 (H-2^b), B10.D2 (H-2^d), B10.M (H-2^f) and B10.A (H-2^a), recombinant strains B10.D2(R101), abbreviated R101 ($K^dI^dD^b$), B10.D2(R107), abbreviated R107 ($K^bI^bD^d$) as well as mutant strains of the K^b allele bm 1 (K^{ba}) and bm 3 (K^{bd}) were bred in the Laboratory of Experimental Biological Models (Yurlovo) and the Cancer Research Centre (Moscow). Mice of BALB/c (H-2^d), DBA/2 (H-2^d) and C57BL/6, abbreviated B6 (H-2^b) were supplied by the "Stolbovaja" farm.

d anti-d CTL, SSTC and MC were induced in spleens of B10.D2 mice by B6 or B10 cells.

The CTL activity was assayed 10 to 11 d. after i.p. injection of $2x10^7$ EL4 leukemia cells, using ^{51}Cr-labeled peritoneal macrophages as TC (seeded $6x10^4$ per well of FB-96-TC microplates and grown for 2 days). Cytotoxic index (CI) was asessed as a-b/c-b x 100, where a, b and c denote ^{51}Cr release from TC after incubation for 16 h. at 37°C with immune, normal lymphocytes (or culture medium), and 2% solution of sodium dodecyl-sulfate, respectively (19).

The SSTC d anti-b obtained 3 to 4 d. after i.v. injection of $9x10^7$ B10 irradiated spleen cells were treated with 50 µg/ml mytomycin C and assayed in one-way three-cell mixed lymphocyte reaction

(MLR) for 5 d. The inhibition index (II) of the DNA synthesis was assessed as a-b/a x 100, where a and b denote ^{3}H-thymidine incorporation in control and experimental cultures, respectively (mytomycin C pretreated normal B10.D2 spleen cells were added to the control MLR, instead of SSTC)(20).

For induction of the MC d anti-b and anti-K^bI^b, mice of B10.D2 and R101 strains, respectively, were injected i.p. with $5x10^7$ B10 spleen cells or $2x10^7$ EL4 leukemia cells. 8 to 10 weeks later, a mixture of $5x10^6$ responder and heated (at 45°C for 1 h) stimulator spleen cells were incubated in a volume of 2.0 ml of RPMI-1640 medium supplemented with 10% fetal calf serum, 2mM L-glutamine $5x10^{-5}$M 2-mercaptoethanol, 10mM HEPES-buffer and gentamycin in 16-24-TC microplates at 37°C for 4 d. in an atmosphere of 5% CO_2 (21). CTL were tested as described above.

Absorption and elution of lymphocytes were performed on macrophage monolayers cultivated for 24 h. in N 3024 or N 3012 flasks (Falcon Plastics), $25x10^6$ or $10x10^6$ per flask, respectively. 2 to $2.8x10^8$ B10.D2 CTL were added to the washed BALB/c or B10.D2 macrophage monolayer grown in the large flasks. After incubation for 2 h. at 30°C 1 to $1.4x10^8$ non-adherent lymphocytes were absorbed repeatedly in the same conditions on different H-2 haplotype macrophage monolayers pretreated with pronase (Calbiochem) 25 μg/ml to reduce non-specific adherence (22). The non-adherent lymphocytes were harvested, and the adherent ones were washed from serum and eluted for 30 min. at 37°C by pronase at the successive concentrations of 25 μg/ml (fr.I), 100 μg/ml (fr.II), and then by 5 mM EDTA (fr.III) with addition of 1% viocase (GIBCO) in both solutions. After each treatment, the flasks were rocked on a New Brunswick shaker, 180 rpm for 5 min. (18). The number of the eluted cells washed from pronase and EDTA was recounted, and the CTL activity was assayed. Absorption and elution of SSTC on allogeneic macrophage monolayers were performed in the same way but without previous incubation on a syngeneic monolayer and using a pool of the fr.I and II of the eluted cells (20). MC were absorbed for 2 h. at 37°C incubation $15-20x10^6$ immune spleen cells on the macrophage monolayers grown in N 3012 flasks.

RESULTS

The cross-lysis value of third-party H-2^a and H-2^f TC amounted to 4-6% of the direct lysis value of H-2^b TC as judged by the anti-b CTL doses required for the same cytotoxicity, H-2^f TC being lysed more than H-2^a TC (Fig. 1). The cross lysis was specific (H-2^d TC were not lysed) and was shown to be caused by T cells: treatment of CTL with anti-Thy-1.2 serum in the presence of low-tox rabbit complement (Cedarlane) prevented lysis of any TC. At the same time, removal of B cells by passing CTL through nylon wool (23) led to a 1.3 to 1.5 fold increase of the cross lysis (24).

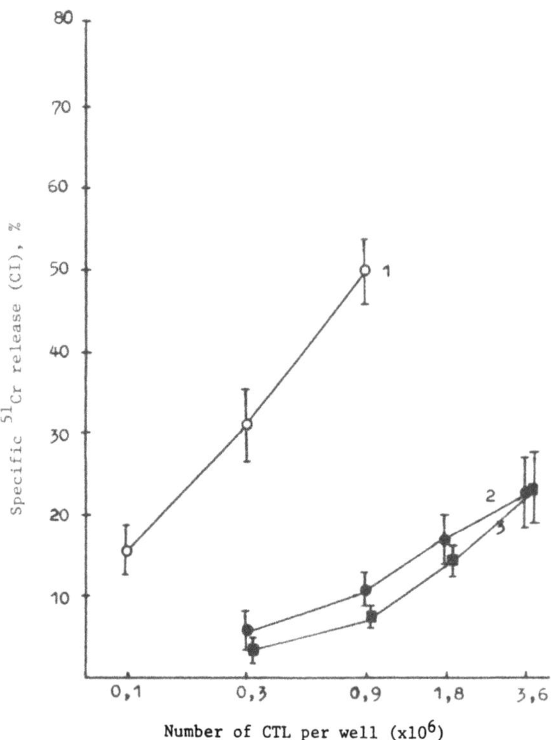

Fig. 1. Direct and cross cytotoxicity of d anti-b CTL as a function of their dose.

TC: B10(1), B10.M(2), B10.A(3). Each point indicates the mean $\pm$ SE of 8 to 14 exps.

Each of CR d anti-b CTL fractions lysing H-2^f TC (Fig. 2b) and H-2^a TC (Fig. 2c), respectively, was found to adhere selectively to the relevant CR haplotype monolayer only. This indicates non-identity of two CR fractions, each of them representing merely a small portion of d anti-b CTL, as judged by the lack of any reduction of the H-2^b TC lysis exerted by CTL non-adherent to H-2^f or H-2^a monolayers. Conversely, the activity of CTL non-adherent to the H-2^b monolayer is reduced similarly (by 54 to 72%) with respect to any TC (Fig. 2 a,b,c). This reduction of the CTL effect was specific, as it was insignificant after two successive absorptions onto BALB/c and B10.D2 monolayers (Fig. 2 a,b,c).

Similar results were obtained when studying the SSTC cross reactivity: each of d anti-b SSTC fractions reacting to H-2^f and H-2^a stimulators, respectively, was found to adhere to the relevant third-party TC in a selective fashion (Table 1). The value of the irrelevant cross SSTC absorption in these cases (when SSTC non-

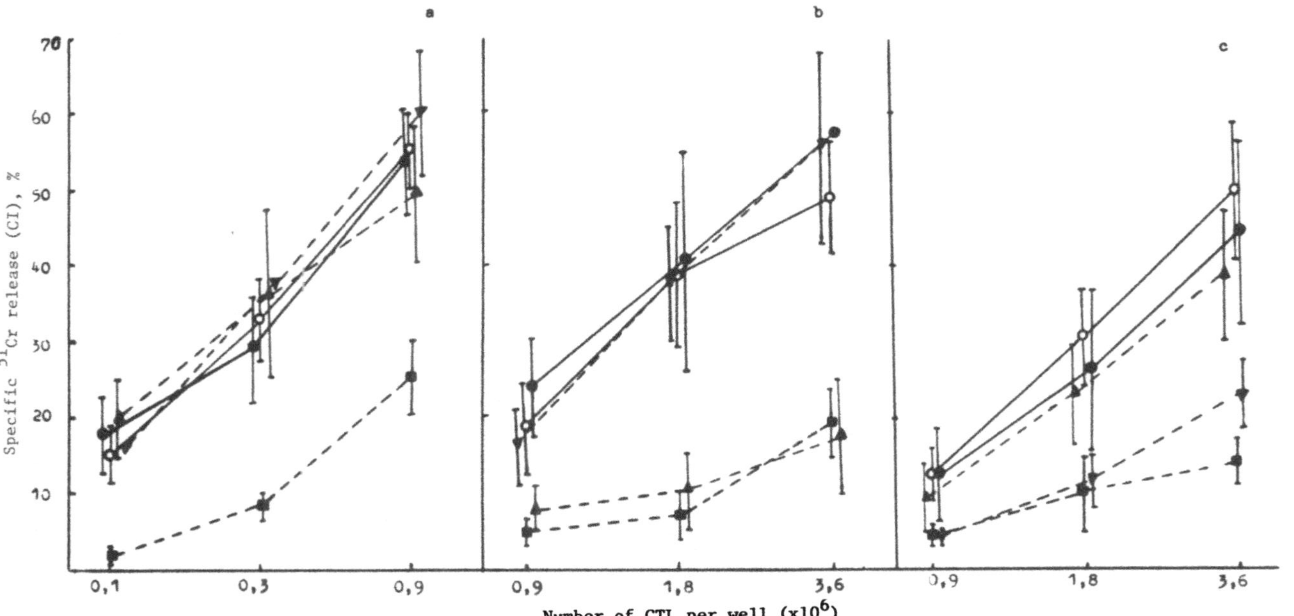

Fig. 2. Absorption of d anti-b CTL on cellular monolayers of different H-2 haplotypes.

TC: B10(a), B10.M(b), B10.A(c). CTL are intact (1) or nonadherent after successive absorption to the macrophage monolayers of BALB/c and B10.D2 (2), BALB/c and B10 (3), BALB/c and B10.M (4), BALB/c and B10.A (5) strains. Each point indicates mean $\pm$ SE of 4 to 8 exps.

TABLE I. Separation of d anti-b SSTC* into two subsets specific to H-2^f and H-2^a

Source of macrophages for SSTC absorption	H-2 specificities**	Stimulators of MLR***	
		B10.M	B10.A
None	-	45.4 ± 2.5	41.5 ± 2.2
B10.D2	-	38.2 ± 5.4 (16.2)	37.8 ± 5.5 (10.3)
B10.M	39,53	7.4 ± 2.6 (84.2)	37.3 ± 4.5 (11.3)
B10.A	5	39.2 ± 3.5 (13.6)	1.3 ± 0.6 (96.8)

* SSTC are enriched by elution from a B10 macrophage monolayer.

** H-2 specificities of monolayer cells potentially capable of reacting to d anti-b SSTC.

*** The figures denote II (%) of ^{3}H-thymidine incorporation (mean ± SE of 5 exp). In parentheses: SSTC absorption index.

adherent to B10.M monolayer were assayed on B10.A stimulators, and vice versa) did not exceed a slight unspecific absorption index on B10.D2 TC (10-16%).

This specific cross absorpton of CTL and SSTC small CR fractions to the relevant third-party TC can be caused by contact of T cell receptors with either serologically defined (SD) public H-2 specificities shared by the immunizing and the CR H-2 haplotypes (Table 1), or the unique CR determinant linked to the private H-2 specificity possessed by the particular third-party H-2 antigen. To resolve this alternative, CR fractions of CTL and SSTC were isolated, and their activity was assayed on TC of different H-2 origin.

Fig. 3. Direct and cross cytotoxicity of d anti-b CTL eluted from macrophage monolayers of B10(a), B10, B10.M and B10.A(b), B10.M(c) and B10.A(d) strains.

TC: B10(o), B10.M(•), B10.A(x). CTL are eluted from B10 (__), B10.M(--), B10.A(-•-) monolayer cells as the fractions II+III (a,c,d). The most active fractions with respect to B10 TC are shown in b: fr. II+III (eluted from B10) and fr.I (eluted from B10.M and B10.A). Each point (here and in Figs. 4 to 6) denotes mean ± SE of 5 to 8 exps or mean of 3 to 4 exps (without vertical bars).

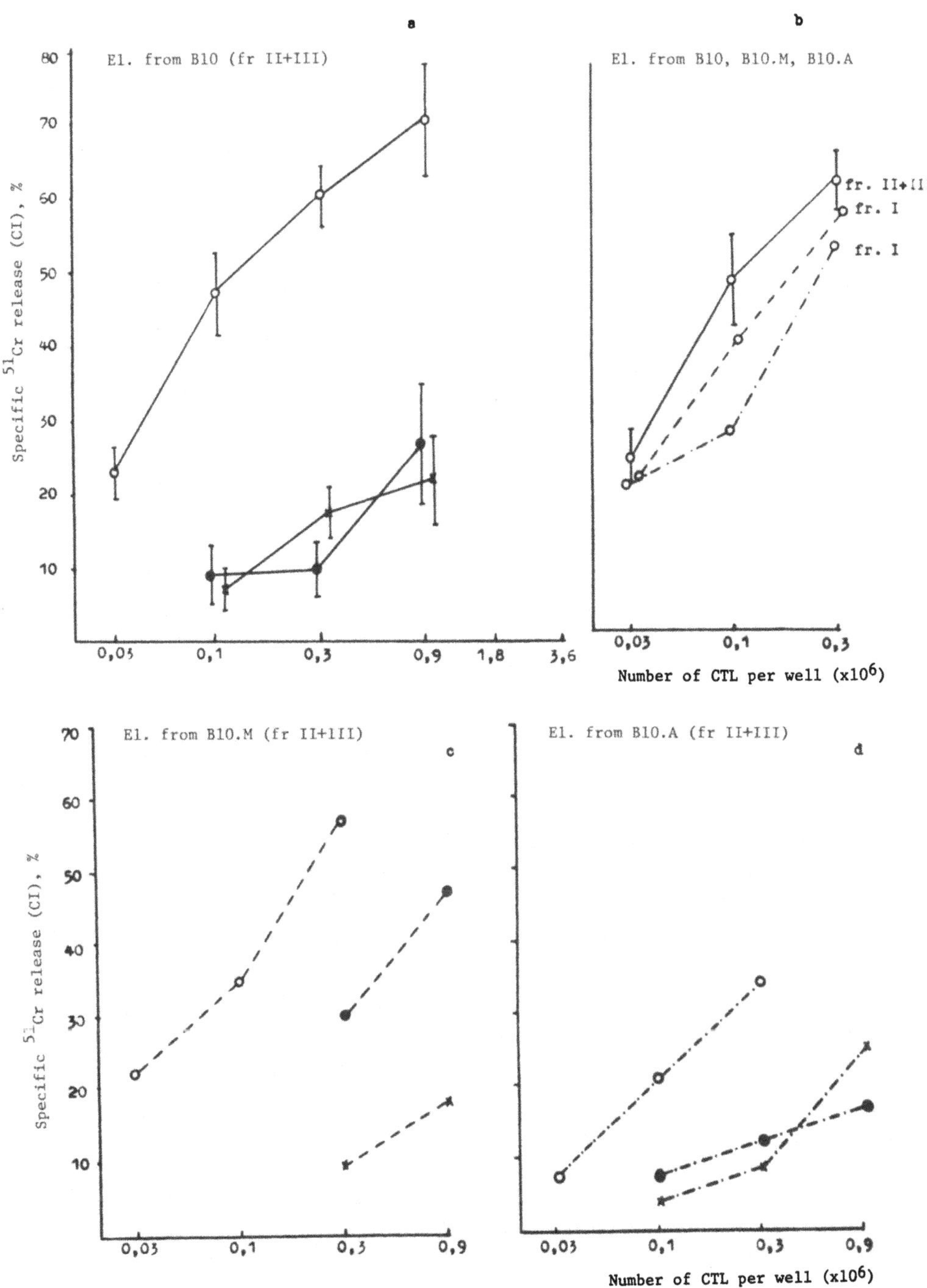
a
b
El. from B10 (fr II+III)
El. from B10, B10.M, B10.A
Specific 51Cr release (CI), %
80
70
60
50
40
30
20
10
0,03
0,1
0,3
0,9
1,8
3,6
fr. II+III
fr. I
fr. I
Number of CTL per well (x10^6)
El. from B10.M (fr II+III)
c
El. from B10.A (fr II+III)
d
Number of CTL per well (x10^6)

Since the CTL enrichment rate detected in a pool of the eluted immune spleen cells appeared to be considerably less as compared to those of the eluted immune lymph node CTL (18), two approaches were employed in this work to increase the elution efficiency: removal of non-specifically "sticky" splenocytes by their previous adherence to the syngeneic (H-2^d) monolayer and separate determination of the CTL activity in each of the eluted fractions. Combination of these methods led to 3-fold and 8-fold CTL enrichment in the fr.I and II+III, respectively (as compared to non-fractionated splenocytes), a sum of fr. II and III lymphocytes accounting for 30-40% of the eluted cells. Similar ratios in the fraction activities were found if d anti-b CTL eluted from H-2^b, H-2^f and H-2^a monolayers were tested on TC of the corresponding haplotypes, although the CTL enrichment rate was shown to be less when CTL were eluted from the H-2^a monolayer (24). Therefore, d anti-b CTL could be enriched by elution of the lymphocytes adherent, not only to the H-2^b monolayer, but to H-2^f and H-2^a CR monolayers as well.

To study the receptor specificity of CR CTL subsets, d anti-b CTL, separated from the lymphocytes non-specifically adherent to the BALB/c cell monolayer, were absorbed on and then eluted from H-2^b, H-2^f and H-2^a cell monolayers and assayed on TC of all three strains.

d anti-b CTL eluted from the H-2^b monolayer (Fig. 3a) as well as intact d anti-b CTL (Fig. 1) are able to lyse H-2^b TC 20 to 30-fold more effectively than H-2^f and H-2^a TC as judged by the lymphocyte number required for the maximum cross lysis. Surprisingly, CR CTL, eluted from H-2^f and H-2^a monolayers, lysed H-2^b TC with almost the same efficiency as CTL eluted from H-2^b monolayer (Fig. 3b). Moreover, each particular CR fraction of d anti-b CTL lysed H-2^b TC considerably more than H-2^f TC (Fig. 3c) and H-2^a TC (Fig. 3d) from which it had been eluted, and displayed cross lysis of the irrelevant third-party TC which was either lower than the lysis of the relevant third-party TC (Fig. 3c), or similar to it (Fig. 3d). In both cases, fr. II+III of the eluted CTL showed 2-to-4-fold gain in cross lysis as compared to the activity of the intact CTL (Fig. 1).

One can see the difference in cytotoxicity between CR CTL eluted from H-2^f monolayer (Fig. 3c) and H-2^a monolayer (Fig. 3d): in the former, CTL lyse H-2^f TC more than H-2^a TC, the difference from the lysis value of H-2^b TC being reduced 5-6-fold for the fr. II+III and 10-12-fold for the fr. I; in the latter, third-party TC of both origins are lysed similarly.

A further peculiarity of CR CTL, isolated by elution from H-2^f and H-2^a monolayers, is that when they were assayed on H-2^b TC, fr. I CTL either did not differ by their activity from fr. II+III CTL, or even exceeded those of fr. II+III CTL (Fig. 4). In all other cases, fr. II+III CTL showed much more cytotoxicity than fr. I CTL.

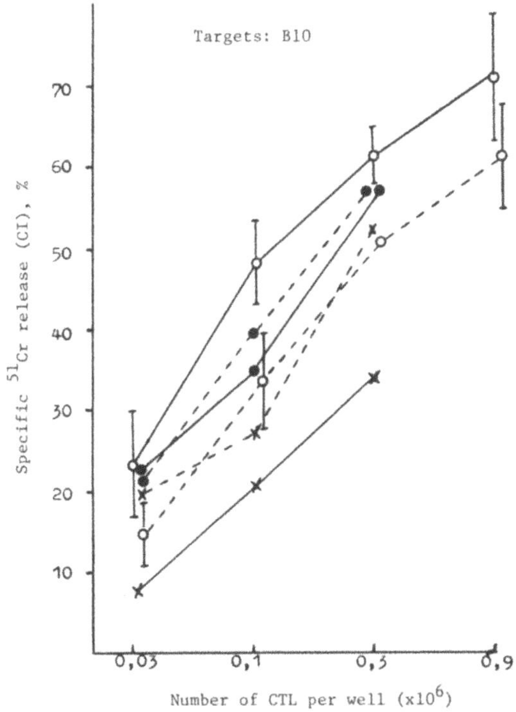

Fig. 4. Comparative cytotoxicity of different CTL fractions eluted from macrophage monolayers of different H-2 haplotypes and assayed on B10 TC. Fractions I (- - -) and II+III (⟵⟶) of the CTL eluted from monolayers of B10(o), B10.M(•) and B10.A(x) cells.

Cross reactivity of d anti-b SSTC appeared to be lower than that of CTL: it was not detected in the intact SSTC but only with SSTC enriched by elution from H-2^b monolayer. In the latter case, the concentration of CR SSTC was found to be about 1/60 out of all SSTC as judged by the increase of the SSTC dose (from 0.6% to 40% with respect to the responders) required for the 50% suppression of MLR triggered by H-2^b stimulators as compared to H-2^f and H-2^a (Fig. 5a).

Further study of the SSTC cross reactivity showed the opposite result as compared to those of CTL. The CR SSTC fractions, isolated by elution from H-2^f and H-2^a monolayers, were found to comprise about 1/60 of SSTC eluted from H-2^b monolayer when they were assayed by suppression of MLR triggered with H-2^b stimulators (Fig. 5b). Moreover, the reactions of the same CR SSTC fractions

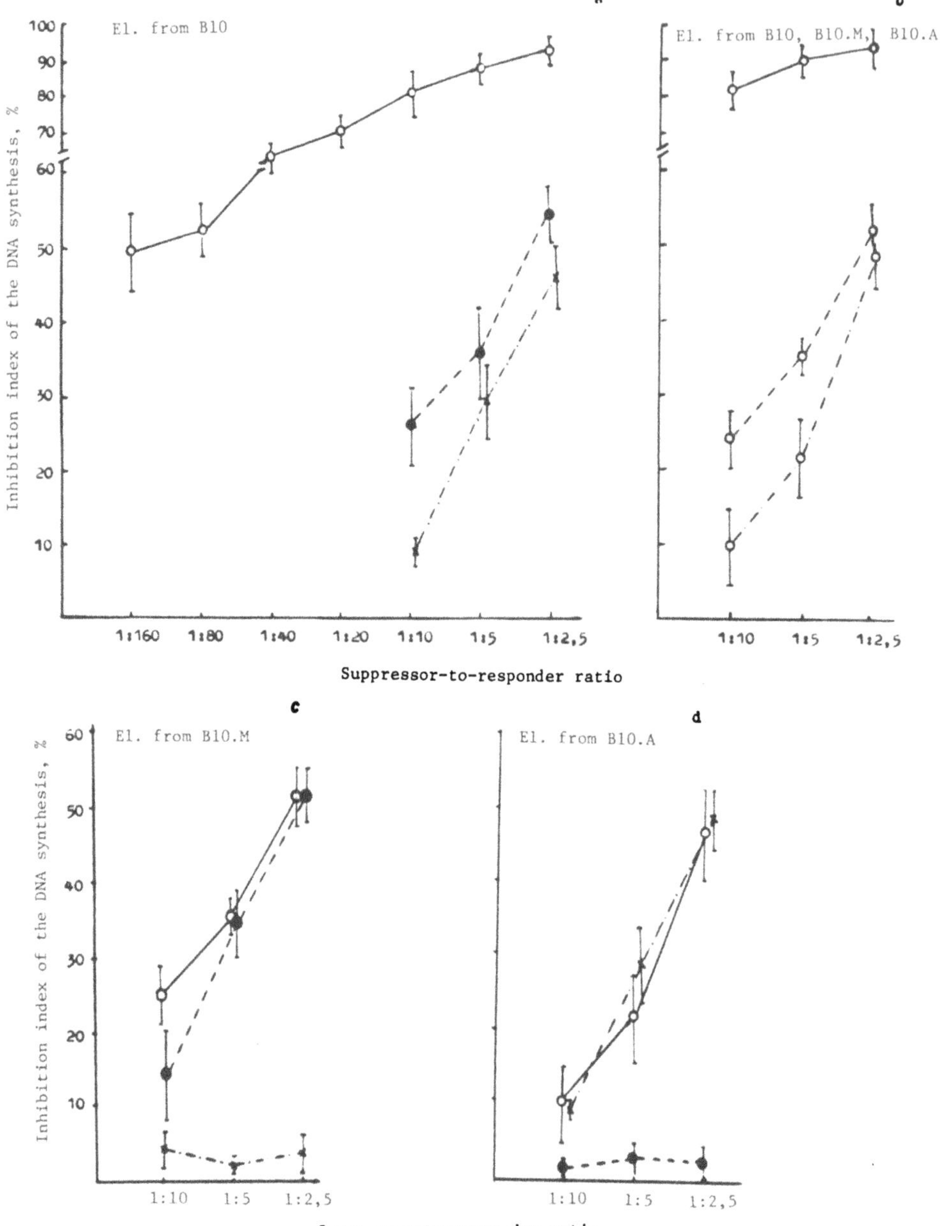

Fig. 5. Direct and cross effects of d anti-b SSTC eluted from macrophage monolayers of B10(a), B10, B10.M and B10.A(b), B10.M(c), B10.A(d) strains. Anti-B10 B10.D2 SSTC eluted from macrophage monolayers of B10 (–), B10.M(––) or B10.A (–•–) strains are pretreated with mitomycin C and mixed with the syngeneic responders triggered in the one-

to H-2^b antigen and to the relevant third-party antigen were found to be equalized, whereas the reaction to the irrelevant third-party antigen disappeared (Fig. 5c and 5d). Therefore, SSTC, unlike CTL, can be suggested to represent a set of narrow-specific clones, each representing about 1.5% of the whole d anti-b SSTC population.

To study clonal structure of d anti-b MC, they were absorbed onto macrophage monolayers bearing either the whole H-2^b haplotype (B10), or the products of K^b and D^b alleles separately, R107 and R101, respectively, or (in controls) the syngeneic H-2^d haplotype (B10.D2). Non-adherent lymphocytes were triggered in MLR by heated B10 cells, and the resulting secondary CTL were assayed on TC of three strains (B10, R107, R101).

Absorption of d anti-b MC by R107 macrophages was found to prevent the secondary CTL generation by the same amount (80 to 90%) as absorption by B10 macrophages. Conversely, absorption of MC by R101 macrophages appeared to be of as low efficiency as the control absorption by B10.D2 macrophages (Fig. 6a). However, when the same secondary CTL were assayed not on B10 TC but on R101 or R107 TC, the CTL generation was prevented only after absorption of MC by macrophages of both B10 origin and the corresponding haplotype, R101 or R107, respectively, but not vice versa (Fig. 6a). Thus, like CTL, MC consist of two populations, at least, each bearing receptors to the products of one of antigens (K or D) of the H-2 complex, but unlike CTL, anti-D^b MC population makes up a minimal portion of MC d anti-b, so that it can be elicited only provided the secondary CTL are assayed on TC devoid of the K^b end.

To study fine receptor structure, anti-B6 R101 MC, directed to the K^b-end only, were absorbed by macrophages of B6 or bm1 mutant. Irrespective of the stimulator origin used for triggering of non-adherent MC, B6 (Fig. 6b) or bm1 (Fig. 6c), absorption of MC by B6 macrophages was shown to prevent the secondary CTL generation with respect to any TC, B6 and bm 1. On the contrary, absorption of the same MC by bm1 macrophages appeared to be either fully non-efficient or highly efficient depending on the TC used for the secondary CTL assay, B6 or bm 1, respectively (Fig. 6 b,c). Unlike bm 1 macrophages, bm 3 macrophages absorbed anti-B6 R101 MC as effectively as B6 macrophages when the secondary CTL were tested on B6 TC (not shown on Fig. 6). In addition, one can notice that the use of bm1 stimulators (Fig. 6c) instead of B6 (Fig. 6b) for MC triggering led to reduction of the efficiency of MC absorption by B6 macrophages, irrespective of the source of TC (B6 or bm1) for secondary CTL.

way MLR by the stimulators of B10(o), B10.M(•) or B10.A(x) origin.

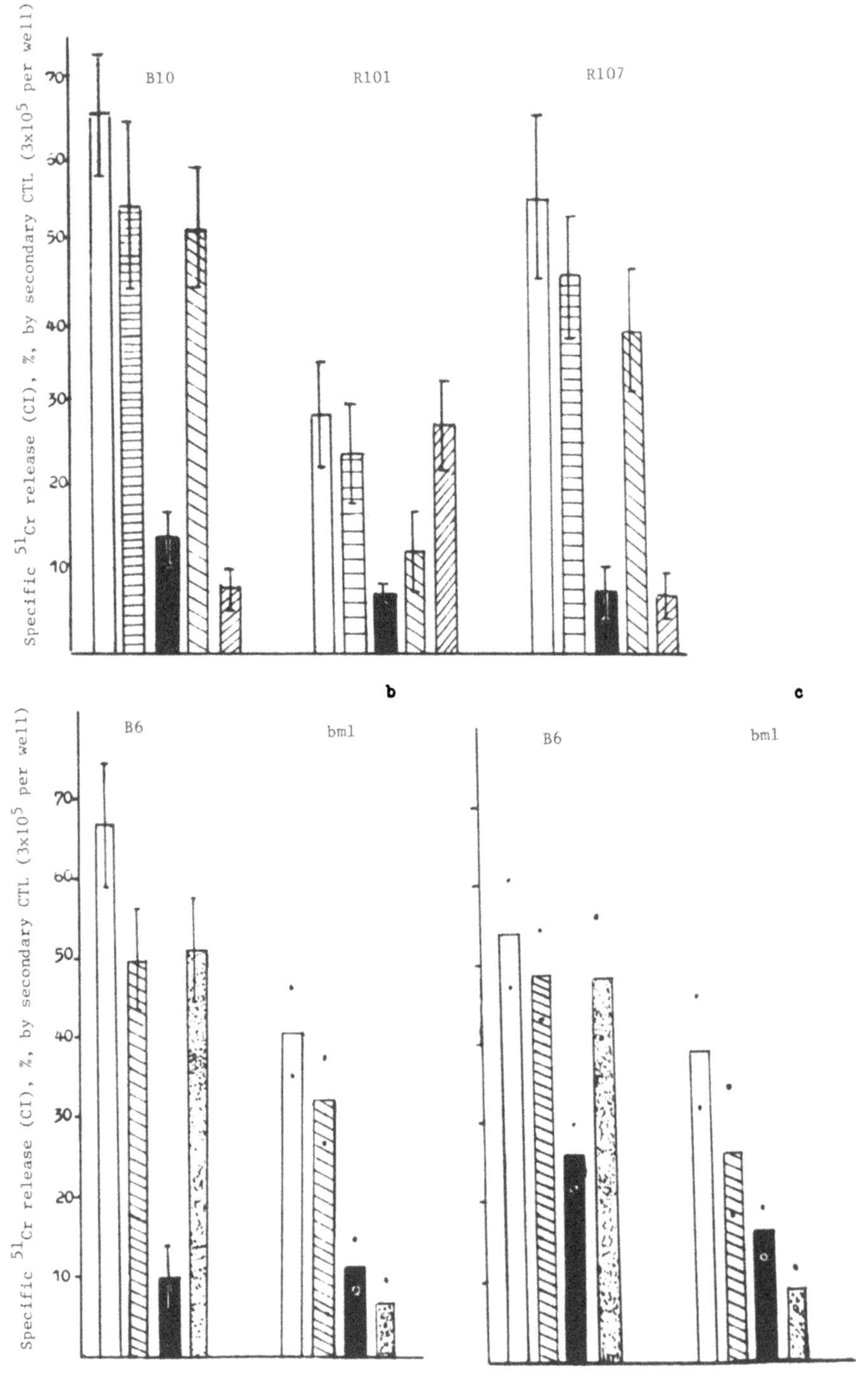
Specific ^{51}Cr release (CI), %, by secondary CTL (3x10^5 per well)
B10
R101
R107
b
c
B6
bm1
B6
bm1

DISCUSSION

H-2 antigens can induce a set of T cell clones which are either non-identical by specificity (each clone bears receptors to the particular SD determinant of the H-2 antigen), or identical by specificity of receptors but differing in affinity or complementarity rate with respect to the immunizing H-2 antigen. In accordance with the former, a single clone only, anti-H-2.5, out of anti-K^b T cell clones bearing receptors to one of SD-specificities, will cross react to H-$2K^k$ antigen of B10.A strain (H-2^a)(Fig. 7a). Alternatively, receptors of all anti-K^b T cells are directed to the unique CTL-determinant of the H-$2K^b$ molecule which represents either the private H-2.33 specificity, or linked to it a serologically silent structure formed by space combination of public SD-specificities foreign for the particular recipient (1). In the latter, those anti-K^b CTL, whose receptors are less complementary to the K^b CTL-determinant and are able to accommodate the K^k CTL-determinant, would be responsible for cross reaction to the H-$2K^k$ antigen (Fig. 7b).

These two alternative T cell clonal structures cannot obviously be distinguished by studies using both direct cross reactions and cross absorption in the H-2 system, since both cross cytotoxicity and selective absorption of the CR CTL fraction on the particular third-party TC would occur in both cases presented in Fig. 7a and 7b, although they would be caused by different mechanisms.

In accordance with previous findings (11-14), the cross reactivity of CTL and SSTC immune to H-2 antigens is shown in the present report to be a consequence of their minor fraction capacity to adhere to the particular CR H-2 antigen in a selective fashion, probably due to pecularities of its receptors differing from those of the rest of the T cell population. The nature of these differences was examined here by assaying the reactivity of the CR CTL and SSTC fractions of the same specificity (d anti-b) isolated by elution from the cellular monolayers bearing third-party H-2 antigens. CTL and SSTC are found to be essentially different in the character of their cross reactivity (see Figs. 5-7).

Fig. 6. Absorption of anti-B10.D2 MC(a) and anti-B6 R101 MC (b,c) on macrophage monolayers bearing the products of K^b or D^b alleles separately (a), or the mutant K^{bm1} antigen (b,c).

Secondary CTL were generated in MLR from MC, intact (□), or non-adherent to macrophage monolayers of B10.D2 (□), B10 (■), R101 (□), R107 (□) and bm1 (▩) origin triggered by the stimulators of B10 (a), B6 (b) or bm1 (c) origin. The source of TC is denoted above.

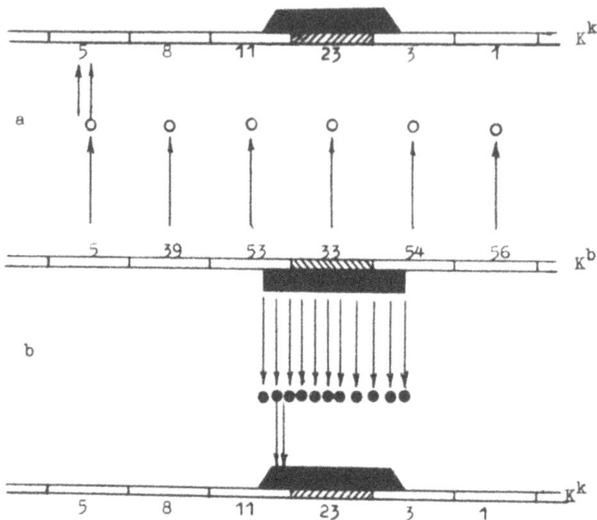

Fig. 7. Scheme of the alternative clonal structure of d anti-b T lymphocytes directed to the K^b antigen and CR to the K^k antigen. Each figure indicates an SD specificity of the K^b and K^k antigens, either public (non-shaded), or private (shaded). The black figures denote the assumed CTL-determinants linked to the private SD specificity. Open and closed circles denote d anti-b lymphocytes of non-identical clonal structure (see text for explanation).

$\longrightarrow$ induction of anti-K^b lymphocytes

$\rightrightarrows$ cross anti-K^b lymphocyte effect to K^k TC.

a: each narrow-specific clone bears receptors to one of SD specificities.

b: all lymphocytes bear receptors to a single CTL-determinant.

The inability of the CR CTL fractions, unlike the CR SSTC ones, to react selectively to the corresponding third-party antigen from which they have been eluted, might result from a non-specific absorption of some d anti-b CTL onto the third-party monolayer contaminating the eluted CTL population. This would give rise to more intensive lysis of H-2^b TC than of CR strain TC. The latter possibility, however, seems unlikely since, firstly, most of the non-specifically "sticky" lymphocytes were removed by a previous absorption onto an

H-2 identical monolayer, and secondly, an appreciable gain in the cytotoxic effect on B10 TC was not found after elution of d anti-b CTL from the syngeneic B10.D2 monolayer as compared to the effect of the intact CTL. Therefore, non-specific absorption did not significantly contribute to the activity of the eluted CTL in our experimental conditions.

One can suppose that, unlike specific SSTC clones (as shown in Fig. 7a), most of the CTL immune to a given H-2 antigen are identical as to the specificity of their receptors, directed to a single CTL-determinant of the H-2 molecule (Fig. 7b). In this case, CTL receptors identical in specificity are different in terms of affinity or flexibility, and therefore, the CTL fraction bearing less complementary (rigid) receptors with lower affinity to the immunizing CTL-determinant, would be capable of accommodating a CTL-determinant of some third-party H-2 antigen. It follows from this suggestion that the CTL fraction I, loosely fixed to the CR antigen is expected to show not lower, but perhaps even more activity with respect to the immunizing antigen than the same CTL fraction II+III firmly adherent to the CR antigen. Just such a result (equalization or inversion of the cytotoxic activity of I and II+III d anti-b CTL fractions eluted from the CR monolayers and assayed on B10 TC) was obtained in this work (Fig. 4). At the same time, non-identity in the activities of the CR CTL eluted from two third-party strains, $H\text{-}2^f$ (Fig. 3b) and $H\text{-}2^a$ (Fig. 3c), with respect to the same strain TC, as well as a selective adherence of the CTL fractions to these two CR strain monolayers (Fig. 2), indicate the non-identity of the CR CTL which presumably are distinguished by the capacity to accommodate their receptors to the particular CR CTL-determinant.

Our findings are in close agreement with the data showing that non-identical CTL immune to a syngeneic H-2 antigen modified with a Sendai virus, give rise to cross lysis of different non-modified allogeneic TC (25) and, conversely, non-identical CTL, induced by an alloantigen give rise to cross lysis of syngeneic TC modified with different haptens (26). The proportion (about 4%) of the CR CTL fractions in these cases, as well as in our experiments seems to reflect a frequency of the corresponding precursors (27). Receptors of the CR CTL appear to differ from those of the remaining CTL by a lower complementarity (affinity) to the immunizing antigen as has been suggested earlier in view of cross lysis of the cloned CTL immune to the influenza virus-modified syngeneic cells (28) and cross binding of third-party H-2 antigens by MLR-induced CTL (29). It is tempting to believe that the diversity of monospecific CTL receptors in the complementarity rate with respect to the single (for a given system) CTL-determinant reflects a general rule related to the structure of CTL receptors.

The study on the cross lysis of d anti-b clones with the use of a set of seven K^b allele mutants as TC, allowed us to suggest multiple (about 23) K^b-antigen determinants recognized by different anti-K^b CTL clonotypes (30). This assumption, however, is at variance with the data that the CR anti-K^b CTL fraction isolated by elution from the bm1 mutant cell monolayer does not differ in the character of its cytotoxicity from all anti-K^b CTL eluted from the K^b-bearing cell monolayer (22). Hence, different anti-K^b CTL clonotypes are expected to bear receptors to a single CTL determinant and to be unable to recognize SD public specificities of the H-2 molecule.

Unlike CTL, SSTC immune to a given H-2 antigen appear to represent, as do B lymphocytes, a set of clones narrowly specific for one out of multiple (presumably SD) determinants of this antigen. They also do not see serologically "silent" mutant antigens of the K^b allele and do not discriminate between bm1 and bm3 mutants (14). Similar data were found upon immunization of mice with syngeneic tumors: SSTC were proved to differ from CTL by the ability to recognize more accurately the specificity of a tumor antigen and by a lower cross reactivity (15,16). It is tempting to suggest that CTL and SSTC essentially differ from each other by their clonal structure, and that their receptors, non-identical by nature, recognize non-identical determinants of the same antigenic molecule. As SSTC have been proved unable to kill TC (20,31,32), triggering of the membrane molecules responsible for killing seems to require the occupation of those T cell receptors only which see the unique (complex?) CTL-determinant of TC.

Transformation of CTL into MC seems to be followed by a change of receptor specificity: when differences in the whole H-2 complex are involved, the fraction of MC with receptors to the D-end products is considerably reduced as compared to those of CTL, while most of the MC induced by the K^b antigen, unlike anti-K^b CTL, prove to be unable to cross react to the bm1 antigen and to discriminate between bm1 and bm3 antigens.

Nonetheless, minor MC subsets may be identified in both cases, bearing receptors to the D^b and bm1 antigens, respectively (Fig. 6). Hence, receptors of most MC can be suggested to differ from those of CTL by more strict specificity, which may be a consequence of a reduced discriminative capacity related to a lower flexibility of the receptors. A similar phenomenon has been shown earlier when CTL and MC immune to virus-modified syngeneic cells were compared (17). These differences in the specificity of CTL and MC receptors could be a consequence of some alteration at the level of either the cell populations or the receptor structures. This question is the subject of our further study.

ACKNOWLEDGEMENTS

The authors with to thank Miss G.N. Vornakova for excellent technical assistance, and Drs. A.P. Suslov and A.V. Chervonsky for valuable critical discussion. The work was partially supported by a WHO grant.

REFERENCES

1. Brondz, B.D., and O.V. Rochlin. Molecular and Cellular Bases of Immunological Recognition (Russian). Nauka, Moscow (1978).
2. Parker, W.L., and E. Martz. Lectin-induced non-lethal adhesion between cytolytic T lymphocytes and antigenically unrecognizable tumor cells and nonspecific "triggering" of cytolysis. J. Immunol. 124:25 (1980).
3. Wei, W.Z., and R.R. Lindgnist. Alloimmune cytolytic T-lymphocyte activity: triggering and expression of killing mechanisms in cytolytic lymphocytes. J. Immunol. 126:513 (1981).
4. Brondz, B.D, and A.E. Snegirova. Interaction of immune lymphocytes with the mixture of target cells possessing selected specificities of the H-2 immunizing allele. Immunology 20:457 (1971).
5. Golstein, P., E.A. Svedmyr, and H. Wigzell. Cell mediating specific in vitro cytotoxicity. I. Detection of receptor-bearing lymphocytes. J. Exp. Med. 134:1385 (1971).
6. Forman, J., and G. Moller. Generation of cytotoxic lymphocytes in mixed lymphocyte reaction. II. Importance of private and public H-2 alloantigens on the expression of cytotoxicity. Immunogenetics 3:211 (1974).
7. Brondz, B.D., I.K. Egorov, and G.I. Drizlikh. Private H-2 specificities as possible selective target for cell-mediated immunity. J. Exp. Med. 141:11 (1975).
8. Forman, J., and J. Klein. Analysis of H-2 mutants. Evidence for multiple CMC target specificities controlled by the $H\text{-}2K^b$ gene. Immunogenetics 1:469 (1975).
9. Melief, C.J.M., deWaal, L.P., van der Meulen, Melvold, R.W., and H.I. Kohn. Fine specificity of alloimmune cytotoxic T lymphocytes directed against H-2K. A study with K^b mutants. J. Exp. Med. 151:993 (1980).
10. Vazquez, A.A., Senyk, Fridman, W.H., and C. Neauport-Sautes. Public H-2 specificities are target determinants for alloreactive cytotoxic T-lymphocytes. J. Immunogen. 7:107 (1980).
11. Andreev, A.V., Drizlikh, G.I., and B.D. Brondz. Interction of anti-K^b and anti-D^d effector lymphocytes with target cells of mutant haplotypes. Bull. Exp. Biol. Med. (Russian) 8: 710 (1976).
12. Geib, R., Ching, C., and J. Klein. Evidence for multiple clones of cytotoxic T cells responding to antigenic determinants on the same molecule. J. Immunol. 120:340 (1978).

13. Vazquez, A., Neauport-Sautes, C., and A. Senik. Separate cyto-T-lymphocyte subsets recognize the different H-2 specificities. J. Exp. Med. 151:776 (1980).
14. Brondz, B.D., Karaulov, A.V., Abronina, I.F., and Z.K. Blandova. Biological immunological and genetic characterization of specific suppressor T cells and their receptors immune to antigens of the H-2 complex. Clonal structure, narrow specificity of receptor and genetic restriction by specific T-suppressor function. Molec. Immunol. 17:833 (1980).
15. Fujimoto, S., Matsuzawa, T., Nakagawa, K., and I. Tada. Cellular interaction between cytotoxic and suppressor T cells against syngeneic tumor in the mouse. Cell. Immunol. 38:378 (1978).
16. Greene, M.I., and L.L. Perry. Population of the immune response to tumor antigens. IV. Differential specificities of suppressor T cells or their products and effector T cells. J. Immunol. 121:63 (1978).
17. Mulbacher, A., and R.V. Blanden. Cross-reactivity patterns of murine cytotoxic T lymphocytes. Cell. Immunol. 43:70 (1979).
18. Brondz, B.D., Egorova, S.G., and I.F. Kotomina. Enrichment of effector T lymphocytes specific to H-2 antigens by elution from allogeneic target cells and characterization of the eluted lymphocyte population. Eur. J. Immunol. 5:734 (1975).
19. Drizlikh, G.I., Andreev, A.V., Kotomina, I.F., and B.D. Brondz. Quantitative estimation of cytotoxic activity of immune lymphocytes using ^{51}Cr-labeled peritoneal macrophages as target cells. J. Immunol. Meth. 8:383 (1975).
20. Brondz, B.D., Karaulov, A.V., Abronina, I.F., and Z.K. Blandova. Requirements for induction of specific suppressor T cells and detection of their H-2 antigen-binding receptors by fractionation on target cell monolayers. Scand. J. Immunol. 13:517 (1981).
21. Rollinghoff, M., and H. Wagner. Secondary cytotoxic allograft response in vitro. I. Antigenic requirements. Eur. J. Immunol. 5:875 (1975).
22. Brondz, B.D., Andreev, A.V., Egorova, S.G., and G.I. Drizlikh. Cross reaction of cytotoxic T lymphocyte antigen-binding receptors immune to antigens of the H-2 system. Scand. J. Immunol. 10:195 (1979).
23. Julius, M.H., Simpson, E., and L.A. Herzenberg. A rapid method for the isolation of functional thymus-derived murine lymphocytes. Eur. J. Immunol. 3:645 (1973).
24. Brondz, B.D., Pimenov, A.A., Blandova, Z.K., and G.N. Vornakova. study on the nature of cross reactivity of cytotoxic T lymphocyte receptors immune to the antigens of the H-2 complex by their fractionation on target-cell monolayers. Molec. Biol. (Russian) 16:000 (1982).
25. Finberg, R., Burakoff, S.J., Cantor, H., and B. Benacerraf. Biological significance of alloreactivity: T cells stimulated by Sendai virus-coated syngeneic cells specifically lyse allo-

geneic target cells. Proc. Natl. Acad. Sci. USA 75:5145 (1978).
26. Levy, R.B., Gilheany, P.E., and G.M. Shearer. Role of self and foreign antigeneic determinants in allogeneic and self-restricted cytotoxic T cell recognition. J. Exp. Med. 152: 405 (1980).
27. Teh, H.S., Phillips, R.A., and R.G. Miller. Quantitative studies on the precursors of cytotoxic lymphocytes. IV. Specificity and cross reactivity of cytotoxic clones. J. Immunol. 120:425 (1978).
28. Komatsu, Y., Nawa, Y., Ballamy, A.K., and J. Marbrook. Clones of cytotoxic lymphocytes can recognize uninfected cells in a primary response against influenza virus. Nature 274:802 (1978).
29. Nagy, Z.A., and B.E. Elliott. The receptor specificity of alloreactive T cells. Distinction between stimulator K I and D region products and degeneracy of third-party H-2 recognition by low-affinity T cells. J. Exp. Med. 150:1520 (1979).
30. Sherman, L.A. Dissection of the B10.D2 anti-H-2K^b cytolytic T lymphocyte receptor repertoire. J. Exp. Med. 151:1386 (1980).
31. Orosz, C.G., and F.H. Bach. Alloantigen-activated CML suppression independent of cytotoxic activity. J. Immunol. 123: 1419 (1979).
32. Brondz, B.D., Karaulov, A.V., Chervonsky, A.V., and Z.K. Blandova. Requirement of the localization of both appropriate and irrelevant H-2 antigens on the same stimulator cell for unspecific DNA synthesis inhibition caused by the H-2 antigen-primed specific suppressor T cells. Immunogenetics 14:000 (1981).

SECTION II. LYSIS BY NON-T CELLS AND BY COMPLEMENT

INTRODUCTION

Could lysis be exclusively caused by a soluble product secreted by the effector cell upon recognition of the target cell? Evidence for this in the T cell system is scarce, and objections are many, but in NK-mediated lysis and in antibody-dependent cell-mediated cytolysis (briefly dicussed by Perlmann) ring-shaped structures were observed by electron microscopy, which could represent pore-forming substances transferred from the effector cell into the target cell membrane (Henkart and Henkart). This hypothesis comes very close to assimilating at least in part the mechanisms of cell- and complement-mediated cytolysis. Whether this assimilation is feasible is discussed, together with some of the characteristics of the latter system (Lachmann; Mayer).

Of the cellular cytotoxicity systems discussed in this volume, the lytic mechanism involved in macrophage killing of target cells is probably the closest to being understood. But, as pointed out by Mike Hanna's group, there may not be a unique mechanism by which macrophage cytolysis is carried out. Both phagocytic and non-phagocytic (extracellular) processes can be involved, sometimes in combination. The localized secretion of granular contents onto target cells, generally thought to be unique to macrophages, was suggested earlier in this volume by Zagury to be involved in CTL killing as well. Some parallels, at least at the morphological level, may also be seen between extracellular macrophage cytotoxicity and K cell killing, as suggested by the Henkarts. Investigators in the field of lymphocyte mediated cytotoxicity may thus find renewed interest in the study of extracellular killing by macrophages.

Yet another possible mechanism by which macrophages perturb and perhaps kill target cells is discussed in John Hibb's review. His group has found that cytotoxic "activated" macrophages inhibit metabolic pathways in target cell membranous organelles, e.g., DNA synthesis in nuclei and respiration in mitochondria. This review includes speculations on the relation of macrophage killing of certain target cells to normal tissue degenerative processes, and to other modes of cell-mediated cytotoxicity.

The mechanisms by which NK cells kill appropriate target cells, and the relationship of these mechanisms (and indeed, of NK cells themselves) to other lymphocyte effector systems, are questions very much in the forefront of immunological research. The scope of this research is indicated in the review by Herberman's group. Henney comments on the relation of NK cells to CTL, and discusses his findings on the target antigens recognized by NK effectors. NK target antigens are also the topic of Rolf Kiessling's paper. He presents additional evidence that NK targets may have something in common with stem cells that occur naturally in the body. Possible mechanisms are discussed by Ron Goldfarb, who reviews in some detail his and others findings on the involvement of proteases and phospholipases in various lytic systems, but particularly NKCC. A particularly intriguing possible mechanism is suggested by Bonavida, who summarizes his evidence for involvement of a soluble factor mediating NK killing of target cells. Targan describes a mAb specific for NK cells that appears to block lysis at a post-recognition stage.

MEMBRANE ATTACK BY COMPLEMENT (WITH COMMENTS ON CELL-MEDIATED CYTOTOXICITY)

Manfred M. Mayer

Johns Hopkins University School of Medicine
Department of Molecular Biology and Genetics
Baltimore, MD 21205

ENZYMATIC ACTIVATION OF THE COMPLEMENT SYSTEM

As shown in the simplified scheme in Fig. 1, the complement system comprises two routes of activation, the classical and the alternative activation pathways, and a single membrane attack sequence which can be initiated by either one of the activating pathways.

The Classical Activation Pathway

This pathway comprises Clq, Clr, Cls, C4,C2, C3 and C5. Activation is initiated when Clq combines with two Fc segments of immunoglobin G or M in an antigen-antibody complex. This leads to activation of the enzymes Clr and Cls. (Activation can also be mediated by agents other than antigen-antibody complexes, for example, RNA tumor viruses, central nervous system myelin, or the lipid A component of lipopolysaccharides.) When activated, Cls can split a susceptible peptide bond in the alpha chain of the C4 molecule, thus producing fragments C4a and C4b. In this process, an internal thioester is cleaved generating a transiently reactive carboxyl group on the C4b molecules, some of which then become esterified with hydroxyl groups on a nearby cell surface. In this way C4b molecules become covalently bound on the surface of a cell under attack by complement.

Activated Cls also cleaves the C2 molecule, producing fragments, C2a and C2b. In the presence of Mg^{++}, the former combines non-covalently with the bound C4b, thus generating C4b,2a, an enzyme complex which is called "C3 convertase" because the catalytic site on the C2a fragment cleaves a susceptible peptide bond in the alpha chain of the C3 protein.

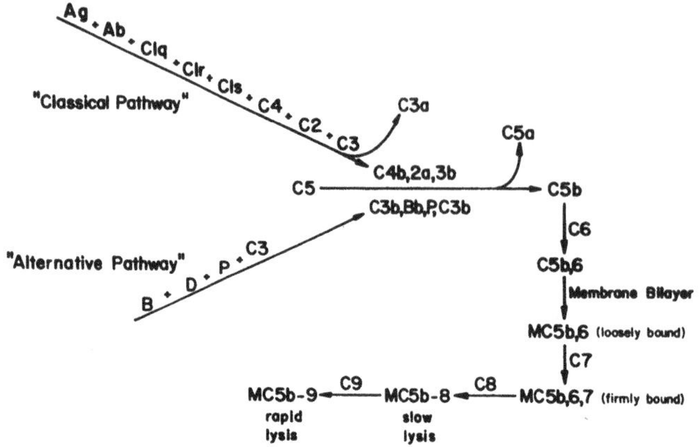

Fig. 1. Schematic representation of the reaction pathways of the complement system. This scheme summarizes the classical and alternative pathways of C activation leading to the assembly of the C5 cleaving enzymes C4b,2a,3b and C3b, Bb,P,C3b. Antigen and antibody are represented by Ag and Ab. C1, C2, B, P, etc. stand for C proteins. The letters a and b, as in C4b or C2a, indicate fragments of their respective components. The C5b-9 sequence, the final common pathways, begins with the cleavage of C5. The C5b fragment complexes with C6 and is thus stabilized. The C5b6 complex combines reversibly with membranes but its binding affinity is very low. Cell-bound C3b enhances the binding affinity of C5b6 and thus increases the efficiency of the membrane attack process. Reaction of C5b6 with C7 leads to deep insertion of hydrophobic peptides from these proteins into the membrane bilayer. When inserted C5b6,7 reacts with C8, a hydrophobic peptide from this protein becomes exposed and is inserted into the bilayer. This leads to formation of small channels that cause slow lysis. When the inserted C5b-8 reacts with C9, a hydrophobic peptide from this protein is exposed and becomes inserted into the lipid bilayer. This causes formation of stable channels, some of which are quite large, with consequent rapid lysis.

The cleavage of C3 is similar to that of C4. A small fragment, C3a, is released and a transiently reactive carboxyl group is activated on C3b, the remainder of the molecule. This group may then become esterified with a hydroxyl group on a nearby cell surface. When a C3b fagment becomes bound in the correct stereochemical configuration in the vicinity of a C4b,2a complex, a new complex, C4b, 2a,3b, is generated which is designated "C5 convertase" because it cleaves the C5 molecule. In this enzyme, the C3b subunit contributes a binding site for the substrate, C5, and C2a supplies the catalytic site.

The Alternative Activation Pathway

This pathway comprises C3 and three other proteins designated by the letters B, D and P. It can be activated on the surfaces of numerous microbes, even without antibody and thus serves as an important protective mechanism during the early stages of an infectious process when a specific immune response has not yet developed.

The alternative pathway is activated when Factor D, an active enzyme in blood, cleaves molecules of B that are transiently associated with C3, thus generating a small amount of C3-cleaving enzyme designated C3,Bb. This enzyme produces C3b in normal blood serum, though at a low rate. Like native C3, the C3b fragment can associate transiently with B, which is then cleaved by D, yielding a second C3-cleaving enzyme, designated C3b,Bb. Both C3,Bb and C3b,Bb are unstable since they are subject to spontaneous dissociation. Their stability is influenced positively by a protein called properdin (P), and negatively by a protein called H and an enzyme designated I (C3b inactivator). Under normal physiologic conditions, the C3-cleaving enzymes of the alternative pathway in the fluid phase of blood or tissue fluids are held at a very low level due to these control processes. By contrast, on certain microbes a substantial amount of C3-cleaving enzyme of the composition C3b,Bb,P can be formed because the microbial surface protects the complex against breakdown by H and I. The C3b subunit in C3b,Bb,P serves as a ligand to cell surfaces and P functions as a stabilizer. The Bb subunit is an analog of the C2a subunit in the C4b,2a enzyme of the classical pathway, both structurally and enzymatically.

The alternative pathway C3 convertase can become a C5 convertase by uptake of an additional C3b fragment which supplies a binding site for the substrate, C5.

The Enzymatic Cleavage Products of the Classical and Alternative Pathways

C4a and C3a are peptides that cause release of histamine and other factors from cells such as basophilic leukocytes, mast cells and platelets. As noted already, the large fragments, C4b and C3b, have the capacity, when freshly generated, to esterify with hydroxyl groups on a cell surface. Cells carrying C4b or C3b adhere to leukocytes or other cells that possess receptors. This "immune adherence" promotes phagocytosis.

Cleavage of C5 by the C5 convertases produces C5a, a peptide of about 11,000 daltons, which is a chemotactic factor. Also, like C4a and C3a, it releases histamine from cells that store this substance.

The large fragment, C5b, about 190,000 daltons, initiates a series of reactions with the other terminal complement proteins (C6, C7, C8 and C9) that mediate the process of membrane attack against targets such as envelope viruses, bacteria, protozoa, fungi and cells of higher organisms. (For detailed background review, cf. Ref. 1.)

THE MEMBRANE ATTACK PATHWAY

The membrane attack pathway is initiated when C5 is cleaved into C5a and C5b by the C5 convertases of the classical or alternative activation pathways. The C5b fragment decays to a cytolytically inactive form immediately after its release from the convertase into the fluid phase. The mechanism of this decay is unknown. However, if C5b combines with C6 while it is still associated with the convertase, its cytolytic capacity becomes stabilized. As a consequence, when the C5b6 complex dissociates from the convertse and diffuses into the fluid phase, its C5b subunit remains in the "activated" state, i.e., capable of initiating the cytolytic process. Hence, C5b6 may be regarded as a stable form of "activated" C5b. When C5b6 is added to a membrane, a very small proportion of it becomes reversibly adsorbed. The reversible adsorption of C5b6 is substantially increased by membrane-bound C3b. On addition of C7, the complex C5b6,7 is formed which binds firmly and irreversibly to the membrane. This is attributed to conformational changes and consequent insertion of hydrophobic peptides from C5b, C6 and C7 into the hydrocarbon of the bilayer membrane. On addition of C8, the complex C5b6,7,8 (abbreviated C5b-8) is formed. This reaction presumably involves a conformational change in the C8 molecule which exposes a hydrophobic peptide that becomes inserted in the hydrocarbon core of the lipid bilayer. Small unstable hydrophilic passages across the membrane appear at this stage. On reaction of C5b-8 with C9, a hydrophobic peptide from this protein is inserted into the hydrocarbon core of the lipid bilayer and large stable trans-membrane channels are formed.

The concept that the lipid bilayer of cell membranes is the target of complement attack originated in studies by Haxby et al. (2) in which it was shown that complement activation on the surface of liposomes made with phospholipid and cholesterol releases glucose that had been trapped in the aqueous compartments (Fig. 2). Subsequent studies showed that complement can release trapped marker from liposomes made with phospholipid analogs that are not susceptible to phospholipases (3). Therefore, an enzymatic mode of membrane damage was excluded and, instead, a detergent-like mechanism was suggested by Kinsky (3). However, lysis by a detergent substance of low molecular weight is a highly cooperative process, as evidenced by the sigmoidal shape of the dose-response curve, and thus conflicts directly with the well-known non-cooperative or one-hit characteristic of complement-mediated hemolysis (4). In view of this, and in light

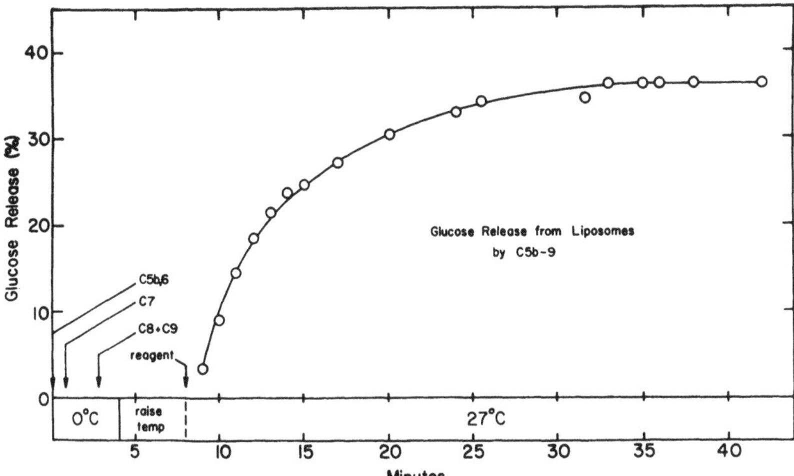

Fig. 2. Release of glucose from liposomes by C5b-9. Multilamellar lecithin liposomes containing glucose trapped in their aqueous compartments were treated sequentially with C5b6 + C7 + C8 + C9, as indicated (unpublished data from experiment by M.L. Shin).

of the development of the Singer-Nicolson fluid mosaic model of membrane structure (5), I proposed about ten years ago that complement causes membrane damage by formation of channels (6). In essence, this hypothesis describes a trans-membrane channel that has a stable, hollow structure with a hydrophobic exterior face and a hydrophilic interior surface. It was pointed out that the terminal complement proteins, C5, C6, C7, C8 and C9 are the most probable source of the structural components of such a channel. Furthermore, it was suggested that the formation of the channel proceeds in three stages: (1) A series of successive interactions among the terminal complement proteins which lead to exposure of hydrophobic peptides; (2) insertion of these peptides into a nearby lipid bilayer, and (3) assembly into trans-membrane channels. Since then, numerous experimental investigations in several laboratories have addressed these processes.

Three Stages of Channel Formation

(1) Hydrophobic exposure: It has been shown in several ways that activation of the terminal complement proteins, C5 - C9, leads to exposure of lipid binding sites. Thus, binding of phospholipid was demonstrated by Shin et al. (7) and confirmed by Podack et al. (8). (Cf. Ref. 9 for detailed comment.) Furthermore, binding of Triton (10) and of desoxycholate (11) have been reported. Also, charge-shift electrophoresis experiments indicate a change from hydrophilic to amphiphilic behavior during the terminal reaction sequence (10,

11). As a result of these investigations, consensus has developed on the issue of hydrophobic exposure.

(2) Insertion into the lipid bilayer: Experimental studies aimed at demonstrating insertion of complement proteins into lipid bilayer membranes have followed approaches that were pioneered in studies of membrane proteins. Thus, integral or intrinsic membrane proteins, like glycophorin, resist elution from membranes by ionic manipulations with various solvents and are refractory to enzymatic stripping by proteases. On the other hand, peripheral membrane proteins, like cytochrome c, can often be removed by the above treatments. The first positive experimental indications for the insertion hypothesis came from tests by Hammer et al. on elution of ^{125}I-C5b (12). A striking difference was observed between elution experiments with EAC1-6 (erythrocytes carrying antibody and complement proteins C1 through C6) and EAC1-7, both containing ^{125}I-C5b. Thus, radioiodinated C5b eluted readily with 0.3 M NaCl from EAC1-6, but not from EAC1-7. This observation was interpreted as a possible indication that C5b had become inserted into the membrane during the conversion of EAC1-6 to EAC1-7 by reaction with C7. Experiments on elution of radioiodinated C9 from EAC1-9 have also yielded results suggesting insertion (13). (Cf. also Refs. 14 and 11).

The issue of insertion has also been investigated by proteolytic stripping experiments with radioiodinated C3, C5, C7, C8 and C9 on various erythrocyte intermediates. Trypsinization removed practically all of the ^{125}I-C3 from the intermediate EAC1-6 and EAC1-7 (12)(Fig. 3). Similarly, radioiodinated C5 was removed completely from EAC1-6 by trypsinization (12)(Fig. 4). On the other hand, only about one-half of the ^{125}I-C5 could be stripped from the intermediate EAC1-7(12)(Fig. 4). This difference, which corresponds to that in the elution experiments, was taken as a possible indication that part of the C5 molecule had become inserted in the lipid bilayer during the formation of EAC1-7 from EAC1-6. Similar experiments with radioiodinated C7, C8 and C9 also may be interpreted as an indication of insertion (12,13)(Fig. 4). It should be emphasized that the evidence provided by the proteolytic stripping experiments is unidirectional. While it rules out insertion of C3, it does not rigorously prove insertion of C5, C7, C8 and C9 because the resistance to stripping by proteases might be due to a cause other than insertion.

Convincing evidence supporting the insertion concept has become available in a recent study with the membrane-restricted photoreactive glycolipid probe 12-(4-azido-2-nitrophenoxyl) stearoyl [I-^{14}C] glucosamine, which only labels integral membrane proteins. By use of this probe, V.W. Hu et al. (15) have demonstrated directly that C5b, C6, C7, C8 and C9 enter the hydrophobic milieu of the lipid bilayer during membrane attack by complement (Fig. 5). These observations have been confirmed in experiments by Podack et al. (16).

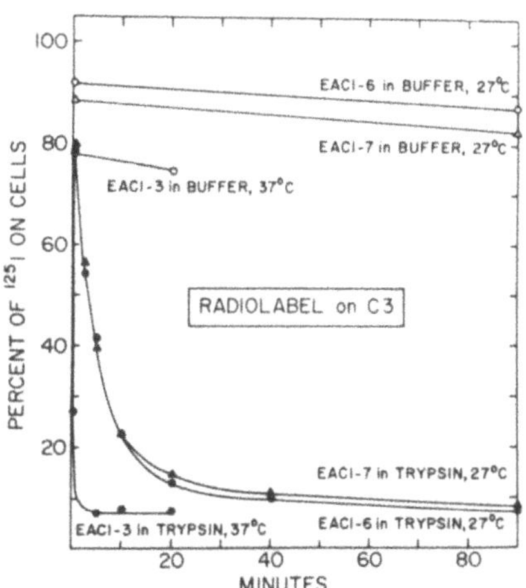

Fig. 3. Kinetics of tryptic removal of ^{125}I from EAC1-3 (⬢) EAC1-6 (●) and EAC1-7 (▲) carrying ^{125}I-C3b. The intermediates EAC1-3, EAC1-6 and EAC1-7 were prepared with radioiodinated C3. (For example, EAC1-3 refers to erythrocytes carrying antibody and all of the complement proteins up to and including C3.) The enzymatic digestion was performed with 0.1% trypsin at pH 7.4 and ionic strength 0.075. Buffer controls for each of these intermediates are shown by corresponding open symbols. The sudden initial release of ^{125}I in the controls was due to temperature and ionic strength shift.

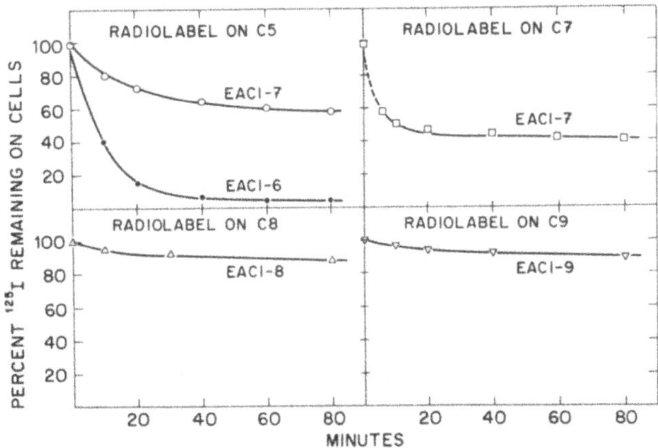

Fig. 4. Kinetics of tryptic removal of ^{125}I from EAC1-6 (●) of EAC1-7 (○) carrying ^{125}I-C5b, or from EAC1-7 carrying ^{125}I-C7 (□); or from EAC1-8 carrying ^{125}I-C8 (△), or from EAC1-9 carrying ^{125}I-C9 (▽).

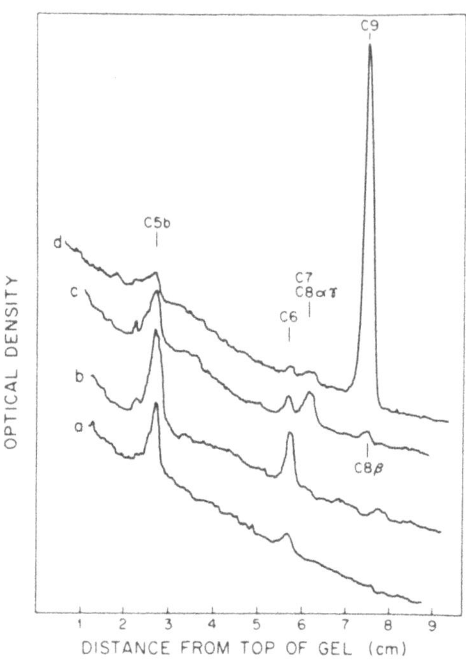

Fig. 5. Photolabeling of C components as a function of complex assembly. Densitometric scans of radioautograms from gels show protoactivated probe association with individual complement proteins. The gels were loaded with lecithin vesicles carrying complement complexes that had been irradiated at the following stages: (a) C5b6, (b) C5b-7, (c) C5b-8, (d) C5b-9. (From Hu et al., Ref. 15.)

I regard the insertion of complement peptides as a manifestation of a partition which occurs during the interaction of activated complement with nearby lipid bilayers. In this process, some of the hydrophobic peptides become inserted into the membrane and form channels, while others bind phospholipid molecules from the membrane and form lipoprotein complexes in the aqueous phase.

(3) Formation of Trans-Membrane Channels: The fact that the hemolytic action of complement conforms to a non-cooperative or one-hit mechanism is a direct indication that channels are formed because mechanisms causing membrane disintegration would display cooperative or multi-hit characteristics. Further evidence indicating channel formation has come from molecular sieving experiments with resealed erythrocyte ghosts containing markers of appropriate molecular dimensions. Fig. 6 shows a series of kinetic experiments with marker molecules ranging from raffinose (1.1 nm diameter) to human serum albumin (ellipsoid, 3.1 x 15.3 nm; twice Stokes' radius = 7.1 nm). It is evident that all of the markers up to and

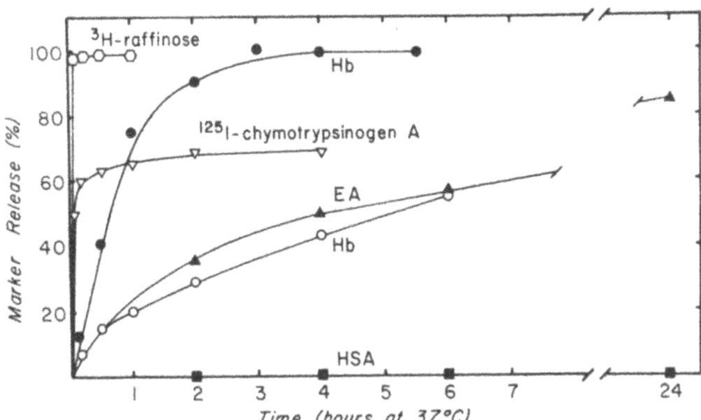

Fig. 6. Release of various marker proteins from ghosts treated with antibody and whole serum C. Release of ovalbumin (EA) and human serum albumin (HSA) was measured by radial immunodiffusion with antisera against these proteins. ^{3}H-raffinose and ^{125}I-chymotrypsinogen A were measured by radioactivity. The latter marker is included to illustrate the aberrant behavior of a radioiodinated protein. Hb release was measured spectrophotometrically at 412 nm. The open symbols indicate experiments in which the ghosts were treated with 16.7 µl of serum C per ml. The closed symbols represent experiments with 66.7 µl of serum C per ml.

including ovalbumin (5.5 nm diameter) were released from the complement-treated ghosts, while human serum albumin was not (17). Obviously, the demonstration of an upper size limit beyond which marker molecules are not released constitutes evidence that in erythrocyte ghosts complement mediates channel formation rather than membrane disintegration. There are cases in which complement causes membrane disintegration. For example, large doses of complement disassemble the envelope membrane of murine leukemia viruses (18); similarly, complement disintegrates the outer membrane of *E. coli* (19-21).

More recent experiments (22) by double marker molecular sieving with resealed erythrocyte ghosts have shown that whole serum complement forms a series of well-defined trans-membrane channels that fall into three size ranges, namely 0.5-0.9 nm, 1.1-3 nm, 3-7 nm. (The demonstration of these size ranges represents a minimal estimate.) It is likely that all of these are attributable to C5b-9 complexes. (Also, cf. Ref. 29.)

Channel stability

In the experiments cited in the preceding paragraph, the release of the markers after complement attack was followed until a state of equilibrium between the ghosts and the surrounding fluid was obtained. No channels were lost during this period (ca. 3 hr) indicating channel stability. With certain marker pairs (e.g., inositol and sucrose), it was found that the proportion of ghosts releasing the smaller (inositol, 0.7 nm molecular diameter) was somewhat larger than that releasing the bigger marker (sucrose, 0.9 nm molecular diameter). This means that a sub-population of the ghosts contained a channel capable of discriminating between the two markers and, hence, possessing an effective diameter intermediate between the molecular diameters of the two markers. In the present example this channel lies between 0.7 and 0.9 nm. These observations also indicate stability because fluctuations in channel diameter sufficient to encompass the differential in marker size (0.2 nm) would have led to identical marker release from all of the ghosts. The lack of fluctuation in these studies agrees with electrical conductance experiments on lipid bilayer membranes in which Michaels observed that C5b-9 channels do not fluctuate and are not polarity dependent (30). By contrast, he found that C5b-8 channels fluctuate and are sensitive to electrical polarity (30).

Structure of the Complement Channels

There has been disagreement on the nature of the hydrophilic passages across the membrane that are produced by the terminal complement proteins. In my view, as well as that of Bhakdi et al., the C5b-9 passage is a protein channel located within the interior of the C5b-9 complex. The initial proposal of this concept (6) was based on the one-hit theory (4) and on the stability of the membrane lesions (6) produced by complement, because only a rigid channel structure could satisfy these requirements. By contrast, the Müller-Eberhard group has proposed a hydrophilic lipid channel that is formed by head groups of reoriented phospholipid molecules around the periphery of inserted complement protein (8,23). Several reasons for rejecting this proposal have been detailed in a review article (9). More recently, they have put forward a "leaky patch" model (25) involving formation of a ring of several C5b-9 complexes (dimers of C5b-9, in their view, Ref. 24), the center of which becomes leaky and thus forms a hydrophilic passage across the membrane (26). They have suggested that the heterogeneity of channel size is due to variation in size of the ring depending on the number of constituent putative $(C5b\text{-}9)_2$ complexes. However, this model is in conflict with unpublished measurements by Louise Ramm in this laboratory which show that the channel through which a large marker (inulin, 3 nm molecular diameter) is released from resealed erythrocyte ghosts contains only one molecule each of C5 and C6. This experiment indicates that even large channels exist in the membrane as C5b-9 monomers (27), rather than dimers or higher polymers.

However, the disputes on the structure of the hydrophilic transmembrane passage are now approaching resolution. In a recent paper of the Müller-Eberhard group (28) they consider it likely that the membrane-associated C5b-9 contains some form of internal protein channel. (This view was reaffirmed at the Ninth International Complement Workshop, November 22-24, 1981 at Key Biscayne, Fla.)

Factors Influencing Channel Formation

In studies with phospholipid/cholesterol liposomes by M. Shin et al. (31) it has been found that the release of trapped marker by complement is inversely related to the length of the phospholipid acyl chains. A corresponding effect has been observed in BLM experiments by Michaels. Presumably, this reflects the greater probability of spanning the bilayer by complement peptides when the acyl chains are relatively short.

It has been shown that the release of trapped marker from liposomes, or of hemoglobin from erythrocytes, varies inversely with the concentration of membrane cholesterol (31). Also, sheep erythrocytes can be rendered more susceptible to complement attack by increasing the ratio of lecithin to sphingomyelin in their membranes (33). These observations have been interpreted as an indication that increased membrane fluidity exerts a promoting effect on the efficiency of complement attack.

Similarly, incorporation of A2C [2-(2-methoxy-ethoxy)-ethyl-8-(cis-2-n-octyl-cyclopropyl)-octanoate], a fluidizing and fusogenic agent, into the membranes of sheep erythrocytes greatly increases their susceptiblity to lysis by C5b6 + C7 + C8 + C9. The enhancing effect of A2C on complement efficiency is operative in the formation of EC5b6,7 as well as in the subsequent reactions with C8 and C9 · (33,34). Parenthetically, it should be noted that enhancement of the terminal complement pathway is not a general property of amphiphiles. Thus, the detergents SDS, melittin and Triton X-100 do not act like A2C in tests for complement enhancement. The effectiveness of A2C is attributed to the cyclopropyl ring in the middle of the acyl chain. This ring gives rise to a pronounced bend in the acyl chain which causes disorder in the bilayer lipids. A similar effect has been noted with myristoleyl alcohol, the cis isomer of a C14:1 aliphatic alcohol (34).

The susceptibility of cells to lysis by complement is not only dependent upon the properties of the hydrophobic part of the membrane, but modulation of the hydrophilic structures of membranes also affects the efficiency of complement attack. For example, it has been reported that treatment of erythrocytes with neuraminidase increased their susceptibility (35). Similarly, treatment of Line 10 guinea pig hepatoma cells with various proteolytic enzymes rendered them sensitive to complement (36). In the case of rat mast cells it has been reported that cytolysis by complement can be prevented by raising the intracellular concentration of cycic AMP (37).

Complement Attack on Nucleated Cells

In comparison with the extensive studies of complement attack on erythrocyte membranes, relatively little work has been done on complement attack against the membranes of other kinds of cells. There is need for information on channel size, and especially on channel life-time in the membranes of metabolically active nucleated cells. It is conceivable, and even likely, that such cells may have the capacity to defend themselves against complement attack by removal of inserted trans-membrane channels, perhaps by endocytosis or exocytosis of membrane regions containing channels. The Borsos group has reported a rise in lipid synthesis that occurs within minutes of attack by complement (38). They have shown that certain drugs, e.g., adriamycin, render tumor cells more susceptible to lysis by complement (39). A correlation was found between the adriamycin-induced increase in sensitivity and the loss of the cell's ability to incorporate fatty acids into complex cellular lipids (39). Conversely, they observed a reduction in sensitivity to complement after treatement of tumor cells with certain hormones, e.g., cortical steroids, which elevate lipid synthesis (39). While these correlations are of interest in relation to cell sensitivity, their interpretation is complicated because the substances under study exert diverse physiological effects. Finally, it should be noted in this context that certain cells vary in their susceptibility to complement in different stages of their growth cycle (40,41).

Membrane Destruction by Complement-Mediated Phospholipid Removal

In the late 1960's it was observed by Wilson and Spitznagel (19, 20) that complement activation on the surface of Escherichia coli causes release of about 60-70% of the bacterial phospholipid into the medium. Electron micrographs showed indications of damage to the outer bacterial membrane. Extensive studies of this problem have also been reported by the Inoue group (21) during the past ten years. In addition to confirming the release of phospholipid from bacteria into the fluid medium as a consequence of complement attack, they demonstrated release of the periplasmic enzyme alkaline phosphatase. This observation indicates that the outer membrane was disrupted because the enzyme molecule is too large to diffuse through the 5.5 nm complement channel. However, the outer membrane does not function as an osmotic barrier, since it has natural channels that are formed by porin (42). Therefore, the formation of trans-membrane channels by complement would not be expected to cause colloid-osmotic rupture. While there is no direct evidence to explain the apparent contradiction of alkaline phosphatase release, we suspect that this could be due to disassembly of the outer membrane by complement-mediated phospholipid removal.

In discussing this issue it is necessary to keep in mind, as noted earlier, that substantial removal of phospholipid from membranes requires the use of large doses of complement, whereas colloid-osmotic membrane disruption and consequent cell lysis can be accomplished with relatively small doses. This quantitative aspect of the problem is important in considering recent studies by Esser et al. (18) in which it was reported that a large dose of complement disassembled the envelope membrane of murine leukemia viruses. In parallel experiments they showed that melittin, an amphiphile from bee venom, also disintegrates the viral envelope membrane and they concluded from this that complement attacks membranes like a detergent, rather than by channel formation. It should be emphasized that this interpretation is applicable only to membranes like the outer membrane of *E. coli*, which does not function as an osmotic barrier, or to organisms like the murine leukemia viruses which are not susceptible to colloid-osmotic lysis. In these situations the formation of channels, which can be achieved with small doses of complement, is irrelevant; membrane disruption can be accomplished only through massive phospholipid removal by large doses of complement.

This issue is also relevant to studies with liposomes. While there is no direct evidence, we suspect that treatment of these vesicles with large doses of complement causes bilayer disassembly. Under these conditions, markers trapped in the aqueous compartment would be released regardless of their molecular dimensions in relation to the size of the complement channel. This could explain some of the experiments by Kinsky's group in which complement caused release of trapped enzymes of large molecular dimensions from liposomes (43).

In summary, there is sufficient information to support the view that both channel formation and detergent action play a role in complement-mediated membrane damage. The relative importance of one or the other is believed to depend on the properties of the target membrane, i.e., whether it functions as an osmotic barrier and whether its structure permits disassembly by phospholipid removal. Channel formation is a more efficient mechanism from a quantitative standpoint, and in the case of cells that are subject to colloid-osmotic lysis it is likely that only the channel mechanism is relevant because it requires much less complement than phospholipid removal.

In addition, in studying cytotoxicity against metabolically active nucleated cells, it should be kept in mind that in some cases death may be caused by metabolic disturbances. For example, there is reason to believe that the killing of *E. coli* by complement involves metabolic causes (44,32).

HOW DOES A COMPLEMENT CHANNEL CAUSE CYTOLYSIS?

The Colloid-Osmotic Mechanism

Mammalian cells suspended in an isotonic medium, such as 0.15 M NaCl or 0.3 M glucose solution, are in osmotic equilibrium. This means that the concentration (or activity) of water is the same on both sides of the plasma membrane. Under these conditions there is no net flow of water in either direction. However, since plasma membranes are freely permeable to water, a change in the water activity of the suspending medium or of the cytoplasmic fluid, will cause net water flow from the compartment of higher to that of lower activity.

Before discussing further the action of factors that disturb the osmotic equilibrium of cells, it will be helpful to consider the behavior of artificial semi-permeable membranes, like dialysis membranes, which are freely permeable to water and salts, but not macromolecules. If a two-compartment system divided by such a membrane is set up with macromolecules on only one side, but water and salt on both, an osmotic imbalance will develop due to the osmotic contribution of the macromolecules and, consequently, water will flow into the macromolecular compartment. If the impermeant macromolecule is a polyelectrolyte, the osmotic imbalance will be greater than that caused by a neutral macromolecule due to a shift of salt into the macromolecular compartment. Consequently even more water will flow into the macromolecular compartment. In effect, the osmotic contribution of polyelectrolytes, such as proteins, is greater than that expected from uncharged macromolecules. (This phenomenon is known as the Donnan effect.) It should be emphasized that two-compartment systems of this kind cannot attain osmotic equilibrium and, therefore, the net water flux into the macromolecular compartment continues, unless a mechanical force is exerted to prevent infinite expansion.

By contrast, living cells are able to maintain osmotic equilibrium in an isotonic medium. This is due to the fact that their plasma membranes, unlike artificial semi-permeable membranes, are not freely permeable to cations, such as Na^+ and K^+. Instead, the net flux of cations across plasma membranes is controlled by pumps. As a consequence, the activity of water inside the cell can be balanced against that of the outside medium and no net water flow occurs.

When a complement channel is formed across a cell membrane, this osmotic equilibrium is destroyed because cations, but not proteins, can flow freely through the channel. In effect, a plasma membrane carrying a complement channel behaves like the artificial semi-permeable membranes discussed above in the sense that water will flow unchecked into the cell (the protein compartment) which

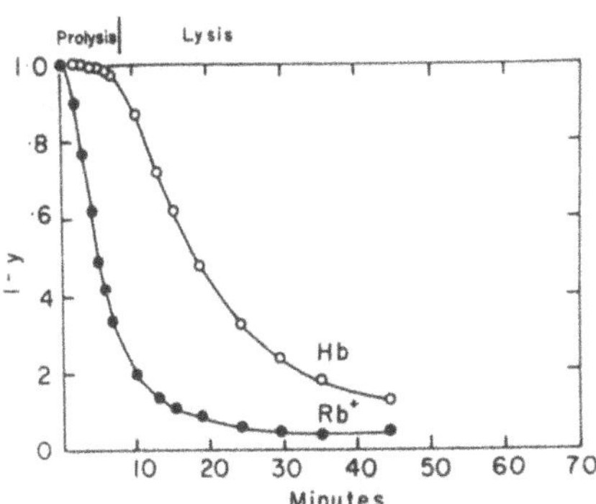

Fig. 7. Time course of $^{86}Rb^+$ (closed circles) and Hb (open circles) release from red cells treated with C. Value of z (average number of channels per cell) was about 3. The reaction mixture contained 10 ml sensitized red cells (EAC1,4b) and 10 ml of C2 dilution (1/250). After 8 min (t_{max}) incubation at 30°C, (zero time on graph), 27 ml of C-EDTA (1/37.5 dilution) were added to supply excess C3, C5, C6, C7, C8 and C9. Rapid sampling of the extracellular fluid then commenced, by a special filtration method. One ml samples were assayed for hemoglobin and $^{86}Rb^+$. (56)

causes it to swell and, eventually, to burst. This phenomenon is known as colloid-osmotic lysis.

These events are illustrated in Fig. 7 which shows the time course of the release of $^{86}Rb^+$ (a measure of channel formation) and hemoglobin (a measure of cell bursting) from erythrocytes after complement attack. The lag between these release curves represents the time required for erythrocytes to swell and burst. The experiment in Fig. 7 was done with about three channels per cell. When the number of channels per cell is increased, less time is required for swelling and bursting because ion and water flow is more rapid.

In order to avoid possible confusion, it should be noted that the resealed erythrocyte ghosts used in the marker release experiments in Fig. 6, contained too little residual protein to cause colloid-osmotic lysis after channel formation by complement. Therefore, the slow release of ovalbumin and hemoglobin (the hemoglobin dimer, 34,000 daltons) shown in this figure is due to diffusion through the 5.5-7 nm complement channels. This is the reason why the release of these proteins from ghosts is extremely slow compared to the hemoglobin release from cells shown in Fig. 7, despite the fact that the ghosts in Fig. 6 carried many more channels than cells in Fig. 7.

It should be stressed also that complement attack on metabolically active nucleated cells need not necessarily cause colloid-osmotic lysis in all cases. The outcome of complement channel formation will depend on the capacity of a cell to repair the damage, on the concentration of macromolecules in the cytoplasm, on the susceptibility of the membrane to rupture and on the rate of channel formation. In cases where the colloid-osmotic mechanism is not operative, other causes of cytotoxicity must be sought, e.g., membrane disassembly or metabolic disturbances.

COMMENTS ON CYTOTOXICITY OF LYMPHOID CELLS

Does Cell-Mediated Cytotoxicity Involve Formation of Trans-Membrane Channels?

Since some lymphoid cells, notably macrophages, have the capacity to synthesize complement proteins, attempts have been made to implicate the complement system in cell-mediated cytotoxicity, but these efforts have not been successful. However, in view of the widespread distribution of amphiphilic mechanisms of membrane attack among bacteria, fungi and lower animals, the possible applicability of this kind of mechanism to cell-mediated cytotoxicity need not be restricted to the complement system. It is quite possible that lymphoid cells possess the capacity to produce amphiphilic molecules other than complement that can attack the membranes of target cells.

Cell-mediated cytotoxicity by amphiphiles would not necessarily require the high complexity and sophistication of complement. These attributes reflect the necessity of focusing the killing mechanism of a fluid phase system on selected targets in order to spare bystander cells. This is accomplished by fixation of the early complement proteins, notably the covalent binding of C3 and C4 through esterification to hydroxyl groups on the membrane surface. As a consequence, the enzymatic generation of the C5b6 complex, which initiates the process of membrane attack, takes place in the immediate vicinity of the membrane. This promotes the subsequent reactions with C7, C8 and C9 that culminate in channel formation or phospholipid removal.

In the case of cell-mediated cytotoxicity, the direct and intimate contact between killer and target cells may suffice to focus the attack on the membrane of the target so as to spare bystander cells. Conceivably, appropriate cell-cell contact could cause a conformational change in a single species of protein on the killer cell surface, leading to exposure of hydrophobic peptides that can then become inserted in the lipid bilayer of the target cell. It is possible that an activating protease is required for the conformational change that converts the putative "attack" protein from the hydrophilic to the amphiphilic state; moreover, a protease may be required to cleave the hydrophobic peptide from the remainder of this protein so that it may remain inserted in the target cell membrane after separation of the killer and target cells. Thus, the entire attack process may require only two or three components, compared to the fourteen proteins that make up the complement system.

Since the great majority of mechanistic complement studies has been made with erythrocytes, which are metabolically passive cells, or with artificial bilayers, we do not have adequate information on the role of channel formation and colloid-osmotic lysis in complement attack on metabolically active nucleated cells. Nor is it known to what extent phospholipid removal from the membrane or metabolic disturbances contribute to cytotoxicity. Therefore, information transfer to the cell-mediated cytotoxocity field from complement studies has been limited to methodology and general concepts. Specifically, I refer to several publications that directly implicate a channel-forming mode of attack by lymphoid cells.

The earliest indication that the lipid bilayer of the cell membrane may be the target of cell-mediated attack came from an experiment by Henkart and Blumenthal (45) in which lymphocytes produced ion flow across a membrane of "oxidized cholesterol" in which DNP-phosphatidylethanolamine was incorporated. The bilayer was treated with antibody against TNP antigen. About 30-40 minutes after addition of non-immune splenic lymphoid cells, the time required for them to settle on the membrane, ion flow across the membrane, as measured electrically, began to increase significantly and rose several hundred-fold over the next hour. This effect was observed only when the membranes were treated with antibody and lymphoid cells. No substantial increase of conductance was produced by lymphoid cells alone. Nor did treatment of the membranes with antibody alone change their electrical conductance. Another important control involved the use of $(Fab)_2$, instead of intact antibody. Treatment of membranes with this fragment plus lymphocytes did not increase the trans-membrane conductance. This indicates that the Fc segment of the antibody is necessary for binding to the Fc receptor of lymphocytes.

It is also of interest that the change of conductance produced by antibody and lymphocytes was found to be dependent on electrical polarity. The same phenomenon was observed in studies of the effect of C5b-8 on the electrical conductance of planar lecithin bilayers. This probably indicates that the electric field can cause conformational changes in the proteins associated with the membrane, or can effect an electrostatic association between two or more components within the membrane. Conceivably, electrically mediated changes of this kind could be so extreme as to close down existing channels or to open up new channels depending on the direction of the electric field.

The second indication that the lipid bilayer is the target of attack derives from experiments reported by Frye and Friou (46) that Rosenthal's inhibitor, a synthetic analog of lecithin and inhibitor of phospholipase A, as well as lecithin itself, have the capacity to inhibit ADCC. The authors interpreted this effect as an indication that ADCC involves phospholipase activity. However, I do not share this interpretation because attack by phosphoipase is not an effective cytolytic mechanism, especially when the enzyme is restricted to a small area of contact between the cytotoxic lymphocyte and the target cell. Rather it is preferable to interpret Frye and Friou's results as competition of Rosenthal's inhibitor or phosphatidylcholine for hydrophobic peptides that form channels in lipid bilayers after insertion. Thus, the phosphatidylcholine inhibition experiments tend to support the electrical ion flow studies of Henkart and Blumenthal.

A third way of approaching this issue involves the use of liposomes as targets. As reviewed by Mayer et al. (47) this approach has been explored by several investigators, but the results, though encouraging, were not conclusive, probably for technical reasons.

Strong evidence implicating the lipid bilayer as the target has come from experiments by Willoughby and Mayer (48) in which it was shown that incorporation of additional cholesterol into sheep or chicken erythrocyte membranes caused a substantial decrease in the susceptibility of these cells to ADCC (Figs. 8 and 9). The same effect has been demonstrated in experiments on complement-mediated hemolysis, both with antibody and whole serum complement, and with the C5b-9 membrane attack sequence (Fig. 8). There is good reason to attribute the depressing effect of cholesterol to the well-known capacity of this substance for tightening the packing of the lipid bilayer which would be expected to decrease the probability of insertion of hydrophobic peptides. In the case of complement, it also has been possible to demonstrate the opposite effect, namely, that agents which increase membrane disorder exert a potentiating effect on the efficiency of complement-mediated cytolysis.

The most direct evidence for channel formation has emerged from experiments by Simone and Henkart (49) in which it was shown that channels exhibiting a minimal diameter of about 12 nm are formed in the membranes of resealed erythrocyte ghosts by ADCC. It is of interest in this context that Dourmashkin et al., (50) have recently reported electron microscopic observations showing uniformly shaped circular lesions of this approximate magnitude on the membrane of erythrocyte ghosts after attack by antibody and lymphocytes.

In addition, there is some evidence in favor of the colloid-osmotic type of lysis by lymphocytes. Rosenow (51) has reported that treatment of target cells with immune T cells causes swelling. Similarly, Biberfeld and Perlmann (52) have observed that chicken

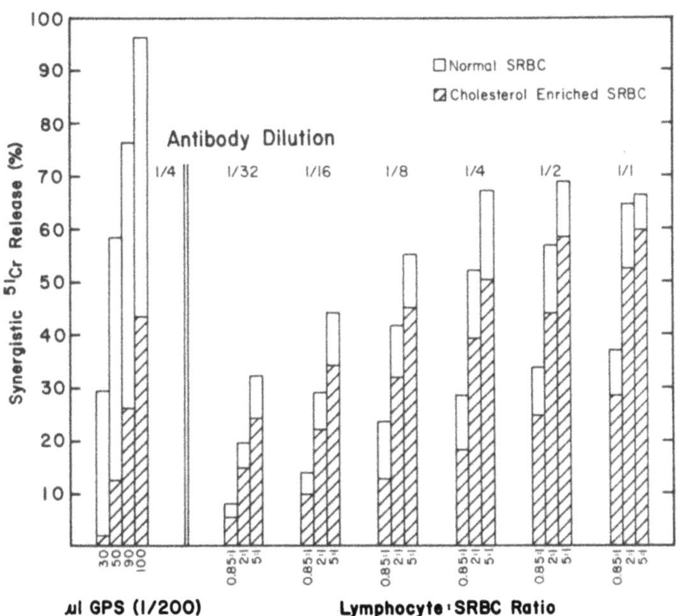

Fig. 8. Effect of cholesterol incorporation into SRBC membranes on cytolysis by lymphocytes in ADCC. Cholesterol-enriched (▨) or normal (□) ^{51}Cr-labeled SRBC (5×10^5 cells in 0.1 ml) were sensitized with 0.1 ml of the designated dilutions of an anti-Forssman IgG stock preparation (1/1) containing 0.6 µg IgG protein/ml. The desired number of human PBL were then added in 0.2 ml and the incubation continued at 37°C for 4 hr. Indicated amounts of a 1/200 dilution of GPS, rather than lymphocytes, were added in some cases. The degree of cytolysis is expressed as % synergistic ^{51}Cr release, defined as that percentage of the maximum releasable ^{51}Cr which was released into the supernatant fluid in the presence of both antibody and PBL, minus that due to spontaneous leakage, or to antibody or PBL interacting with the SRBC separately. Spontaneous ^{51}Cr leakage from cholesterol-enriched and normal SRBC was 1.5% and 6.5% of the maximum value, respectively, and no additional marker release was caused by the separate additions of IgG or PBL.

erythrocytes swell during ADCC. Furthermore, experiments by Ferluga and Allison (53), as well as Henney (54), indicate that macromolecular substances block lymphocyte-mediated lysis. Collectively, these observations support the trans-membrane channel hypothesis, although metabolic effects would also be consistent.

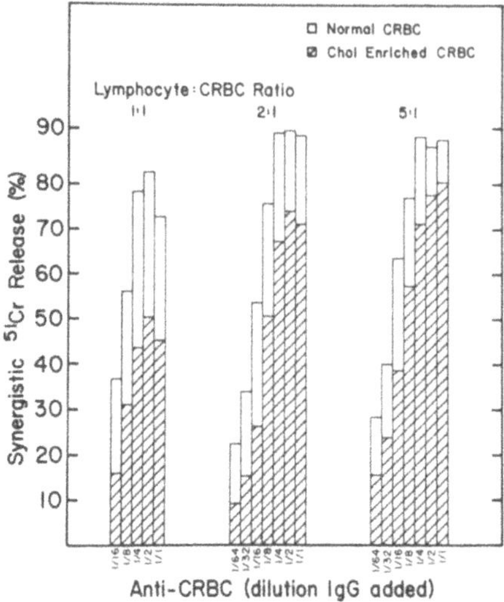

Fig. 9. Effect of cholesterol incorporation into CRBC membranes on cytolysis by lymphocytes in ADCC. The experimental format was as described for Fig. 8 except that designated dilutions of a stock preparation (1/1) of anti-CRBC IgG containing 3.75 μg IgG protein/ml were used to sensitize the cholesterol-enriched (▨) or normal (□) CRBC. Release of ^{51}Cr from target CRBC was measured after a 6 hr. incubation period at 37°C and is expressed as % synergistic release. Cholesterol-enriched CRBC incorporated 14.2 μg cholesterol/10^8 cells, as estimated from tracer ^{14}C-cholesterol uptake.

On the Relation Between Specific Recognition and the Killing Mechanism

In the case of complement, the mechanism of cytotoxicity is not dependent on specific recognition by antibody since the cytotoxic process can be initiated non-specifically either at the beginning of the reaction sequence, i.e., by non-specific activation of C1, or in the middle of the cascade by enzymatic or non-enzymatic activation of C5. By analogy, in cell-mediated cytotoxicity, it should not be assumed that specific recognition necessarily plays a direct role in the mechanism of attack.

However, complement cytotoxicity in the absence of antibody is not devoid of specificity. Thus in studies of hemolysis by C5b-9, it has been shown recently by Hänsch et al. (55) that C8 and C9 from a given mammalian species act very inefficiently against erythrocytes of the same species. This species restriction is not due to the membrane lipids but probably reflects recognition involving membrane glycoproteins.

REFERENCES

1. Mayer, M.M. Complement, Past and Present. The Harvey Lectures, Series 72, Academic Press, p. 159 (1978).
2. Haxby, J.A., Kinsky, C.B., and S.C. Kinsky. Immune response of a liposomal model membrane. Proc. Natl. Acad. Sci. USA 61:300 (1968).
3. Kinsky, S.C., Bonsen, P.P.M., Kinsky, C.B., Van Deenen L.L.M., and A.F. Rosenthal. Preparation of immunologically responsive liposomes with phophonyl and phosphinyl analogs of lecithin. Biochim. Biophys. Acta. 233:815 (1971).
4. Mayer, M.M. In "Immunochemical Approaches to Problems in Microbiology. Heidelberger, M., and Plescia, O.J., Eds., Rutgers Univ. Press, New Brunswick, NJ, p 268 (1961).
5. Singer, S.J., and G.L. Nicholson. The fluid mosaic model of the structure of cell membranes. Science 175:720 (1972).
6. Mayer M.M. Mechanism of cytolysis by complement. Proc. Natl. Acad. Sci. USA 69:2954 (1972).
7. Shin, M.L., Paznekas, W.A., Abramovitz, A.S., and M.M. Mayer. On the mechanism of membrane damage by C: exposure of hydrophobic sites on activated C proteins. J. Immunol. 119:1358 (1977).
8. Podack, E.R., Biesecker, G., and H.J. Müller-Eberhard. Membrane attack complex of complement: generation of high-affinity phospholipid binding sites by fusion of five hydrophilic plasma proteins. Proc. Natl. Acad. Sci. USA 76:897 (1979).
9. Mayer, M.M., Michaels, D.W., Ramm, L.E., Whitlow, M.B., Willoughby, J.B., and M.L. Shin. Membrane damage by complement. Criitical Reviews in Immunology 2:133 (1981).
10. Bhakdi, S., Bjerrum, O.J., Bhakdi-Lennen, B., and J. Tranum-Jensen. Complement lysis: evidence for an amphiphilic nature of the terminal membrane C5b-9 complex of human complement. J. Immunol. 121:2526 (1978).
11. Podack, E.R., and H.J. Müller-Eberhard. Binding of desoxycholate, phosphatidylcholine vesicles, lipoprotein, and of the S-protein to complexes of terminal complement components. J. Immunol. 121:1025 (1978).
12. Hammer, C.H., Nicholson, A., and M.M. Mayer. On the mechanism of cytolysis by complement: evidence on insertion of C5b and C7 subunits of the C5b,6,7 complex into phospholipid bilayers of erythrocyte membranes. Proc. Natl. Acad. Sci. USA 72:5076 (1975).
13. Hammer, C.H., Shin, M.L. Abramovitz, A.S., and M.M. Mayer. On the mechanism of cell membrane damage by complement: evidence on insertion of polypeptide chains from C8 and C9 into the lipid bilayer of erythrocytes. J. Immunol. 119:1 (1977).
14. Bhakdi, S., Bjerrum, O.J., Rother, U., Knüfermann, H., and D.F.H. Wallach. Immunochemical analyses of membrane-bound complement. Detection of the terminal complement complex and its similarity to "intrinsic" erythrocyte membrane proteins.

Biochim. Biophys. Acta 406:21 (1975).
15. Hu, V.W., Esser, A.F., Podack, E.R., and B.J. Wisnieski. The membrane attack mechanism of complement: Photolabeling reveals insertion of terminal proteins into target membrane. J. Immunol. 127:380 (1981).
16. Podack, E.R., Stoffel, W., Esser, A.F., and H.J. Müller-Eberhard. Membrane attack complex of complement: Distribution of subunits between the hydrocarbon phase of target membranes and water. Proc. Natl. Acad. Sci. USA 78:4544 (1981).
17. Ramm, L.E., and M.M. Mayer. Life-span and size of the trans-membrane channel formed by large doses of complement. J. Immunol. 124:2281 (1980).
18. Esser, A.F., Bartholomew, R.M., Jensen, F.C., and H.J. Müller-Eberhard. Disassembly of viral membranes by complement independent of channel formation. Proc. Soc. Natl. Acad. Sci. USA 76:5843 (1979).
19. Wilson, L.A., and J.K. Spitznagel. Molecular and structural damage to Escherichia coli produced by antibody, complement, and lysozyme systems. J. Bacteriol. 96:1339 (1968).
20. Wilson, L.A. and J.K. Spitznagel. Characteristics of complement-dependent release of phospholipid from Escherichia coli. Infect. Immun. 4:23 (1971).
21. Inoue, K., Kinoshita, T., Okada, M., and Y. Akiyama. Release of phospholipids from complement-mediated lesions on the surface structure of Escherichia coli. J. Immunol. 119:65 (1977).
22. Ramm, L.E., and M.M. Mayer. Size comparison of the trans-membrane channels formed by C5b-8 and C5b-9. Molecular Immunology. In press (1981).
23. Esser, A.F., Kolb, W.P., Podack, E.R., and H.J. Müller-Eberhard. Molecular reorganization of lipid bilayers by complement. A possible mechanism for membranolysis. Proc. Natl. Acad. Sci. USA 76:1410 (1979).
24. Biesecker, G., Podack, E.R., Halverson, C.A., and H.J. Müller-Eberhard. C5b-9 dimer: isolation from complement, lysed cells and ultrastructural identification with complement-dependent membrane lesions. J. Exp. Med. 149:448 (1979).
25. Sims, P.J. Permeability characteristics of complement-damaged membranes: evaluation of the membrane leak generated by the complement proteins C5b-9. Proc. Natl. Acad. Sci. USA 78: 1838 (1981).
26. Esser, A.F. Interactions between complement proteins and biological and model membranes. Vol. 4, "Biological Membranes," Dennis Chapman, Ed., Academic Press, NY (1981).
27. Bhakdi, S., and J. Tranum-Jensen. Molecular weight of the membrane C5b-9 complex of human complement: Characterization of the terminal complex as a C5b-9 monomer. Proc. Nat. Acad. Sci. USA 78:1818 (1981).
28. Podack, E.R., Esser, A.F., Biesecker, G., and H.J. Müller-Eberhard. Membrane attack complex of complement. A structural analysis of its assembly. J. Exp. Med. 151:301 (1980).

29. Sims, P.J., and P.K. Lauf. Analysis of solute diffusion across the C5b-9 membrane lesion of complement: evidence that individual C5b-9 complexes do not function as discrete, uniform pores. J. Immunol. 125:2617 (1980).
30. Michaels, D.W., Abramovitz, A.S., Hammer, C.H., and M.M. Mayer. Characterization of the complement lesion: the formation of trans-membrane channels and their mechanism of assembly. (Abstract) J. Immunol 120:1785 (1978).
31. Shin, M.L., Paznekas, W.A., and M.M. Mayer. On the mechanism of membrane damage by complement: the effect of length and unsaturation of the acyl chains in liposomal bilayers and the effect of cholesterol concentration in sheep erythrocyte and liposomal membranes. J. Immunol. 120:1996 (1978)
32. Wright, S.K., and R.P. Levine. How complement kills E. coli. II. The apparent two-hit nature of the lethal event. J. Immunol. 127:1152 (1981).
33. Shin, M.L., Paznekas, W.A., and M.M. Mayer. Effect of membrane fluidity on efficiency of sheep erythrocyte lysis by terminal complement proteins. Fed. Proc. 38:1468 (1979).
34. Shin, M.L., Hansch, G., and M.M. Mayer. Effect of agents that produce membrane disorder on lysis of erythrocytes by complement. Proc. Nat. Acad. Sci. USA 78:2522 (1981).
35. Lauf, P.K. Immunological and physiological characteristics of the rapid immune hemolysis of neuraminidase-treated sheep red cells produced by fresh guinea pig serum. J. Exp. Med. 142:974 (1975).
36. Boyle, M.D.P., Ohanian, S.H., and T. Borsos. Lysis of tumor cells by antibody and complement. VI. Enhanced killing of enzyme-pretreated tumor cells. J. Immunol. 116:661 (1976).
37. Kaliner, M., and K.F. Austen. Adenosine 3',5'-monophosphate: inhibition of complement-mediated cell lysis. Science 183: 659 (1974).
38. Schlager S.I., Ohanian, S.H., and T. Borsos. Stimulation of the synthesis and release of lipids in tumor cells under attack by antibody and C. J. Immunol. 120:895 (1978).
39. Schlager, S.I., Ohanian, S.H., and T. Borsos. Correlation between the ability of tumor cells to resist humoral immune attack and their ability to synthesize lipid. J. Immunol. 120:463 (1978).
40. Shipley, W.U. Immune cytolysis in relation to the growth cycle of Chinese hamster cells. Cancer Res. 31:1925 (1971).
41. Cooper, N.R., Polley, M.J., and M.B.A. Oldstone. Failure of terminal complement components to induce lysis of Moloney Virus transformed lymphocytes. J. Immunol. 112:866 (1974).
42. von Myenburg, K., and H. Nikaido. Outer membrane of gram-negative bacteria. XVII. Specificity of transport process catalyzed by the λ-receptor protein in Escherichia coli. Biochem. Biophys. Res. Commun. 78:1100 (1977).
43. Kataoka, T., Williamson, J.R., and S.C. Kinsky. Release of macro-molecular markers (enzymes) from liposomes treated with

antibody and complement. An attempt at correlation with electron microscopic observations. Biochim. Biophys. Acta. 298: 158 (1973).
44. Wright, S.D., and R.P. Levine. How complement kills _E. coli_. I. Location of the lethal lesion. J. Immunol. 127:1146 (1981).
45. Henkart, P., and R. Blumenthal. Interaction of lymphocytes with lipid bilayer membranes: a model of lymphocyte-mediated lysis of target cells. Proc. Natl. Acad. Sci. USA 72:2789 (1975).
46. Frye, L.D., and G.J. Friou. Inhibition of mammalian cytotoxic cells by phosphatidylcholine and its analogue. Nature 258: 333 (1975).
47. Mayer, M.M. Hammer, C.H., Michaels, D.W., and M.L. Shin. Immunologically mediated membrane damage: the mechanism of complement action and the similarity of lymphocyte-mediated cytotoxicity. Immunochem. 15:813 (1979).
48. Willoughby, J.B., and M.M. Mayer. Effect of target cell membrane cholesterol on susceptibility to ADCC. Fourth International Congress of Immunology. Paris, No. 11.5.35 (1980).
49. Simone, C.B., and P. Henkart. Permeability changes induced in erythrocyte ghost targets by antibody-dependent cytotoxic effector cells: evidence for membrane pores. J. Immunol. 124:954 (1980).
50. Dourmashkin, R.R., Deteix, P., Simone, C.B., and P. Henkart. Electron microscopic demonstration of lesions in target cell membranes associated with antibody-dependent cellular cytotoxicity. Clin. and Exp. Immunol. 42:554 (1980).
51. Rosenau, W. Target cell destruction. Fed. Proc. 27:34 (1968).
52. Biberfeld, P., and P. Perlmann. Morphological observations on the cytotoxicity of human blood lymphocytes for antibody-coated chicken erythrocytes. Exp. Cell Res. 62:433 (1970).
53. Ferluga, J., and A.C. Allison. Observations on the mechanism by which T-lymphocytes exert cytotoxic effects. Nature 250: 673 (1974).
54. Henney, C.S. Estimation of the size of a T-cell-induced lytic lesion. Nature 249:456 (1974).
55. Hänsch, G.M., Hammer, C.H., Vanguri, P., and M.L. Shin. Homologous species restriction in lysis of erythrocytes by terminal complement proteins. Proc. Natl. Acad. Sci. USA 78:5118 (1981).
56. Hingson, D.J., Massengill, R.K., and M.M. Mayer. The Kinetics of Release of ^{86}Rubidium and Hemoglobin from Erythrocytes Damaged by Antibody and Complement. Immunochemistry 6:295 (1969).

DISCUSSION

M. Mayer

I think there are three issues that are important from the standpoint of this discussion. The first one is the issue of hydrophobic exposure, which is what happens as the terminal complement proteins interact sequentially with one another, i.e., they undergo a conformational change, that exposes varied hydrophobic residues to the aqueous environment. The second issue is that of insertion of these hydrophobic peptides into the membrane, which is essentially due to the fact that the hydrophobic peptides are repelled by water, and it is the water that drives them into the membrane. That will only happen if the membrane is really close by. If it's more than a few Angstrom units away, it is not likely to happen because under those circumstances, these exposed hydrophobic structures undergo aggregation, unless the S-protein or other acceptors are present. The third issue is that of channel formation, i.e., following insertion these peptides appear to undergo a polymerization, which leads to the formation of the channel structure. In the case of complement, the subunits are distinct. 5, 6, 7, 8 and 9 polymerize to form the channel structure.

If a large amount of the terminal complement proteins is applied to a membrane, phopholipid is actually pulled out of the membrane and ends up in the aqueous phase in the form of lipoprotein, so that the properties and composition of the membrane lipids are changed as a consequence. I think it's fair to say that there is complete agreement among different investigators as to the matter of hydrophobic exposure. To demonstrate insertion into the membrane proved much more difficult and, in fact, clear cut evidence became available only recently from the work of Valerie Hu.

Valerie Hu

The idea is to insert a probe into a membrane which can report on events that happen at and within the membrane (J. Immunol. 127: 380, 1981). The probe is essentially a fatty acid molecule that has been modified to include a photoreactive group which upon irradiation will nonspecifically crosslink any molecule that happens to be in the vicinity, within the hydrophobic region of the membrane. We can monitor events occuring within a single monolayer of the target membrane. Using this protocol, we asked the question, can we detect any of the complement components within the hydrophobic region of the target membranes during complement attack, and if so, what are the molecular interactions involved between these proteins and phospholipid molecules? Initially, we looked at the reaction at two stages, the prelysis stage, i.e., at the C7 stage, and at the terminal stage, that is building up the complex to C9. What we found at the prelysis stage is that we were able to label all three of the complement proteins, 5b, 6 and 7, within the membrane. However, to our surprise, when we built up the complex to C9 we noticed the disappearance of label in the earlier components and we appear to label only the C9. We subsequently looked at intermediate stages of complement attack and we found, in fact, that up to the C8 stage, we find that we label both C5b and 6, and this labeling is enhanced upon addition of C7, which suggests that C7 might serve to anchor the C5b-6 complex deeper into the membrane. Upon the addition of C8, we noted a decrease in the labeling of the first three companents, 5, 6 and 7, and C8 also becomes labeled. This we interpret as C8, which is the stage at which lysis begins, initiating a reordering of the earlier proteins within the target membrane.

Upon addition of C9, we get enhanced lysis and in addition, a labeling pattern in which the radioactivity in all of the earlier components has disappeared and we only seem to be labelling C9, which implies that only C9 is in direct contact with the lipid bilayer, at least at the depth at which our probe is sensing, within the target membrane.

Thus, we conclude that a molecular rearrangement has occurred in going from the C8 to C9 stage, such that ultimately the only protein of the complex in contact with the lipid is C9. This can be explained either by vertical displacement of the earlier proteins, either upwards, i.e., towards the external surface of the bilayer or perhaps into the inner monolayer, which in these experiments our probe does not sense. Another possibility is a shielding of earlier components by C9. We conclude that the mechanism of complement lysis involves substantial changes in the protein-lipid as well as protein-protein interactions in the developing complex.

I would like to suggest that this type of approach might also be used to study cell-mediated lysis. I would design the experiment by putting this probe into the target membrane and subjecting the target cells to killer cells. What we would need is a mechanism to arrest the process after the lethal hit, and then try to isolate the target affected by the killer but not yet disintegrated. We would then assay for new components within the membrane. That is, to look for inserted molecules.

C. Henney

Whichever way you do it,. it's going to be a fairly heroic experiment. I would like, before encouraging anyone to do it, to ask what is the experimental basis for doing it.

M. Mayer

There are so many amphiphiles that can insert into membranes. It's quite possible that a system other than complement in the killers may do it. So, it's a broad general question.

W. Clark

The problem with that experiment may be that, if you see a lipid of the target cell interacting with a new protein, it may come from the effector cell, or it may just be due to new lipid-protein interactions in the target cell.

P. Henkart

I will show later some data which indicates that we have some evidence that in ADCC one has an insertion of a pore-forming substance into the target cell. In thinking about how one can get convincing evidence that this comes from the effector cell, and how it is really operating on a molecular basis, we also have considered possibilities of looking for transfer of labeled moieties from the effector cell into the target cell. We have always been rather concerned about interpreting data of this sort. What you have, in the case of an effector cell-target cell interaction, is a very tight adhesion and there is bound to be some slopping off of components from cells, and exchange of materials. It is not going to be easy to decide whether some components that transfer are, in fact, physiologically relevant, i.e., do they do anything to membrane permeability of the target cell? We are using resealed erythrocyte ghosts and looking at permeability of various markers into resealed erythrocyte ghosts. What we are able to do is to measure the flux of markers added from the outside into the internal space of the ghost. We have some data now with this system using complement and asking questions about permeability, which we believe to be the damage caused by the complement system, and also the ADCC system.

E. Martz

I'd like to ask Dr. Hu if there is any evidence whether the probe that you described, if put into a target cell membrane for the experiment you proposed, would flip into the killer, and thereby label the killer proteins without them being actually transferred.

Valerie Hu

There is that possibility and I have started some probe transfer studies to see how likely that is. It's very easy to get lipid molecules to flip between vesicles. I don't know how easily they would flip between cells. If we could get it into the inner monolayer and keep it there, on the inside of the target membrane, then I think the possibility of transfer to the killer cell would be very low.

P. Lachmann

I would like to ask those who investigate T cell lysis whether they know of data to contradict the idea that lymphocyte toxicity results from the insertion of a hydrophobic "plug" which causes the membrane of the target cell to leak?

C. Sanderson

I'd like to respond to this point. Firstly, there are the morphological differences between complement and T cell or K cell killing. I remain completely unconvinced by anything that has been said here or published, that complement has anything to do with lysis by T cells or K cells. I restrict myself to lymphocyte killing of tumor cells. There is a danger here of getting confused about ADCC. People talk about lysis without defining target cells, red cell targets or others, and not defining the effector cells. I think it's very important because there are many cells capable of causing ADCC, when you use erythrocytes as targets. Could I just take this opportunity to criticize the work that Peter Lachmann quoted from Dourmashkin. I thought this was interesting until I read the Materials and Methods. What Dourmashkin (Clin. Exp. Immunol. 1980, 42:554) is doing is incubating for four hours. From our kinetic studies, it is known that K cells inflict the lethal damage within a few minutes, say 15 minutes, so there is a four hour incubation period, in which autolysis could well be taking place. Membranes may develop these patterned structures as a result of zeiosis. So, I think Dourmashkin's experiment needs to be repeated within the first few minutes of killing and not after a four hour incubation period.

P. Henkart

I can speak to some of these experiments that were done in my laboratory in which erythrocyte ghosts were used as targets. These experiments were made with three hour incubation periods. All of that time is required for endpoint release of the markers from those ghosts. So, I think that part of your criticism is justified with regard to the experiments that Dourmashkin did while he was in London in which nucleated target cells were used. I can speak, though, to the experiments that were done in my laboratory and as I say we actually did side-by-side marker release in the kinetics. We did require that long a time period to see release. You have to appreciate the fact that it is not easy to see these structures. You do not see them in every cell, and it is obvious when you think about the geometry and the problems of finding this "needle in the haystack". It is not likely that you will always find the lesion for a particular damaged cell. Therefore, we have to try to maximize the chances.

C. Sanderson

We have to be careful about bringing in erythrocytes when we are talking about tumor cells. I think we must be clear about this. I think there is a good possibility that the mechanism of killing of erythrocytes is quite different from that of tumor cells.

M. Mayer

Quite possibly, but the point has to be emphasized that the functional definition of a channel is the formation of a well-defined leak. Defined with respect to size, and Pierre Henkart's experiments show that there is a leak corresponding to a 120 Angstrom diameter lesion. So, that indeed would support those rings seen by Dourmashkin.

C. Henney

Let's address the hypothesis that complement components might be involved in T cell killing. While I too subscribe to the notion that complement components are not involved, let's review the evidence.

You can carry out T cell-mediated lysis in serum-free medium and the addition of fresh serum as a complement source affects neither the rate nor the extent of lysis that's observed. Now, that in itself, certainly doesn't rule out the notion that complement components might be synthesized in vitro and be contributing. Dr. Mayer and I, about a decade ago, tried sequentially to add antibodies against complement components and look for their consumption and also for effects on T cell killing. Again, we found no evidence that such antibodies affected either the rate or the extent of killing. As far I know those are the only pieces of evidence that bear on the issue. I'd like to hear some additions to that list.

M. Mayer

But Chris, they do not bear on the possibility that another amphiphile may be involved.

C. Henney

Oh, absolutely not, but I thought before we get to that general hypothetical case we could address complement.

Eric Martz

What we are asking is really two questions. One is, whether complement, as we know it, may be involved in T cell-mediated killing and the other is, whether a similar, as you say, amphipathic channel is occurring. I think many of us in CTL-mediated killing will favor the idea of insertion of some sort of amphiphile. Not all of us, as we have heard today, but many would favor the idea of the insertion of a channel of some sort. As to arguments that would disfavor the direct involvement of complement as we know it in T cell killing, I think there are two additional functional pieces of evidence that distinguish complement-mediated lysis from T cell-mediated lysis. One is Colin Sanderson's observation of the difference in morphology of the dying target cell in the two cases, which has been underemphasized and should be more carefully followed up. The other, that the effect of the two attack mechanisms on the mast cell is so drastically different.

Peter Lachmann

I too have reservations about ascribing T cell killing to complement. For example, complement deficient subjects seem to have normal lymphocytotoxic reactions. The more general hypothesis is that complement provides a model for the mechanism of lymphocyte killing. Perhaps the killer cell, like complement, inserts into the target cell.

M. Mayer

The reason why complement people favor this type of insertion channel-forming mechanism is two-fold. One, that this is a type of mechanism that is very widely distributed in nature, throughout all forms of life. Second, specific attacks on membranes that are localized, as these are, are difficult to mediate. It is difficult to imagine mechanisms other than pore insertion.

Gideon Berke

An approach that could resolve the question whether the complement components have a role would be to see whether cloned CTL lines or CTL hybrids synthesize any of the complement components. Once this has been eliminated, I think we have no discussion about complement being involved. The question of whether there is another type of plug would of course still be open.

Peter Lachmann

I am not sure whether such data would be a help. You may well find that cloned CTL make small quantities of complement components, because many cell lines do so. Complement synthesis seems not to be a deeply repressed activity. For example, HeLa cells are found to make some complement components under certain culture conditions and so do fibroblasts. Macrophages seem to make nearly all complement components. But it doesn't really answer the question of whether such molecules are involved in cell killing.

Manfred Mayer

I feel rather strongly that if methods could be developed to look for channels and characterize them in CTL killing, that would help. But that may be very difficult.

Pierre Golstein

Is it possible, when you have two cells very near one another, like a killer and a target cell, that a channel would be inserted into one and not into the other?

M. Mayer

Yes, and the first thing to point out relates to insertion of hydrophobic complement proteins. Let's say you have a hydrophobic peptide. It's been exposed. It is repelled by water. If it has been generated on the surface of a membrane and if another membrane is nearby, it will be driven into that membrane. Now, you're asking, is it going to turn around and hit its own membrane? Well, that depends on what's there. If you have membrane proteins sitting in the membrane of the CTL that are closely clustered and you haven't got much accessible lipid bilayer, it couldn't insert. So, you need to make the assumption that the CTL has a cluster of membrane proteins at the site of "plug" generation that are pretty tightly packed. The other assumption would be that the target cell has a patch of accessible bilayer. Purely imaginary, of course. But it presents no difficulty.

W. Clark

One problem is that membranes aren't nice discrete two-dimensional layers. They fold back on themselves, have numerous processes, and are tremendously complex. It seems to me that the likelihood of one of those hydrophobic molecules hitting a target cell is perhaps not that much greater than hitting another process of the same effector cell.

M. Mayer

This is debatable.

Matt Mescher

One possibility is to use liposomes as they have been used to study complement lytic mechanisms. What you would obviously want is a way of directing the killer cell to those liposomes, which would mean the insertion of the appropriate MHC antigens. We've done a lot of work looking at stimulation of a CTL response using H2 containing liposomes (PNAS, 1981, 7:2488). Those antigens on the liposomes can clearly be recognized by the pre-cytolytic T lymphocyte and trigger those cells to differentiate to active killers. H. McConnell's lab has reported some results using large liposomes as targets for CTL (PNAS, 1979, 76:4042). There are some problems with those experiments in terms of reproducibility and possibly specificity. But there is at least a bit of an indication that it might, in fact, be possible to lyse liposomes with CTL.

M. Mayer

That sounds like a good approach.

C. Henney

We can't let that go so easily. There must be at least seven people here whose laboratories have spent many man-years on that approach, with no concrete results. The issue is whether liposomes bearing MHC products can serve as targets for CTL attack. With the exception of that one series of experiments from McConnell's laboratory involving an eye muscle protein as a "stabilizer" or whatever, such experiments have not been successful to my knowledge.

M. Mescher

But are those attempts to actually lyse antigen containing liposomes, or to block killing with antigen-containing liposomes? I think there is a big difference in that regard. We've been doing a lot of studies comparing the relative affinity of cytolytic T lymphocytes for various kinds of targets, and one indication from our work is that the size of the target may play a big role in how effectively the CTL interacts with it (J. Immunol. 1981, 127:51). And a point to be made about liposomes being used by McConnell et al is that they were using very large liposomes relative to what can normally be obtained. We've observed that large liposomes containing antigen trigger pre-CTL much more effectively. So, the possibility still exists that that approach may be made feasible.

P. Henkart

I would like, just in a very speculative way, to suggest that one answer to this fascinating problem of the lytic hit mechanism may be to think about the possibility that the lytic moiety may be itself in a lipid vesicle. I will later show some suggestive data that in ADCC this may be so. If that is true, there is a possibility that the recognition unit may reside in the same membrane as the lytic hit mechanism.

W. Clark

In the killer anti-killer experiments (A-anti-B attacking a B-anti-C), both of these cells are killers, and should have hydrophobic attack complexes sitting in their membrane. Yet in that case where you have a very intimate apposition of two killer cell membranes during conjugation, killing only occurs in one direction. The only way you can get around it not being bidirectional is that recognition and insertion of the plug are linked together. That means that the insertion mechanism does not operate unless the MHC receptor of the killer cell is occupied and then you can explain why the plug gets inserted in only one direction. But that's an important boundary condition that we have to keep in mind.

LYMPHOCYTE MEDIATED CYTOLYSIS AS A SECRETORY PHENOMENON

Maryanna P. Henkart and Pierre A. Henkart

Immunology Branch
National Cancer Institute
Bethesda, Maryland 20205

In this paper we would like to develop the idea that lymphocyte-mediated killing of foreign cells is a result of a secretory process by the effector lymphocyte which is triggered by the interaction of cell surface receptors with specific ligand, and that the result of this secretory event is the transfer of a pore-forming substance into the membrane of the target cell. We will discuss the evidence which we have obtained in studying human ADCC and NK systems, but we also believe that this serves as a plausible general model for events in cytolysis mediated by CTL. At present we realize that there remains much work to be done to establish this hypothesis even for the ADCC and NK mechanisms, but we also believe that the time has come to bring together the growing body of evidence which supports this concept.

MEMBRANE DAMAGE IS THE MECHANISM FOR THE LETHAL HIT

We have considered the target cell membrane a likely site of action for the lethal hit in lymphocyte killing for two principal reasons: 1) It is a lytic effect which is exerted quickly, i.e., within a few hours or less after specific contact between the effector cell and the target. This alone makes unlikely many possible types of toxic effects because inhibition of most biochemical pathways by drugs will not result in cell death for many hours. 2) In the case of ADCC by human blood lymphocytes, macrophages, and neutrophils, an extracellular cytotoxic effect is observed even with mammalian red blood cells as targets. These simple cells have no nuclei and are lacking most biochemical synthetic pathways; thus the membrane remains the most obvious target. Furthermore, there are many diverse biological examples of membrane permeability damage being mediated by toxins, beginning with many examples of bacterial toxins (1), continuing with toxins from fungi (2), various invertebrate toxins including some from coelenterates (3) and insects (4), and, of course, the complement systems of vertebrates (4). In most of these biological systems there is a mechanism to protect the effector system from being damaged by its own toxin, a property exquisitely displayed by the lymphocyte killing mechanisms.

In order to study membrane damage in isolation from other events associated with cell death, a number of years ago we began to develop systems for using model membranes which could be recognized as targets by lymphocytes. These studies have utilized antibody dependent cell mediated killing because it appears much easier to obtain recognition (ie., strong and specific binding) between the effector cell Fc receptor and model membranes than between CTL and such membranes. The first model system utilized (6) was the planar lipid bilayer, which has classically been used to study ionic permeability mechanisms by measurement of electrical resistance across the membrane. It was found that specifically under conditions in which target cell lysis occurred, i.e., in the presence of Fc receptor-bearing lymphocytes and antibody-coated lipid bilayers, the electrical resistance of the model membranes decreased by orders of magnitude, indicating an ionic permeability increase. In some instances

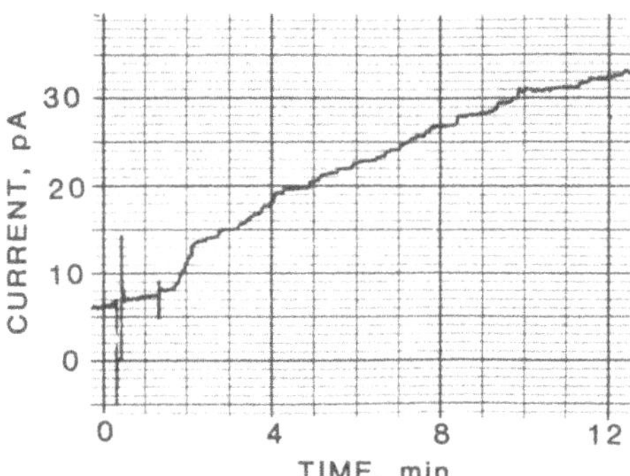

Fig. 1. Discrete conductance increases caused by human peripheral blood lymphocytes in contact with antibody-coated planar lipid bilayer membrane. Effector lymphocytes regularly induced conductance increases of orders of magnitude under conditions where cytotoxicity of cells would have been observed. In this experiment the onset of the conductance increase was slow enough so that the small discrete increases shown here could be observed. Such small discrete conductance changes in bilayer membranes have been shown to be associated with the opening of individual channels induced by a variety of substances. (From Henkart, P. and R. Blumenthal, ref. 6.)

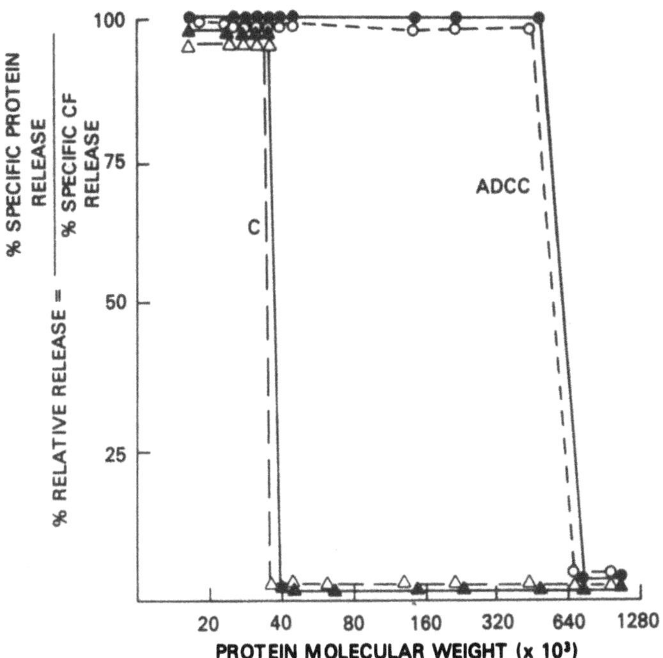

Fig. 2. Size dependence of release of marker proteins from resealed ghosts by lymphocytes in ADCC. Each marker protein tested was rhodamine-labeled and resealed together with the small water-soluble dye carboxyfluorescein (CF) in TNP-modified human erythrocyte ghosts. After addition of anti-TNP and human peripheral blood lymphocytes to the ghosts attached to a monolayer, followed by incubation for 3 hours at 37°C, marker release from the ghosts was monitored by fluorometry of the supernatant and fluoresence microscopy of the ghosts. (Taken from Simone, C.B. and P.A. Henkart, ref. 7.)

the permeability increase could be seen to occur in discrete steps, suggesting that individual pores were inserted into the membrane (Fig. 1). This series of experiments provided evidence that lymphocytes were capable of mediating membrane damage to a pure lipid bilayer. Since the ionic permeability increases observed could hardly have been explained without insertion of some sort of exogenous molecules into the target lipid bilayer, and those could only reasonably have been proposed to come from the lymphocyte, it seemed plausible that the bilayer damage was caused by a secretory product of the lymphocyte.

In order to be able to investigate the nature of the permeability increases induced by lymphocytes in target membranes in more detail we turned to the mammalian red cell ghost membrane and examined the selectivity of the increased permeability (7). We found that ADCC effector cells specifically induced in ghost membranes dramatic increases in permeability to molecules slightly larger than 10 nm in diameter, but the largest molecules utilized, with over 15 nm diameter, did not measurably pass through the affected membrane (Fig. 2). We regard a permeability profile which shows such a sieving property as evidence for membrane pores, in this case with a maximal diameter of about 14 nm. Identical sieving properties were observed for both lymphocytes and neutrophils as effector cells, while monocyte effector cells gave a slightly smaller size cut-off. For all these ADCC systems a non-phagocytic extracellular killing system is operational (8).

How can such large pores be created in a membrane? They are far larger than pores that comprise natural permeability pathways in membranes of normal cells, and it did not seem appealing to postulate that lymphocyte killing works by enlargement of a naturally occurring transport system because the planar lipid bilayer results would not be accounted for. We were, of course, aware of studies on complement which suggested that pores are created by insertion into the membrane of the terminal proteins of the complement pathway. We (7) and others (9) have used the resealed erythrocyte ghost to show that the maximal pore size of the complement channels is about 5 nm (which corresponds to the 40,000 d protein cut-off seen in Fig. 2). While this is considerably smaller than the maximal size of the lymphocyte-induced pores it is, nevertheless, again far larger than most naturally occurring membrane pores. It seemed plausible to consider complement as a model for how large membrane pores can be created, even though there is not presently agreement in the complement field as to the permeability pathway with respect to the inserted C5b-9 complex (10). The analogy with complement was further enhanced as a result of our collaboration with Dr. Robert Dourmashkin, who originally described the presence of "lesions" in negatively stained membranes of complement lysed erythrocytes using the electron microscope (11). He had more recently been looking at negatively stained pieces of membranes present at the end of an ADCC reaction asnd had discovered the presence of ring shaped membrane "lesions" which appeared generally similar to those seen after complement treatment, but which were considerably larger. He had concluded that these were likely to be permeability increasing "lesions." Since the correlation of sizes with respect to complement was in striking agreement with our functional results, he came to NIH where we were able to show that these "lesions" were associated with red cell ghost membranes specifically under conditions where marker release occurred, and were not seen in control incubations of ghosts and effector cells in the absence of antibody (12 and Fig. 3). From this evidence we found it highly likely that the "lesions" seen in negatively stained preparations were associated with membrane damage, and were tempted to speculate that the permeability pathway was an

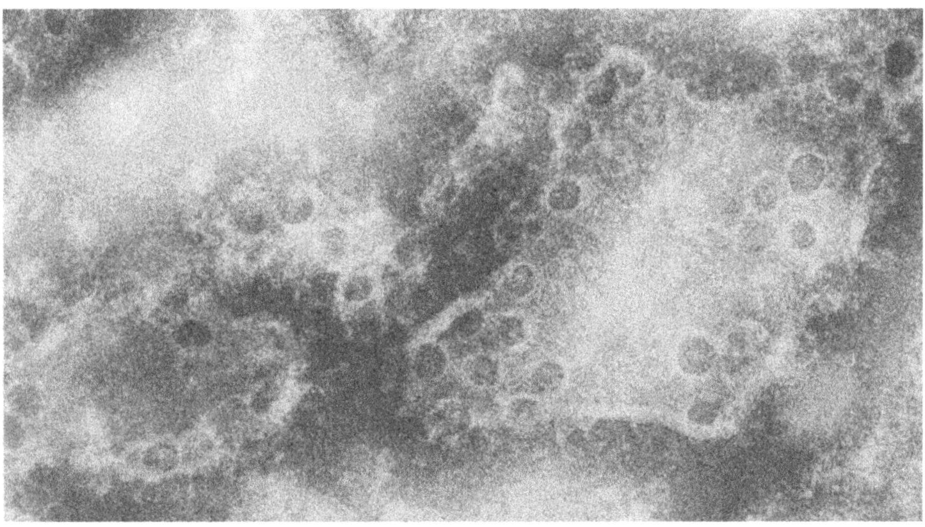

Fig. 3. Negatively stained erythrocyte ghost membrane after attack by ADCC effectors. Human erythrocyte ghosts were TNP-modified and coated with anti-TNP antibody. Human periphal blood lympocytes were added and after 4 hours the effector cells were washed away and the ghosts were negatively stained with 1% phosphotungstic acid. 315,000 X. (From Dourmashkin, R.R. et al, ref. 12.)

aqueous pore down the center similar to Manfred Mayer's vision of the complement pore as a donut (13).

EFFECTOR CELLS ALONE, WHEN APPROPRIATELY TRIGGERED, RELEASE MEMBRANOUS MATERIAL BEARING RING-SHAPED STRUCTURES

During development of model systems for the study of ADCC, we noted that human peripheral blood lymphocytes adherent to surfaces coated with antigen-antibody complexes underwent dramatic changes of shape within a few minutes (14,15). In the electron microscope these lymphocytes were found to contain organelles of various complex shapes and contents, which will be discussed in more detail below. Below or adjacent to some of the cells on the antigen-antibody coated surfaces there were clusters of membranous material, essentially membrane vesicles of various sizes and shapes, which we initially regarded as debris (Fig. 4a). Upon examining this material at higher magnification, it was apparent that these extracellular clumps of membrane bore ring-shaped structures between 10 and 20 nm in internal diameter (Fig. 4b). These corresponded in size to the stain-filled center portions of the "lesions" found by Dourmashkin on negatively stained red cell ghosts after ADCC attack. This indi-

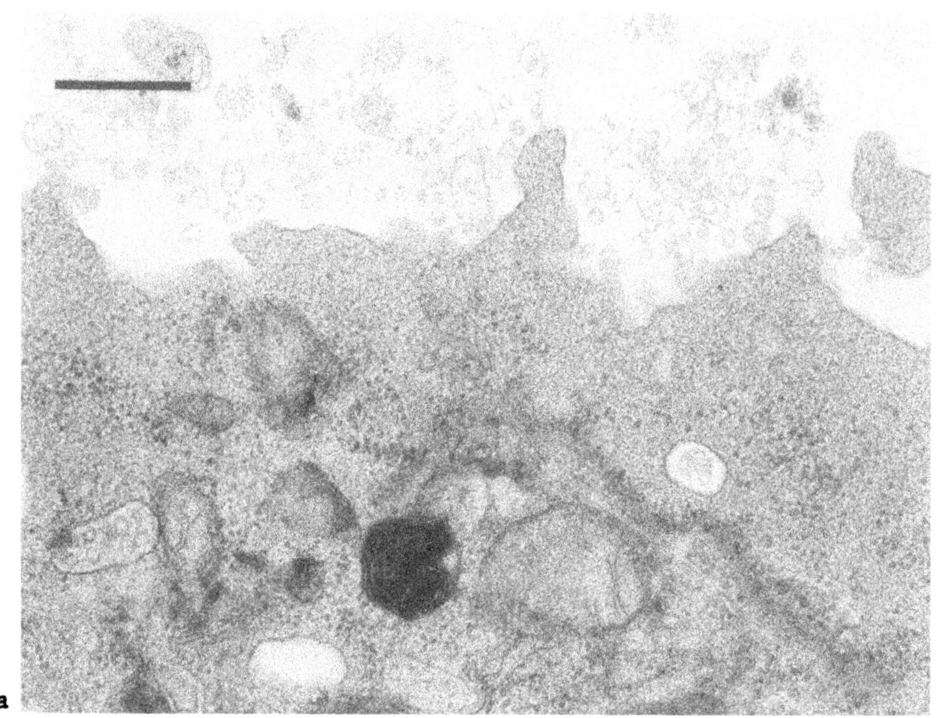

a

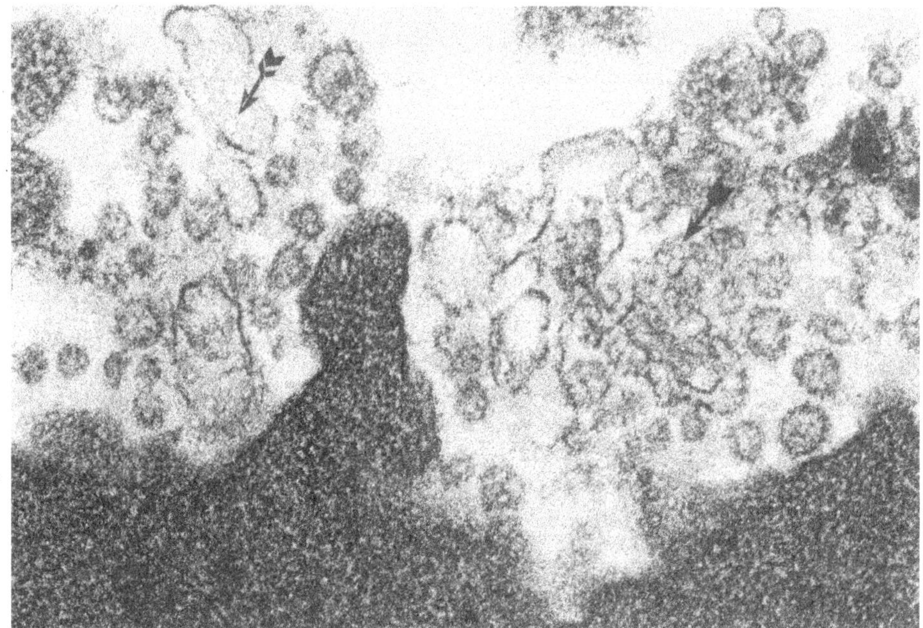

b

cated that the ring-shaped structures borne on membranous material were a product of the lympocytes and could not have been a breakdown product of lysed target cells since in this model system no target cells were present.

Other evidence that the appearance of the ring-shaped structures correlated with cytotoxic action included the observations that: 1) such ring-shaped structures are not a feature of random membrane debris observed in cultures of other cells types. (2) Lymphocytes adherent to antigen-antibody complexes do not elaborate ring-bearing material when incubated at low temperature or in presence of azide. 3) Experiments with natural killer cells (which will be discussed in more detail below) show that in conjugates with appropriate target cells, membranous material bearing rings is seen to be elaborated progressively with time after target cell contact.

It seemed reasonable to postulate that the rings might be patent pores through the membranes constituting channels responsible for increased permeability. The ring-bearing membranous material from the effector cells might then transfer ring-forming material (or fully formed rings) to the target cells either by fusion with them or by some other mechamism.

What is the cellular source of the membranous material bearing rings? The membranes appear not to be shed directly from the lymphocyte surface, but to be formed from material produced and packaged as secretory granules.

GRANULES IN THE EFFECTOR CELL ARE REORGANIZED UPON TARGET CELL CONTACT AND THEIR CONTENTS, INCLUDING MEMBRANOUS MATERIAL BEARING RING-SHAPED STRUCTURES, ARE RELEASED BY EXOCYTOSIS

Lymphocyte effectors of ADCC (K cells) and natural killer (NK) cells belong to highly overlapping populations (16). This is indicated, for example, by the fact that adherence to surfaces coated with antigen-antibody complexes is an effective method for depletion

---

Fig. 4. Electron micrograph of a human peripheral blood lymphocyte adherent to an antigen-antibody coated plastic surface. The surface was coated with TNP-anti-TNP complexes prepared by methods described in ref. 17. This section is parallel to and just above the plane of the complex-coated plastic plate. In the lower magnification view (a) membrane vesicles of various sizes and shapes are seen adjacent to the cell.

An area of the same micrograph enlarged and printed at a higher density is shown in part b. The arrows indicate examples of ring-shaped structures on the membrane vesicles. The mark indicates 0.4 μm.

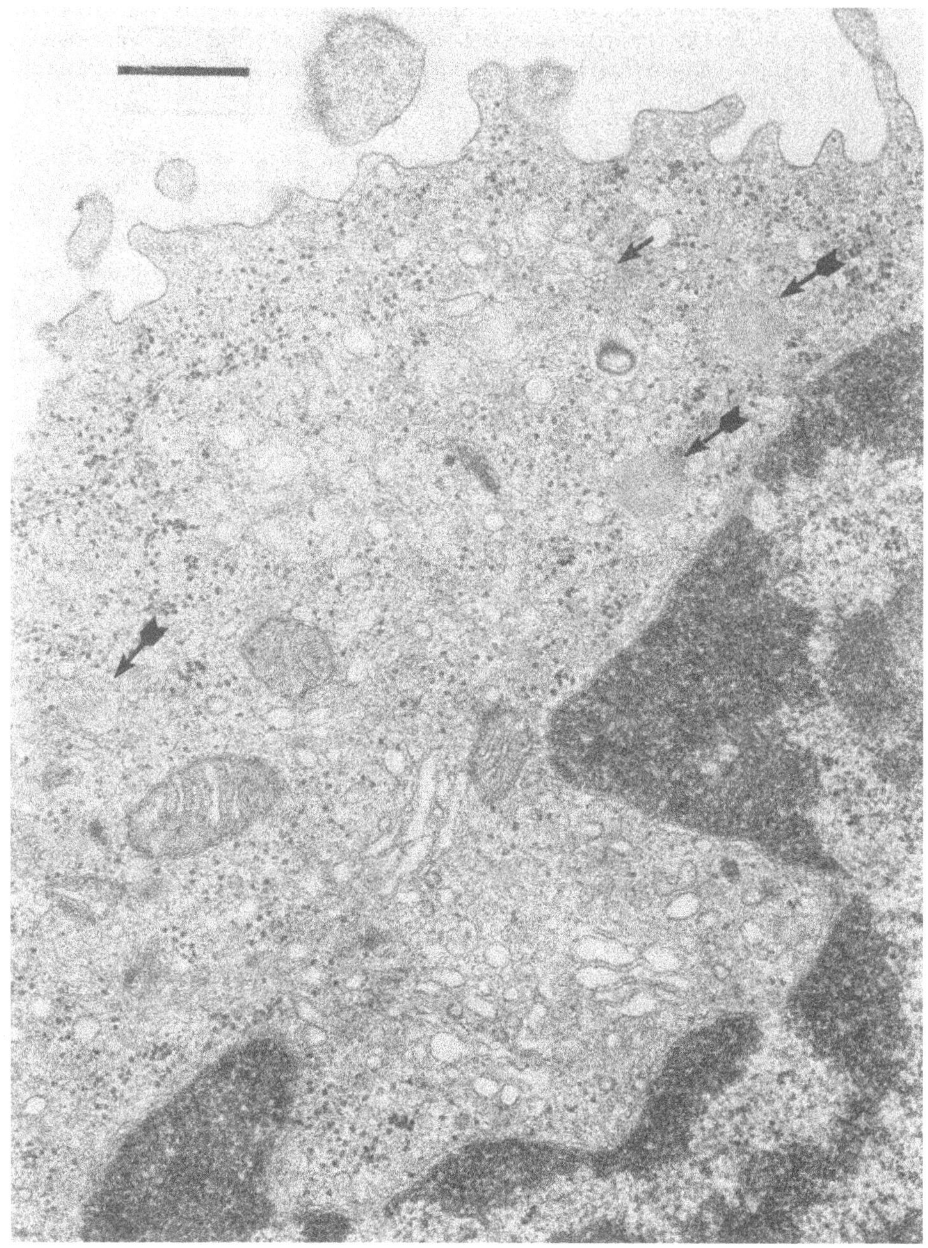

Fig. 5. Electron micrograph of a human large granule lymphocyte. This is a cell typical of those isolated from human peripheral blood in the LGL fraction on Percoll gradients (18). The arrows indicate examples of typical granules. The arrow without a tail indicates a granule in which a small bundle of tubules is cut in cross section. The mark indicates 0.4 μm.

of both types of effectors (16,17). NK and ADCC effectors can be enriched by fractionation of human peripheral blood lymphocytes on Percoll gradients; the fraction enriched for both effectors contains primarily large granular lymphocytes (LGL) (18,19). The electron microscope shows that a high proportion of LGL, as their name would imply, contain discrete membrane bound granules of several types (Fig. 5). The predominant granules are generally spherical and contain uniformly grainy-textured materials which stain to various degrees (appear several shades of grey in micrographs). Another grannule type contains crystalline arrays of tubules or tubule bundles which we had previously found to characteristic of Fc receptor positive lymphocytes (20).

In collaboration with Tuomo Timonen and John Ortaldo in the Laboratory of Immunodiagnosis, NCI, electron microscope studies of NK-target conjugates were done using as effectors LGL that had been pretreated with interferon (21). In this condition, approximately 80% of LGL binding to K-562 targets lyse the target cells in a 4 hour assay (T. Timonen, manuscript in preparation). Conjugates were fixed in suspension. After embedding, individual conjugates were selected and serially sectioned for electron microscopy. We felt confident that by examining serial sections of entire conjugates fixed at different times after target binding we had a high probability of observing events relevant to the lytic mechanism.

At early times (5-10 minutes at room temperature) NK cells bound to targets with random orientation, and both cells contributed interdigitating projections in the region of contact. These identified NK cells contained the several distinct morphologic types of granules including some with the characteristic tubule bundles (22 and manuscript in preparation) which were seen in LGL in suspension and in Fc receptor positive cells. At early times after conjugate formation the granules were still generally discrete and spherical. After incubation for 1 hour at 37°C the NK cells in conjugates tended to be oriented with the centrioles and Golgi apparatus directed toward the target. The granules were no longer discrete and spherical, but when traced through serial sections were found to be continuous with one another, forming complex membrane-bound structures extending through the cytoplasm of the lymphocyte for considerable distances. The contents of the previously distinct granules was seen to mingle and more heterogeneous material was formed. In some areas this appeared as clusters of membrane vesicles, and it was common to find more irregularly shaped membranous forms within the same organelle as pieces of tubule bundles and amorphous darkly-staining materials. These changes in granules gave rise to organelles with complex shapes and contents resembling those seen previously in lymphocytes adherent to antigen-antibody complexes (Fig. 6).

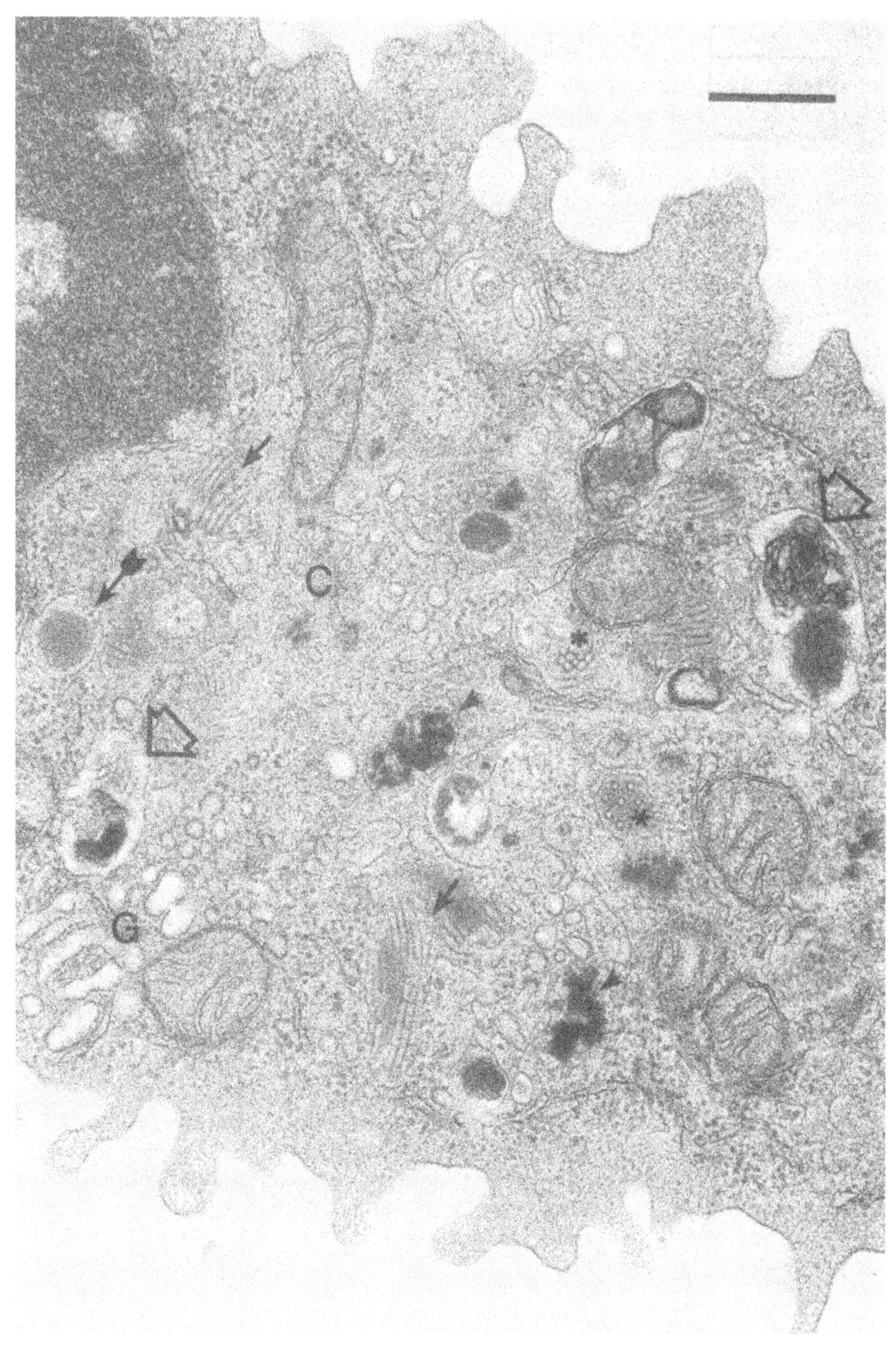
C
G

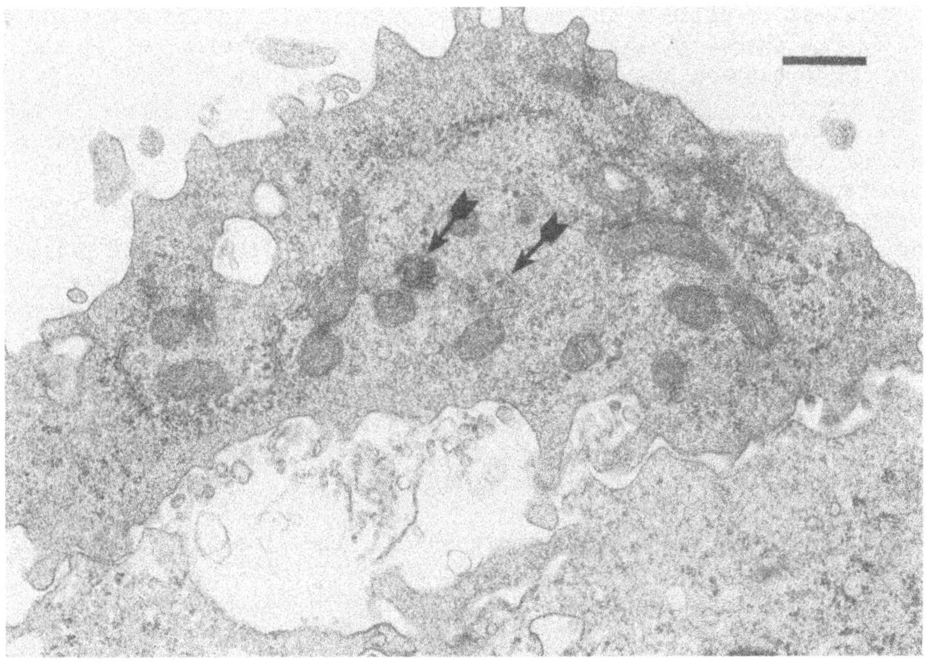

Fig. 7. An NK cell conjugate with a K-562 target after 1 hr at 37°C. In the space between the killer cell (above) and the target there is a cluster of membrane vesicles of various sizes and shapes which had been released from the effector. The arrows indicate regions of fused granules within the effector cell, containing complex materials including longitudinally oriented tubule bundles. The mark indicates 0.4 μm.

Fig. 6. Electron micrograph of a lymphocyte adherent to antigen-antibody complexes. The cell is cut parallel to the surface. The arrow on the left indicates a granule similar to the granules in LGL's fixed in suspension. The arrows without tails point to longitudinal sections through tubule bundles. Asterisks indicate cross sections through tubule-containing structures. Arrow heads point to darkly stained, osmiophilic amorphous material. The large open arrows indicate membrane enclosed structures with heterogeneous contents. The one on the left contains recognizable pieces of tubule bundles. The one on the right contains a grainy-textured material similar to that in the typical LGL granules as well as a clump of complex membranous material. Serial sections of this and other similar cells attached to surfaces via their Fc receptors or NK cells in conjugates show that these various materials are contained within extensive membrane bound strctures having complex shapes. The Golgi apparatus is marked "G" and the edge of the centriolar region is marked "C". Cytoplasmic microtubules radiate from the centriole. The mark indicates 0.4 μm.

Material resembling the complex, fused granule contents was also found in the extracellular space adjacent to the effector cells, and in the space between the killer and target cell (Fig. 7).

A closer look at the material in the extracellular space (Fig. 8) showed that is was made up primarily of membranes in various forms, ranging from small round vesicles approximately 50 nm in diameter to large, irregularly shaped structures with longest dimensions up to a few hundred nm. Occasionally recognizable small pieces of tubule bundles were seen. The various membranous extracellular structures often bore ring-shaped structures superimposed or intercalated in the membranes. The internal diameter of these rings ranged from 10 to 20 nm which, again, corresponded to the range of pore size suggested by the marker release experiments of Simone and Henkart (7) and to the size of the dark centers of the ring shaped "lesions" described by Dourmashkin et al. (12) in red blood cell ghost membranes after attack by ADCC effectors.

In sum, these observations suggest that the lymphocyte reorganized its granule contents to produce and subsequently to secrete clusters of membrane vesicles bearing "lesion"-forming molecules or fabricated "lesions." After their release in proximity to the

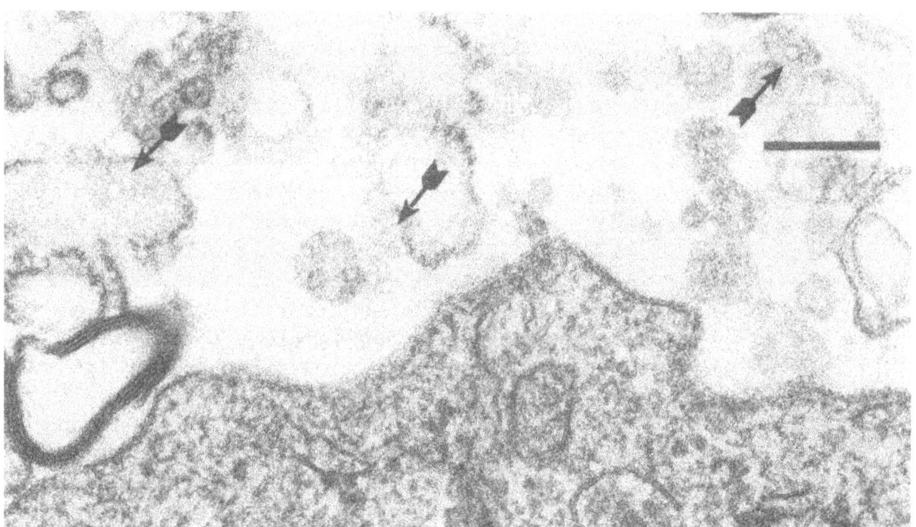

Fig. 8. Membrane vesicles secreted by an NK cell in a conjugate with a K-562 target after 1 hour at 37°C. The arrows indicate ring-shaped structures on the membranes. Lamellar structures such as the one at the left are sometimes associated with the ring-bearing membranous material. The mark indicates 0.4 μm.

target cell they cling to, and probably fuse with, the target cell membrane.

Whether the ring-bearing membranous material actually fuses with the target cell membrane is difficult to establish from the morphology of thin sections. Some images of the edges of target cells suggest that they do. The observations of Dourmashkin on negatively stained red cell ghosts also suggest this.

Are the granules and their products lysosomal? The criteria for identification of lysocomes are the presence of certain hydrolytic enzymes (23). Timonen found at the light microscope level diffuse staining for acid phosphatase in the region of the cell center in LGL (personal communication). It cannot be determined from this result, however, whether the stain was associated with the granules. The histochemical demonstration of lysosomal enzymes at the EM level has certain ambiguities in that the final reaction product of most reactions is a lead salt, and lead tends to bind to a variety of cellular structures in the absence of any lysosomal enzyme reaction product. Thus a certain background is always found against which the specific reaction product must be judged. The tubule bundle containing granules of human peripheral blood lymphocytes have been reported to be negative for acid phosphatase (24). In our initial experiments with lysosomal enzyme histochemistry, there was no more "reaction product" in the complex, fused granules of NK cells than in their mitochondria; this precipitate is probably nonspecific. At present, the question of whether the complex granule contents secreted by stimulated effector cells should be regarded as lysosomal remains open. Detailed analysis of the granule remains to be done by further histochemistry and immunocytochemistry in combination with biochemistry.

Clearly the outstanding morphologic feature of the secreted material is the presence of ring-shaped structures on the surface of the membranous material. The similarity in size of these structures and the ring-shaped "lesions" observed in negative stained red cell ghosts attacked by ADCC effectors and their correspondence to the size of marker release in the sieving experiments of Simone and Henkart (7) makes it attractive to interpret them as the mechanism of delivery of the lethal hit.

Examination of the target cells during the course of NK attack suggests that other, later events could also contribute to target cell death. For example, the target cell may internalize some of the killer cell derived material.

The involvement of secretory events in lymphocyte-mediated killing has been considered previously in the history of this field (reviewed in 25,26). One objection to explaining lymphocyte mediated killing on the basis of a stimulus-secretion model has been that the killing process shows more metabolic complexity than would be predicted from other stimulus-secretion systems (e.g., the mast cell). However, the hypothesis presented here would predict this since our results indicate that a variety of complex cellular functions (reorientation of organelles and reorganization of granule contents) are intermediate between the bindng of the target cell and the secretory event. Even more troubling for a secretory model has been the exquisite specificity of the damage inflicted by the lymphocyte. Not only are "innocent bystanders" in the neighborhood of the target cells not lysed, but from experiments in which one CTL acts on another CTL it is clear that the lytic process is highly directed (polarized) towards the cell recognized as target by receptors on the effector CTL (27). The sort of secretory process we have proposed could account for this since the secreted material is elaborated in high concentration in close proximity to the target cell and seems to cling to the adjacent cell membranes. This would then result in localized transfer to the target cell membrane of the lethal pore-forming material. It is even possible to imagine that the membrane vesicles bearing the lytic moieties may also bear receptors so that there would be two stages of membrane receptor-target antigen recognition: the first one to trigger the secretory process, and the second one to guide the lethal vesicles. Although such ideas are highly speculative at present, hypotheses based upon the results summarized in this paper are subject to testing and suggest several lines of experiments for the near future.

REFERENCES

1. Jelajasjcwicz, J., and T. Wadstrom, editors. Bacterial toxins and Cell Membranes. Academic Press, New York. (1978)
2. Seeger, R., and B. Wachter. Rubescenslysin and phallolysin release marker molecules from phospholipid cholesterol liposomes. Biochem. Biophy. Acta. 645:59. (1981)
3. Michaels, D.W. Membrane damage by a toxin from the sea anemone _Stoihactus helianthus_. I. Formation of transmembrane channels in lipid bilayers. Biochem. Biophy. Acta. 555:67. (1979)
4. Dawson, C.R, A.F. Drake, J. Helliwell, R.C. Hider. The interaction of bee melittin with lipid bilayer membranes. Biochem. Biophy. Acta. 510:75. (1978)
5. Mayer, M.M., D.W. Michaels, L.E. Rammn, M.L. Shin, M.B. Whitlow, and J.B. Willoughby. Membrane damage by complement. CRC Critical Reviews in Immunology 2:133. (1981)
6. Henkart, P. and R. Blumenthal. Interaction of lymphocytes with lipid bilayer membranes: a model for lymphocyte mediated lysis of target cells. Proc. Natl. Acad. Sci. 72:2789. (1975)
7. Simone, C.B., and P. Henkart. Permeability changes induced in erythrocyte ghost targets by antibody-dependent cytotoxic effector cells: evidence for membrane pores. J. Immunol. 124:952. (1980)

8. Katz, P., C.B. Simone, P.A. Henkart, and A.S. Fauci. Mechanisms of antibody-dependent cellular cytotoxicity. The use of effector cells from chronic granulomatous disease patients as investigative probes. J. Clin. Invest. 65:55. (1981)
9. Giavidoni, E.B., Y.M. Chow, and A.P. Dalmasso. The functional size of the primary complement lesion in resealed erythrocyte membrane ghosts. J. Immunol. 122:240. (1979)
10. Podack, E.R., G. Biescher, and E. Muller-Eberhard. Membrane attack complex of complement: Generation of high affinity phospholipid binding sites by fusion of five hydrophilic plasma proteins. Proc. Natl. Acad. Sci. 76:897. (1979)
11. Humphrey, J.H., and R.R. Fourmashkin. The lesions in cell membranes caused by complement. Adv. in Immunol. 11:756. (1969)
12. Dourmashkin, R.R., P. Deteix, C.B. Simone, and P. Henkart. Electron microscopic demonstration of lesions om target cell membranes associated with antibody-dependent cellular cytotoxicity. Clin. Exp. Immunol. 43:554. (1980)
13. Mayer, M.M. Mechanism of cytolysis by complement. Proc. Natl. Acad. Sci. 69:2954. (1972)
14. Alexander E., and P. Henkart. The adherence of human Fc receptor bearing lympocytes to antigen-antibody complexes. II. Morphologic alterations induced by substrate. J. Exp. Med. 143:329. (1976)
15. Henkart, P.A., M.P. Henkart, and E.L. Alexander. Behavior and fine structure of human Fc receptor bearing lymphocytes adherent to immobilized antigen-antibody complexes. Proceedings of the 10th Leucocyte Culture Conference, p. 70. (1975)
16. Kay, H.D., G.D. Bonnard W.H. West, and R.B. Herbermann. A functional comparison of human Fc receptor bearing lymphocytes active in natural cytotoxicity and antibody-dependent cellular cytotoxicity. J. Immunol. 118:2058. (1977)
17. Henkart, P.A., and E. Alexander. The adherence of human Fc receptor bearing lymphocytes to immobilized antigen-antibody complexes. I. Specificity and use as a preparative separation technique. J. Immunol. Meth. 20:155. (1978)
18. Timonen, T., and E. Saksela. Isolation of human natural killer cells by density gradient centrifugation. J. Immunol. Meth. 36:285. (1980)
19. Timonen, T., J.R. Ortaldo, and R.B. Herberman. Characteristics of human large granular lymphocytes and relationship to natural killer and K cells. J. Exp. Med. 153:569. (1981)
20. Henkart, M., and P. Henkart. Macrotubule bundles in human Fc receptor bearing lymphocytes. J. Cell. Biol. 67:166a. (1975)
21. Herberman, R.R., J.R. Ortaldo, and G.D. Bonnard. Augmentation by interferon of human natural and antibody-dependent cell-mediated cytotoxicity. Nature 277:221. (1979)
22. de Duve, C. Exploring cells with a centrifuge. Science 189: 186. (1975)
24. Huhn, D. Neu Organelle im peripheren Lymphozyten? Dtsch. Med.

Wochenschr. 93:2099. (1968)

25. Golstein, P., and E.T. Smith. Mechanism of T-cell-mediated cytolysis: The lethal hit stage. Contemp. Top. in Immunobiol. 7:273. (1977)
26. Carpen, O., Vitanen, I., and E. Saksela. The cytotoxic activity of human natural killer cells requires an intact secretory apparatus. Cell. Immunol. 58:97. (1981)
27. Berke. G. Interaction of cytotoxic T lymphocytes and target cells. Progr. Allergy 27:69. (1980)

ACKNOWLEGEMENTS

We thank Raymnond T. Rusten and Paul J. Millard for excellent technical assistance.

DISCUSSION

Mike Hanna

Microvesiculation of cells, especially cells stimulated under various conditions, is not uncommon. I'd like again to know the size of your vesicular products.

Marianna Henkart

The vesicles are very heterogeneous. The smallest ones are probably in the range of 15 nanometers. They come in all varieties of sizes, in fact, not just vesicles but also irregular membrane sheets which can be tenths of microns.

Mike Hanna

I think that's the part of it that may be a little bit of a bother. What do you think has happened?

Marianna Henkart

What I think is happening, is that all the material that now appears on the outside of the cell as vesicles, was originally contained within an intracellular compartment. You have a vesicle cluster within a vesicle within a cell, which is then exocytosed. I think this is a big massive secretory product out here, not the surface of the cell budding off.

Unknown

Have you ever done a classical organelle separation experiment, taken the granular fraction either with or without solubilization and seen if it's cytotoxic?

P. Henkart

No, I've not done that. It's an interesting approach that we're starting to consider.

R. Herberman

Are the granules you see lysosomes?

M. Henkart

I really can't be sure on the basis of simple morphology. In the light microscope there is definitely staining for acid phosphatase, but it is rather diffuse and as much in mitochondria as in the granules so I'm not sure what to make of it. It's not convincing.

C. Nathan

Among the most cytotoxic things in the granules of other leukocytes are the cationic proteins. I wonder if you had a chance just to see by a variety of techniques, whether these granules are rich for cationic proteins?

M. Henkart

Actually, equating azurophilic granules in the light microscope with granules that I see in EM is probably risky. But azure stain is thought to stain acid muco-substances, which means they probobly have fixed anionic rather than cationic charges.

P. Lachman

I think you're drawing the analogy of these ring-like structures you see with complement lesions. The complement lesion has to be assembled in the membrane in which it is formed, and it cannot be integrated, once it already has a ring-structure, without deoxycholate. I think one possibility you might consider is that what you're seeing is still in the killer cell and not actually the lesions that make it to the target, and lyse it, but those that fail to make it and are then got rid of in some other way.

M. Henkart

That's possible. In fact I rarely see the ring-shaped lesions, if we want to call them that for short-hand, already assembled inside the cell. They are most obvious on this mass of material that's outside the cell.

E. Martz

Can you exclude that what you see between the cells and in the killer cell, is actually subsequent to initial collapse, with pieces of the target cell coming off and then being endocytosed by the killer cell?

M. Henkart

The fact that we see something extremely similar on antigen-antibody complex coated surfaces, where only the Fc receptor-bearing effector cells are present, probably makes that unlikely.

I.C.M. MacLennan

CTL perhaps don't have the same sort of granules. It could also be that these granules are not entirely related to the killing process.

D. Zagury

I have isolated hundreds of killers with ghosts or at different stages from the beginning of the incubation to two hours, either CTL, or K cells, or NK cells, and in all the lysosomal granules were there.

C. Henney

Don't we also agree with Ian that this doesn't necessarily mean that the granules have got anything to do with killing?

D. Zagury

I agree again and again that they just are there. Their presence is one argument for a secretory process, together with the other argument that the metabolic requirements for killing and for exocytosis are the same.

Marianna Henkart

I wanted to address the question of not seeing vesicles and seeing projections. At early time points and in random sections one sees many, many projections and conjugates between K cells or NK cells and targets. As you well know, doing electron microscopy to insure oneself that one is looking at the relevant piece of action is very difficult. One really has to do serial sections and be very sure that the conjugates are likely to be "killing conjugates." When I first started looking at these things, through serial sections, I saw many sections just like the one you showed with projections and interdigitations. Then in some cases, I saw a lot of membranous debris which I ignored for a long time. Then, after I had looked at many cells, I found this membranous debris more a very regular feature of the killing conjugates and I began to pay closer attention to them and then I noticed these ring-shaped structures. I have a question about why you think zeiosis suggests that membrane damage is not a primary effect. All these changes could be perfectly consistent with an initial effect of membrane permeability increase with ionic equilibration which could cause the swelling of internal organelles and the loss of control of the cytoskeleton.

C. Sanderson

Yes, I think that's possible, but these sort of changes have never been described in any situation where you get membrane damage. For example, in complement or granulocyte killing of tumor cells, you don't see zeiosis at all. Zeiosis could be an important clue here and I think many people have overlooked it. If we knew more about zeiosis we might know more about the mechanism of T cell-mediated cytolysis.

G. Berke

Zeiosis could be an event subsequent to early damage. In fact, if you look at the single cell level, the efflux of small molecules precedes zeiosis quite substantially. We used cinematography under a UV microscope to monitor conjugates comprised of fluorescently labeled target cells and non-labeled killer cells. The target cell would usually lose its fluorescent labeling long before it began to show signs of disintegration. So, I think zeiosis is a post-mortem event as far as membrane permeability is concerned.

Manfred Mayer

A disturbance of the ionic enviroment could well lead to the changes you described. Of course, with complement, if the cell explodes before these changes take place, then one wouldn't see zeiosis. It may be that a great many channels are being made in the case of the complement treatment and it just goes too quickly.

C. Sanderson

You're suggesting that if you slow down complement, you should see zeiosis. However, over a range of doses, the morphological changes are identical. The time course is different, that's all.

Ron Herberman

I wonder how sure, in fact, you can be that the cell in a conjugate is a K cell. I raise this question particularly because with an unfractionated human PBL preparation, on a gross level the majority of the cells forming conjugates are not the large granular lymphocytes and these conjugates are non-lytic.

C. Sanderson

In the mouse T cell system, we can actually purify the T cells. You can be absolutely sure when we see the projections there. The K cell work is more a confirmation of the T cell work in that sense.

ASSOCIATIVE RECOGNITION IN ADCC

Peter Perlmann

Wenner-Gren Institute
University of Stockholm
5-113 45 Stockholm, Sweden

In ADCC, recognition of the target cells is mediated by IgG antibodies. Available evidence also suggests that target cell lysis is triggered by the interaction of Fc structures of the inducing IgG with the Fc_{γ}-receptors of the killer cell (1). Target cell recognition and triggering of lysis would thus appear to be linked but independent reactions. In the following I will discuss some additional recognition phenomena which are independent of the inducing antibody but which nevertheless are important in regulating killer cell - target cell interaction ADCC. We call this "associative recognition" and I will discuss four examples, three from our own work and one from the work of others.

Together with Hans Muller-Eberhard and Robert Schreiber we have worked for some time on the importance for ADCC of target cell bound C3-fragments. By using purified human complement components of the alternative pathway, C3 fragments were attached (without antibodies) to the surface of bovine erythrocytes (E_b) which were used as target cells for purified human blood lymphocytes. These target cells carried from 50-100,000 molecules of either C3b, C3bi or C3d. When lymphocytes were added in the absence of IgG anti-E_b antibodies, no lysis ensued, in spite of the fact that 40-50% of the K cells active in this system have receptors for C3 fragments and form stable rosettes with the complement carrying target cells (1). However, upon addition of minute amounts of IgG anti E_b, the target cells were lysed. Even at suboptimal IgG concentrations, giving no ADCC without complement, a strong and IgG-dose dependent ADCC was seen when C3 was attached to the target cell surface. These C3-fragments amplified ADCC solely by improving effector cell-target cell contact. About twice as many of the K cells had C3bi receptors (CR3) as C3b receptors (CR1). These non-cross-reacting receptors were largely expressed on different types of K cells (CR1 mostly on null cells, C3bi on T_γ cells). A minor fraction of the K cells also had receptors for C3d (CR2), but these receptors were probably to a large extent present on the same K cells as CR3 (2).

These experiments were done with the ^{51}Cr release assay. Important additional information was obtained by using the ADCC plaque assay which allows analysis of individual effector cells (3). Table I shows a typical experiment with E_b targets attached as monolayers to poly-L-lsyine coated coverslips.

These targets were either untreated or carried one of the fragments C3b, C3bi or C3d, respectively. To all samples, lymphocytes and a suboptimal amount of rabbit anti-E_b IgG were added. With untreated E_b, about 1.5% of the added lymphocytes were active K cells under these conditions. When C3 was present on the targets, this number was very significantly increased, indicating that the change of the target cell surface due to C3-attachment leads to a recruit-

TABLE I. Surface Markers Profile of K-Cells Before or After C3-Fragment Induced Enhancement of ADCC[1]

Target Cells[2]	% K-Cells[3]	% K-Cells With Surface Marker[4]			
		E_cC3b	E_cC3bi	E_cC3d	HP
E_b	1.5	11	26	9	38
E_bC3b	6.8	69	12	6	20
E_bC3bi	9.5	16	81	59	66
E_bC3d	8.6	5	46	75	57

[1]For details see (4).

[2]Monolayers of bovine erythrocytes carrying human C3-fragments as indicated.

[3]Plaque forming cells as per cent of total no. of lymphocytes added. ADCC was induced with a suboptimal concentration (1.5 μg IgG/ml) of rabbit anti-E_b IgG; 18 h.

[4]Per cent of plaque forming lymphocytes forming rosettes in situ with chicken erythrocytes (E_c) carrying C3 fragments as indicated; or stained with FITC-labeled Helix pomatia hemagglutinin (HP), a T-cell marker.

ment of effector cells. Most importantly, these newly recruited K cells differed, depending on which of the C3 fragments was present. Thus, when the targets carried C3b, the majority of the K cells were $CR2^+/CR3^+$ T_γ cells. Thus, out of a heterogenous population, the target cells select those effector cells which have the corresponding, target-fitting receptors and these K cells will predominate a given cytolytic system (4).

A very similar example of this type of associative recognition is provided by experiments with IgM anti-target cell antibodies. In our hands, carefully purified rabbit IgM anti-E^b, free of trace amounts of IgG, does not induce ADCC against E_b-targets. However, in the presence of suboptmal concentrations of IgG anti-E^b, IgM antibodies very strongly amplify IgG dependent ADCC (5,6). Here, it could be shown that this was entirely due to improved contact between IgM carrying target cells and K cells having both Fc_γ and Fc_γ receptors (5). These $T_{\gamma\mu}$ cells are known to be a minor fraction of the T_γ subset in normal blood (7). Normally, 30-40% of the K cells in an IgG anti-E_b system are of T_γ-type (1). However, when the target surface is modified by IgM adsorption, effector cell recruitment and selection takes place and the majority of the lytic cells are of the $T_{\gamma\mu}$-type.

When human lymphocytes are treated with live or UV-inactivated Paramyxoviruses, e.g., Parotis virus, their natural cytotoxicity to nucleated target cells is strongly enhanced (1). It was found that the only viral component responsible for this enhanced cytotoxicity is the surface glycoprotein bearing viral hemagglutinin and neuraminidase activities (HN)(8,9). When lymphocytes, treated with virus or the HN-glycoprotein were added to E_b target cells, no lysis of the latter occured, in spite of a very conspicuous mixed lymphocyte-E_b agglutination. However, when small amounts of IgG anti-E_b were added, ADCC was strongly enhanced in comparison with that seen with untreated lymphocytes. In addition, experiments at the cellular level by the ADCC-plaque assay revealed that this enhancement was due to a selective recruitment of T_γ-effector cells. A typical experiment is shown in Table II (A. Alsheikhly et al., manuscript in preparation). Thus, in these experiments, some lymphocytes had acquired a new target-recognition factor, the viral hemagglutinin. Obviously, however, although this recognition resulted in strong target cell binding, it was not sufficient for lysis which was triggered by the IgG antibody.

A fourth example indicating that target cell recognition may be brought about by different means but is not sufficient for lysis is provided by the work of Fuson et al. (10). When human lymphocytes were incubated with sheep erythrocytes, no erythrolysis followed. However, addition of immune complexed IgG with no antibody activity to either targets or effector cells resulted in lysis of the sheep erythrocytes, mediated by T-cells. Since it was only erythrocytes

TABLE II. Surface Marker Profile of K-Cells Before or After Parotis Virus Induced Enhancement of ADCC[1]

Lymphocytes	% K-Cells[2]	% K-Cells With Surface Marker[3]	
		CR	ER
Untreated	1.5	31	41
Virus Treated[4]	5.7	24	59

[1]Alsheikhly et al, manuscript in preparation.

[2]Plaque forming cells on E_b monolayers as percent of total no. of lymphocytes added.

[3]Per cent of plaque forming lymphocytes binding Zymosan particles carrying activated human C (CR), or forming rosettes with NANAse treated sheep erythrocytes (ER).

[4]10 μg of purified, UV-inactivated mumps virions /4x10^{-6} lymphocytes/ml, 30 min. 37°C.

from sheep but not from other species which were lysed the results suggested that the sheep erythrocyte receptor on certain lymphocytes ($T\gamma$) served as recognition factor, establishing effector cell-target cell contacts while the immune complexes triggered the cytolytic reaction via the Fc_γ receptor on the receptor cell.

In conclusion, these experiments show that a great variety of "receptor" structures on the lymphocytes may strongly affect cell mediated cytotoxicity by improving target cell recognition but without inducing lysis. Indirectly, these results support the notion of a triggering function of the Fc_γ-receptor in ADCC. In addition they show that the target cell surface is an important factor in the selection of appropriate effector cell subsets. Hence, defined changes of target cell surface structure may also lead to important changes in selection of the effector cell types which will mediate lysis.

REFERENCES

1. Perlmann, P. and J.C. Cerottini. Cytotoxic lymphocytes. In "The Antigens," Vol. 5, M. Sela (ed.), p. 173. Academic Press, Inc., New York (1979).

2. Perlmann, H., Perlmann, P., Schreiber, R.C., and H.G. Muller-Eberhard. Interaction of target cell-bound C3bi and C3d with human lymphocytes receptors. J. Exp. Med. 153:1592 (1981).
3. Wahlin, B., and P. Perlmann. Detection of K-cells by a plaque assay. In "In vitro methods in cell mediated and tumor immunity," B. Bloom and J.R. David (eds.)., p. 523. Academic Press, Inc., New York (1976).
4. Wahlin, B., Perlmann, H., Perlmann, P., Schreiber, R.D., and H.J. Muller-Eberhard. Human K-cells. Distribution of receptors for Ceb, C3bi and C3d and the ADCC regulatory function of these fragments. J. Immunol., submitted (1982).
5. Perlmann, H., Perlmann, P., Moretta, L., and M. Ronnholm. Regulation of IgG antibody-dependent cellular cytotoxicity in vitro by IgM antibodies. Scand. J. Immunol. 14:47 (1981).
6. Ohlander, C., Perlmann, H., and P. Perlmann. Regulation of IgG-IgM interplay by antibody specificity in human K-cell mediated cytotoxicity. Scand. J. Immunol. (in press)(1982).
7. Merrill, J.E., Biberfeld, G., Holmodin, G., Landin, S., and E. Norrby. A T-lymphocyte subpopulation in multiple sclerosis patients bearing Fc-receptors for both IgG and IgM. J. Immunol. 124:2758 (1980).
8. Harfast, B., Orvell, C., Alsheikhly, A., Andersson, T., Perlmann, P. and E. Norrby. The role of viral glycoproteins in mumps-virus dependent lymphocyte mediated cytotoxicity in vitro. Scand. J. Immunol. 11:391 (1980).
9. Alsheikhly, A., Orvell, C., Harfast, B., Andersson, T., Norrby, E., and P. Perlmann. Sendai virus dependent cellular cytotoxicity in vitro. The Role of viral glycoproteins. Scand. J. Immunol. (in press)(1982).
10. Fuson, E.W., Shaw, M.W., Hubbard, R.A., and E.W. Lamon. Antibody-antigen complex stimulated lysis of non-sensitized sheep red blood cells by human lymphocytes. Clin. Exp. Immunol. 38: 158 (1979).

INFLUENCE OF MONOVALENT CATION CONCENTRATIONS ON MONOCYTE-MEDIATED ADCC

Stephan Ladisch, Lisa Ulsh, and Stephen A. Feig

Division of Hematology/Oncology and
Gwynne Hazen Cherny Memorial Laboratories
Dept. of Pediatrics, UCLA School of Medicine
Los Angeles, CA 90024, USA

INTRODUCTION

Studies of effector cell biochemical processes associated with cell-mediated cytolysis have been undertaken by numerous laboratories to define the conditions required for the expression of cytolytic activity, and hopefully to ultimately eludicate mechanisms of cytolysis. By such studies, the requirements for the divalent cations, Ca^{++} and/or Mg^{++}, in T-cell and non-T cell-mediated cytolysis have been demonstrated using chelating agents (1,2). Similar studies of the possible importance of the monovalent cations, Na^+ and K^+, had been impeded by lack of equally selective means of altering their intracellular concentrations. However, inhibition of cytolytic activity by ouabain (3,4), which specifically blocks membrane active transport of Na^+ and K^+ (5), indicates that these cations as well may influence cytolytic activity.

In this presentation, we shall review some of the previous studies we have performed (6) using ouabain as a probe to elucidate monovalent cation requirements for monocyte-mediated ADCC (MMADCC), present additional direct evidence for a modulating effect of extracellular K^+ and/or Na^+ concentrations on MMADCC, and propose a hypothetical schema unifying the above findings with previous observations of an increased rate of glycolytic energy metabolism of monocytes exposed to hyperimmune anti-erythrocyte antiserum in the MMADCC system (7,8).

METHODS

MMADCC, as described by Poplack et al (9) was used as the cytotoxicity system because definitive quantitation of effector cell glycolytic energy metabolism can be made in parallel with the cytotoxicity assay. This is possible because the target in MMADCC is the metabolically relatively inactive human erythocyte and the effector cell population (human PBM) can be enriched for monocytes by adherence. Problems of substantial metabolic contributions of nucleated targets or of very heterogeneous cell populations containing few active effector cells are thereby avoided. Experimental details of the cytotoxicity assay and of the assay of glycolysis (measured as lactate production) are described in reference 7.

To quantitate the inhibition of active transport of monovalent cations by the monocyte we measured the cellular uptake of $^{86}Rb^+$, an analogue of K^+ which is similarly actively transported into the cell. The method of Segal et al (10) was used.

Modification of extracellular concentrations of K^+ and Na^+ was accomplished by the use of specially prepared, HEPES-buffered minimum essential medium in which the usually present Na^+ and K^+ salts were substituted for each other to obtain the desired final concentrations of these catious. The final pH of these media was 7.2-7.4 and osmolality 270-280 mosm/l. Five per cent v/v heat-inactived fetal calf serum which had been dialyzed against the appropriate medium above was added to obtain the final, complete medium used in these studies.

RESULTS AND DISCUSSION

When measured in a 20 hr assay, MMADCC was inhibited by the presence of ouabain (Table I). However, conditions of exposure to ouabain ($5x10^{-6}M$, 30 min preincubation) which caused essentially complete inhibition of active transport of monovalent cations (measured as $^{86}Rb^+$ influx) caused only partial inhibition of MMADCC, even though ouabain was continuously present during the 20 hr assay period (6). These results are similar to those of the two previous reports of ouabain-induced inhibition of cellular cytotoxcity (3, 4) in which only partial inhibition was observed. The findings suggest that monovalent cation transport and the ion fluxes (K^+ into and Na^+ out of the cell) generated by this transport are not essential to the expression of cytolytic activity. If they were, complete inhibition of active transport by ouabain should have immediately resulted in complete inhibition of cytotoxicity.

The incomplete inhibition of MMADCC was further investigated to determine whether residual cytotoxicty represented a depressed but constant rate of lysis or a delayed, eventually complete inhibi-

TABLE I. Effect of ouabain on monocyte active transport of monovalent cations and on MMADCC[a]

Ouabain concentration	$^{86}Rb^{+}$ influx[b]	% inhibition of ADCC[c]
0 (Control)	1267	--
$5x10^{-8}$ M	1200	17
$5x10^{-7}$ M	707	41
$5x10^{-6}$ M	99	50

[a] Experimental details in reference 6.

[b] Measured as cpm $^{86}Rb/10^{6}$ monocytes/min, 30 min after the addition of ouabain.

[c] 20 hr assay.

tion of MMADCC by ouabain. As shown by the selected experiments summarized in Table II, lytic activity in the presence of ouabain was almost normal during the first six hours of a 20 hr assay but thereafter no further lysis was observed (Expt. 1). By increasing the preincubation time in ouabain to six hours (Expt. 2), cytolysis was essentially completely inhibited. This complete inhibition observed following prolonged incubation of the effector cells in ouabain (which was reversible by removal of ouabain) further support the interpretation that an effect other than inhibition of the Na^{+}-K^{+} ATPase by ouabain was responsible for inhibition of MMADCC.

TABLE II. Kinetic characteristics of ouabain-induced inhibition of MMADCC

Preincubation time	Ouabain ($5x10^{-6}$M)	Duration of MMADCC Assay 6 hrs.	20 hrs.
30 min.	-	0.9[a]	2.3
(Expt. 1)	+	0.7	0.7
6 hrs.	-	0.8	N.D.
(Expt. 2)	+	0.1	N.D.

[a] Lytic activity expressed as targets lysed/monocyte.

One delayed effect of ouabain is reduction of the intracellular K^+ concentration (and elevation of Na^+ concentration). That such an effect might be important is suggested by the fact that a number of biochemical processes (such as synthesis of macromolecules) which might be critical to the cytotoxic mechanism are dependent upon maintenance of normal intracellular K^+ concentration (reviewed in ref. 11). To test the possibility that cation concentrations themselves (as opposed to the transport of cations) might influence the expression of cytotoxic activity, we have conducted experiments in which MMADCC was assessed in media containing varying concentrations of K^+ (and Na^+), following a one-hour preincubation of effector cells in these same media (Fig. 1). Optimal lytic activity was observed when the extracellular K^+ concentration ranged between 3 and 15 mEq/l, while both higher ($\geq$ 30 mEl/l) and lower ($\leq$ 1.5 mEq/l) K^+ concentrations and the corresponding changes in Na^+ concentrations were associated with lower levels of target cell lysis. These results would seem to indicate an importance for cytotoxic activity of extracellular concentrations of monovalent cations. However, interpretation of the results must also take into account the effects on intracellular changes in the extracellular concentrations. Direct evidence of whether intracellular or extracellular concentrations of monovalent cations are crucial to MMADCC may be obtainable by sequential measurements of MMADCC and monocyte intracellular cation concentrations under the conditions of the studies summarized in Table I and Figure 1. These studies are in progess.

The ATP utilized in the maintenance of normal intracellular cation concentrations is mainly generated by glycolysis. Since the

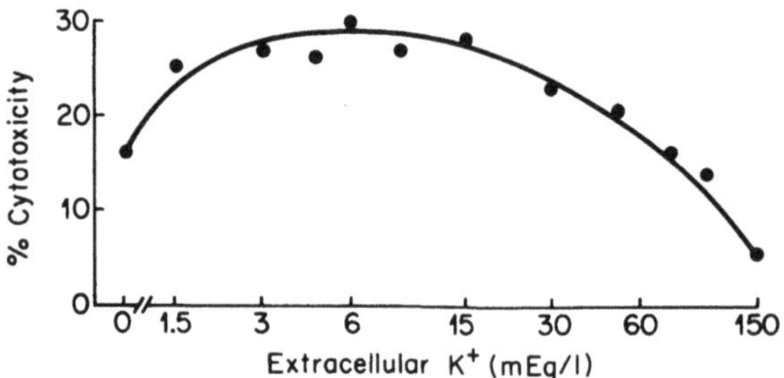

Fig. 1. Effect of extracellular K^+ concentration on MMADCC. Cells were preincubated for one hour in complete medium in which the K^+ concentration was adjusted as shown (see text for details). MMADCC was then quantitated in the same medium. Each point represents the mean specific lysis in two experiments, each performed in triplicate.

rate of glycolysis is increased in monocytes exposed to sensitizing antiserum in the MMADCC system (7,8) and monocyte cytotoxic function is inhibited when glycolysis is inhibited (12), we have also quantitated the monovalent cation transport-related glycolysis of monocytes (6). These measurements are made by completely inhibiting Na^+/K^+ transport by ouabain, and measuring the associated decrease in lactate production, termed ouabain-inhibitable lactate production. In a series of seven experiments, we found that essentially all of a 68% increase in lactate production associated with MMADCC was inhibited by 5×10^{-6}M ouabain, suggesting that the increase in glycolysis associated with MMADCC reflects an increased utilization of glycolysis-derived ATP in the active transport of Na^+ and K^+. Therefore, although the studies summarized by Tables I and II appear to exclude a direct role of monovalent cation transport in the cytotoxic process, an importance of maintenance of cation concentrations (accomplished by active transport) is suggested by the above data and the findings of others. An hypothesis which reconciles the findings is that analogous to an increase in lymphocyte membrane permeability to monovalent cations caused by exposure to phytohemagglutinin (10); exposure of monocytes to sensitizing antiserum also results in a membrane perturbation which increases permeability to monovalent cations. The sequence of events consequent to such a membrane perturbation is shown in Fig. 2. Either interference with cation transport (e.g., ouabain) or energy (ATP) production (by inhibition of glycolysis) could prevent regeneration of normal intracellular cation concentrations postulated to be critical to MMADCC. Since both of the above interferences have been shown to inhibit monocyte cytotoxic function (6,12) studies to prove the postulated increase in monocyte membrane permeability to monovalent cations are in progress.

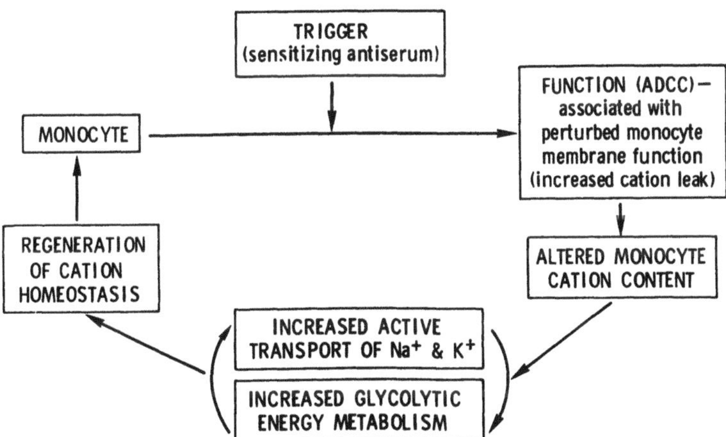

Fig. 2. Proposed relationship between monovalent cation homeostasis and MMADCC.

SUMMARY

Monocyte-mediated ADCC was inhibited by ouabain, which blocks active transport of Na^+ and K^+ by the membrane Na^+K^+-ATPase. Inhibition of ADCC was incomplete, however, even when monovalent cation transport was completely inhibited. On the other hand, increasing the duration of exposure to ouabain did result in complete inhibition of ADCC. ADCC wa also depressed by incubation of monocytes in media with low ($\leq$ 1.5 mEq/l) or high ($\geq$ 30 mEq/l) K^+ concentrations. The results suggest that monocyte ADCC is dependent upon monovalent cation concentrations (secondarily altered by ouabain exposure) but not upon active Na^+K^+ transport *per se*. Finally, since monovalent cation transport-related glycolysis accounted for esentially all of the previously observed increase in monocyte glycolysis associated with monocyte ADCC, we hypothesize that exposure of monocytes to sensitizing antiserum in the ADCC assay results in increased monocyte membrane permeability to monovalent cations.

ACKNOWLEDGEMENT

These studies were supported in part by an NIH Biomedical Research Support Grant and grant CH-159 from the American Cancer Society.

REFERENCES

1. Golstein, P., and E.T. Smith. The lethal hit stage of mouse T and non-T cell mediated cytolysis: differences in cation requirements and characterization on an analytical "cation pulse" method. Eur. J. Immunol. 6:31 (1976).
2. Plaut, M., Bubbers, J.E., and C.S. Henney. Studies on the mechanism of lymphocyte-mediated cytolysis. VII. Two stages in the T cell-mediated lytic cycle with distinct cation requirements. J. Immunol. 116:150 (1976).
3. Lawrence, E.C., Muchmore, A.V., Dooley, N.J. and R.M. Blaese. Differential effects of ouabain on human cell-mediated cytotoxicity. Cell. Immunol. 46:100 (1979).
4. Wright, P., and M. De Marchi. Ouabain inhibition of human lymphocyte cytotoxicity. Cell. Immunol. 45:318 (1979).
5. Skou, J.C. Enzymatic basis for active transport of Na^+ and K^+ across cell membrane. Physiol. Rev. 45:596 (1965).
6. Ladisch, S., and S.A. Feig. Submitted, J. Immunol.
7. Ladisch, S., Feig, S.A., Henderso, T., and B. Berman. Submitted, J. Immunol. Meth.
8. Kragballe, K., Beck-Nielsen, W., Pedrsen, O., Ellegaard, J., and N.S. Sorensen. Monocyte-mediated antibody-dependent cytotoxicity. Modulation by glycolysis and insulin. Scand.

J. Haematol. 26:137 (1981).
9. Poplack, D.G., Bonnard, g.d., Holiman, B.J., and R.M. Blaese. Monocyte-mediated antibody-dependent cellular cytotoxicity. A clinical test of monocyte function. Blood 48:809 (1976).
10. Segel, G.B. and M.A. Lichtman. Potassium transport in human blood lymphocytes treated with phytohemagglutinin. J. Clin. Invest. 58:1358 (1976).
11. Kernan, R.P. Cell K. Butterworth, Washington, pp. 121-141 (1965).
12. Koller, C.A., Laufman, H.B., and A.F. Lo Buglio. Characterization of monocyte antibody dependent cellular cytotoxicity (ADCC) against RBC targets. Blod 51:152a (1978).

DISCUSSION

R. Herberman

I'd like to raise an alternative hypothesis. Ouabain will also interfere with binding of interferon to the interferon receptor on cells. I wonder whether you might interpet the results that you've seen as some later requirement for endogenous interferon in the system to keep the activity of the monocytes going? The kind of pattern that you see is somewhat reminiscent of what John Artaldo in my lab saw when he exposed NK cells to ouabain. It did not interfere with spontaneous NK activity, but it interfered with the boosting of NK by interferon.

S. Ladisch

We thought of this possibility in terms of whether this effect is on recycling or on recruitment of effector cells, since it was a delayed effect. So we preincubated effector cells in ouabain for longer periods of time before the addition of antibody and targets and in fact finally were able to obtain complete inhibition of cytotoxocity. So it was not something that was occurring only after exposure to sensitizing antibody on the target cell.

I. MacLennan

Were you able to reduce the effect of ouabain at a given concentration by increasing the extracellular potassium concentration? Certainly for CTL lysis, which is highly dependent upon extracellular potassium, ouabain is only inhibitory when in reduced potassium concentration.

S. Ladisch

I think that is really two questions in one. The first would be, what is the effect of potassium concentration on cytotoxic capacity of the cell? The second part is, what is the effect of ouabain at different potassium concentrations? Since ouabain binds to the receptor on the enzyme for potassium, it is a competitive inhibitor, so that it's a very complex study that you're doing if you vary both. You're in fact inhibiting, or augmenting the binding of, ouabain or of potassium to the cell.

I. MacLennan

The point is, you can probably exclude the interferon effect by showing the potassium dependence of the ouabain effect. If you increase the potassium concentration to say 15 millimolar you might then require really a lot more ouabain to get, say, 50% inhibition. And I think that would be the way of answering your question. I think there is a fairly striking difference, from what you say, between the potassium depletion effect on CTL and on macrophage-mediated kill, because it's more or less instantaneous in the CTL system (the effect of potassium depletion).

S. Ladisch

We would calculate in terms of saturating the potassium binding sites that the level of intracellular potassium necessary for expression of lytic function is approximately 70 to 80 mill-equivalent per liter based on a 4-6 hour time necessary for the evolution of activity.

MECHANISMS OF MACROPHAGE-MEDIATED TUMOR CYTOLYSIS

M. E. Key, L. Hoyer, C. Bucana, and M. G. Hanna, Jr.

Cancer Metastasis and Treatment Laboratory
NCI-Frederick, Cancer Research Facility
Frederick, Maryland 21701

INTRODUCTION

Important roles have been proposed for both cellular (1,2) and humoral (3-5) immunity in the complex host reaction to neoplastic growth. Killing of syngeneic tumor cells, at least *in vitro*, can be mediated by many different host cell types either alone or in combination with humoral factors. The mechanisms of tumor cell destruction by macrophages in particular have been studied extensively because of the known tumoricidal properties of macrophages (6-8) and the histological observation that these cells are capable of infiltrating various solid tumors in several different species (9).

Evidence that mononuclear phagocytes are uniquely endowed with the properties necessary to generate potent cytotoxic responses is derived, in part, from studies of their antimicrobial functions. Macrophages possess a primitive mechanism for distinguishing foreignness, they are actively phagocytic, and they can destroy phagocytosed materials by a remarkable sequence of lytic events. All of these functions that macrophages can generate toward microorganisms also can be mediated against neoplastic cells. These similarities prompted Mackaness (10) to speculate that "there is an almost perfect parallel between cell-mediated antimicrobial immunity and resistance to neoplasia." Only the observation that macrophages also kill tumor cells by nonphagocytic processes serves to distinguish tumoricidal from antimicrobial functions.

We review here our studies of the mechanisms of macrophage-mediated cytotoxicity against two very different kinds of tumors, the T1699 mammary adenocarcinoma of DBA/2 mice (11) and the Line 10 (L10) hepatocarcinoma of strain 2 guinea pigs (12). In both of these systems, tumor regression can occur in vivo; the T1699 tumor often undergoes spontaneous regression, whereas the L10 tumor can be induced to regress following immune stimulation of tumor-bearing animals. There is evidence in both of these tumor systems that tumor-associated macrophages participate in the process of tumor regression. Macrophages contained within T1699 tumors can kill tumor cells by both intracellular (phagocytic) and extracellular (nonphagocytic) processes (13), whereas macrophages from guinea pigs immunotherapeutically cured of L10 tumors kill exclusively by extracellular means (14). Despite these apparent differences, our studies show that the subcellular events involved in the killing of tumor cells, whether by intracellular or extracellular means, are essentially the same. In recent years, there has been a proliferation of reports on the various mechanisms by which macrophages kill tumor cells. By reviewing our studies and the extensive related work of others, we hope to identify some unifying concepts to explain how macrophages accomplish this task. In the process, we also will explore some interesting similarities between the antimicrobial and antitumor properties of macrophages.

CELLULAR EVENTS OF MACROPHAGE-MEDIATED CYTOTOXICITY

The Biology of Macrophage Activation

In the pioneering studies of Hibbs (15,16) on the tumoricidal functions of macrophages, it was observed that macrophages derived from mice chronically infected with particular intracellular parasites could destroy neoplastic target cells in vitro. Target cell killing was selective in that contact-inhibited allogeneic target cells of kidney cells were spared, whereas both syngeneic and allogeneic tumor cells were killed. Because all the neoplastic cells tested were susceptible to killing by macrophages, this suggested that macrophages recognized neoplastic cells by a nonimmunologic means, possibly by surface modifications of the malignant cells. Thus, in these in vitro studies, macrophages demonstrated a primitive mechanism for discriminating foreignness from self. In contrast to the cytotoxic activity displayed by macrophages from mice infected with certain intracellular microorganisms, resident murine peritoneal macrophages (PM) obtained from unstressed animals are not tumoricidal when tested in vitro. Macrophages that express enhanced tumoricidal activity have been described as "activated", a term originally used by Mackaness to describe macrophages with enhanced microbicidal properties.

Despite the immunlogically nonspecific manner in which activated macrophages express their cytotoxic effects, the sequence of events leading to macrophage activation may initially require the interaction of specifically sensitized lymphocytes with appropriate antigen (17). Studies have shown that the lymphokine containing macrophage-activating factor (MAF) is responsible for this effect (18). Incubation of macrophages with MAF-rich lymphocyte supernatants induces a number of morphologic, metabolic, and functional changes including enhanced microbicidal and tumoricidal activity. In a manner similar to that of macrophages obtained from mice chronically infected with certain intracellular parasites, macrophages activated *in vitro* with MAF are cytotoxic only to malignant target cells but not to syngeneic fibroblasts or kidney cells (18).

Activation of macrophages has been explained by Ruco and Meltzer (19) to be the final result of at least two signals presented in a specific order. The first signal was induced by the interaction of macrophages with lymphokines containing MAF. Lymphokine-primed macrophages that progressed through this initial induction stage could develop further into cytotoxic macrophages only after exposure to a second signal of lipopolysaccharide. In a similar experiment, it was shown by Sone and Fidler (20) that rat alveolar macrophages could respond to a single activating signal of either MAF or the microbial product, muramyl dipeptide (MDP). Unlike the PM in the system of Ruco and Meltzer (19), rat alveolar macrophages did not require combined treatment with lymphokines and a bacterial product; however, a synergistic activation of tumoricidal properties did occur when both signals were simultaneously introduced or when MAF was given before MDP. As in the studies of Ruco and Meltzer (19), exposure to the bacterial signal before exposure to MAF was ineffective in augmenting macrophage activation. Thus, it appears that the major pathways for macrophage activation are through the interaction of macrophages with lymphokines containing MAF or through the direct interaction of macrophages with microorganisms or their products. However, activation by both pathways simultaneously may have a synergistic effect.

Recently, Sone et al. (21) and Sone and Fidler (22) reported that normal mouse or rat alveolar macrophages could be directly activated by the phagocytic uptake of liposomes containing either MAF or synthetic MDP. These studies added two important new pieces of information to our knowledge concerning mechanisms of macrophage activation. First, the activating agent did not have to interact directly with the macrophage membrane since internalization of the activating agents encapsulated in liposomes was an effective stimulus for activation, and second, macrophages could be activated directly by the bacterial product, MDP, without the requirement for T lymphocyte participation.

The Requirement for Effector Cell-to-Target Cell Contact

The interaction *in vitro* between activated macrophages and target cells often leads to the selective destruction of the neoplastic targets (16,18). Hibbs (23) has shown that when activated macrophages are plated on coverslips and then overlaid with tumor cells, the tumor cells will grow on all cell-free portions of the coverslip up to and adjacent to the macrophage areas but will not invade into the macrophage areas. In this system, the growth of tumor cells was not inhibited at sites adjacent to the activated macrophages, suggesting that, unless tumor cells were in actual physical contact with macrophages, their growth was not inhibited. Several other studies have also confirmed that cytolysis of tumor cells is restricted to the immediate vicinity of the macrophages (7,8,14). Some studies, however, have reported that secreted factors from macrophages may also mediate these cytotoxic effects (24-26). Perhaps these apparently discrepant findings can be reconciled by assuming that macrophages release labile cytolytic substances that need to be focused and concentrated onto the surface of susceptible target cells (26).

Killing of tumor cells _in vivo_ may also require direct effector cell-to-target cell contact. Fidler et al. (27) have shown that established lymph node and pulmonary metastases were eradicated in mice bearing the B16-Bladder 6 malignant melanoma when liposomes containing the macrophage-activator MDP were injected i.v. into the mice. If macrophage-mediated tumor killing requires intimate effector cell-to-target cell contact, then infiltration of activated macrophages into metastases must be a prerequisite for the destruction of the lesions, assuming the effect is dependent upon macrophage cytolytic activity. We have recently been able to identify within metastases macrophages that have taken up liposomes containing MDP. Mice were injected i.v. with the B16-Bladder 6 (28) spontaneously metastatic melanoma of C57BL/6 mice to induce experimental pulmonary metastases. Fluorescently labeled liposomes containing MDP were prepared according to the method of Fidler et al. (29) and injected i.v. into the tumor-bearing animals. Macrophages containing the fluorescent label were found at various anatomic sites, but, most importantly, they were found within the pulmonary tumors (Table 1). Fluorescently labeled cells obtained from tumor digests were identified as macrophages by their ability to form rosettes with antibody-coated sheep erythrocytes. Parallel examination of cell preparations stained with Giemsa confirmed that 90% of the cells with macrophage morphology also formed rosettes. Macrophages from the tumor digests were isolated by brief adherence to plastic and then recovered with a rubber policeman. When these isolated macrophages were tested _in vitro_ for tumoricidal activity, only those macrophages from mice treated with liposomes containing MDP were cytotoxic, whereas macrophages from tumors of untreated mice or from mice treated with empty liposomes were not cytotoxic (Table 1). This demonstrated that after the systemic administration of liposomes containing macrophage-activating substances, liposomes were taken up by tumor-infiltrating macrophages resulting in their activation. Thus, the therapeutic effectiveness of this treatment modality in tumor-bearing mice could be explained on the basis of activation of macrophages residing within tumor deposits.

TABLE 1. Uptake of liposomes and *in situ* activation of tumor-associated macrophages in pulmonary metastases[a]

Treatment[b]	Macrophages/ total cells (%)[c]	Macrophages containing liposomes/total macrophages (%)[d]	Cytotoxicity (%)[e]
None	11	0	0 ± 2.5
Liposomes + free MDP	11	5	5 ± 2.4
Liposome-encapsulated MDP	13	5	40 ± 2.0

[a]Experimental pulmonary metastases were induced by the i.v. injection of 2.5×10^4 B16-BL6 cells into syngeneic C57BL/6 mice.

[b]28 days after tumor injection, mice received no further treatment or were treated on 3 consecutive days by the i.v. injection of liposomes (5 µmol of phosphatidyl choline and phosphatidyl serine at a 7:3 mol ratio) suspended in 25 µg MDP or liposomes containing 25 µg MDP as previously described (27). The final injection on day 3 was with fluorescently labeled liposomes (29).

[c]Pulmonary metastases were recovered and pooled (3 mice/group). Tumor macrophages were identified in single cell suspensions of the enzymatically dissociated tumors by their ability to phagocytose india ink and form rosettes with sensitized sheep red blood cells.

[d]Percentage of macrophages containing liposomes was assessed by the number of cells that contained both fluorescent material and formed rosettes with sensitized sheep red blood cells.

[e]Macrophages were recovered from tumor digests by adherence to plastic and tested *in vitro* for cytotoxicity as previously described (29) against B16-BL6 target cells grown *in vitro* at an effector: target cell ratio of 10:1. Value equals percentage of cytotoxicity ± SD for triplicate assays.

Recent studies by Marino and Adams (30,31) have shown that contact between murine *Bacillus Calmette Guérin* (BCG)-activated PM and neoplastic target cells resulted in a physical binding between effector and target cells. This binding was selective in that the binding of tumor cells to resident or elicited PM from normal mice was considerably less than that to activated macrophages. These studies further showed that the binding of target cells to activated macrophages required the presence of divalent cations and trypsin-sensitive structures on macrophages. The dependency of tumor cytolysis on binding was suggested by the observation that increased or decreased tumor cell killing could be achieved by treatments which either increased (Con A or neuraminidase and galactose oxidase) or decreased (chelators or trypsinization) binding of macrophages to target cells. The recognition and binding _in vitro_ of activated macrophages to target cells may be one mechanism by which activated macrophages, but not normal macrophages, are able to kill tumor cells.

These findings support our own observations on the mechanisms of macrophage killing of L10 tumor cells (32). The interactions of PM and L10 tumor cells were examined _in vitro_ by electron microscopy. These studies showed a marked increase in the binding to tumor cells of macrophages obtained from BCG-treated guinea pigs compared to those obtained from normal guinea pigs. These interactions were also studied by time-lapse cinematography which revealed that normal macrophages from BCG-tumor-cured animals remained closely associated with tumor cells for long periods of time followed by eventual cytolysis of the tumor cell.

Antibody Regulation of Macrophage-Mediated Cytotoxicity

Another mechanism that facilitates macrophage contact with target cells is the ability of cytophilic antibody to bind to both Fc-receptor-positive effector cells and antigen-positive tumor cells. Macrophages that bind cytophilic antibody possessing antitumor specificity are capable of the specific immunological recognition of the antigenically appropriate tumor cells. Such macrophages have been termed "armed" (33) to distinguish them from "activated" macrophages which kill neoplastic cells in an immunologically nonspecific manner. An alternative hypothesis is that macrophages can be specifically armed by a T lymphocyte product termed "specific macrophage-arming factor" which endows macrophages with a specificity similar to that of antibody. However, the interpretation of these experiments is complicated by the fact that T cells can also activate macrophages nonspecifically to kill tumor cells and by the extreme difficulty of excluding all antibody-secreting cells from the _in vitro_ systems.

Mechanisms of antibody-dependent macrophage-mediated cytotoxicity have been studied extensively _in vitro_ (5,34). There is now evidence that suggests that immunoglobulin with antitumor specificity can localize within many solid tumors (3-5). The observation that tumors may contain both immunoglobulin as well as macrophages suggests that the potential for macrophage-mediated antibody-dependent cellular cytotoxicity (ADCC) exists _in situ_ as well.

A second important role for antibody may be the triggering of the cytolytic event. In adition to macrophage activation by lymphokines and bacterial products, there are indications that macrophages can also be activated after they interact with antibody or antigen-antibody complexes (35). Again, there may be a synergistic effect if macrophages are activated both by the interaction with MAF or microbial products followed by a second activation sequence initiated by antibody (36).

In our studies of the immunologicaly controlled regression of the T1699 murine mammary adenocarcinoma, we have accumulated evidence suggesting that macrophage-mediated ADCC participates in this regression process. Using an immunoperoxidase staining technique, we have studied the pattern and degree of macrophage infiltration and immunoglobulin deposition within regressing tumors. The tumor-associated macrophage (TuM) is highly reactive with an antimacrophage serum produced in rabbits against murine macrophages grown _in vitro_ from bone-marrow precursors. The reactivity of the anti-macrophage serum with TuM provides an excellent means of identifying these cells both in cell suspensions and histological sections of tumors. _In vitro_ studies of tumor cell killing by TuM show that these cells kill by an apparent phagocytic mechanism and only in the presence of antibody (37). From these studies, it was not possible to determine the exact moment when irreparable damage had been inflicted on the tumor cells. Whether this occurred before or after complete closure of the phagocytic vacuole could not be determined from the data. What is important, however, is that phagocytosis can provide a readily identifiable feature indicating that a killing event has occurred and may be of value in identifying tumor cell killing _in vivo_ as well. In fact, within histological sections of regressing T1699 tumors, it has been possible to identify phagocytosed tumor cells at areas of contact between macrophages and tumor cells. T1699 tumors, obtained from tumor-bearing animals that had received a prior pulse with ^{3}H-thymidine, possessed numerous macrophages containing phagocytosed, labeled tumor cells (37). These findings suggest that the labeled tumor cells were fully capable of synthesizing new nuclear material immediately preceding phagocytosis and also that phagocytosis is not limited solely to the removal of dead and degenerating tumor cells.

An analogous situation exists under physiologic conditions within germinal centers of mice where tingible body macrophages are observed containing phagocytosed lymphocytes. When mice are pulsed with ^{3}H-thymidine, autoradiographic analysis of germinal centers shows replicating lymphocytes (positive nuclear labeling) within tingible body macrophages. This suggests that the elimination of lymphoid elements by macrophages is not limited to senescent cells (38). The mechanisms of recognition and phagocytosis are not clear. However, because of the known stimulating effect of antibody on phagocytic responses (39), it is possible that certain types of antibody, such as anti-idiotypic antibody, could stimulate the phagocytic removal of particular B lymphocyte populations thus limiting a specific immune response. The capacity of macrophges to remove antibody-coated senescent or nonessential cellular elements from the body has, in fact, been postulated to be a physiological role for autoantibody (40).

In the T1699 system, TuM isolated from tumors phagocytose tumor cells in vitro only in the presence of immune serum. It appears likely that phagocytosis in situ also requires the presence of antibody since parallel analysis of serial sections of the same T1699 tumor shows that TuM and tumor-associated immunoglobulin are not distributed randomly throughout the whole tumor but show specific areas of concentration and that both macrophages and immunoglobulin show similar distribution patterns. Phagocytosis of tumor cells is observed in areas where both macrophages and immunoglobulin are localized but rarely in areas where immunoglobulin is absent (41).

Antibody may also facilitate macrophage-mediated killing of L10 tumor cells. Guinea pigs immunotherapeutically cured of L10 tumors have high titers of circulating anti-L10 antibody as detected by immunofluoresence against L10 tumor cells (42). When serum from cured L10 tumor bearers is added to in vitro cytotoxicity assays, killing of L10 tumor cells by macrophages is facilitated (43).

The role that antibody plays in the mediation of tumor cell killing by macrophages is strikingly similar in many respects to the role that antibody plays in the destruction of microbes by macrophages. Bacteria opsonized with antibody are rapidly bound and internalized by macrophages. The antibody itself not only facilitates the contact but also enhances the process of phagocytosis (39). Furthermore, the interaction of antibody with both macrophages and neutrophils stimulates the production of toxic enzymes which mediate the rapid intracellular destruction and degradation of the endocytosed organisms (35,44).

SUBCELLULAR EVENTS IN MACROPHAGE-MEDIATED CYTOTOXICITY

Exocytosis of Lysosomes

Electron microscopy studies have shown that, after phagocytosis of bacteria, the specific granules of the phagocyte fuse with the phagosome presumably releasing digestive enzymes and other antimicrobial substances. Attempts to identify similar subcellular mechanisms of macrophage-mediated killing of tumor cells have, in general, been overlooked since phagocytosis does not precede tumor cell killing in most cases. However, in the absence of phagocytosis, it is still possible that macrophages may transfer their lysosomal enzymes to tumor cells by a process of exocytosis. The possibility that transfer of lysosomes or lysosomal products of macrophage origin into susceptible tumor cells would result in their lysis was originally proposed by Hibbs (23) and subsequently by us (32). Hibbs (23) has shown that preincubation of macrophages with dextran sulfate resulted in the uptake, concentration, and storage of dextran sulfate within secondary lysosomes, thus allowing macrophage lysosomal organelles to be labeled. After co-cultivation of labeled macrophages with tumor cells, transfer of the marker to tumor cells was observed followed by tumor cell cytolysis. Agents that interfered with exocytosis of macrophage lysosomes, such as hydrocortisone, or agents that inactivated macrophage lysosomal enzymes, such as trypan blue, inhibited macrophage-mediated killing.

Although some studies have proposed that secreted cytolytic factors provide the means by which activated macrophages kill tumor cells, most studies have suggested that intimate contact between macrophages and tumor cells is required (7,8,14,30,31). In fact, both models of macrophage killing may be partially correct. The macrophage may release labile cytolytic factors contained within lysosomes which need to be focused by the macrophage onto the tumor cell surface. This possibility is supported by our observations that during killing of tumor cells, the membranes of the macrophage and tumor cell are closely apposed (32). Electron microscopic analysis shows that these contacts appear to create protected spaces between the macrophage and tumor cell in which secretion or exocytosis can take place in an environment with limited interference from extracellular components.

Exocytosis of macrophage lysosomal enzymes does not appear to be limited to macrophage-tumor cell interactions but appears to occur also in other situations in which phagocytosis is absent or incomplete (45-47). For example, Carr et al. (45) have described the accumulation of macrophages around lipid globules in artificially induced rat granulomas. In these studies electron-dense materials, presumably lysosomes derived from macrophages, collected on the surface of the lipid by a process morphologically suggestive of exocytosis. The extracellular release of lysosomes from macrophages as reported in these studies, may represent a common alternative mechanism of enzymatic degradation operative in the absence of phagocytosis. In these cases of extracellular degradation, the fusion of lysosomes with the outer cell membrane of the macrophage occurs by a process analogous to the fusion of lysosomes with phagosomes.

The T1699 Tumor System

In the T1699 tumor system, we have investigated the possibility that transfer of macrophage lysosomal enzymes into tumor target cells occurs *in vitro* and is the mechanism of macrophage-mediated target cell destruction. In this system, we utilized as effector cells bone-marrow-derived macrophages (BMM) grown *in vitro* since these cells have been shown to be antigenically and functionally similar to TuM (37,48). Like the TuM, BMM kill target cells _in vitro_ by a phagocytic process. Macrophages were labeled _in vitro_ with dextran sulfate by 48-hour incubation in media containing 30 μg/ml dextran sulfate. Uptake of dextran sulfate by macrophages has been shown to be nontoxic and does not interfere with the expression of cytolytic activity (23). Dextran sulfate is concentrated into secondary lysosomes and can be detected by its metachromatic staining with the Azure A stain for sulfated mucosubstances. Figure 1 shows that macrophages stained with Azure A contain numerous metachromatic granules. When labeled macrophages are cultured with tumor cells in acrylamide dishes (37), cells do not adhere to the vessel surface and can be removed periodically for morphological observation. When these macrophages are incubated with tumor cells in the presence of specific tumor antibody (derived from serum from tumor-bearing animals), the macrophages adhere vigorously to the tumor cells. Even when macrophages and tumor cells are removed from cultures and cytocentrifuge preparations are made, most of these adhesions remain intact. When macrophages and antibody are incubated with tumor cells, several events are observed (Fig. 1): a) macrophages make contact with tumor cells; b) following contact, increased amounts of dextran sulfate-positive material become polarized near the macrophage-tumor cell junction; c) metachromatic granules are detected within the cytoplasm of tumor cells; d) macrophages extend processes around the tumor cell eventually completely enclosing it; e) tumor cells are lysed intracellularly; and f) after lysis is complete, a large clear vacuole remains which contains undigested dextran sulfate-positive material. When macrophages are incubated

Fig. 1. Macrophage-mediated cytotoxicity against T1699 tumor cells. BMM were labeled with dextran sulfate and incubated with tumor cells at a ratio of 10:1 either with a 1:40 dilution of tumor-bearer sera (a and b) or normal mouse sera (c). a) Macrophage (M) in contact with two tumor cells (T) 1 hour after initiation of assay. Dextran sulfate-positive staining material within macrophage is polarized (arrows) toward areas of contact between the macrophage and tumor cells. b) Single dextran sulfate-labeled macrophage containing two phagocytic vacuoles 4 hours after initiation of assay. In one vacuole, a recently phagocytosed tumor cell (not digested) shows an accumulation of dextran sulfate-positive material (white arrow). In the other vacuole, the phagocytosed tumor cell has been completely digested and only nondigestible dextran sulfate remains (black arrow). c) Control cytotoxicity assay at 1 hour (incubated with normal mouse sera) showing two macrophages (M) in contact with a single tumor cell (T). Note the absence of polarization of dextran sulfate material toward areas of contact. X 800.

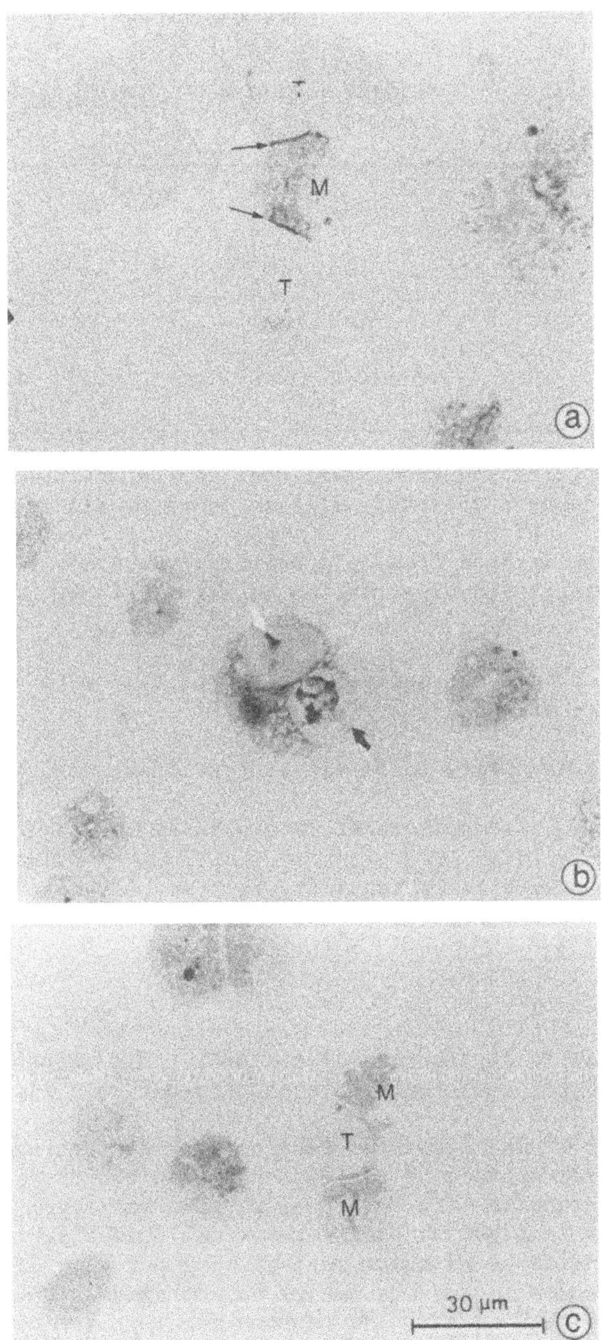
T
M
T
a
b
M
T
M
30 µm
c

TABLE 2. BMM-Mediated Killing of T1699 Tumor Cells

Effectors[a]	Antibody[b]	Dextran sulfate-positive tumor cells (%)[c]	Cytotoxicity (%)[d]	
			2 hr	24 hr
BMM, cells	+	26	77	96
	-	12	0	0
BMM, sonicated	+	30	0	0
	-	28	0	0

[a]BMM were grown *in vitro* from mouse bone marrow precursors and labeled with dextran sulfate. Effector:target cell ratio = 20:1.

[b]A pool of serum derived from mice bearing tumors for 15 days as a source of antibody (+) or normal mouse serum (-) was used (diluted 1:40).

[c]Percentage of free tumor cells staining positive with Azure A for dextran sulfate at 4 hr.

[d]Cytotoxicity assays were performed as previously described (37).

Percentage of cytotoxicity =

$$1 - \frac{\text{No. tumor cells remaining in test cultures}}{\text{No. tumor cells cultured alone}} \times 100$$

with tumor cells in the absence of antibody, this sequence of events is not observed and tumor cells are not lysed (Table 2).

In another study, lysosomes labeled with dextran sulfate were released from macrophages by sonication. When the crude sonicated material was incubated with tumor cells, some positively staining material was again taken up by the tumor cells (Table 2). However, under these conditions no tumor cell killing occurs. Thus, the uptake of lysosomes in the absence of macrophages is not sufficient to induce tumor cell death. The reasons for this are not immediately apparent. It could mean that uptake of lysosomes is not associated with cell death or that, in addition to the uptake of lysosomes, other macrophage functions are required to generate a cytotoxic

TABLE 3. PM-Mediated Killing of T1699 Tumor Cells

Effector cell[a]	Antibody[b]	Dextran sulfate-positive tumor cells (%)[c]		Cytotoxicity (%)[d]	
		6 hr	24 hr	24 hr	48 hr
PM	+	52	95	23	41
	-	18	16	0	12
None	+	0	0	0	0
	-	0	0	0	0

[a]Resident PM were labeled with dextran sulfate and incubated with target cells at a ratio of 20:1.

[b]A pool of serum derived from mice bearing tumors for 15 days as a source of antibody (+) or normal mouse serum (-) was used (diluted 1:40).

[c]Percentage of tumor cells staining positively with Azure A for dextran sulfate.

[d]Cytotoxicity assays were performed as previously described (37).

$$\text{Percentage of cytotoxicity} = 1 - \frac{\text{No. tumor cells remaining in test cultures}}{\text{No. tumor cells cultures alone}} \times 100$$

effect. Other possibilities are that lysosomes are nonfunctional following sonication or exposure to the extracellular environment or that lysosomes may not gain their full complement of toxic enzymes until after contact with tumor cells or tumor cells and antibody occurs (35). However, these studies do show, a) that with intact macrophages, lysosomal organelles polarize toward areas of contact with tumor cells and, b) that the uptake of lysosomes by tumor cells may be, in some instances, a tumor cell-mediated process.

In a similar experiment, normal mouse PM were utilized as effector cells (Table 3). In contrast to BMM, PM are less dependent upon phagocytic killing and more dependent upon extracellular lysis of tumor cells (13). Mouse PM were labeled *in vitro* with dextran sulfate as previously described. PM in the presence of antibody efficiently transferred dextran sulfate-positive material to tumor cells as early as 6 hours, whereas in the absence of antibody, transfer was less apparent (Table 3). When cell samples were removed from the assays at 6 hours and stained for dextran sulfate, it was found that as with BMM, PM in contact with tumor cells showed polarization of dextran sulfate particles toward the areas of tumor cell contact. By 24 hours, 95% of the remaining tumor cells in the cultures containing PM and antibody were labeled with dextran sulfate, whereas in cultures without antibody there was no further increase in the percentage of labeled tumor cells above that seen at 6 hours. By 48 hours, 41% of the tumor cells had been lysed in the cultures containing PM and antibody compared to only 12% killing in the assays without antibody.

To determine whether this process of exocytosis of lysosomes into tumor cells had any relevance _in vivo_ for killing of tumor cells, the following experiments were performed. A) BMM and tumor-associated macrophages were stained by an immunoperoxidase technique with an antimacrophage reagent, and a granular staining pattern throughout the cytoplasm was seen. Tests of the antimacrophage serum revealed that it could specifically inhibit the lytic activity of murine lysozyme on _Micrococcus lysodicticus_, suggesting that part of the reactivity of the antimacrophage serum was against lysozyme, a

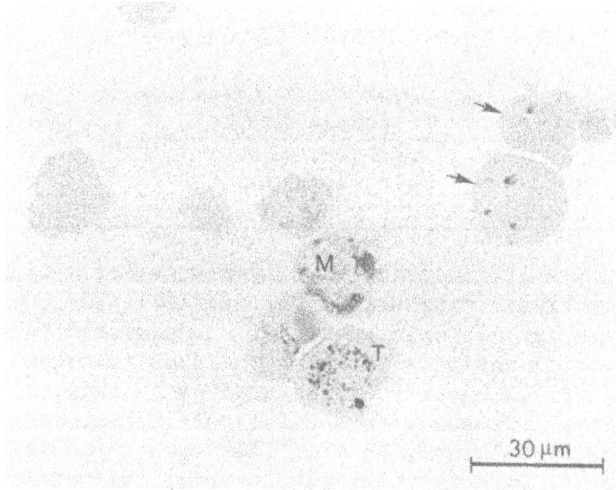

Fig. 2. Cytocentrifuge preparation of T1699 tumor digest on day 14 stained with the antimacrophage reagent and developed for autoradiography. Macrophage (M) shows positive staining with the antimacrophage reagent. One tumor cell (T) shows positive nuclear labeling with ^{3}H-thymidine. Other unlabeled tumor cells (arrows) show discrete granules of macrophage-derived material. X 800.

presumed component of certain macrophage lysosomes (45). Thus, it appeared that this antiserum could label macrophage lysosomal organelles. B) Tumor cells were incubated in vitro with BMM in the presence of immune serum. Some of the tumor cells contained discrete bodies of material which stained positively with antimacrophage reagent, whereas tumor cells incubated in the absence of macrophages never stained positively. As with the dextran sulfate studies, transfer of macrophage-derived material as detected by the antimacrophage reagent was facilitated when specific tumor antibody was incorporated into the assay system. More importantly, tumor cells derived from in vivo tumors often showed macrophage-derived material apparently within the cytoplasm of the tumor cell (Fig. 2). Tumor cells were isolated from solid tumors derived from animals that had received a prior pulse with ^{3}H-thymidine and then were analyzed for macrophage-derived material. A striking inverse correlation (r = -0.87) was observed between the proliferative capacity of the tumor cells, as measured by the incorporation of ^{3}H-thymidine by autoradiography and the number of macrophage-derived granules per tumor cell (Fig. 3). These data are compatible with the hypothesis that inhibition of tumor cell proliferation in vivo may be associated with the transfer or uptake by tumor cells of lysosomes or lysosomal enzymes of macrophage origin.

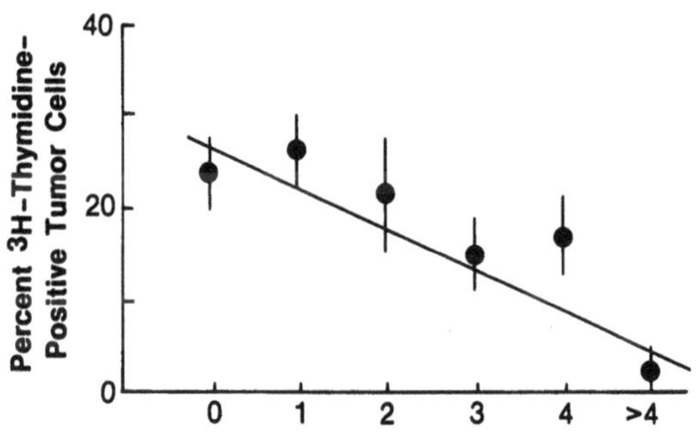

Fig. 3. Correlation of the nuclear-labeling index of T1699 tumor cells with the amount of macrophage-derived material which they contain. Tumors were obtained on day 14 from animals previously pulsed with ^{3}H-thymidine. Cell suspensions of enzymatically dissociated tumors were stained with the antimacrophage reagent and developed for autoradiography. The labeling index of tumor cells is inversely correlated with the accumulation of macrophage-derived material (r = -0.87).

The L10 Tumor System

Histopathological and ultrastructural studies of BCG-mediated regression of dermal L10 tumors in guinea pigs have suggested that infiltrating cells of the macrophage compartment are the primary effector cells of the antitumor response (14,49,50). Both at the tumor site and in the regional lymph nodes, tumor cell destruction occurs within a BCG-induced granulomatous reaction. Using strain 2 guinea pigs with transplanted syngeneic L10 tumors, we evaluated morphologically and functionally the interactions between macro-

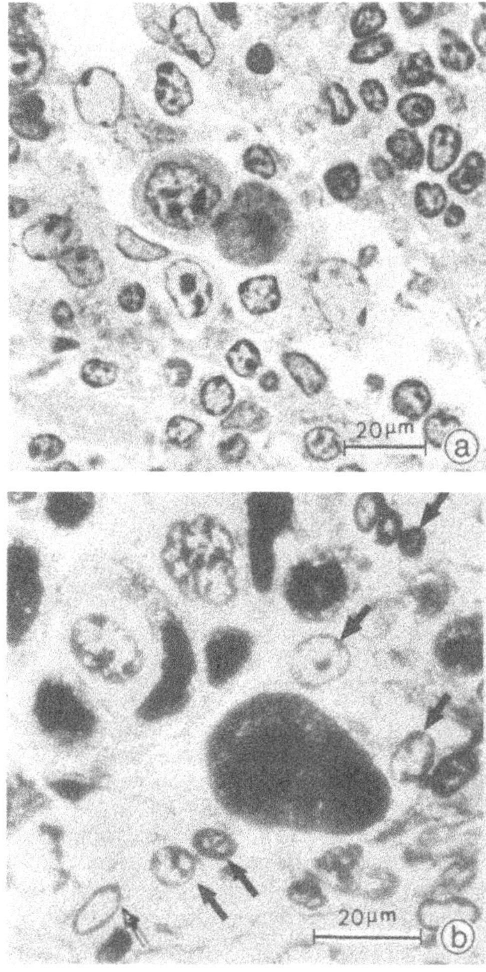

Fig. 4. a) Macrophages in contact with 2 metastatic tumor cells 8 days after treatment. x 950. b) Macrophages (arrows) among hepatocarcinoma cells 8 days after treatment. Both mitotic and degenerate tumor cells are present. x 950.

phages and tumor cells during the course of BCG-mediated tumor regression.

Interaction in vivo of cells of the macrophage-histiocyte compartment with tumor cells during BCG-mediated tumor regression. Between 4 and 16 days after intratumoral injection of BCG, numerous examples of interactions between macrophages and tumor cells were observed at the tumor site, as well as in various regions of the draining lymph nodes. In many cases we observed degeneration of tumor cells associated with or surrounded by macrophages. The association of tumor cells and macrophages in the subcapsular marginal sinus of the regional lymph nodes, as observed from 1 μm sections, is shown in Figure 4a. Several macrophages are associated with the surface of the tumor cells and the latter are dark and pyknotic, indicative of cell degeneration. Such "rosette" formations of tumor cells surrounded by macrophages and occasional lymphocytes (Fig. 4b) were commonly observed in lymph nodes and in the skin

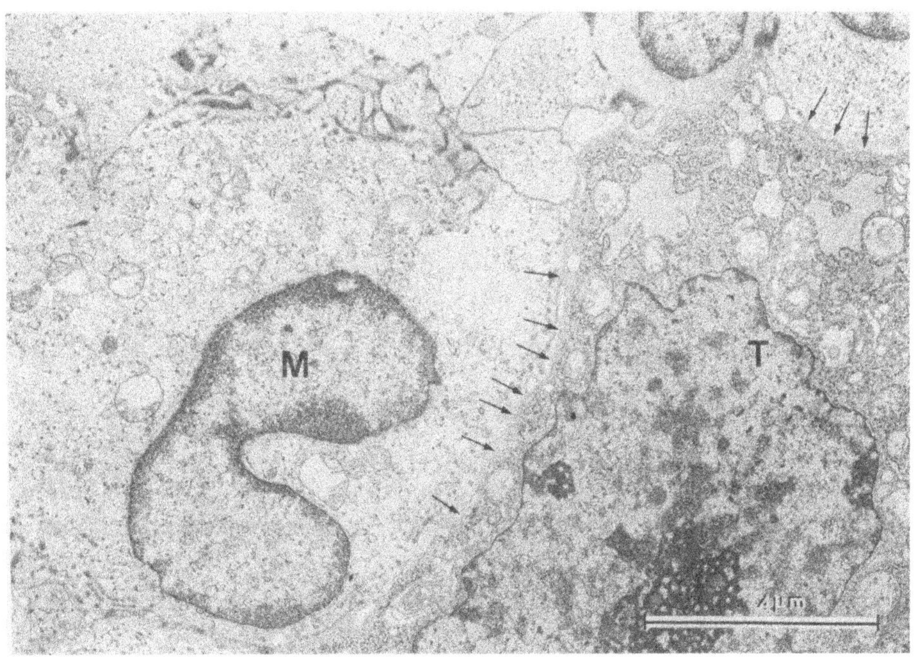

Fig. 5. Areas of apparent fusion (arrows) of the plasmalemmae of macrophages (M) and an electron-dense hepatocarcinoma cell (T) 8 days after treatment. Note that the macrophages have numerous intracytoplasmic channels containing electron-dense material, which is also found extracellularly around these cells. x 11,000.

tumor during the couse of BCG-mediated tumor regression. The plasmalemmae of the L10 tumor cell and the macrophage are generally very closely apposed, the distortion of the cytoplasm of macrophages, in an atempt to make contact with the tumor cells, indicates that this is an active rather than a passive function of the macrophage (Fig. 4a).

The interaction of macrophages and L10 tumor cells in the regional lymph node of BCG-treated guinea pigs is shown on the ultrastructural level in Fig. 5. Numerous electron-dense, round bodies and intracellular tubules containing electron-dense material were observed in the macrophage cytoplasm. Often these were polarized in the region of cell surface contact. The cytoplasm of the tumor cell is dark (electron dense) and contains numerous irregular vesicles and ribosomes that appear to have lost their normal polysomal organization. The mitochondria are severely disrupted and the pleomorphic, pyknotic nucleus contains several nucleoli. Although morphology alone cannot ascertain the functional mechanism of the cellular interaction, the ultrastructure shown in Figure 5 shows areas of apparent intercellular bridges between the membranes of macrophages and tumor cells. These areas are observed with regularity in tissue samples obtained from the regional lymph nodes and the skin tumor sites and seem to be an integral part of the mechanism by which BCG-activated macrophages destroy the tumor cells. As seen in Figure 5, adjacent to these apposed cell surface regions, the macrophages have numerous intracytoplasmic channels containing electron-dense material that is also found extracellularly. Higher magnification of the intercellular bridges between macrophages and tumor cells are shown in Figure 6. Morphologically, these cell bridges are distinct from the electron-dense "tight junctions" which can be observed within homogenous L10 cell populations.

Interaction in vitro of L10 cells and cells of the macrophage compartment. Purified preparations of mineral-oil-induced PM obtained from animals that had undergone BCG-mediated regression of intradermally transplanted L10 tumors and had eliminated regional lymph node metastases were tested in vitro for cytotoxicity against L10 cells. Comparative studies were also performed with similarly isolated macrophages obtained from normal and L10-tumor-bearing guinea pigs.

In the absence of serum, macrophages from normal guinea pigs showed no cytotoxic effect against L10 cells, whereas macrophages from tumor-bearing guinea pigs showed a significant cytotoxic effect against L10 cells at an effector-to-target cell ratio of 100:1 (Table 4). Macrophages from tumor-bearing guinea pigs were also cytotoxic in the presence of various test sera; however, only sera from BCG-tumor-cured guinea pigs markedly increased the cytotoxicity of these macrophages. BCG-tumor-cured guinea pig macrophages in the absence of serum produced approximately 37% cytotoxicity against

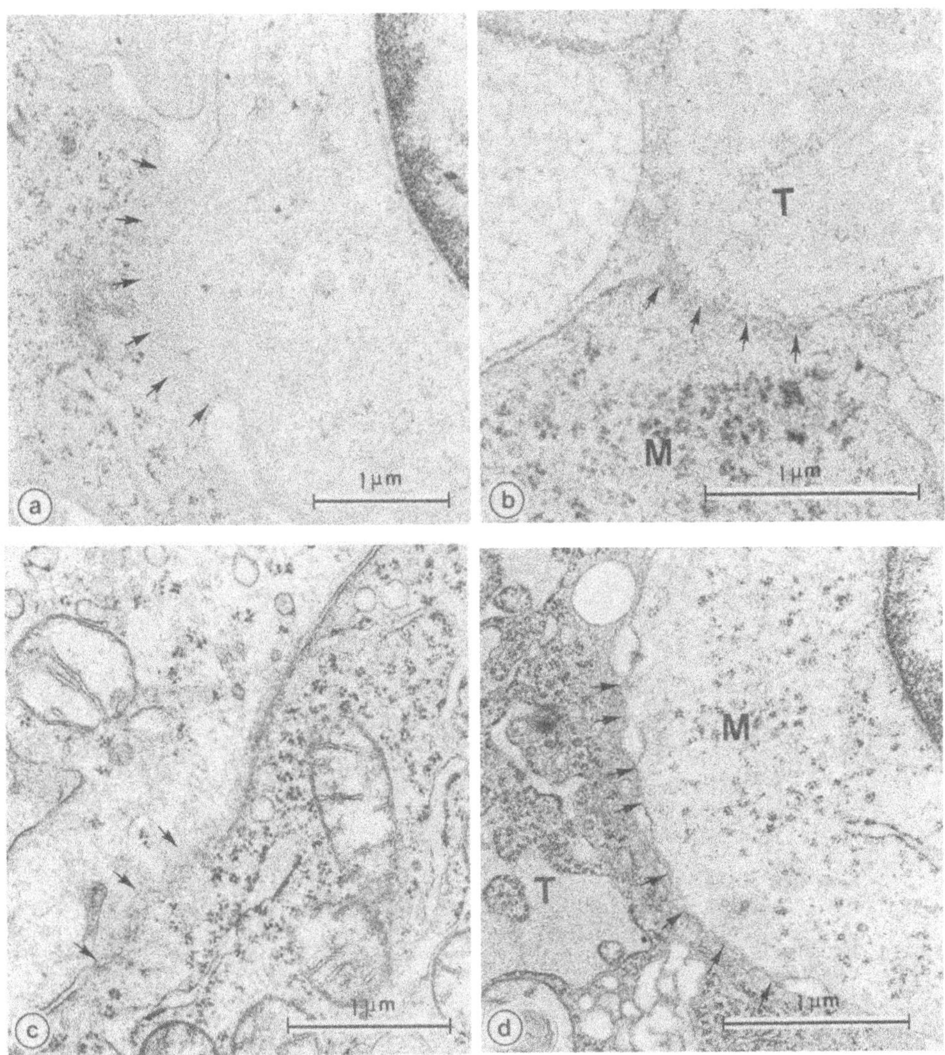

Fig. 6. Areas of apparent adhesion (arrows) between the plasmalemmae of macrophages (M) and hepatocarcinoma cells (T). a and b) Subcapsular sinus of the SDA lymph node 8 days after BCG treatment. x 25,000 and 40,000, respectively. c and d) The s.c. tumor transplantation site 8 and 16 days after BCG treatment. x 30,000 and 35,000, respectively.

L10 cells at an effector-to-target cell ratio of 10:1 and 44.6% cytotoxicity at a ratio of 100:1. The addition of serum from tumor-bearing or BCG-tumor-cured guinea pigs enhanced the cytotoxicity of BCG-tumor-cured guinea pig macrophages at ratios of 10:1 (Table 4).

TABLE 4. *In Vitro* Cytotoxicity of Macrophages From Normal, Tumor-Bearing or BCG-Tumor-Cured Strain 2 Guinea Pigs in the Presence or Absence of Serum

Source of macrophages	Source of serum	Average radioactivity of L10 target cells[a] at a ratio of macrophages:target cells of		
		0	10:1	100:1
None	None	16.6 ± 3.4	-	-
	Normal	15.0 ± 2.9	-	-
	Tumor-bearing	14.7 ± 2.6	-	-
	BCG-tumor-cured	15.0 ± 1.7	-	-
Normal	None	-	15.4 ± 0.9	14.8 ± 1.9
	Normal	-	14.3 ± 3.0	12.1 ± 1.7
	Tumor-bearing	-	12.7 ± 3.0	11.4 ± 3.0
	BCG-tumor-cured	-	13.9 ± 0.5	10.4 ± 2.0 (30.6)[b]
Tumor-bearing[c]	None	-	12.7 ± 2.0	10.3 ± 1.5 (37.9)
	Normal	-	11.0 ± 3.0	9.4 ± 1.3 (37.3)
	Tumor-bearing	-	10.8 ± 2.0	8.9 ± 1.8 (39.5)
	BCG-tumor-cured	-	8.4 ± 0.8 (44.0)	7.9 ± 1.9 (47.3)
BCG-tumor-cured	None	-	10.4 ± 3.3 (37.3)	9.2 ± 2.9 (44.6)
	Normal	-	9.4 ± 3.5 (37.3)	6.5 ± 2.0 (56.7)
	Tumor-bearing	-	6.8 ± 2.5 (53.7)	6.5 ± 2.2 (55.8)
	BCG-tumor-cured	-	7.0 ± 2.1 (53.3)	5.9 ± 1.3 (60.7)

[a]1000 L10 hepatocarcinoma cells plated, labeled, and counted at day 5 as controls. Mean cpm x 10^2 ± SD of triplicate cultures made from a pooled macrophage preparation taken from 2 to 3 guinea pigs per group.

[b]Statistically significant % cytotoxicity ($p < 0.05 - p < 0.01$) in parenthesis.

[c]Animals bearing L10 skin tumors for a period of 8 weeks prior to *in vitro* assay.

Data taken in part from (43).

Several observations can be made from the *in vitro* data. A) Macrophages from BCG-tumor-cured guinea pigs at effector-to-target cell ratios of 10:1 and 100:1 are cytotoxic to L10 tumor cells. B) Macrophages from tumor-bearing guinea pigs, i.e., animals that had borne L10 skin tumors for a period of 5 or 8 weeks, are cytotoxic to L10 cells only at ratios of 100:1. C) The cytotoxicity of effector macrophages was potentiated by BCG-tumor-cured guinea pig sera. The possibility that the potentiation of macrophage-mediated cytotoxicity by serum from cured tumor-bearers is due to antibody is suggested by other studies which have shown that sera from cured tumor-bearers possess high titers of circulating anti-L10 antibody (42).

The significant cytotoxicity achieved with macrophages from BCG-tumor-cured guinea pigs and the potentiation of this cytotoxic response in the presence of autologous serum would suggest that cytotoxic macrophages in these guinea pigs could play a major role in BCG-mediated destruction of L10 tumors. These results are in agreement with the histological and ultrastructural studies of the cytotoxic effector cell as previously discussed.

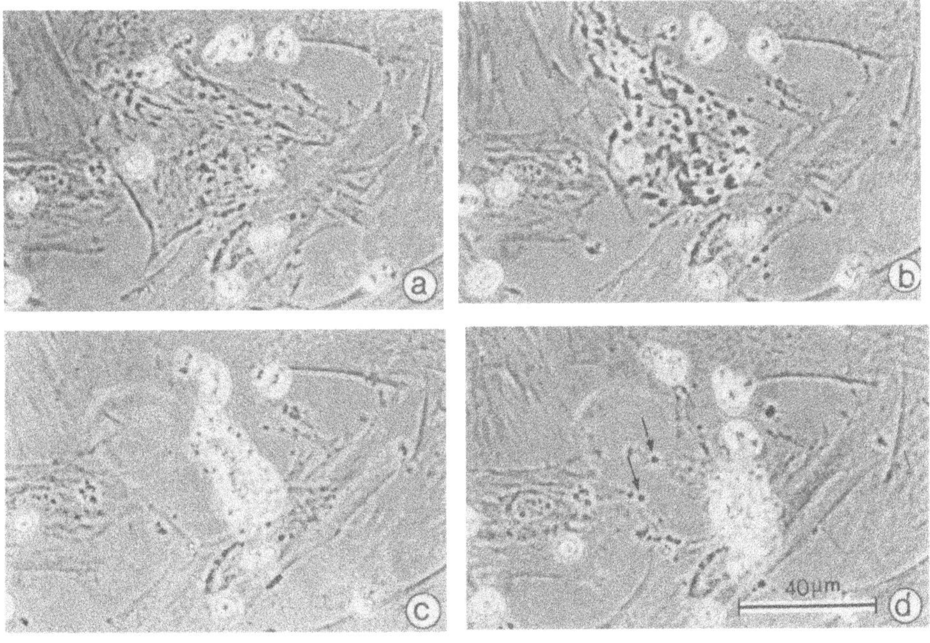

Fig. 7. Time lapse sequence of macrophage-tumor interaction showing tumor cell death. The time interval between a and b is 80 minutes, between b and c it is 60 minutes, and between c and d it is 140 minutes. x 645. Arrows indicate apoptotic bodies.

<u>Time-lapse cinematography</u>. Morphological studies of <u>in vitro</u> cytotoxicity assays were performed by time lapse cinematography. When mineral-oil-induced peritoneal exudate cells (PEC) were incubated <u>in vitro</u> with L10 tumor cells, the events recorded ranged from precytolytic changes to complete cytolysis of the tumor target cells (Fig. 7). The sequence of tumor cell cytotoxicity consisted of an initial ruffling and detachment of the adherent edges of the target cell from the glass (Fig. 7a), followed by condensation of intracellular material, giving the appearance of highly refractile cytoplasmic components (Fig. 7b). Following this condensation, the tumor cell contracted and rounded (Fig. 7c). During this phase there was mild blebbing following by target cell fragmentation. Apoptotic bodies were released from damaged tumor cells and appeared to be taken up by PEC in the proximity of the dying tumor cell (Fig. 7d). The activity of adherent PEC markedly increased before the contraction of the tumor cell, and at the time of cytolysis the PEC often migrated a short distance away from the target cell. After tumor cell cytolysis, distinct migration of other PEC to the area was observed.

Since it is unlikely that all macrophages from BCG-tumor-cured guinea pigs are cytotoxic, only prolonged macrophage-tumor cell interactions that resulted in precytolytic changes in the tumor cell were studied. A typical example is shown in Figure 8, a to g. The sequence occurred over a 2-hour period, and during this time the PEC remained adherent to the surface of the tumor cell. The activity associated with the adherent PEC occurred via the cytoplasmic processes of the PEC (Fig. 8, a to g). There was active extension and retraction of these cytoplasmic processes throughout the 2-hour interval. A PEC beneath the tumor cell showed considerable lateral movement within the area of the overlying tumor cell. Such movement was not seen with surface-adherent PEC. The early contraction of the tumor target cell was the first sign of tumor cell cytolysis, and at that point the cells were fixed with glutaraldehyde in preparation for immunofluoresence.

Fig. 8. a to g) Time lapse sequence of macrophage-tumor interaction from 17 to 19 hours after addition of macrophages to L10 tumor cells. Note the changes in the relative positions of the macrophage underneath the tumor cell (black arrow) compared with the fixed macrophages on top of the tumor cell (white arrows). These sequences show the active extension and contraction of cytoplasmic processes of the adherent macrophages. Early phases of tumor cell retraction are noted in e and g (white arrowhead). x 645. h) Fluorescence micrograph of the cell shown in a to g after reaction with goat anti-guinea pig macrophage serum. The L10 cell as well as the macrophage underneath showed background fluorescence only. x 640.

The positive immunofluoresence of adherent PEC with goat anti-guinea pig macrophage sera identified the adherent PEC as macrophages. A comparison of the time-lapse (Fig. 8g) and the immuno-

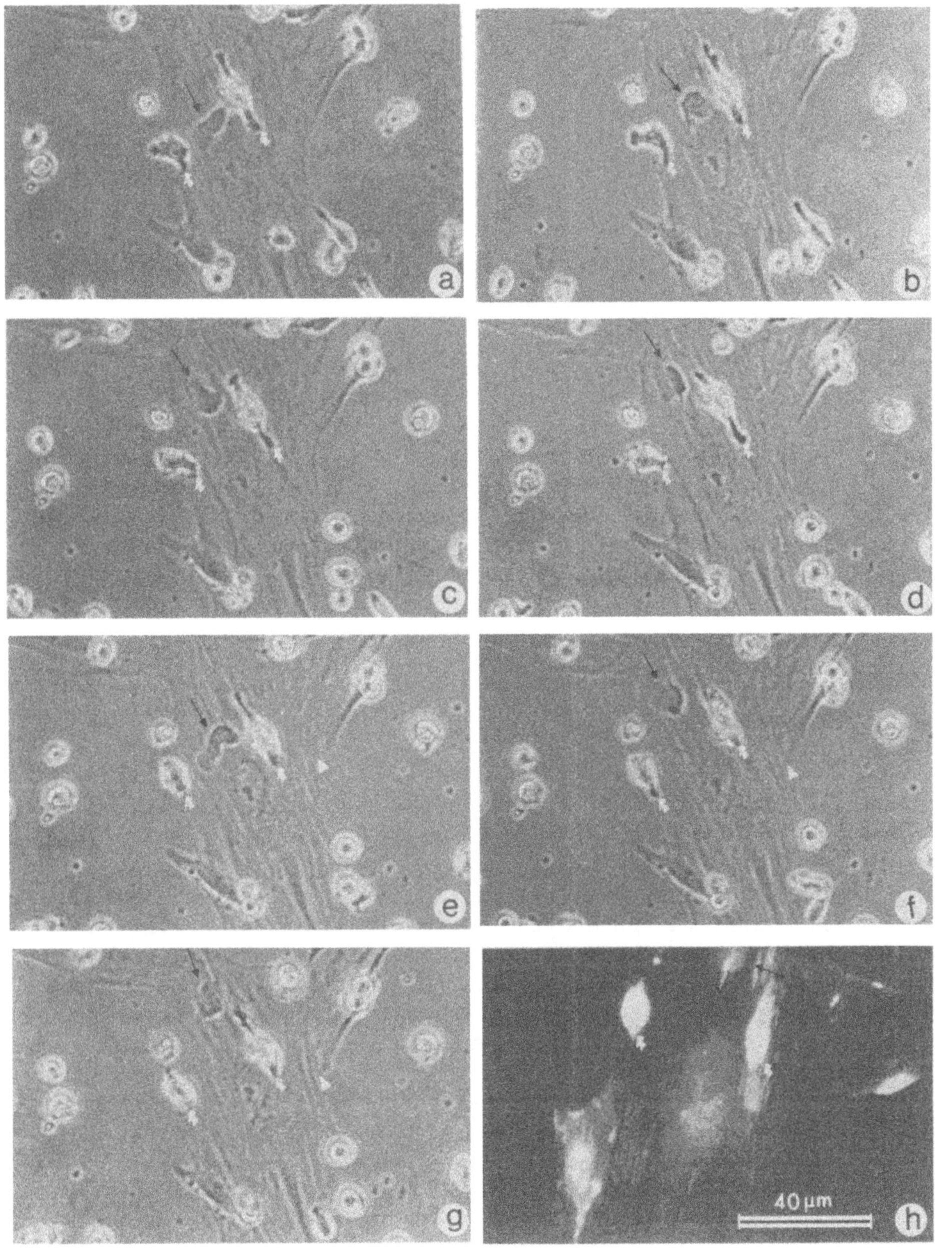

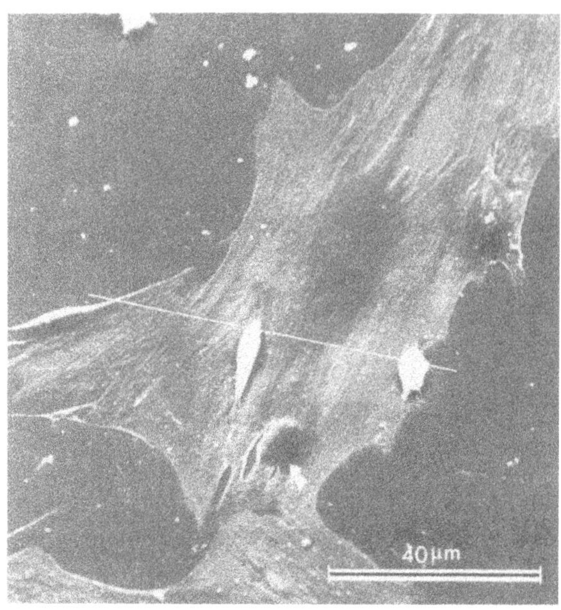

Fig. 9. SEM micrograph of the cell shown in Fig. 8. Note the 2 macrophages on top of the tumor cell and the macrophage underneath the tumor cell (arrow). White line, plane of sectioning for TEM. This particular area was examined by TEM. (See Figure 12.) x 510.

fluorescence (Fig. 8h) photomicrographs shows clearly that the fixation and preparation for immunofluoresence eliminated many of the loosely attached cells.

Scanning electron microscopy (SEM) and transmission electron microscopy (TEM). The same tumor target cell described above was observed by SEM (Fig. 9). The 2 macrophages attached to the tumor cell surface and the macrophage beneath the tumor cell surface were identified. Higher magnification of the elongated adherent macrophage showed multiple cytoplasmic extensions extending to and across the tumor cell surface (Figs. 10 and 11). These processes contained numerous internal bodies. Detachment of entire lengths of these cytoplasmic processes, presumably a result of their rapid extension and contraction, is shown in Fig. 11. We often observed this clasmatosis by SEM.

Fig. 11. SEM micrograph of the long processes of the macrophage shown in Fig. 10. Note the presence of spherical or ovoid knobs (160 to 400 nm diameter) along and at the tip of the processes. Arrow, remnant of a cytoplasmic process. x 65,000.

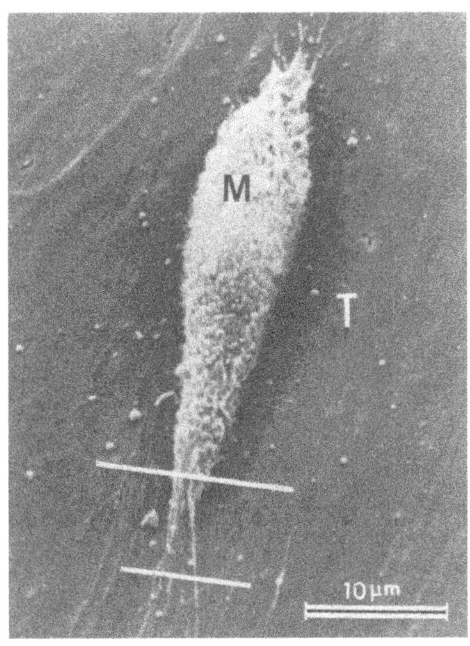

Fig. 10. SEM micrograph of an elongated macrophage (M) on L10 tumor (T) cell shown in Fig. 9. Long slender processes are observed on both poles of the cell. White lines, area examined by TEM in Fig. 14. x 2,600.

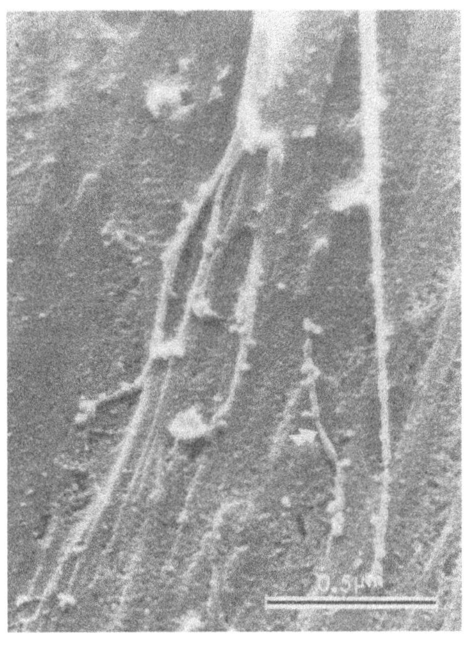

Fig. 12. TEM micrograph of the area indicated in Fig. 9. A cross-section of the 2 macrophages (M) on the top of the L10 cell (T) can be seen. Gold coating used in SEM preparation can be seen on the surface of the cells. x 16,000.

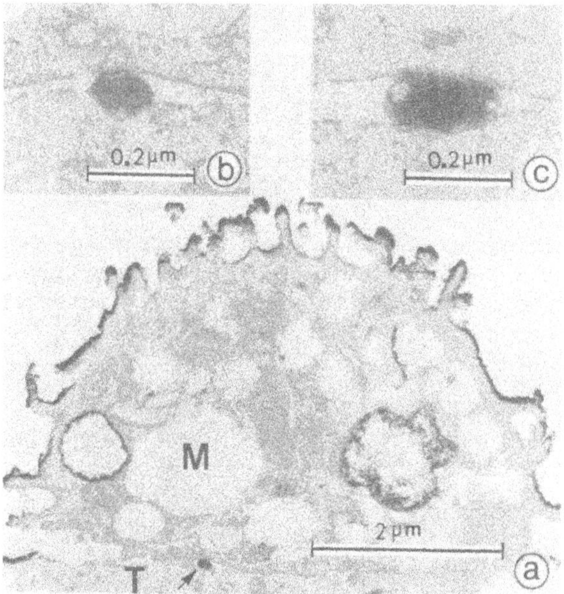

Fig. 13. a) Serial section of one of the macrophages shown in Fig. 12 showing an electron-dense body (arrow) between the macrophage (M) and tumor cell (T). x 17,500. b) High magnification of the electron-dense body. x 100,000. The large vacuoles in the macrophages are due to the phagocytosed mineral oil.

Serial sections through the main body of the 2 macrophages and the tumor cell, including the nucleus, are shown in Figure 12. Numerous mineral-oil-induced vacuoles can be seen in both of the adherent macrophages. In subsequent serial sections of these effector cells, electron-dense bodies (Fig. 13) were observed in

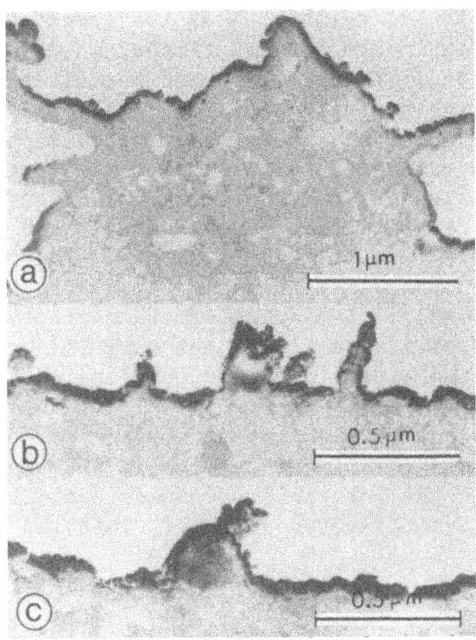

Fig. 14. a) TEM micrograph of macrophage and L10 tumor cell at the area indicated in Fig. 10. One of the processes of the macrophage has 3 discrete knobs at the end. x 27,500.
b) TEM micrograph of a section from an area containing long slender processes of the macrophage. x 57,000.
c) Serial section of the area shown in Fig. 10. x 52,500.

the intercellular space between macrophage and tumor cell. Some of these electron-dense bodies were observed partially embedded in the tumor cell surface (Fig. 13, a and b).

High-magnification SEM of the tumor-adherent cells reveals long slender processes extending from both poles of the macrophage to the tumor (Fig. 10). Blebs, ranging in size from 120 to 500 nm, were observed along the main body as well as at the tip of these cytoplasmic extensions (Fig. 11). TEM micrographs of the serial sections of this particular region of the macrophage are shown in Figure 14. Although dense granular material was observed at the tip of a macrophage process, as well as on the tumor cell, positive identification of these bodies could not be made morphologically.

Samples of macrophage-tumor cell interactions examined by SEM and TEM showed a marked difference in the ability of macrophages isolated from BCG-tumor-cured and normal animals to bind to tumor cells. Four to 13 hours after macrophages from BCG-tumor-cured animals were added to L10 cells, 90% of the tumor cells had 3 or more macrophages adhering to their surfaces, whereas only 45% of tumor cells incubated with macrophages of normal animals had 1 or 2 macrophages adhering to their surfaces. Macrophages obtained from tumor-cured animals and placed on tumor cells were predominantly spread, with extensive ruffling of the cytoplasm in long slender processes extending to the tumor cell (Fig. 15). In contrast, macrophages obtained from normal animals and placed on tumor cells were predominantly spherical (Fig. 16). This morphological difference was also observed with macrophages attached to the cover glass (Figs. 17 and 18); 85% or more of the macrophages from BCG-tumor-cured animals spread on glass, but only 15% or less of the macrophages from normal animals spread on glass.

A major difference between the macrophage-tumor cell interactions of BCG-tumor-cured and normal guinea pigs is the presence of electron-dense bodies in the intercellular space between L10 cells and macrophages from BCG-tumor-cured animals. This was noted in numerous

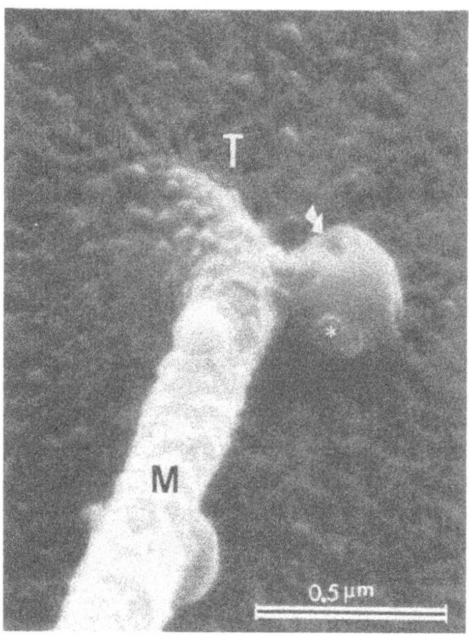

Fig. 15. SEM micrograph of one area of contact between macrophage (M) cytoplasmic process and L10 tumor cell (T). The spherical knob at the end of the macrophage process has a diameter of 500 nm (arrow) and the smaller knob attached to it (*) measures 200 nm in diameter. x 70,000.

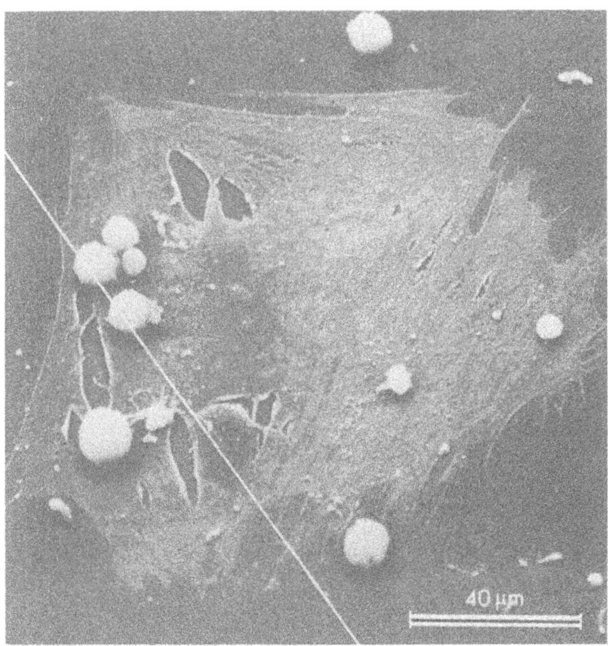

Fig. 16. SEM micrograph of L10 tumor cell that has been incubated with peritoneal macrophages from normal guinea pigs. The normal macrophages on the tumor cell are round. White line, plane of sectioning for TEM. x 800.

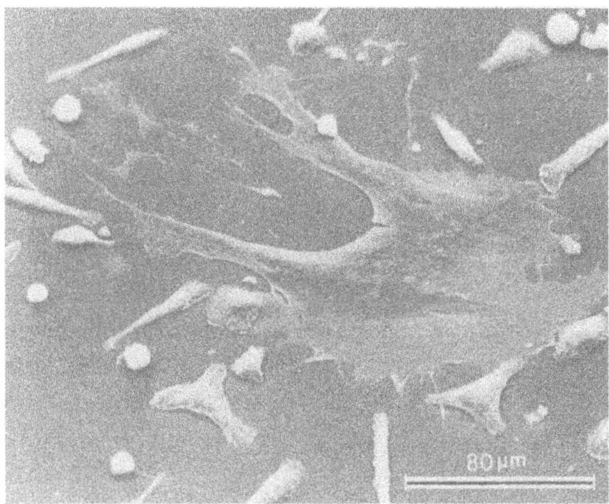

Fig. 17. SEM micrograph of L10 tumor cell and peritoneal macrophages from immune guinea pigs. Note the predominance of pleomorphic forms of macrophages spread on glass. x 440.

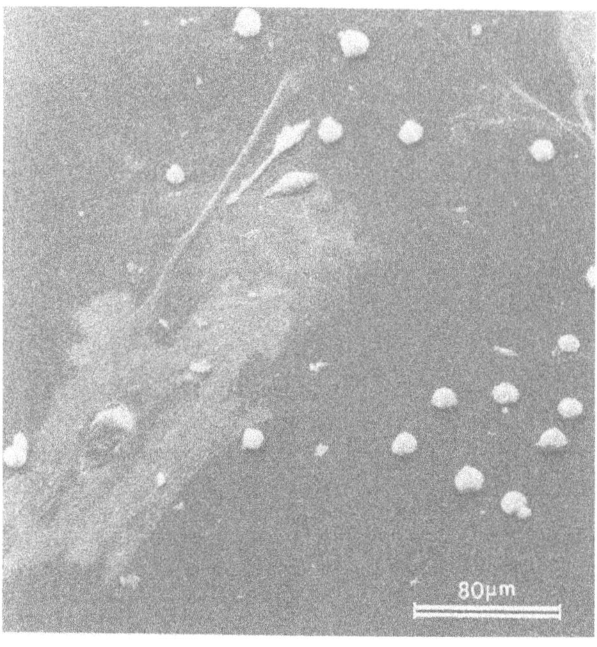

Fig. 18. SEM micrograph of L10 tumor cell and peritoneal macrophages from normal guinea pigs. The macrophages assume a predominantly round shape as shown here and in Fig. 16. x 337.

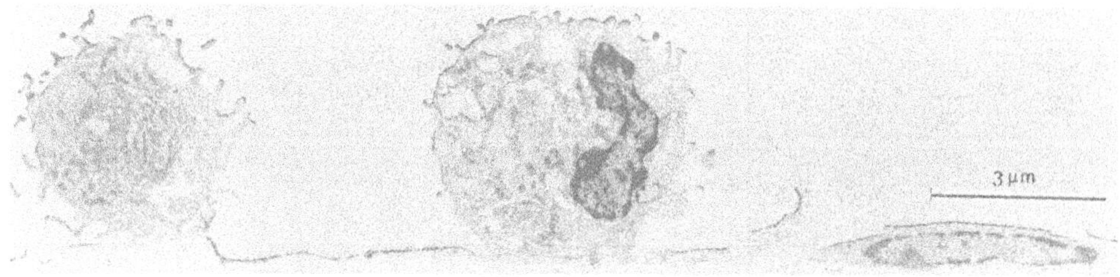

Fig. 19. TEM micrograph of the area indicated in Fig. 16. Right, a cross-section of the macrophage underneath the tumor cell. x 12,000.

samples studied. The electron-dense bodies were observed as early as 4 hours after activated macrophages were added to L10 cells. In contrast, serial sections of L10 cells plus normal macrophages or normal syngeneic guinea pig embryo cells incubated with activated macrophages showed no electron-dense bodies in the intercellular space between macrophage and target cell (Fig. 19). These results

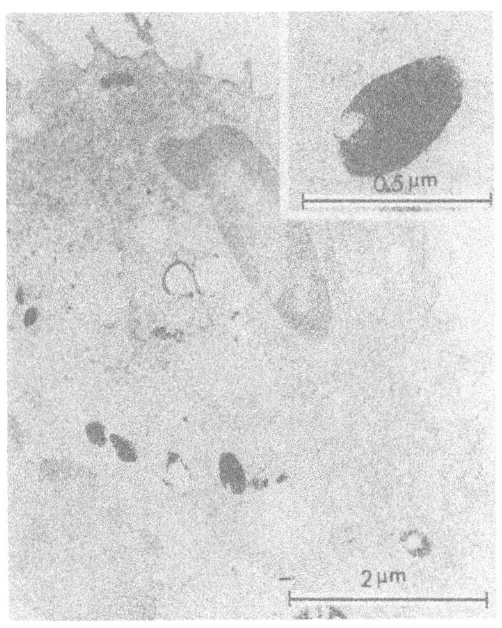

Fig. 20. Acid phosphatase reaction of immune peritoneal macrophages at the ultrastructural level is localized in lysosomes. The cells were not fixed with OsO_4 to eliminate other osmiophilic organelles from the micrograph. x 18,400. Inset, high magnification of a lysosome that is positive for acid phosphatase. Note granular appearance of a lysosome. x 70,000.

are in agreement with the finding that cytotoxic macrophages discriminate between neoplastic and non-neoplastic cells (16,18).

Accepting the fact that morphological classifications are not unequivocal, we tentatively classified the intercellular, electron-dense bodies as lysosomal organelles of macrophage origin since they closely resembled the intracellular lysosomes of PM that exhibited acid phosphatase reactivity (Fig. 20). The extracellular, electron-dense bodies possessed a granular matrix and a "halo" or eccentric clear region, and they were approximately the size of lysosomal organelles. They were often associated with cytoplasmic extensions of macrophages (Figs. 21 and 22) or sandwiched between the macrophage and tumor cell (Fig. 23). These lysosomes were also observed in L10 cells at regions closely apposed to the macrophage surface (Figs. 23 and 24). Also, intact lysosomes were often associated with a macrophage process as well as the tumor cell (Fig. 25).

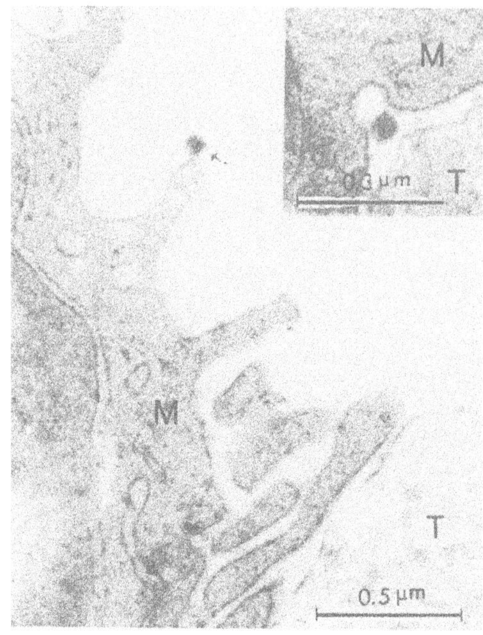

Fig. 21. TEM micrograph of a macrophage (M) from immune guinea pigs on a tumor cell (T). An electron-dense body (80 nm) is seen associated with one of the processes of the macrophage (arrow). x 52,500. Frequently, the dense body (80 nm) is seen between the macrophage and tumor cell (inset). x 74,000.

In many instances, the penetrations of lysosomes within the tumor cell surface suggested that an active or passive transport process on the part of the tumor cell might participate in the lysosomal translocation. Uptake of exocytosed lysosomes of macrophage origin at the intercellular space between macrophages and L10 tumor cells could be achieved through endocytosis. The endocytic capacity of tumor cell surfaces has been described elsewhere (51) and may be requisite to the translocation of lysosomes from macrophages to tumor cells.

The extracellular lysosomes were extremely pleomorphic varying from disrupted, dense, granular particles to intact lysosomes with single limiting membranes (Fig. 26). Membrane-associated lysosomes appeared to be enclosed in cytoplasmic material and may be within the detached processes of macrophages (Fig. 26, c and d). Clasmatosis of macrophage processes containing these intracellular organelles would result in these structures remaining attached at the tumor cell surface. Since the macrophages utilized in this study were isolated from tumor-immune animals, they may also be "armed" as well as "activated," as described by Evans and Alexander (33). The question whether or not we are dealing with specific tumor cytotoxicity, however, was not approached in this study. Nevertheless,

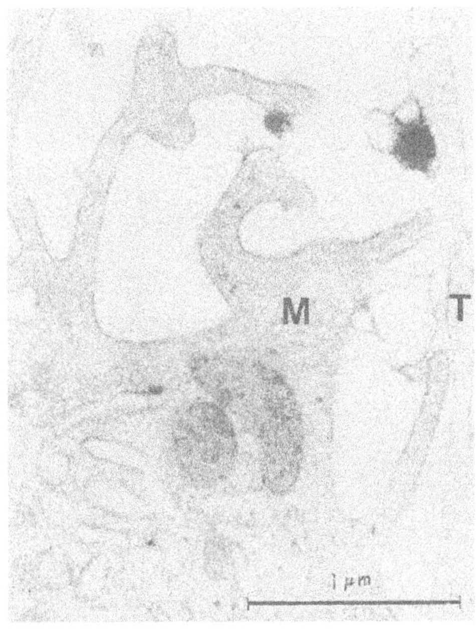

Fig. 22. TEM micrograph of a macrophage (M) on a tumor cell (T). A dense body is associated with one of the processes of the macrophage and another dense body is associated with the L10 tumor cell. x 40,000.

our results suggest that the cytotoxic reaction has both an effector cell recognition and a target cell susceptibility component. The macrophage-tumor cell interaction initiating the recognition phase may result in the extracellular release of lysosomes, the exocytosis phase of this cytotoxic reaction. The susceptibility of the neoplastic cells to these events appears to be the result of an active or passive uptake of lysosomes by the tumor cells ultimately resulting in cytolysis.

Comparison of Macrophage-Mediated Cytotoxicity in the L10 and T1699 Tumor Systems

Killing of T1699 tumor cells *in vitro* has been shown to be mediated by functionally and morphologically different types of macrophages (13,37). The large TuM kills by an apparent phagocytic mechanism both *in vitro* and *in vivo*, whereas other smaller macrophage effector cells appear to kill *in vitro* by nonphagocytic means. In most other reported cases of macrophage-mediated cytotoxicity, nonphagocytic killing of tumor cells appears to be the more commonly observed pathway. Such would appear to be the case for the macrophage-mediated killing of L10 tumor cells, since phagocytosis of intact cells has not been observed. Despite these obvious morpholog-

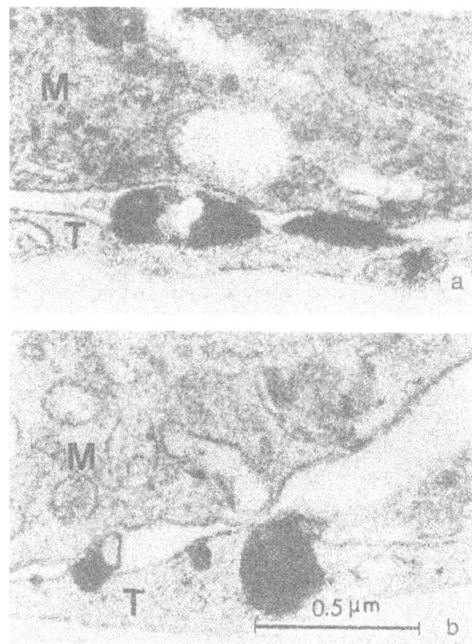

Fig. 23. a) Granular electron-dense bodies (ca. 450 nm) were frequently found between macrophages (M) from immune animals and tumor cells (T). x 60,000. b) Electron-dense bodies were also found in the tumor cells (T) at points of contact between macrophage (M) and tumor cell (T). x 60,000.

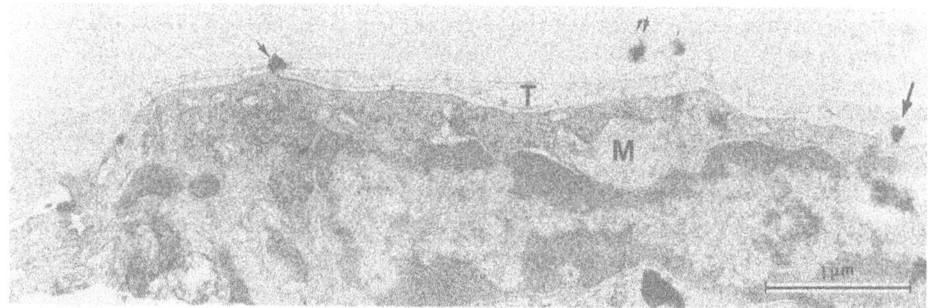

Fig. 24. TEM micrograph of a macrophage that is completely underneath the tumor cell. Note the presence of electron-dense bodies in the macrophage (white arrow), in the tumor at a point of contact between macrophage and tumor cell (black arrow), between the tumor cell and the macrophage (black arrow, white border), and in the vicinity or in contact with the tumor cell (double black arrows). x 35,000.

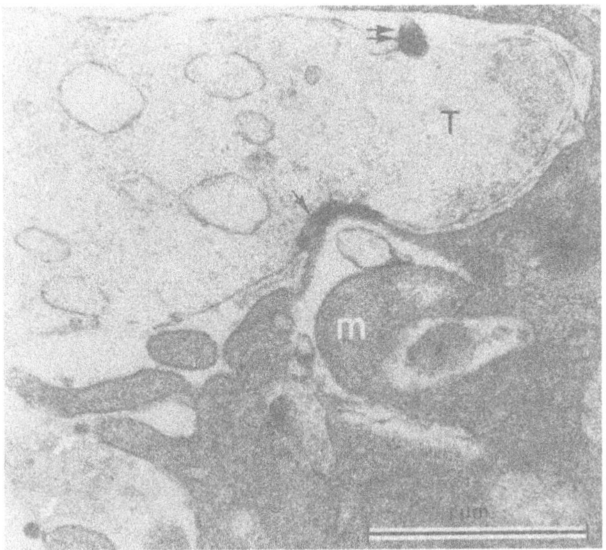

Fig. 25. Pleomorphic dense bodies were frequently observed associated with the macrophage process (white arrows) between macrophage (M) and tumor (T) (black arrow) and with tumor alone (double black arrow). Fuzzy osmiophilic material was also observed at areas of close association between the macrophage and tumor cell. The macrophage process has partially enveloped the tumor cell at one end (*). x 41,000.

ical differences between intracellular and extracellular killing of tumor cells, the subcellular events involved may, in fact, be quite similar.

In the L10 tumor system, we have studied the events surrounding macrophage-mediated killing of tumor cells by electron microscopy. These studies showed that tumor cell cytolysis was preceded by macrophage-to-tumor cell contact, polarization of electron-dense granules, presumably lysosomes, to the areas of contact, and transfer of granules to tumor cells. The transfer of lysosomes to tumor cells was by either an exocytic process or by breaking off of macrophage cytoplasmic processes containing lysosomes onto the surfaces of tumor cells. After transfer, the uptake of lysosomes by the tumor cells may have been accomplished by endocytosis.

In the T1699 tumor system, the sequence of events of tumor cell killing was studied by light microscopy utilizing a technique of labeling secondary lysosomes of macrophages with dextran sulfate,

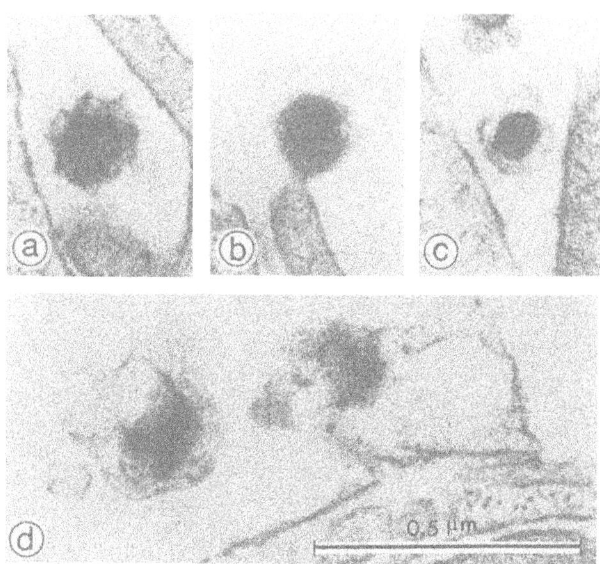

Fig. 26. High magnification of some of the electron-dense bodies found between or associated with either the macrophage or the L10 cell. a) Dense body with loose granular and filamentous internal structure. x 100,000. b) Dense body with homogeneous granular internal structure. x 100,000. c) Dense body with homogeneous granular internal structure and a loosely arranged limiting membrane. x 100,000. d) Dense body with granular internal structure and associate membrane. x100,000

thereby making them discernible by light microscopy. These studies revealed that cytolysis of tumor cells was preceded by a sequence of interactions between macrophages and tumor cells. Following contact between macrophage and tumor cell, polarization of dextran sulfate-positive material toward the areas of contact was observed. On some portions of tumor cell surfaces where macrophages were not in direct contact, it was possible to identify dextran sulfate-positive staining material associated with strands of membranous materials suggestive of macrophage membranes. In other tumor cells, discrete granules of dextran sulfate material was observed within the cytoplasm of the tumor cell. Under conditions where tumor cells were phagocytosed, the release of dextran sulfate into the phagosome was observed. Following the digestion of tumor cells, large deposits of undigested dextran sulfate remained within the digestive vacuole. In studies where crude sonicates of macrophages were applied to tumor cells, we found that the tumor cells could take up the dextran sulfate-labeled subcellular structures apparently by an endocytic process.

The sequence of events for macrophage killing in both tumor systems can be summarized as follows: a) contact occurs between macrophages and target cells; b) lysosomal enzymes of macrophages are polarized toward tumor cells; c) spreading of macrophages at the tumor cell surface occurs; d) tumor cells are lysed. If spreading of macrophages is quite rapid, for example when tumor cells are coated with antibody, then phagocytosis may predominate if the tumor cell is sufficiently small enough to be accommodated within the macrophage. If the lytic process is more rapid, then extracellular killing will predominate followed by phagocytosis of dead tumor cells. When phagocytosis does not or cannot occur, killing is entirely extracellular without subsequent phagocytosis. We are just beginning to understand the factors that determine which mechanism will predominate. Most studies that have described phagocytosis of tumor cells have also shown that antibody is required for phagocytosis to proceed (37,52-54). Antibody not only provides the mechanism necessary to initiate contact between phagocytes and tumor cells, but also stimulates phagocytic activity (39). Only certain subclasses of antibody will trigger the phagocytic response (55), and even then not all classes of macrophages will respond to these triggers to the same extent (13).

Electron microscopy studies of cells have revealed that various membranes permeate throughout every part of the cytoplasm. Certain exoplasmic components of the cell, such as lysosomes, phagosomes, and secretory granules, are separated by these membranes from other intracytoplasmic (endoplasmic) portions. Phagocytosed materials generally stay within these exoplasmic structures which are topologically equivalent to the extracellular spaces. Thus, in cases where tumor cells are not, or cannot be phagocytosed, killing of tumor cells can proceed extracellularly by the release of lysosomal enzymes, at the point where the tumor cell contacts the macrophage surface membrane rather than into the phagocytic vacuole, as is the case in phagocytosis. In fact, certain biochemical changes which have been detected in the cell membrane of activated macrophages, such as an increase in 5'-nucleotidase, are similar to changes detected in the membrane of the phagosome (56). Perhaps these or similar membrane changes are related to the capacity of the membrane for lysosomal fusion.

BIOCHEMICAL EVENTS IN MACROPHAGE-MEDIATED TUMOR CELL CYTOTOXICITY

Despite considerable research the biochemical and molecular nature of macrophage activation is, as yet, little understood. Changes in the biochemistry of activated macrophages compared to normal or elicited macrophages have been reported (57). For example, the activated macrophage contains increased levels of acid hydrolases (58,59), increased respiratory activity (60), increased glucose metabolism (61), and a decrease in membrane associated ecto-5'-

nucleotidase (62). However, which of these biochemical alterations, if any, relate to the tumoricidal activity of macrophages is still unknown. Several substances have been proposed to mediate the cytotoxic effects of macrophages toward tumor cells including thymidine (63), arginase (64), complement products (65), proteases (25,26), peroxidase (66), lysozyme (67), and hydrogen peroxide (H_2O_2) or other reduced species of oxygen (68). However, at present, evidence supporting any of these proposed mechanisms is inconclusive.

Nathan et al. (68) has suggested that an oxidative mechanism may provide the means by which activated macrophages kill tumor cells. Conceptually, an oxidative mechanism is attractive because of the known similarities to the biochemical mechanisms of microbial killing (69), but this concept has been difficult to prove. In fact, other studies have concluded that macrophage-mediated cytotoxicity is independent of oxygen, H_2O_2, or superoxide anions (O_2^-) (70). In these studies, the cytotoxic effects of macrophages on tumor cells were unaffected in cultures containing free catalase or superoxide dismutase, two enzymes capable of inactivating O_2^- and H_2O_2. However, the absence of an inhibitory effect in these studies could have been because of the failure of these exogenous enzymes to cross cell membranes or localize within the lysosomes of macrophages. For example, studies in which phagocyte-mediated bacterial killing was measured in media containing catalase and superoxide dismutase showed that microbial killing could be only partially inhibited by these enzymes (71). However, when latex particles were added to the cultures to aid in the transfer of exogenous enzymes into secondary lysosomes of the phagocytes, the killing of bacteria was virtually eliminated. This suggests that, at least for bacterial killing, the inhibitory effects of catalase and superoxide dismutase were optimally effective only when these enzymes were concentrated into secondary lysosomes of the phagocytes and not when the enzymes were free in the media.

In the bacterial killing systems of phagocytes, H_2O_2 has been shown to be a component of a potent killing system in conjunction with myeloperoxidase and halide ions (69). A possible role for myeloperoxidase in the killing of tumor cells by macrophages has also been suggested (66,72). Although most mature macrophages are peroxidase negative, Ruco and Meltzer (72) have suggested that perhaps the immature macrophage mediates tumor cell killing. The recruitment of immature, peroxidase-positive macrophages into the peritoneal cavity of mice infected with BCG was coincident with the development of tumoricidal macrophages. However, other studies have shown that mature macrophages (presumably peroxidase negative) also can be activated *in vitro* to the tumoricidal state (20-22). Thus, the role of myeloperoxidase in these killing systems is unclear. Other oxidative killing systems not dependent upon myeloperoxidase have also been proposed, although their operation is poorly understood (69).

Several investigators have reported that the antibody-mediated killing of tumor cells by both granulocytes and macrophages occurs by oxidative processes (73-75). Thus, at least in two instances, an oxidative mechanism of tumor cell killing has been reported: a) in the presence of certain drugs that trigger a respiratory burst (68), and b) in the presence of antibody directed against tumor cell surface antigens (74). Another possible biochemical mechanism by which macrophages kill tumor cells has been reported to involve secretion by macrophages of neutral proteases (25,26). Murine BCG-activated PM secrete more neutral proteases than do unactivated PM. The possibility that these proteases are involved in the cytolysis of neoplastic cells was suggested by data which showed that protease inhibitors could block the cytotoxic effects of macrophages on target cells (25). Whether the relationship between production of proteases and lysis of tumor cells was direct or indirect ws not determined. The possibility that proteases could act as intermediaries in a reaction sequence is suggested by observations that neutral proteases also participate in the production of O_2^- by both neutrophils and monocytes (76). This compound, under catalysis by superoxide dismutase, forms H_2O_2, and H_2O_2 or other oxygen intermediaries may mediate the toxic effects of macrophages on tumor cells either directly (68) or in combination with myeloperoxidase (66).

This discussion has indicated that a number of different biochemical mechanisms may operate in the process of tumor cell killing. The most obvious question is, which of these proposed pathways is most relevant? In fact, the death of a tumor cell may not be the result of a single cytotoxic event but the cumulative effect of multiple lesions, each inflicted by a different agent. For example, the studies of Sorrell et al. (70), showed that the toxic effects of macrophages toward target cells were significantly reduced but not eliminated when cells were cultured under anaerobic conditions, suggesting that killing was partially, but not wholly, dependent upon the presence of free oxygen. Perhaps the macrophage should be regarded as a cell having a high degree of functional redundancy, such that it can generate its cytotoxic effects against a wide variety of targets in a number of different environments and situations.

CONCLUSIONS

Although macrophages isolated from tumors may be cytotoxic to tumor cells *in vitro* (77-79), they apparently are unable, in most cases, to alter progressive tumor growth *in vivo*. The probable exceptions to these observations are those tumors capable of undergoing immunologically induced regression. In these tumors, many histiocytes have been found and have been associated with the process of tumor regression (14,37,80), and, in these systems, it may be possible to correlate *in vitro* data of tumor cell killing with events occurring *in vivo*.

We have investigated two widely different tumor systems, both of which undergo immunologically controlled regression and have compared the cellular and subcellular events associated with the macrophage-mediated killing of tumor cells. In the T1699 murine tumor system, cytotoxic activity of macrophages can be mediated by either phagocytic or nonphagocytic mechanisms, depending in part on the class of macrophage involved, whereas in the L10 guinea pig tumor system only nonphagocytic killing by macrophages is observed. Despite these apparently different methods of killing, we have found that the subcellular mechanisms appear to be fundamentally the same. We base these conclusions on the following observations. In both tumor systems, a) target cell-to-effector cell contact preceded the cytotoxic event; b) Lysosomes within macrophages were polarized toward tumor cells; c) Macrophages spread over tumor cell surfaces and then destroyed the tumor cell. At the moment that the tumor cell is killed, the phagocytic process may or may not be complete depending upon a number of factors, such as the rapidity with which macrophage spreading occurs in relation to the rapidity of the lytic process, the type of tumor involved, the type of macrophage involved, the presence or absence of antibody, or the subclass of antibody present. Regardless of whether the phagocytic process is successful, the underlying subcellular events of tumor cell killing can proceed with or without the formation of a phagocytic vacuole.

The killing of tumor cells by macrophages, whether by phagocytic or nonphagocytic means, appears to have many features in common with microbial killing such as recognition, attachment, and perhaps even the susceptibility of tumor cells and microorganisms to similar biochemical toxins. From the contributions of numerous researchers over the past decade, it can reasonably be concluded that the macrophage is well equipped for its accessory role in maintaining the body's defenses. The ability of macrophages to distinguish self from nonself and their capacity to undergo changes in form and function in almost endless variations suggest that the macrophage is uniquely equipped to express their cytotoxic effects in many diverse ways and situations.

REFERENCES

1. Haskill, J.S., Häyry, P., and L.A. Radov. Systemic and local immunity in allograft and cancer rejection. Contemp. Top. Immunobiol. 8:107-170 (1978).
2. Herberman, R.B., Holder, H.T., Varesio, L., Taniyama, T., Puccetti, P., Kirchner, H., Gerson, J., White, S., Keisari, Y., and J.S. Haskill. Immunologic reactivity of lymphoid cells in tumors. Contemp. Top. Immunobiol. 10:61-78 (1980).
3. Witz, I.P. Tumor-bound immunoglobulins: In situ expressions of humoral immunity. Adv. Cancer Res. 25:95-141 (1977).
4. Von Kleist, S., King, M., and C. Huet. Evidence for membrane-

bound antibodies directed against antigens expressed on tumors. Contemp. Top. Immunobiol. 10:177-189 (1980).
5. Shin, H.S. Johnson, R.J., Pasternack, G.R., and J.S. Economou. Mechanisms of tumor immunity: The role of antibody and non-immune effectors. Prog. Allergy 25:163-210 (1978).
6. Fidler, I.J., and A. Raz. The induction of tumoricidal capacities in mouse and rat macrophages by lymphokines. Lymphokines 3:345-363 (1981).
7. Evans, R., and P. Alexander. Mechanism of extracellular killing of nucleated mammalian cells by macrophages. In "Immunobiology of the Macrophage," D.S. Nelson, ed., Academic Press, New York, pp. 535-576 (1976).
8. Hibbs, J.B., Jr. Role of macrophages in resistance to cancer. In "Immunologic Aspects of Neoplasia," M. D. Anderson Hospital and Tumor Institute, Williams and Williams Co., Baltimore, pp. 305-327 (1975).
9. Evans, R. Macrophages in syngeneic animal tumors. Transplantation 14:468-473 (1972).
10. Mackaness, G.B. Role of macrophages in host defense mechanisms. In "The Macrophage in Neoplasia," M.A. Fink, Ed., Academic Press (1976).
11. Haskill, J.S. A micro-colony-inhibition method for quantitation of tumor immunity. J. Natl. Cancer Inst. 51:1581-1588 (1973).
12. Zbar, B., Wepsic, H.T., Rapp, H.J., Whang-Peng, J., and T. Borsos. Transplantable hepatomas induced in strain-2 guinea pigs by diethylnitrosamine: characterization by histology, growth, and chromosomes. J. Natl. Cancer Inst. 43:821-831 (1969).
13. Haskill, J.S., Key, M.E., Radov, L.A., Parthenais, E., Korn, J.H., Fett, J.W., Yamamura, Y., DeLustro, F., Vesley, J., and G. Gant. The importance of antibody and macrophages in spontaneous and drug-induced regression of the T1699 mammary adenocarcinoma. J. Reticuloendothel. Soc. 26:417-425 (1979).
14. Hanna, M.G., Jr., Bucana, C., Hobbs, B., and Fidler, I.J. Morphological aspects of tumor cell cytotoxicity by effector cells of the macrophage-histiocyte compartment: In vitro and in vivo studies in BCG-mediated tumor regression. In "The Macrophage in Neoplasia," M. Fink, Ed., Academic Press, New York, pp. 113-133 (1976).
15. Hibbs, J.B., Jr., Lambert, L.H., Jr., and J.S. Remington. Resistance to murine tumors conferred by chronic infection with intracellular protozoa, Toxoplasma gondii and Besnoitia jellisoni. J. Infect. Dis. 124:587-592 (1971).
16. Hibbs, J.R., Jr. Discrimination between neoplastic and non-neoplastic cells in vitro by activated macrophages. J. Natl. Cancer Inst. 53:1487-1492 (1974).
17. Churchill, W.H., Jr., Piessens, W.F., Sulis, C.A., and J.R. David. Macrophages activated as suspension cultures with lymphocyte mediators devoid of antigen become cytotoxic for

tumor cells. J. Immunol. 115:781-786 (1975).
18. Piessens, W.F., Churchill, W.H., Jr., and J.R. David. Macrophages activated in vitro with lymphocyte mediators kill neoplastic but not normal cells. J. Immunol. 114:293-299 (1975).
19. Ruco, L.P., and M.S. Meltzer. Macrophage activation for tumor cytotoxicity: tumoricidal activity by macrophages from C3H/HeJ mice requires at least two activation stimuli. Cell. Immunol. 41:35-51 (1978).
20. Sone, S., and I.J. Fidler. Syngergistic activation by lymphokines and muramyl dipeptide of tumoricidal properties in rat alveolar macrophages. J. Immunol. 125:2454-2460 (1980).
21. Sone, S., Poste, G., and Fidler, I.J. Rat alveolar macrophages are susceptible to activation by free and liposome-encapsulated lymphokines. J. Immunol. 124:2197-2202 (1980).
22. Sone, S., and I.J. Fidler. In vitro activation of tumoricidal properties in rat alveolar macrophages by synthetic muramyl dipeptide encapsultated in liposomes. Cell. Immunol. 57:42-50 (1981).
23. Hibbs, J.B., Jr. Heterocytolysis by macrophages activated by Bacillus Calmette-Guérin: Lysosome exocytosis into tumor cells Science 184:468-471 (1974).
24. Kramer, J.J., and G.A. Granger. In vitro induction and release of a cell toxin by immune C57/BL6 mouse peritoneal macrophages. Cell. Immunol. 3:88-100 (1972).
25. Adams, D.O. Effector mechanisms of cytolytically activated macrophages. I. Secretion of neutral proteases and effect of protease inhibitors. J. Immunol. 124:286-292 (1980).
26. Adams, D.O., Kao, K., Farb, R., and S.V. Pizzo. Effector mechanisms of cytolytically activated macrophages. II. Secretion of a cytolytic factor by activated macrophages and its relationship to secreted neutral proteases. J. Immunol. 124:293-300 (1980).
27. Fidler, I.J., Sone, S., Fogler, W.E., and Z.L. Barnes. Eradication of spontaneous metastases and activation of alveolar macrophages by intravenous injection of liposomes containing muramyl dipeptide. Proc. Natl. Acad. Sci. USA 78:1680-1684 (1981).
28. Hart, I.R. The selection and characterization of an invasive variant of the B16 melanoma. Am. J. Pathol. 97:587-600 (1979).
29. Fidler, I.J., Raz, A., Fogler, W.E., Kirsh, R., Bugelski, P., and G. Poste. Design of liposomes to improve delivery of macrophage-augmenting agents to alveolar macrophages. Cancer Res. 40:4460-4466 (1980).
30. Marino, P.A., and D.O. Adams. Interaction of Bacillus Calmette-Guérin-activated macrophages and neoplastic cells in vitro. I. Conditions of binding and its selectivity. Cell. Immunol. 54: 11-25 (1980).
31. Marino, P.A., and D.O. Adams. Interaction of Bacillus Calmette-Guérin-activated macropahges and neoplastic cells in vitro. II. The relationship of selective binding to cytolysis. Cell. Immu-

nol. 54:26-35 (1980).
32. Bucana, C., Hoyer, L.C., Hobbs, B., Breesman, S., McDaniel, M., and M.G. Hanna, Jr. Morphological evidence for the translocation of lysosomal organelles from cytotoxic macrophages into the cytoplasm of tumor target cells. Cancer Res. 36:4444-4458. (1976).
33. Evans, R., and P. Alexander. Rendering macrophages specifically cytotoxic by a factor released from immune lymphoid cells. Transplantation 12:227-229 (1971).
34. Pearson, G.R. In vitro and in vivo investigations on antibody-dependent cellular cytotoxicity. Cur. Top. Microbiol. Immunol. 80:65-96 (1978).
35. Johnston, R.B., Jr., Lehmeyer, J.E., and L.A. Guthrie. Generation of superoxide anion and chemiluminescence by human monocytes during phagocytosis and on contact with surface-bound immunoglobulin G. J. Exp. Med. 143:1551-1556 (1976).
36. Yamazaki, M., Shinoda, H., Suzuki, Y., and D. Mizuno. Two-step mechanism of macrophage-mediated tumor lysis in vitro. Gann. 67:741-745 (1976).
37. Key, M., and J.S. Haskill. Macrophage-mediated antibody-dependent destruction of tumor cells in DBA/2 mice: In vitro identification of an in situ mechanism. J. Natl. Cancer Inst. 66:103-110 (1981).
38. Odartchenko, N., Sordat, B., Pavillard, M., and H. Cottier. Cytokinetic studies on tingible bodies in germinal centers of Peyer's patches in mice. In "Lymphatic tissue and germinal centers in immune response," L. Fiore-Donati and M.G. Hanna, Jr., Eds., Plenum Press, New York, pp. 93-100 (1969).
39. Griffin, F.M., Jr., Griffin, J.A., Leider, J.E., and S.C. Silverstein. Studies on the mechanism of phagocytosis. I. Requirements of circumferential attachment of particle-bound ligands to specific receptors on the macrophage plasma membrane. J. Exp. Med. 142:1263-1282 (1975).
40. Kay, M.M.B. Mechanism of removal of senescent cells by human macrophages in vitro. Proc. Natl. Acad. Sci. USA 72:3521-3525 (1975).
41. Key, M.E., and J.S. Haskill. Immunohistologic evidence for the role of antibody and macrophages in regression of the murine T1699 mammary adenocarcinoma. Int. J. Cancer 28:225-236 (1981).
42. Hanna, M.G., Jr., Snodgrass, M.J., Zbar, B., and H.J. Rapp. Histopathology of tumor regression after intralesional injection of Mycobacterium bovis. IV. Development of immunity to tumor cells and BCG. J. Natl. Cancer Inst. 51:1897-1908 (1973).
43. Fidler, I.J., Budmen, M.B., and M.G. Hanna, Jr. Characterization of in vitro reactivity by BCG-treated guinea pigs on syngeneic Line-10 hepatocarcinoma. Cancer Immunol. Immunother. 1:179-186 (1979).
44. Henson, P.M., and Z.G. Oades. Stimulation of human neutro-

phils by soluble and insoluble immunoglobulin aggregates: Secretion of granule constituents and increased oxidation of glucose. J. Clin. Invest. 56:1053-1059 (1975).
45. Carr, I., Carr, J., Trew, J.A., Lobo, A., and P.K. Chattopadhyay. Lysozyme production by a granuloma in vivo: Output in blood and lymph in relation to ultrastructure and immunochemistry. J. Pathol. 132:105-119 (1980).
46. Cohn, Z.A. Macrophage physiology. Federation Proc. 34:1725-1729 (1975).
47. Gallin, J.I., Wright, D.E., and E. Schiffmann. Role of secretory events in modulating human neutrophil chemotaxis. J. Clin. Invest. 62:1364-1374 (1978).
48. Haskill, J.S. ADCC effector cells in a murine adenocarcinoma. I. Evidence for blood-borne bone-marrow-derived monocytes. Int. J. Cancer 20:432-440 (1977).
49. Snodgrass, M.J., and M.G. Hanna, Jr. Ultrastructural studies of histiocyte-tumor cell interactions during tumor regression after intralesional injection of Mycobacterium bovis. Cancer Res. 33:701-716 (1973).
50. Hanna, M.G., Jr., Zbar, B., and H.J. Rapp. Histopathology of tumor regression after intralesional injectional of Mycobacterium bovis. I. Tumor growth and metastasis. J. Natl. Cancer Inst. 48:1441-1455 (1972).
51. Nicolson, G.L. Transmembrane control of the receptors on normal and tumor cells and some surface changes associated with transformation and malignancy. Biochim. Biophys. Acta 458:1-72 (1976).
52. Amos, D.B. Possible relationships between cytotoxic effects of isoantibody and host cell function. Ann. N.Y. Acad. Sci. 87:273-292 (1960).
53. Bennett, B. Phagocytosis of mouse tumor cells in vitro by various homologous and heterologous cells. J. Immunol. 95: 80-86 (1965).
54. The, H.T., Eibergen, R., Lamberts, H.B., Oldhoff, J., Ploeg, E., Schrafford-Keops, H., and H.O. Neiweg. Immune phagocytosis in vivo of human malignant melanoma cells. Acta Med. Scand. 192:141-144 (1972).
55. Walker, W.S. Mediation of macrophage cytolytic and phagocytic activities by antibodies of different classes and class-specific Fc-receptors. J. Immunol. 119:367-373 (1977).
56. Werb, Z., and Z.A. Cohn. Plasma membrane synthesis in the macrophage following phagocytosis of polystyrene latex particles. J. Biol. Chem. 247:2439-2446 (1972).
57. Karnovsky, M.L., and J.K. Lazdins. Biochemical criteria for activated macrophages. J. Immunol. 121:809-813 (1978).
58. Saito, K., and E. Suter. Lysosomal acid hydrolases in mice infected with BCG. J. Exp. Med. 121:727-749 (1965).
59. Hard, G.C. Some biochemical aspects of the immune macrophage. Br. J. Exp. Pathol. 51:97-105 (1970).
60. Karnovsky, M.L., Lazdins, J., and S.R. Simmons. Metabolism

of activated mononuclear phagocytes at rest and during phagocytosis. In "Mononuclear Phagocytes in Immunity, Infection, and Pathology," R. Van Furth, Ed., Blackwell Scientific Publications, Oxford, Edinburgh, and Melbourne, pp. 423-439 (1975).
61. Riisgaard, S., Bennedsen, J., and J.M. Rhodes. In vitro studies on normal, stimulated and immunologically activated mouse macrophages. I. Oxidation of 1-^{14}C-glucose by macrophages in monolayer cultures. Acta Pathol. Microbiol. Scand. [C]. 85:233-238 (1977).
62. Karnovsky, M.L., Lazdins, J., Drath, D., and A. Harper. Biochemical characteristics of activated macrophages. Ann. N.Y. Acad. Sci. 256:266-274 (1975).
63. Stadecker, M.J., Calderon, J., Karnovsky, M.L., and E.R. Unanue. Synthesis and release of thymidine by macrophages. J. Immunol. 119:1738-1743 (1977).
64. Currie, G.A., and C. Basham. Differential arginine dependence and the selective cytotoxic effects of activated macrophages for malignant cells in vitro. Br. J. Cancer 38:653-659 (1978).
65. Ferluga, J., Schorlemmer, H.J., Baptista, L.C., and A.C. Allison. Production of the complement cleavage product, C3a, by activated macrophages and its tumorolytic effects. Clin. Exp. Immunol. 31:512-517 (1978).
66. Clark, R.A., Klebanoff, S.J., Einstein, A.B., and A. Fefer. Peroxidase-H_2O_2-halide system: Cytotoxic effect on mammalian tumor cells. Blood 45:161-170 (1975).
67. Osserman, E.F., Klockars, M., Halper, J., and R.S. Fischel. Effects of lysozyme on normal and transformed mammalian cells. Nature 243:331-225 ((1973).
68. Nathan, C.F., Brukner, L.H., Silverstein, S.C., and Z.A. Cohn. Extracellular cytolysis by activated macrophages and granulocytes. I. Pharmacologic triggering of effector cells and the release of hydrogen peroxide. J. Exp. Med. 149:84-99 (1979).
69. Babior, B.M. Oxygen-dependent microbial killing by phagocytes. N. Engl. J. Med. 298:659-668 (1978).
70. Sorrell, T.C., Lehrer, R.I., and M.J. Cline. Mechanism of nonspecific macrophage-mediated cytotoxicity: Evidence for lack of dependence upon oxygen. J. Immunol. 120:347-352 (1978).
71. Johnson, R.B., Jr., Keele, B.B., Jr., and H.P. Misra. The role of superoxide anion generation in phagocytic bactericidal activity: studies with normal and chronic granulomatous disease leukocytes. J. Clin. Invest. 55:1357-1372 (1975).
72. Ruco, L.P., and M.S. Meltzer. Macrophage activation for tumor cytotoxicity: Induction of tumoricidal macrophages by supernatants of PPD-stimulated Bacillus Calmette-Guérin-immune spleen cell cultures. J. Immunol. 119:889-896 (1977).
73. Hafeman, D.G., and Z.J. Lucas. Polymorphonuclear leukocyte-mediated, antibody-dependent, cellular cytotoxicity against tumor cells: Dependence on oxygen and the respiratory burst. J. Immunol. 123:55-62 (1979).
74. Nathan, C., and Z. Cohn. Role of oxygen-dependent mechanisms

in antibody-induced lysis of tumor cells by activated macrophages. J. Exp. Med. 152:198-208 (1980).

75. Nathan, C., Brukner, L., Kaplan, G., Unkeless, J., and Z. Cohn. Role of activated macrophages in antibody-dependent lysis of tumor cells. J. Exp. Med. 152:183-197 (1980).
76. Kitagawa, S., Takaku, F., and S. Sakamoto. Evidence that proteases are involved in superoxide production by human polymorphonuclear leukocytes and monocytes. J. Clin. Invest. 65: 74-81 (1980).
77. Evans, R., Booth, C.G., and F. Spencer. Lack of correlation between _in vivo_ rejection of syngeneic fibrosarcomas and nonspecific macrophage cytotoxicity. Br. J. Cancer 38:583-590 (1978).
78. Mantovani, A., Polentarutti, N., Peri, G., Shavit, Z., Vecchi, A., Bolis, G., and C. Mangioni. Cytotoxocity on tumor cells of peripheral blood monocytes and tumor-associated macrophages in patients with ascites ovarian tumors. J. Natl. Cancer Inst. 64:1307-1315 (1980).
79. Vose, B.M. Cytotoxicity of adherent cells associated with some human tumors and lung tissues. Cancer Immunol. Immunother. 5:173-179 (1978).
80. Russell, S.W., and C.G. Cochrane. The cellular events associated with regression and progression of murine (Moloney) sarcoma. Int. J. Cancer 13:54-63 (1974).

ACKNOWLEDGEMENTS

Figures 4-6 are from Hanna, M.G., Jr., Bucana, C., Hobbs, B., and I.J. Fidler. Morphologic aspects of tumor cell cytotoxicity by effector cells of the macrophage-histiocyte compartment: _In vitro_ and _in vivo_ studies in BCG-mediated tumor regression. _In_ "The Macrophage in Neoplasia," M. Fink, Ed., Academic Press, New York, pp. 113-133 (1976). By permission.

Figures 7-26 are from Bucana, C., Hoyer, L.C., Hobbs, B., Bressman, S., McDaniel, S., and M.G. Hanna, Jr. Morphologic evidence for the translocation of lysosomal organelles from cytotoxic macrophages into the cytoplasm of tumor target cells. Cancer Res. 36: 4444-4449 (1976). By permission.

DISCUSSION

P. Henkart

I'd like to ask a question, which is reminiscent of a perennial family discussion: how do you know that what you see has got anything to do with the actual killing?

M. Hanna

You don't. You really don't. You do the best you can with the technology that's available. We had seen all of this by simply taking transmission, scanning and time-lapse pictures of any cells we were able to find in the grids. First you mark a macrophage effector cell, and then you come off the time-lapse and look and see what is there at the point of contact with the target. What we see at the point of contact are lysosomes. It could very well be that those lysosomes had nothing to do with cytolysis of that tumor cell. However, I find it very difficult to believe that lysosomes transmitted or translocated in that manner do not do some damage to the cell surface. Now that may not have been all the damage that was required, but you can see in the electron microscope they do do some damage. This is about as much as you can do. There might be better ways of approaching it. I leave that for other morphologists.

R. Goldfarb

You depicted one target cell that underwent repair and appeared to be, in the time frame we saw, resistant to macrophage lysis. Do you feel that it was in fact resistant to macrophage kill?

M. Hanna

No, it started to undergo the same kind of events that we see that often proceed to lysis. I think that this is what you would expect. They don't sit there passively and expect to be killed. They try to repair their surfaces. Some make it and survive; others don't.

R. Herberman

Mike, about this generalization that has been around for a long time, that all tumor cells are susceptible and perhaps equally susceptible to killing by macrophages. This doesn't fit too well with some experiments by Robert Wiltrout in my laboratory, looking at a series of suspension target cells. He could see about 100-fold difference in susceptibility to killing of some of the tumor targets compared to others.

M. Hanna

Are you talking about quantitative or qualitative differences?

R. Herberman

Large quantitative differences.

M. Hanna

We didn't say there aren't quantitative differences. We're just saying with activated macrophages we can get killing. We didn't say that it's always ten-to-one for all tumor cells. In some cases you have to go as high as 100-to-one but they will always recognize and kill, and a number of people have done this. It's very interesting that you can take a population of activated macrophages and plate them on a variety of different tumor cell lines and kill the majority of them with the same macrophage population. That's not true for T lymphocytes. The only point I want to make is that there does seem to be a tumor cell susceptibility and it doesn't have the kind of exquisite specificity that we've learned to expect for T cells, and I think that's very interesting.

R. Herberman

Well, I'd like to pursue this a little bit more. In terms of the relative selectivity of activated macrophages versus NK cells, my impression is that they are about comparable. Clearly, there's not as much selectivity as one sees with CTL but I think that's for obvious reasons.

A further point, perhaps suggesting some selectivity of the interaction of macrophages with tumor targets - Bob Wiltrout has been doing some experiments recently, examining the possible inhibiting effects of simple sugars on cytotoxicity against about five or six different tumor targets. He finds that the patterns of inhibition of the sugars varies with each of the different tumor targets that are being used. For example, with one target mannose may be very efficient but for another target mannose might not be inhibitory.

M. Hanna

And what does that mean to you?

R. Herberman

It suggests that things are not just so black and white in terms of one non-specific mechanism by which macrophages can recognize all tumor target cells. Rather there may, in fact, be some kind of specific receptor interaction. The other thing that I'm concerned about is just how conclusive the evidence is for this inability of the macrophage to interact or kill normal targets? There's been some controversy in the literature about the killing of 3T3.

M. Hanna

You go to 1,000-to-one, you can get some normal target killing. If you go high enough you can deprive the medium and you can do a lot of things. Again, it's not absolute. But you have to go very high to get normal cell killing.

R. Herberman

With human monocytes at least, with some short-term cultures of normal fibroblasts even at 50-to-1 you can show low levels of cytolysis of untransformed fibroblasts. This susceptibility is clearly less than that of the transformed partner, but that is most likely a quantitative difference.

M. Hanna

Clearly. And that's the important point. And what I described here could very well happen to normal targets. That's an important point. But the point is, it doesn't.

D. Zagury

Regarding comparison with the model we used with T lymphocytes, if I understood we have absolute analogy of results. Both involve lysosomal granules. The differences occur at the level of the number of effectors needed to lyse one target, because with CTL we are working one-to-one. I guess you're working at hundred-to-one.

M. Hanna

Yes, there appears to be some similarity in our morphologic studies. I've never seen one-to-one effective in the microscope. I've spent a lot of time looking.

D. Zagury

I appreciate also that you point out the concept of tumor cell susceptibility in order to get lysis. Do you have other comparative comments on those two systems? CTL and macrophage?

M. Hanna

I hadn't really thought about it. The first evidence I had seen of T cell killing, where someone indicated that it could be lysosomal organelles being translocated, was what I saw in your film last night. I'm sure others have postulated this. I just don't remember seeing this. I'm really surprised that T cells would use that mechanism. I thought they'd be much more sophisticated.

G. Berke

Just to give the other side of the coin, I think there isn't a consensus that T cells kill by means of lysosomes...

M. Hanna

I'm absolutely sure of that, but I'd never heard it presented. It would be interesting if some of them can. I think that what Zagury showed last night was that T cells have lysosomes in them. I think what we need to do is to show that those things actually do move into the other cells.

ACTIVATED MACROPHAGE MEDIATED CYTOTOXICITY FOR TRANSFORMED TARGET CELLS

John B. Hibbs, Jr.[1], Donald L. Granger[2], James L. Cook[3], and Andrew M. Lewis, Jr.[4]

[1]Veterans Administration Medical Center and
Department of Medicine, Division of Infectious Diseases
University of Utah School of Medicine
Salt Lake City, UT 84148

[2]Department of Physiological Chemistry
Johns Hopkins University
School of Medicine
Baltimore, MD 21205

[3]National Jewish Hospital and Research Center
3800 East Colfax Avenue
Denver, CO 80206

[4]National Institute of Allergy and Infectious Diseases
National Institutes of Health
Bethesda, MD 20205

INTRODUCTION

The biochemical mechanisms that induce target cell lysis in cell mediated cytotoxicity systems--cytotoxic T-lymphocytes, natural killer cells, natural cytotoxicity cells, antibody dependent cell mediated cytotoxicity systems, and cytotoxic activated macrophages--are unknown. Identification of the biochemical effector mechanism(s) utilized by activated macrophages to induce stasis and lysis of transformed target cells is complicated by the large armamentarium of potential cytotoxic effector molecules that can be elaborated by macrophages. Evidence of activated macrophage mediated target cell cytotoxicity-cytostasis and cytolysis--has been observed and documented most extensively with techniques suitable for analysis of biologic phenomena at the cellular level. Observation at the cellular level has not provided evidence that demonstrates, in a definitive way, which potential effector molecules, among the many elaborated by macrophages, are relevant to the destruction of nucleated mammalian cells or to control of abnormal proliferation of mammalian cells in vivo.

Cytostatis and cytolysis develop slowly following contact of transformed target cells with activated macophages (1-3). This provides an opportunity to examine biochemical perturbations that are the cause of activated macrophage induced target cell cytostatis and cytolysis. Studies have documented that cytotoxic activated macrophages cause inhibition of DNA replication and cell division (4-6). In addition, the activated macrophage cytotoxic mechanism deprives transformed target cells of mitochondrial respiration, the metabolic pathway which is the most efficient source of ATP and a major regulator of intracellular redox balance (1). Cytotoxic activated macrophages caused inhibition of DNA replication and inhibition of mitochondrial respiration in all transformed cell targets of activated macrophages that we have tested in vitro. Identification of the pattern of activated macrophage induced metabolic perturbation in transformed target cells is of interest because of its relevance to the general problem of control of cell proliferation. Furthermore, as elucidation of the pattern of activated macrophage induced metabolic perturbation progresses, it should become more obvious which of the many potential effector molecules elaborated by macrophages are causally related to the development of target cell cytostasis and cytolysis.

CYTOTOXIC ACTIVATED MACROPHAGES INHIBIT METABOLIC PATHWAYS IN THE NUCLEUS OF TRANSFORMED TARGET CELLS

Cytotoxic activated macrophages inhibit proliferation and can cause eventual destruction of a wide variety of target cells (1-6). In parallel with inhibition of proliferation, there is, in a population of unsynchronized target cells, inhibition of DNA synthesis (3-6). Krahenbuhl, using EMT-6 adenosarcoma target cells synchronized in discrete phases of the cell cycle, showed that inhibition of DNA synthesis is not an obligatory prerequisite for inhibition of proliferation (6). He showed that when activated macrophages were added to EMT-6 cells synchronized in the late S of G2 phase, many of the target cells which had already completed DNA replication failed to undergo mitosis and cytokinesis. Regardless of the region of the cell cycle in which synchronized EMT-6 cells were at the time of contact with cytotoxic activated macrophages, the proliferation of the target cells was blocked. Synchronized EMT-6 cells continued forward through the cell cycle for 2-6 hours after contact with cytotoxic activated macrophages and then further progression ceased. Kaplan et al. have provided further evidence of dysfunction within the nucleus of transformed cells cocultivated with cytotoxic activated macrophages (7). Using the technique of microfluorometry, these investigators showed that Lewis lung carcinoma cells, in contact with activated macrophages, undergo one round of cytokinesis in the absence of DNA replication ("reductive" cell division) before progressing to eventual lysis.

It has been documented that cytotoxic activated macrophage induced cytostasis of certain transformed target cells can be long lasting. Cytotoxic activated macrophages harvested from the peritoneal cavity of mice with chronic Mycobacterium bovis (strain BCG) infection induce prolonged cytostasis of murine lymphoma target cells (L1210 cells) that have been removed from the macrophage monolayer and resuspended in fresh culture medium (see Figure 1). To show this, L1210 cells, which are non-adherent cells, were removed from cytotoxic activated macrophages after 40 hours of cocultivation, washed 3X and then suspended in fresh medium for a second incubation. Figure 2A shows that L1210 cells that had been cocultivated with cytotoxic activated macrophages failed to divide for an additional 50 hours despite removal from activated macrophages and addition of fresh growth factors. Hence, cytotoxic activated macrophage-induced inhibition of L1210 cell proliferation persists for many hours beyond the time of removal from contact with activated macrophages (1). Although replication is suppressed, L1210 cells maintain almost complete viability for 90 hours as assessed by trypan blue exclusion. Taken together, these results suggest that cytotoxic activated macrophages, in a dramatic way, are capable of having a prolonged effect on metabolic pathways functioning in the nucleus of transformed target cells.

EVIDENCE THAT CYTOTOXIC ACTIVATED MACROPHAGES CAUSE PERTURBATION OF ENERGY HOMEOSTASIS IN MURINE L1210 LEUKEMIA CELLS

The nucleus is not the only targt cell organelle whose function is affected by cytotoxic activated macrophages. They cause equally dramatic inhibiton of mitochondrial respiration in transformed target cells (1). Indeed, thus far, cytotoxic activated macrophage-induced inhibition of mitochondrial respiration has occurred without exception in all transformed cells we have tested. Inhibition of O_2 consumption occurred regardless of species, tissue of origin, or whether the transformation event was spontaneous, induced by radiation, by a chemical carcinogen, or by an oncogenic virus. It is of interest that the pattern of organelle dysfunction (inhibition of DNA replicaiton within the nucleus and inhibition of mitochondrial respiration) induced by cytotoxic activated macrophages in transformed target cells is so constant in all target cells we have tested and from experiment to experiment.

Non-adherent L1210 cells were used to study bioenergetic changes that occur in neoplastic cells after prolonged cocultivation with cytotoxic activated macrophages harvested from the peritoneal

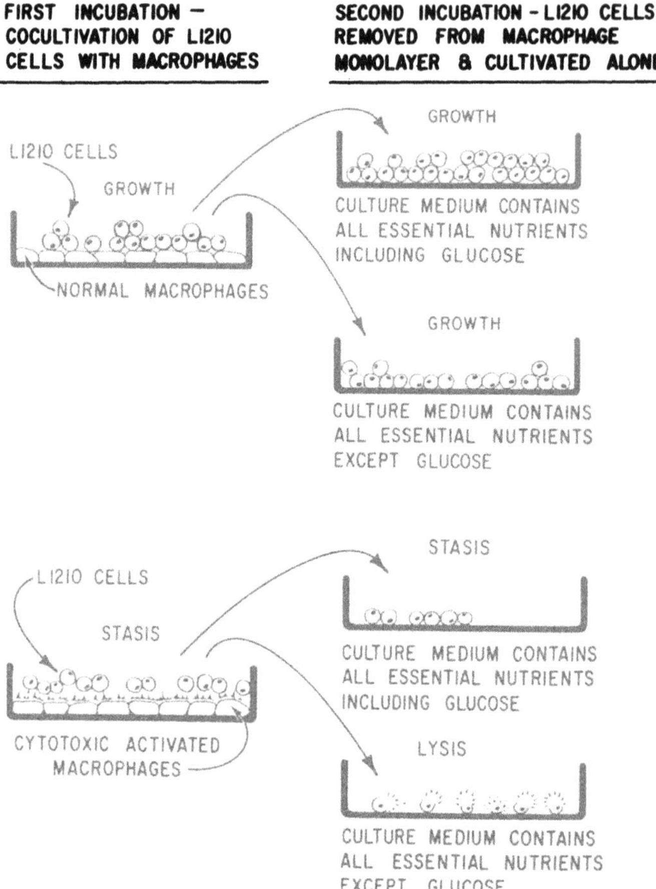

Fig. 1. Diagrammatic representation of the two-step in vitro culture system used to study energy metabolism in transformed target cells of cytotoxic activated macrophages. The scheme shows the glucose requirement for survival of transformed cells with the nonlytic phenotype (L1210 cells) after a period of co-cultivation with cytotoxic activated macrophages. L1210 cells do not develop a similar requirement for glucose after a period of co-cultivation with normal macrophages. See reference 1 for experimental details.

cavity of mice with chronic BCG infection. L1210 cells are highly tumorigenic *in vivo* (<10 cells are lethal for syngeneic mice (8) and L1210 cell grafts are refractory to manipulations that increase nonspecific resistance and long term survival to neoplasia *in vivo* (9). In addition, L1210 cells do not adhere to the substrate when they are grown *in vitro*, and this property was exploited in studies designed to examine metabolic perturbations that occur in transformed

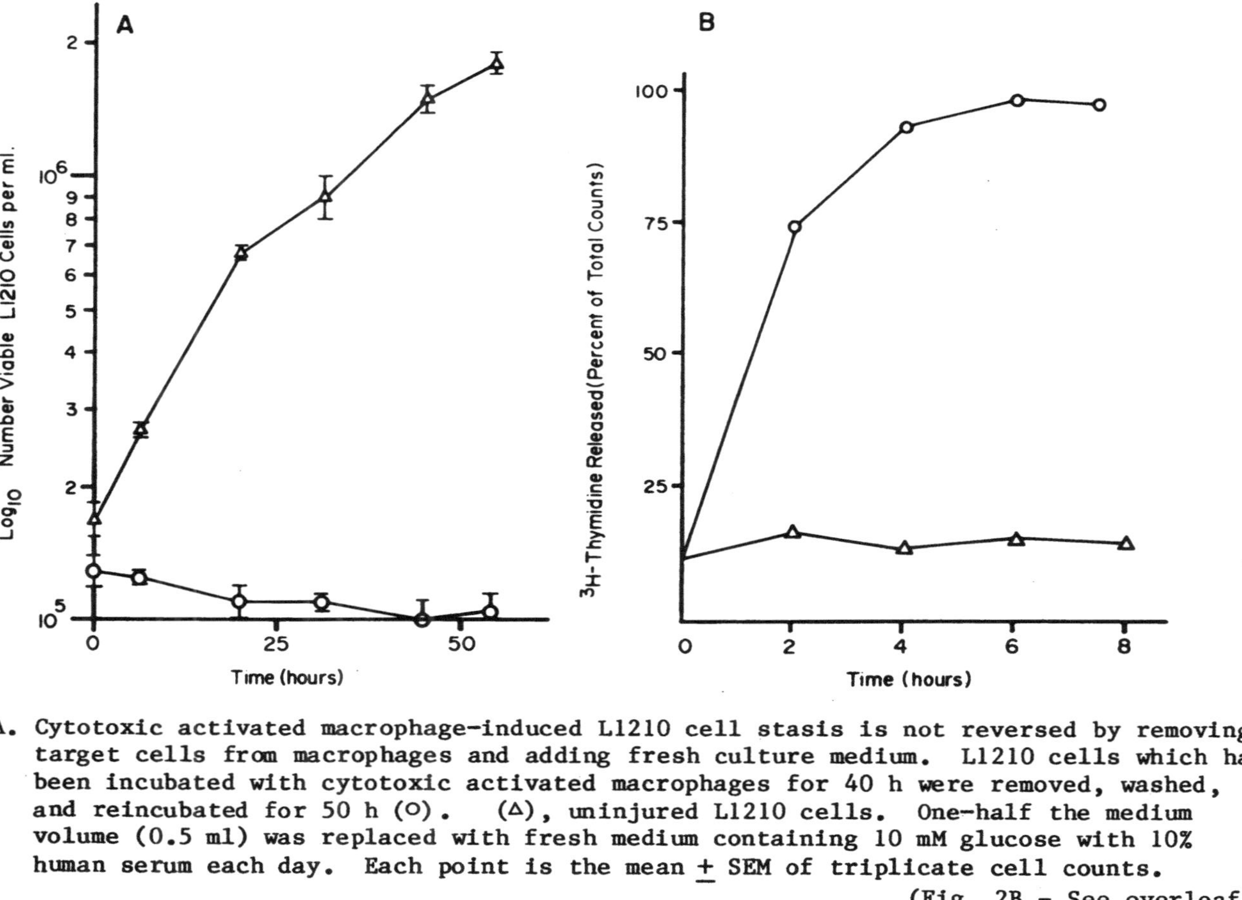

Fig. 2A. Cytotoxic activated macrophage-induced L1210 cell stasis is not reversed by removing target cells from macrophages and adding fresh culture medium. L1210 cells which had been incubated with cytotoxic activated macrophages for 40 h were removed, washed, and reincubated for 50 h (○). (Δ), uninjured L1210 cells. One-half the medium volume (0.5 ml) was replaced with fresh medium containing 10 mM glucose with 10% human serum each day. Each point is the mean ± SEM of triplicate cell counts.

(Fig. 2B - See overleaf)

Fig. 2B. Cytotoxic activated macrophage-injured L1210 cells require glucose to remain viable. Cytotoxic activated macrophage-injured L1210 cells incubated with culture medium minus glucose (○) or culture medium containing 10 mM glucose (Δ).

See reference 1 for experimental details (adapted from reference, with permission of the publisher).

---

cells after a period of contact with activated macrophages (see Figure 1). Because L1210 cells are in contact with but not strongly adherent to macrophage monolayers, they can be removed from the macrophage monolayer after a period of cocultivation by gentle washing. They can then be washed, resuspended in fresh culture medium and added to another tissue culture chamber for a second incubation. At this time, and free from the cytotoxic activated macrophage effector cells, biochemical changes that occur as a result of contact with activated macrophages can be measured. Since the results of these experiments show that cytotoxic activated macrophages cause a profound perturbation of energy metabolism in transformed target cells, cellular energy metabolism under conditions in which molecular oxygen can and cannot be used as the terminal electron acceptor is summarized in Figure 3 (10).

L1210 cells were incubated with cytotoxic activated macrophages for 24 hours with a nonlimiting glucose supply (20 mM under conditions of the assay). After the first incubation, L1210 cells were removed from activated macrophages and reincubated in the absence of macrophages (second incubation) in a culture medium with or without glucose (1). Cytotoxic activated macrophage-injured L1210 cells died within six hours when glucose was omitted from the culture medium of the second incubation (Figures 1 and 2B). As little as 0.25 mM glucose prevented lysis for six hours. Of numerous saccharides tested, only the sugars capable of supporting glycolysis, D-glucose (5 or 50 mM), D-mannose (5 or 50 mM), and fructose (50 mM) prevented lysis of cytotoxic activated macrophage-injured L1210 cells during the second incubation period. If glycolysis was inhibited by 2-deoxy-D-glucose (20 mM inhibitor; 2 mM substrate), cytotoxic activated macrophage-injured L1210 cells died in the presence of glucose or mannose. Substrates for mitochondrial oxidative phosphorylation, pyruvate and glycerol (up to 50 mM each), did not prevent lysis of cytotoxic activated macrophage-injured L1210 cells. Control L1210 cells maintain viability in culture medium without glucose or with 2-deoxy-D-glucose. Thus, cytotoxic activated macrophage-injured L1210 cells require a sugar capable of maintaining glycolysis to remain viable (1).

Dependence on glycolysis for energy production could occur if cytotoxic activated macrophages interfered with mitochondrial oxidative phosphorylation. This was tested by measuring oxygen consumption of L1210 cells removed from activated macrophages after a 24-40 hour period of cocultivation (Table 1). Endogenous respiration of cytotoxic activated macrophage-injured L1210 cells was consistently decreased six to seven-fold compared to control cells (1). This effect did not occur following cocultivation of L1210 cells with macrophages that had not differentiated to the cytotoxic activated stage. Decreased O_2 consumption of cytotoxic activated macrophage-injured L1210 cells was not due to cell death because cell viability was > 90%. Cytotoxic activated macrophage-induced inhibition of O_2 consumption reflects L1210 cell mitochondrial dysfunction because the bulk of O_2 consumed by uninjured L1210 cells was inhibited by either antimycin A or oligomycin (Table 2). Antimycin A inhibits mitochondrial electron transport at the level of cytochrome b-c_1 (11) and oligomycin acts on the mitochondrial ATP synthetase complex (12). The degree of inhibition by cytotoxic activated macrophages (85%) was almost the same as maximal inhibition by oligomycin (87%). If activated macrophages selectively inhibit mitochondrial respiration in L1210 target cells, the prediction would be that they would lose their Pasteur effect (depression of glycolysis upon exposure of anaerobically cultured cells to O_2) and exhibit an inappropriately high rate of glycolysis with O_2 present. Glycolytic rates of cytotoxic activated macrophage-injured L1210 cells conform to this pattern (1). These findings provide an explanation for the death-preventing effect of glucose on cytotoxic activated macrophage-injured L1210 cells. Because activated macrophages caused almost complete inhibition of L1210 respiration, and hence mitochondrial ATP production, injured L1210 cells become dependent on glycolysis for chemical energy production.

Therefore, for L1210 cells, complete inhibition of proliferation and mitochondrial respiration is not a lethal event (1,13). Indeed, transformed cells with the nonlytic phenotype, such as L1210 cells recover from cytotoxic activated macrophage-induced inhibition of DNA replication and inhibition of mitochondrial respiration and begin proliferating at their characteristic rate (13).

THERE ARE AT LEAST TWO TRANSFORMED CELL PHENOTYPIC RESPONSES TO CYTOTOXIC ACTIVATED MACROPAHGES

An intriguing pattern of target cell susceptibility has emerged from these studies. There are at least two target cell phenotypic responses to activated macrophage-induced metabolic perturbation: stasis without progression to lysis (L1210 cells are an example of the nonlytic phenotype) and stasis followed by lysis (P815 murine mastocytoma cells are an example of the lytic phenotype). As described above, L1210 cells do not die following activated macrophage-induced inhibition of mitochondrial respiration. They undergo a prolonged period of cytostasis but remain viable as long as the culture medium contains glucose or another sugar capable of support-

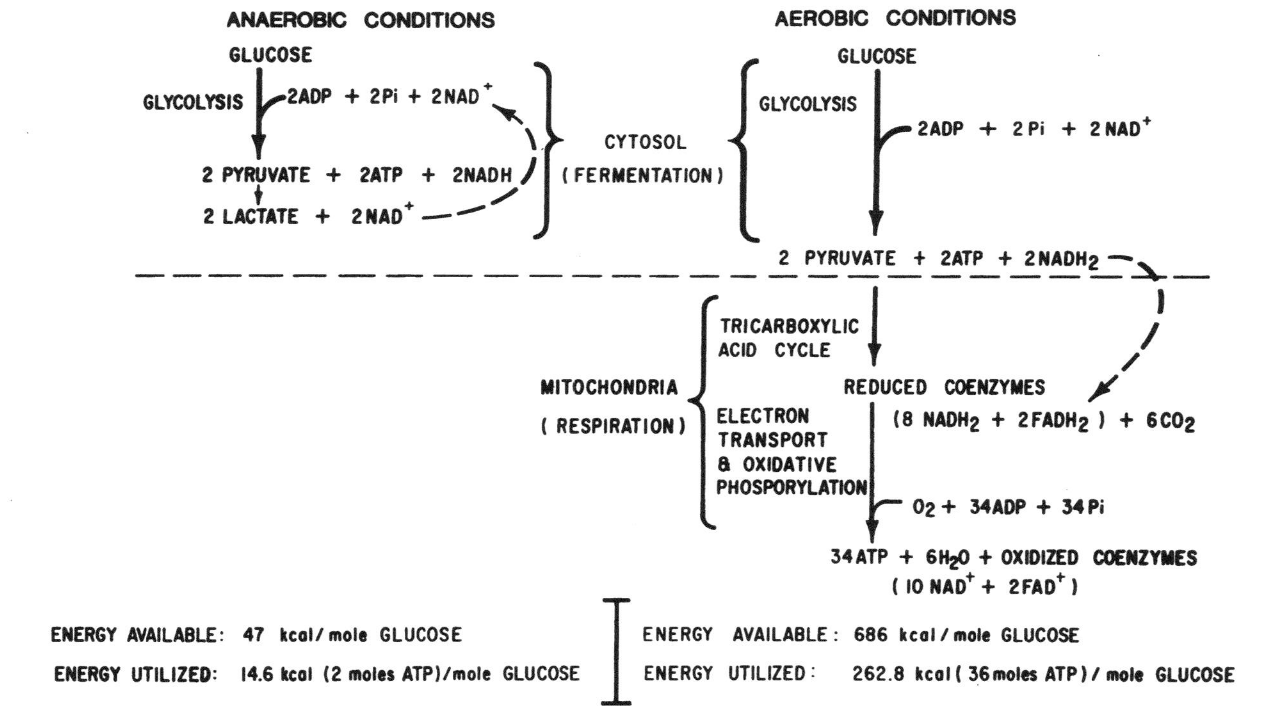

Fig. 3. Cellular energy production when oxygen can and cannot be used as a terminal electron acceptor. Maximal energy yields from oxidizable organic substrates, including glucose, are realized only when oxygen is the terminal electron acceptor (10). When oxygen is not available as the terminal electron acceptor, all ATP required to maintain cellular metabolism must be produced by the relatively inefficient glycolytic pathway which can anaerobically mobilize the free energy intrinsic to the chemical bonds of glucose. Under anaerobic conditions, or when oxygen cannot be used as a terminal electron acceptor, glucose or sugars that can be readily converted to glucose, must be present in the environment or glycolysis ceases and cell death ensues.

Fig. 3 (cont.) However, when oxygen is present and can be utilized as an electron acceptor, the glycolytic breakdown of glucose, which occurs in the cytoplasm, is merely a preparatory step for further catabolism of pyruvate to CO_2 and H_2O. This occurs in the mitochondrial compartment by the combined activities of the tricarboxylic acid cycle and the electron transport chain. These two mitochondrial pathways couple the complete aerobic oxidation of glucose to the phosphorylation of ADP to ATP. The efficient utilization of the free energy intrinsic to the glucose molecule via conversion to pyruvate and subsequent mitochondrial oxidative phosphorylation (respiration) produces 36 moles ATP/mole glucose while the relatively inefficient production of ATP via glycolysis yields only two moles ATP/mole glucose.

---

ing glycolysis. Unlike L1210 cells, however, P815 cells that have been cocultivated with cytotoxic activated macrophages, after an initial period of cytostasis, progress to lysis even in culture medium containing an adequate supply of glucose. It was important to document that similar inhibiton of cellular proliferation and changes in cellular energy homeostasis occur in both the lytic and nonlytic transformed cell phenotypes. To do this we examined, after a period of cocultivation with cytotoxic activated macrophages, the rate of cellular proliferation, whether or not significant cell death occurred O_2 consumption, and lactate production in L1210 cells with the nonlytic phenotype and in P815 cells with the lytic phenotype (Granger, D.L., and J.B. Hibbs, Jr., unpublished observations).

When compared to control cells endogenous respiration of both L1210 and P815 cells was decreased after removal from cytotoxic activated macrophages (Table 2). This effect depended on contact with activated macrophages. It did not occur following cocultivation with peptone stimulated normal macrophages. Trypan blue cell counts were made following all respiration measurements. Decreased O_2 consumption of L1210 and P815 cells that had been cocultivated with cytotoxic activated macrophages was not due to cell death since there was always > 90% viability at the completion of the oxygen consumption measurements. By 10 hours, P815 cell death had begun to occur; however, most cells were still viable. Twenty hour measurements were not made on P815 cells because most of the cells had lysed.

Glycolysis rates were also determined for the nonlytic transformed cell phenotype (L1210 cells) and the lytic transformed cell phenotype (P815 cells)(Table 3). Both L1210 and P815 cells had increased aerobic glycolysis following a period of cocultivation with cytotoxic activated macrophages when compared to control cells, and the Pasteur effect was absent. Although L1210 cells achieve a greater glycolytic rate compared to P815 cells following cocülti-

TABLE 1. Endogenous Respiration of Cytotoxic Activated Macrophage-injured L1210 Cells

No. of Experiments	L_{1210} cells cultured with:[a]	O_2 Consumption[b]
		µl·h·10^6 cells
6	Alone	7.4 ± 0.3
4	Alone + ET (200 ng/ml)	7.2 ± 0.4
2	Aloe + MAF (10% vol/vol)	7.2 ± 0.9
4	SM	6.9 ± 0.7
6	CM	1.1 ± 0.1
2	CM (MAF)	1.7 ± 0.4
3	Alone (oligomycin inhibited)[c]	0.9 ± 0.1
3	Alone (antimycin A inhibited)[c]	0.3 ± 0.1

[a] For these experiments, L1210 cells were cultured alone or with macrophages for 24-40 h before respiration measurements. Cytotoxic activated macrophages (CM), peritoneal macrophages from mice infected intraperitoneally with 0.2 mg Mycobacterium bovis, strain BCG, 17-22 d before harvest and injected with 1 ml of 10% protease peptone 3 d before harvest. Final differentiation stimulus was provided by 20-200 ng ml^{-1} endotoxin. CM (MAF), same as CM except that the final differentiation stimulus was provided by a lymphokine preparation with macrophage activating factor activity. SM, peritoneal macrophages from normal mice injected intraperitoneally with 1 ml 10% protease peptone 3 d before harvest.

[b] Values are the mean ± SEM for the number of experiments shown.

[c] The effects of oligomycin and antimycin A were determined by injection into the respiration vessel to a final concentration of 0.1 and 0.01 µM, respectively. Previous experiments showed that these concentrations produced maximal inhibition of uninjured L1210 cell respiration at 2 x 10^6 cells/ml. See reference 9 for experimental details.

(Adapted from reference 1, with permission of the publisher.)

vation with cytotoxic activated macrophages, the difference is small and the percent increase of glycolytic rate in P815 cells (ca. 70%) is greater than the percent increase of glycolytic rate in L1210 cells (ca. 50%). The results of these experiments do not explain why P815 cells die and L1210 cells do not die following a period of cocultivation with cytotoxic activated macrophages. It is possible

TABLE 2. Endogenous and uncoupled respiration of L1210 and P815 cells that have been co-cultivated with cytotoxic activated macrophages

Cell line	Time of co-cultivation with activated macrophages (endotoxin) prior to respiration measurement (hours)[a]	Oxygen consumption (μl O_2 per hour per 10^6 cells)[a] endogenous
L1210	0	7.2 ± 0.5
	10	3.8 ± 0.3
	20	1.0 ± 0.2
P815	0	5.9 ± 0.3
	10	2.0 ± 0.5

[a] See footnote [a] and [b]Table 1.

(D.L. Granger and J.B. Hibbs, Jr., unpublished data.)

that P815 cells utilize their glycolytically-produced ATP less efficiently than L1210 cells and hence, are unable to survive once inhibition of mitochondrial respiration has occurred. It is also possible that cytotoxic activated macrophage-mediated cytolysis of P815 cells occurs as a result of inhibition of other metabolic pathways not measured in these studies.

These experiments show there are two transformed cell phenotypic responses to metabolic perturbations induced by cytotoxic activated macrophages. The nonlytic transformed cell phenotype (L1210 cells) responds to cocultivation with cytotoxic activated macrophages by prolonged cytostasis but does not die as long as the culture medium contains glucose or other sugars supporting glycolysis. On the other hand, the lytic transformed cell phenotype (P815 cells) responds to cocultivation with cytotoxic activated macrophages by initial cytostasis followed by cytolysis even in culture medium containing an adequate supply of glucose.

An important point made by these experiments is that the pattern of metablic changes seen in both the nonlytic and lytic transformed cell phenotypes following a period of cocultivation with cytotoxic activated macrophages is similar. The results show a pattern of metabolic dysfunction in both transformed cell phenotypes that does not appear to be random and indiscriminate but which, in a reproducible fashion, causes complete inhibition of certain metabolic pathways (i.e., DNA replication and mitochondrial respiration) while apparently sparing other metabolic pathways (i.e., glycolysis).

EVIDENCE THAT THE NONLYTIC TRANSFORMED CELL PHENOTYPE MAY BE A MARKER FOR INCREASED TUMORIGENIC VIRULENCE

Evidence exists that suggests expression of the nonlytic transformed cell phenotype confers increased resistance to host mediated antineoplastic surveillance. This correlation was possible because of the availability of a series of cells transformed by oncogenic DNA viruses (SV40 and adenovirus 2) whose *in vivo* biology was being studied by Lewis and Cook. They observed that SV40-transformed inbred LSH hamster cells grafted in histoincompatible adult CB hamsters induced tumors almost as efficiently as in syngeneic animals (14).

Efforts to induce tumors in mice, rats, guinea pigs, rabbits, and primates by inoculating SV40 subcutaneously has been unsuccessful. Although not causing tumors when injected *in vivo*, SV40 does transform cells from these species growing in tissue culture. The hamster is the exception to the rule that SV40 is nontumorigenic (15). SV40 inoculated subcutaneously into newborn hamsters induces tumors after a latent period of three to nine months. Likewise, hamster cells transformed *in vitro* by SV40 are highly tumorigenic when transplanted into adult syngeneic immunocompetent hosts. In fact, in sharp contrast to the other species the tumorigenic potential of SV40 transformed hamster cells is quite remarkable. SV40-transformed inbred LSH hamster cells grafted in histoincompatible adult CB hamsters induced tumors almost as efficiently as in syngeneic animals (14). It should be mentioned parenthetically that the immunocompetence of the hamster has been found to be equivalent to that of other species when carefully evaluated (16). Therefore, the evidence is that in the hamster, SV40 infection, either *in vitro* or *in vivo*, produces transformed cells with increased tumorigenic potential or "virulence" when compared to *in vitro* or *in vivo* SV40 induced transformation events in other species. The point for emphasis is that cells from species such as the mouse and rat possess *in vitro* abnormal growth characteristics of transformed cells after infection with SV40 and yet are not tumorigenic in syngeneic immunocompetent adult animals. SV40 transformed hamster cells have the same abnormal *in vitro* growth characteristics as SV40 transformed cells from other rodent species but in addition have high tumorigenic potential.

Recent experiments show that mouse and hamster peritonal activated macrophages were cytolytic for nontumorigenic SV40 transformed mouse and rat cells (17). However, the highly tumorigenic SV40-

TABLE 3. Aerobic and anaerobic glycolysis of L1210 and P815 cells that have been co-cultivated with cytotoxic activated macrophages

Cell line	Culture environment prior to glycolysis measurement[a]	Lactate produced (μmoles per hour per 10^5 cells)[b] aerobic	anaerobic
L1210	Medium alone	33 $\pm$ 5	91 $\pm$ 8
	Medium + activated macrophages	65 $\pm$ 6	65 $\pm$ 4
P815	Medium alone	17 $\pm$ 2	42 $\pm$ 4
	Medium + activated macrophages	54 $\pm$ 10	47 $\pm$ 10

[a] See footnote [a] Table 1. L1210 cells were co-cultivated alone or with activated macrophages for 20 hours, and P815 cells, with activated macrophages for 10 hours, prior to removal. Removed target cells were washed three times with medium without serum prior to glycolysis incubation.

[b] See reference 1 for experimental details.

(D.L. Granger and J.B. Hibbs, Jr., unpublished data.)

transformed hamster fibroblasts, as defined by their ability to grow in allogeneic animals, were relatively resistant to the cytolytic effect of cytotoxic activated macrophages (17). These experiments demonstrate that SV40-transformed hamster fibroblasts have the same phenotypic response to the activated macrophage induced cytotoxic effect as another highly malignant cell, the L1210 mouse lymphoma which include (i) resistance to the lytic injury induced in neoplastic target cells by activated macrophages; (ii) susceptibility to a reversible cytostasis that persists for a variable period of time (48-120 hours) before cell proliferation resumes; (iii) respiration is markedly reduced making them dependent on glycolysis for ATP generation. These experiments show that four different lines of SV40 transformed hamster cells (SV40HE1, SV40HE2, SV4HE3, and THK-1t) which have enhanced malignancy as demonstrated by the capability of growing progressively in allogeneic hosts, in addition, have the nonlytic response to cytotoxic activated macrophage induced injury (see Table 4).

TABLE 4. Tumor-inducing capacity and response to cocultivation with cytotoxic activated macrophages of virus-transformed rodent cells

Cell line	Species, strain of origin	Cells (log)/TPD_{50}*: Host of origin	Histoincompatible host (strain)†	Response to cocultivation with cytotoxic activated macrophages: cytostasis	cytolysis
TCMK-1	Mouse, C3H/Mai	> 8.5		+	+
SV40RE1	Rat, Sprague-Dawley	> 8.5		+	+
SV40RE2	Rat, Sprague-Dawley	> 8.5		+	+
SV40HE1	Hamster, LSH	4.2	5.0 (CB)	+	0
SV40HE2	Hamster, LSH	3.6	5.5 (CB)	+	0
SV40HE3	Hamster, LSH	3.5	3.5 (CB)	+	0
$THK-1_t$	Hamster, LSH	< 2.5	< 2.5 (CB)	+	0
Ad2HE7	Hamster, LSH	> 8.5		+	+
Ad2HTL3-1	Hamster, LSH	4.1	> 7.5 (CB)	+	+

* Cells (log)/TPD_{50}, logarithm of number of tissue culture cells required to produce subcutaneous tumors in 50% of the surviving adult animals. TPD, tumor producing dose. $TPD_{50} > 8.5$ = no tumors developed during a 3-month observation period after subcutaneous challenge with 10^8 tissue culture cells. For tumor challenge procedure, see reference 17.

† The inbred CB strain of hamster differs from the LSH strain at a major histoincompatibility locus.

Adapted from reference 17.

It is important to emphasize that the nonlytic transformed phenotype appears to be a marker for enhanced tumorigenicity and not tumorigenicity per se. Transformed but nontumorigenic target cells or transformed cells of low tumorigenicity are highly sensitive to lysis induced by cytotoxic activated macrophages. Examples include TCMK, SV40RE1, SV40RE2, and Ad2HE7 cells (see Table 4). However, other transformed cells that are clearly tumorigenic in adult syngeneic immunocompetent animals also have the lytic phenotype, i.e., respond to activated macrophage-induced inhibition of proliferation and inhibition of mitochondrial respiration by lysis in culture medium containing an adequate supply of glucose (1,17). Examples include a line of Ad2-transformed hamster cells (Ad2HTL3-1), a diethylnitrosamine induced guinea pig hepatoma (L10) and the mouse mastocytoma (P815). Ad2HTL3-1 cells, although tumorigenic in syngeneic adult hamsters, are nontumorigenic in allogeneic hamsters (Table 4). The guinea pig L10 hepatoma, a lytic transformed cell phenotype, is responsive to BCG stimulated nonspecific active immunotherapy. In fact, the guinea pig - L10 system is the classic immunotherapy model used by Zbar, Rapp, and their colleagues to define many of the basic principles of nonspecific active immunotherapy (18). Therefore, these experiments suggest that expression of the nonlytic phenotype may be a marker for increased *in vivo* virulence of transformed cells, i.e., an increased ability to resist destruction by the host cell-mediated response to neoplastic cells.

CONCLUSION

The organizers of the workshop asked that we give a speculative view concerning the possible mechanism of the activated macrophage cytotoxic reaction. Our thinking and the direction of our experimental work has been influenced by the hypothesis that activated macrophage-induced cytotoxicity is related to tissue destruction that occurs during normal embryonic and normal post-embryonic growth and development in metazoans (19-21). We believe it is possible that the highly reproducible pattern of metabolic inhibition that is induced in transformed target cells by activated macrophages will be similar to a yet undefined pattern of metabolic inhibition that may occur in certain types of programmed cell destruction during normal growth and development.

Although the actual molecular effectors of activated macrophage induced cytostasis and cytolysis are not known, an effector mechanism with sufficient specificity to reproducibly inhibit certain metabolic pathways while sparing other metabolic pathways must be seriously considered. We demonstrated earlier that material sequestered in the vacuolar system of cytotoxic activated macrophages was translocated to the cytoplasm of transformed target cells (21). Bucana et al. also showed transfer of material from macrophage cytoplasmic vesicles, with characteristics of lysosomes, to the cytoplasm of tumor target cells using the combined techniques of cinemicrography, scanning electron microscopy, and transmission electron microscopy (22, and see chapter in this volume by M.G. Hanna). The cause and effect relationship between the observations reported in these studies and development of target cell cytotoxicity is difficult to interpret. However, the macrophage vacuolar system contains proteinases with a high degree of substrate specificity (23). Adams has provided evidence that activated macrophages secrete a proteinase, of unknown substrate specificity, capable of producing lysis of transformed cells. Effector proteinases derived from cytoplasmic vesicles of activated macrophages and with acid or neutral pH optima as well as with relatively limited substrate specificity could cause a reproducible pattern of selective and potentially reversible target cell metabolic inhibition.

It also seems possible to us that there may be more underlying similarity and unity to the molecular mechanisms of the different effectors of cell-mediated cytotoxicity than may be apparent at present. For example, the expression of cytotoxicity by activated macrophages, cytotoxic T-lymphocytes, and NK cells is inhibited by tosyl-lysyl-chloromethylketone (25,26 and see chapter by Ron Goldfarb, this workshop). Trypan blue inhibits cytotoxic activated macrophages and cytotoxic T-lymphocytes (21,27). In addition, close contact between effector cells and target cells is critical for the expression of cell-mediated cytotoxicity under usual *in vitro* assay conditions in all systems. There is also circumstantial evidence that lysosomal enzymes could be the final effectors of NK mediated target cell lysis (28).

The involvement of lysosomal enzymes, even in a partial role, in the activated macrophage cytotoxic effector mechanism causing cytostasis and cytolysis of nucleated mammalian cells remains speculation at the present time. It will be important for future experiments to elucidate the molecular basis of the activated macrophage effector mechanism and determine similarities and differences with other cell-mediated cytotoxicity systems.

ACKNOWLEDGEMENTS

We are grateful to Gwenevere Shaw for typing the manuscript. Supported by the Veterans Administration, Washington, D.C., and American Cancer Society Grant CH-139.

REFERENCES

1. Granger, D.L., Taintor, R.R., Cook, J.L., and J.B. Hibbs, Jr. Injury of neoplatic cells by murine macrophages leads to inhibition of mitochondrial respiration. J. Clin. Invest. 65:357 (1980).
2. Hibbs, J.B., Jr., Lambert, L.H., Jr., and J.S. Remington. Control of carcinogenesis: A possible role for the activated macrophage. Science 177:998 (1972).
3. Meltzer, M.S., Tucker, R.W., and A.C. Breur. Interaction of BCG-activated macrophages with neoplastic and nonneoplastic cell lines - in vitro: Cinemicrographic analysis. Cell. Immunol. 17:30 (1975).
4. Keller, R. Cytostatic elimination of syngeneic rat tumor cells in vitro by nonspecifically activated macrophages. J. Exp. Med. 138:625 (1973).
5. Krahenbuhl, J.L., and J.S. Remington. The role of activated marcophages in specific and nonspecific cytostasis of tumor cells. J. Immunol. 113:507 (1974).
6. Krahenbuhl, J.L. Effects of activated macrophages of tumor target cells in discrete phases of the cell cycle. Cancer Res. 40:4622 (1980).
7. Kaplan, A.M., Brown, J., Collins, J.M., Morahan, P.S., and M.J. Snodgrass. Mechanism of macrophage-mediated tumor cell cytotoxicity. J. Immunol. 121:1781 (1978).
8. Skipper, H.E., Schabel, F.M., Jr., and W.S. Wilcox. Experimental evaluation of potential anticancer agents. XIII. On the criteria and kinetics associated with "curability" of experimental leukemia. Cancer Chemother. Rep. 35:1 (1964).
9. Hibbs, J.B., Jr., Lambert, L.H., Jr., and J.S. Remington. Resistance to murine tumors conferred by chronic infection with intracellular protozoa, Toxoplasma gondii and Bemitia jellisonii. J. Infect. Dis. 124:587 (1971).
10. Lehninger, A.L. Biochemistry. Worth Publishers, Inc., New York, p. 387 (1975).
11. Slater, E.C. Application of inhbitors and uncouplers for study of oxidastive phosphorylation. Methods Enzymol. 10: 48 (1967).
12. Racker, E. Lecture 4: The coupling device: In "A New Look at Mechanisms in Bioenergetics," Academic Press, Inc., New York, p. 67 (1976).
13. Granger, D.L., and J.B. Hibbs, Jr. Recovery from injury incurred by leukemia cells in contact with activated macrophages. Fed. Proc. 40:761 (1981).
14. Lewis, A.M., Jr., and J.L. Cook. Presence of allograft-rejection resistance in simian virus 40-transformed hamster cells and its possible role in tumor development. Proc. Natl. Acad. Sci. USA 77:2889 (1980)
15. Butel, J.S., Tenethia, S.S., and J.L. Melnick. Oncogenicity and cell transformation by papovavirus SV40: The role the viral

genome. Adv. in Cancer Res. 15:1 (1972).
16. Duncan, W.R., and J.W. Streilein. Analysis of the major histocompatibility complex in Syrian hamsters. Transplantation 25: 12 (1978).
17. Cook J.L., Hibbs, J.B., Jr., and A.M. Lewis, Jr. Resistance of simian virus 40-transformed hamster cells to the cytolytic. effect of activated macrophages: A possible factor in species-specific viral oncogenicity. Proc. Natl. Acad. Sci. USA 77:6773 (1980).
18. Zbar, B., Wepsic, H.T., Borsos, T., and H.J. Rapp. Tumor graft rejection in syngeneic guinea pigs: Evidence for a two-step mechanism. J. Nat. Cancer Inst. 44:473 (1970).
19. Hibbs, J.B., Jr. Macrophage nonimmunologic recognition: Target cell factors related to contact inhibition. Science 180:868 (1973).
20. Hibbs, J.B., Jr., Chapman, H.A., Jr., and J.B. Weinberg. The macrophage as an antineoplastic surveillance cell: Biologic perspectives. J. Reticuloendothelial Soc. 24:549 (1978).
21. Hibbs, J.B., Jr. Heterocytolysis by macrophages activated by bacillus Calmette-Guerin: Lysosome exocytosis into tumor cells. Science 184:468 (1974).
22. Bucana, C., Hoyer, L.C., Hobbs, B., Breesman, S., McDaniel, M., and M.G. Hanna. Morphological evidence for the translocation of lysosomal organelles from cytotoxic macrophages into the cytoplasm of tumor target cells. Cancer Res. 36:4444 (1976).
23. Otto, K. Cathespins B_1 and B_2. In "Tissue Proteinases," edited by A.J. Barrett and J.T. Dingle. North-Holland Publishing Co., Amsterdam, p. 1 (1971).
24. Adams, D.O. Effector mechanism of cytolytically activated macrophages. I. Secretion of neutral proteases and effect of protease inhibitors. J. Immunol. 124:286 (1980).
25. Hibbs, J.B., Jr., Taintor, R.R., Chapman, H.A., Jr., and J.B. Weinberg. Macrophage tumor cell killing: Influence of the local environment. Science 197:279 (1977).
26. Chang, T.W., and H.N. Eisen. Effects of TLCK on the activity of cytotoxic lymphocytes. J. Immunol. 124:1028 (1980).
27. Martz, E. Mechanism of specific tumor cell lysis by allo-immune T-lymphocytes: Resolution and characterization of discrete steps in the cellular interaction. Contemp. Top. Immunol. 7:301 (1977).
28. Roder, JC., Argov, S., Klein, M., Petersson, C., Kiessling, R., Anderson, K., and M. Hansson. Target-effector cell interaction in the natural killer cell system. V. Energy requirements, membrane integrity, and the possible involvement of lysosomal enzymes. Immunology 40:107 (1980).

DISCUSSION

W. Clark

I'm sort of curious about the difference in the time span between what you were talking about and what Mike Hanna was talking about. What was the time-scale of your assays, Michael?

M. Hanna

We find that, on the average, it's six to eight hours, before we see anything happen.

W. Clark

But we're talking about 60 to 80 hours in John's experiments. What's the difference?

J. Hibbs

The cell that lyses quickest in our system is a P815. It begins to lyse at about 8-10 hours. It extends through about 24 hours. Most cells lyse around 24 to 60 hours.

M. Hanna

I'm talking about being able to see something happening in the microscope. And we usually run 24 hour shifts. Of course we grabbed the first one we saw at 8 hours. You usually do talk about 72 hour assays for the best overall quantitative results. The assay I showed was 72 hours, sometimes as much as four-day assays. It's long. This is in range. I mean, to see the effect in terms of the entire population.

G. Berke

It may be useful to keep in mind that in terms of time-scale, the generation time of the target cell that is being studied is perhaps 12 hours. In assays performed over 72 hours, there is a great deal of additional things that may defer or delay its replication which may be far more important than perhaps the parameter that is actually being measured.

M. Hanna

That's right. What I showed in terms of the cells being blocked and not going into S after they've had interaction with macrophage, that doesn't mean that they can't sit there in a suspended state for several days before they actually do something.

C. Nathan

I think it would probably be fair to point out that many workers have observed the enhancement of proliferation of tumor cells by macrophages, usually normal ones but sometimes also those which can be shown to be activated. This appears to be particularly prominent with myeloma cells and with a variety of lymphomas, especially those that are 2 mercaptoethanol-dependent and in culture, which may be a reflection of the supportive role macrophages sometimes show toward normal lymphoid cells in culture.

J. Hibbs

That's true and I think, as you noticed on the first slide I showed, that the malignant cells actually grew better over macrophages than they did over the plain dish. This is a common observation, as Carl points out. I think whether you see enhancement of growth or inhibition of growth and induction of lysis, depends upon the density of the macrophage monolayer. If you have a confluent monolayer of macrophages that are adequately differentiated and truly activated, to the cytotoxic stage of differentiation, the target cells will undergo a prolonged period of cytostasis or they will lyse.

C.Nathan

I think there also needs to be mentioned at least, that the effect on inhibition of DNA synthesis is not that closely linked to lysis either. For example, in contrast to the effect between transformed versus untransformed cells, I think there's fairly good evidence that macrophages, particularly activated ones, can inhibit DNA synthesis of PHA blasts and yet they don't lyse them.

J. Hibbs

That's right. Macrophages can inhibit the proliferation of both T cells and B cells. And indeed they can inhibit DNA synthesis in other normal cells. However, normal cells, with the exception of lymphocytes, are more resistant to the inhibition of DNA synthesis than are tumor cells. In many experiments in which we used normal target cells, we observed that the normal target cells form a confluent monolayer after 72-80 hours of cocultivation with activated macrophages, whereas, transformed target cells lyse under idenical *in vitro* conditions. It is important to emphasize that normal target cells are very resistant to activated macrophage induced lysis.

OVERVIEW ON NK CELLS AND POSSIBLE MECHANISMS FOR THEIR CYTOTOXIC ACTIVITY

Ronald B. Herberman

Laboratory of Immunodiagnosis
National Cancer Institute
Bethesda, MD 20205

INTRODUCTION

As evidenced by the strong emphasis of this volume on T cells, there has been a long-standing interest in determining the mechanism of cytolysis by immune T cells. Similarly, much attention has been devoted to the mechanism of cytotoxicity by macrophages, as summarized well here by Key et al (1). During the past few years, natural killer (NK) cells have attracted considerable attention as particularly important elements in natural resistance against tumors and possibly against some microbial infections (2). It therefore is of equal concern to elucidate the mechanism of lysis of target cells by NK cells. A further intriguing question that can be raised, in light of the extensive research on mechanisms of lysis by other effector cells, is whether the mechanism of lysis by NK cells is unique or whether it is similar or even identical to that of one or more of the other cell types. Much of the available evidence on these issues is summarized in the manuscript by Goldfarb et al. in this volume (3). Here it seems more appropriate to emphasize the approaches which have been taken to study the mechanism of lysis by NK cells, and to point out current gaps in our knowledge and possible ways to obtain more definitive indications of the critical processes involved in the interaction between NK cells and their target cells.

One of the main limitations to detailed dissection of the mechanisms involved in cell-mediated cytotoxicity has been the difficulty in obtaining highly purified populations of effector cells, separated from a variety of other lymphoid cells that might, on the one hand, simply dilute out the relevant cells and confuse some studies on characterization, and more importantly, on the other hand, might be involved in regulating the levels of activity of the effector cell or have cytotoxic activity of their own. As illustrated by the recent studies on clones of immune cytotoxic T cells, much of the recent advances in our dissection of these complex problems in relation to NK cells may be expected to come from the use of highly purified populations, and ultimately clones, of NK cells.

MORPHOLOGIC IDENTIFICATION AND ISOLATION OF NK CELLS

The need for purification of NK cells has been particularly critical, since these effector cells appear to be present as a relatively low percentage of cells in such heterogeneous lymphoid organs as the spleen or peripheral blood. Therefore, much effort has been directed toward identification of markers restricted to, or at least highly selective for, NK cells. The best such marker to date has been a morphological one: recent evidence indicates that virtually all human and rat NK activity is mediated by large granular lymphocytes (LGL)(4,5) which comprise only about 5% of the peripheral blood or splenic leukocytes in man and other species. Although the evidence is not yet so clear, it also seems likely that such cells are responsible for mouse NK activity (6). LGL can be readily identified in Giemsa-stained lymphoid cells prepared on slides in a cytocentrifuge, and they can be highly enriched by centrifugation on density gradients of Percoll (4,5,7). It now appears that LGL account for a high proportion of human T_G cells (8), whose relation to typical T cells has recently been questioned (9). A monoclonal antibody, OKT10, reacts with most human LGL but not with other peripheral blood leukocytes (10). However, this antigen is not entirely specific for LGL, since it is also expressed on most thymocytes and a small subpopulation of bone marrow cells (11). Several surface antigens are also expressed, with some selectivity, on most or all mouse NK cells (12-16); however, none of these markers is restricted to only NK cells. Further, in contrast to LGL, which account for virtually all of the natural cytotoxic reactivity against a wide range of target cells (4,17), most of the alloantigenic markers on mouse NK cells have not been found on the related natural cytotoxic (NC) effector cells that react with some solid tumor target cells (18,19).

Another useful procedure for obtaining pure populations of NK cells has come from the observation that NK cells can grow in culture in response to interleukin-2 (IL-2). Several groups have now reported the isolation of mouse clones with NK activity (20-22). With human NK cells, efforts at culturing have been aided considerably by the ability to initiate cultures with purified populations of LGL. It has been possible to consistently grow LGL on IL-2 (23). However, it has been very difficult to obtain and maintain functionally active clones of such cells. This may be due to the relatively low frequency of progenitor cells in the LGL preparations, along with the limited knowledge of the culture conditions required for prolonged growth of such cells, particularly at very low cell concentrations required for successful cloning.

APPROACHES TO THE DETERMINATION OF THE MECHANISM OF LYSIS BY NK CELLS

Among the possible mechanisms for lysis of target cells by NK cells, four main candidates have been considered: secretion of soluble factors, with a likely involvement of lysosomal enzymes; proteases; phospholipase A_2; and oxidative burst. At least some suggestive evidence has been offered for most of these possibilities. How might we be expected to proceed and obtain more definitive identification of the sequence of processes required for a lytic interaction between NK cells and target cells? One approach would be to separately analyze the various major phases of this interaction (Table 1). It is generally agreed that the initial step required for NK activity is a physical binding of the NK cell to the target cell. As discussed in detail elsewhere in this volume by Henney (24) and by Kiessling (25), this interaction appears to depend on particular receptors on the surface of the NK cells, which recognize certain structures on the surface on susceptible target cells. Further, it appears that during the usual cytotoxic assays, NK cells can recycle, i.e., dissociate from the initially bound target cell and then move on to similarly interact with other target cells. After binding of NK cells to targets, additional events appear to be required for lysis of the targets to occur. Not all binding interactions lead to lysis and one may hope to separately analyze the various stages of post-binding events that are required for lysis.

One major approach to gain insight into mechanisms of lysis by NK cells has been to examine the effects of a variety of agents on levels of NK activity. On the one hand, understandng of the

TABLE 1. ANALYSIS OF SITES OF ACTION OF VARIOUS AGENTS

Binding of LGL to targets
Recycling of binders
Post-binding events
Percent of binders with lytic activity
Kinetics of lysis
Secretion of soluble, lytic factors
Degree of secretion
Effect of soluble factors on target cells

mechanisms by which some treatments can lead to activation or augmentation of NK activity might help to identify important positive signals, or rate-limiting phases in the lytic process. On the other hand, treatments which lead to inhibition of NK activity also would be expected to point to events or metabolic steps required for lysis. With the currently available procedures, it should be possible to at least determine whether augmenting or inhibiting agents are affecting initial binding recycling, or post-binding events, and thus the focus for the relevant steps that are affected can be narrowed considerably. The initial, binding phase can be well studied by mixing purified populations of NK cells with target cells, centrifuging them together, and then determining the proportion of effector cells that bind to targets, either in suspension or by preparing cytocentrifuge slides (4,5). Recycling has been studied indirectly (26) and, more recently, by directly separating conjugates and examining the proportion of cells that rebind after initially dissociating from the target cells (27). Effects on post-binding events can be carefully studied by the single cell agarose assay of Grimm and Bonavida (28). However, in order to clearly determine whether a treatment which inhibits binding would also intefere with post-binding events, it would be necessary to begin the treatment once binding has already taken place, and such a protocol has not yet been commonly utilized.

If the interaction of NK cells with susceptible target cells leads to secretion of a soluble mediator(s) that is then capable of effecting lysis, as suggested particularly by Bonavida (29), then one might try to distinguish between treatments or agents which affect secretion of the active soluble factors and those which affect the action of these factors on the target cells. It should be possible to set up quantitative assays for the amount of cytotoxic factor(s) produced, and also to focus on the interaction between standard preparations of cytotoxic factor and target cells, and further to characterize and isolate the soluble factors involved in lysis (e.g., determine the possible presence of proteases, phospholipase A_2, other enzymes, separate them, and evaluate whether one or more are in fact involved in the induction of lysis of target cells).

Within the context of the above approaches, it is now of interest to consider the various agents or treatments which have been shown to augment or inhibit NK activity. In regard to augmentation (Table 2), interferon clearly has been the most extensively studied agent and there is the most insight into the mechanisms of its effects. However, the effects of interferon have been amply documented to be exceedingly pleiotropic. Depending on the target cell used in the study, augmentation of NK activity has been associated with significant increases in the percent of NK cells able to bind to the targets (27,30) to increased recycling of NK cells (26,27), and in regard to post-binding events, to be able to switch on some

TABLE 2. AUGMENTATION OF NK ACTIVITY

Interferon

- Binding
- Recycling of binders
- Lytically inactive → active
- Kinetics of lysis
- Proliferation of NK cells
  - Augmented response to IL-2
  - Activation of suppressor cells

Others

- Antibodies to NK cells
- Lectins
- Retinoic acid
- IL-2
- Enzymes:
  - Neuraminidase
  - Low concentration of trypsin, chymotrypsin, phospholipase A_2
- ? cyclic GMP

lytically inactive cells (27,28,30,31) or to accelerate the rate of already active NK cells (27). In addition, interferon has been found to affect the responsiveness of NK cells to IL-2 (27), perhaps by increasing the number of receptors for IL-2 or by otherwise increasing the number of NK cell progenitors susceptible to IL-2, and also to be able to stimulate T cell-dependent suppressors of the growth of NK cells (33). Although such detailed information is highly interesting and some aspects of it may eventually lead to important insights into the mechanism of lysis by NK cells, the heterogeneity of effects have thus far limited the mechanistic value of this approach.

Until recently, it was thought that interferon might be the sole positive signal for NK activity, with other augmenting agents mediating their effects by their ability to induce interferon. However, there are several augmenting agents or treatments which appear to act independently of interferon (Table 2). Antibodies to histocompatibility antigens and to other antigens on the surface of NK cells (34-36), and lectins reactive with NK cells (35,36) have been shown to augment NK activity and these effects appear to be interferon-independent, since inhibitors of protein synthesis do not interfere with augmentation. Similarly, retinoic acid, which generally inhibits interferon production (38), has been shown to augment both mouse and human NK activity (37). Recently, treatment of mouse (32) and human (39) NK cells with IL-2 has been shown to augment NK activity. However, it has not yet been determined whether the IL-2 is acting by stimulating the production of gamma-interferon. Timonen (unpublished observations) has recently found that pretreatment of NK cells or of target cells with neuraminidase leads to increased conjugate formation and lysis, and Goldfarb et al. (3) have found that addition of low concentrations of various enzymes (trypsin, chymotrypsin, or phospholipase A_2) to the NK assay leads to augmented cytotoxicity. Roder et al. (40) have also reported that stimulation of cyclic GMP levels in mouse NK cells caused moderate elevations in NK activity. However, various investigators in my laboratory have failed to confirm such observations with either mouse or human NK cells.

Hopefully, when the phases affected by each of these treatments have been determined, it should be possible to identify those agents with the most selective effects and use them for more intensive dissection of the mechanism of lysis.

A wide variety of agents or treatments has been shown to inhibit NK activity (Table 3). With many of these, it is already possible to state whether they affect initial recognition or whether they

TABLE 3. INHIBITORS OF NK ACTIVITY

Binding	Lysis
Trypsin, 100 μg/ml	Low temperature + other energy blocks
Pronase, 100 μg/ml	cAMP, 10^{-4}M
EDTA, 10 mM	PGE, 10^{-6}M
PMA 100 ng/ml	Cholera toxin, 10^{-9}M
Cytochalasin B	ATP, 10^{-5}M
Membrane Extracts	Man-6-P, .05M
	Gal-6-P, .05M
	Fru-6-P, .05M
	Monomeric, cytophilic IgG

? site
IBMX, 10^{-4}M
NH_4Cl
Tetracaine, 10^{-3}M
Quinacine, 10^{-3}M
DZA, 10^{-4}M + homocysteine, 10^{-4}M
Rosenthal's inhibitor, 10^{-3}M
Hydrocortisone, 10^{-5}M
Antibodies to human NK cells (9.6 and OKT11a) or mouse NK cells (Ly 5)

only inhibit some post-binding events. However, it should be noted that the currently available information would not allow one to conclude that agents shown to inhibit binding have no effect on post-binding events, since the latter have not been separately analyzed by the procedures discussed above. Even this initial categorization of effects, into binding and post-binding events, has been very helpful in some instances. For example, when Stutman and his colleagues (41) first reported that various simple sugars could inhibit mouse NK and NC activities, it was assumed that this was indicative of a lectin-like recognition process. However, since sugars which can inhibit human NK activity have not been found to inhibit binding (42) it seems more likely that some post-binding metabolic events are being affected. It is intriguing in this regard that phosphorylated sugars have been particularly inhibitory (42), and such sugars have been shown to interfere with the binding of lysosomal enzymes to membrane receptors (43). Further, it is of interest that sugars have been shown to inhibit the activity of the soluble factor described by Wright and Bonavida (29,44). This would suggest that secretion of some protein, with subsequent binding and/or uptake by the target cell is a key process for lysis. Such a hypothesis is quite consistent with the observations that beige mice and patients with Chediak-Higashi syndrome, with known defects in lysosomal enzymes and related secretion, have impaired NK activity (45,46). The inhibition of NK activity by ammonium chloride and various other amines could be interpreted along the same lines, since these have been shown to be lysosomotropic and inhibitory of secretory processes. It is intriguing that the electron microscope studies described elsewhere in this volume by Henkart and Henkart (47) also suggest secretion of granular contents from human LGL.

Several of the post-binding inhibitory treatments seem to be associated with increases in levels of cyclic AMP. Dibutryl cyclic AMP has been shown to inhibit human NK activity, without affecting binding to target cells (42). Both cholera toxin and prostaglandin E have been shown in other cellular systems to elevate cyclic AMP levels, and in a recent study by Goto et al (48) it has been possible to demonstrate that treatment of human LGL with prostaglandin E_1 or E_2 leads to appreciable elevations of cyclic AMP levels and that, as would be expected if the mechanism for inhibition by PGE was mediated by its affect on adenyl cyclase, simultaneous treatment with inhibitors of phosphodiesterase produced synergistic depression of NK activity as well as elevation of cyclic AMP levels. It has also recently been found that binding of monomeric, cytophilic IgG will inhibit human NK activity (49), and preliminary studies suggest that this may also be a signal for elevation of intracellular cyclic AMP levels (Goto, T., Sulica, A., and R.B. Herberman, unpublished observations).

It has also been of interest that treatment of human LGL with ATP causes inhibition of NK activity (50). It appears that the effects of such treatment occur at the surface of the NK cell and that the inhibitory activity is restricted to ATP and not shared by other nucleotides. The mechanism for such inhibition has not yet been elucidated but several possibilities have been considered: this treatment might lead to phosphorylation of some important surface carbohydrates or proteins; it might lead to the formation of channels and consequent increased permeability of the cells (51); or it might lead to alterations in intracellular cyclic nucleotide metabolism.

SUMMARY OF EVIDENCE FOR INVOLVEMENT OF VARIOUS BIOCHEMICAL PATHWAYS

The present evidence in support of an involvement of proteases, phospholipase A_2, or oxidative burst is presented in detail in the manuscript by Goldfarb et al. in this volume (3). Therefore, it should suffice here to just briefly summarize the main pieces of evidence for or against each possibility. The direct involvement of reactive oxygen species in NK activity seems unlikely, in view of the failure to detect an oxidative burst in purified human LGL (52). Thus, we may mainly consider the weight of available evidence in favor of the involvement of phospholipid metabolism or of proteases.

TABLE 4. EVIDENCE FOR ROLE OF PHOSPHOLIPID METABOLISM IN HUMAN NK ACTIVITY

1. Methylation
    a. Increased methylation upon contact with NK-susceptible target.
    b. Inhibition of NK by DZA + homocysteine.
2. Phospholipase A_2
    a. Apparent increase in activity upon contact with NK-susceptible target.
    b. Inhibition of NK by Rosenthal's inhibitor, corticosteroids, tetracaine and quinacine.
    c. Increased cytolysis by LGL in presence of exogenous phospholipase A_2.

Regarding phospholipid metabolism, two aspects have been associated with human NK activity (53)(Table 4). Upon contact of human peripheral blood mononuclear cells with an NK susceptible target cell, increased phospholipid methylation was detected (53). In contrast, no such increase in methylation was seen upon incubation of the effector cells with a resistant target cell. In addition, the widely used procedure for inhibition of phospholipid methylation, with deazo adenosine (DZA) plus homocysteine, was found to inhibit NK activity (53). However, some very recent studies in my laboratory (P. Bougnoux and T. Hoffman, unpublished observations) have raised some questions about this association. Treatment of human effector cells with one preparation of recombinant leukocyte interferon or with a partially purified preparation of beta interferon, which lead to augmented NK activity, was associated with a decrease in methylation. Also, other interferon preparations that boosted NK activity had no detectable effect on methylation. Such observations would be difficult to explain if phospholipid methylation were intimately associated with the degree of activation of NK cells. It should be noted that the current evidence for a requirement for this metabolic process rests on the inhibition of activity of DZA and homocysteine. However, such treatment may not be entirely selective for the methylation reaction and the inhibition of NK activity may in fact be due to another metabolic consequence of such treatment.

Evidence has also been obtained for a role of phospholipase A_2 in human NK activity (53). However, at the moment, this evidence is largely indirect or circumstantial. There was an apparent increase in phospholipase A_2 activity upon contact with an NK-susceptible target cell. However, the assay used, the release of arachidonic acid, is not an entirely reliable procedure for measuring this enzyme. Current studies are in progress in my laboratory to examine this point more closely (P. Bougnoux and T. Hoffman, unpublished observations). The use of various inhibitors of phospholipase A_2 activity has revealed an inhibition of NK activity. Again, however, it is not clear just how selective these agents are and their inhibitory effects may be related to other metabolic processes.

There also is increasing evidence for a role of proteases in NK activity, especially with human NK cells (Table 5). As described by Goldfarb et al.(3), purified preparations of LGL have been shown to have detectable protease activity, with the enzyme having the general features of plasminogen activator. However, to date, there is no indication as to whether such an enzme is in fact involved in the lytic process. A more direct indication for a role of protease(s) in human NK activity has come from observations in several laboratories that inhibitors of proteases, particularly those with chymotryptic characteristics, strongly inhibit NK activity (54,55). Conversely, as noted above, increased NK

TABLE 5. EVIDENCE FOR ROLE OF PROTEASE(S) IN NK ACTIVITY

1. Detectable protease(s) associated with purified LGL: plasminogen activator-like.

   ? protease with lytic activity on targets.

2. Inhibition of NK activity by inhibitors of proteases: chymotryptic profile.

3. Increased NK in presence of ng amounts of trypsin or chymotrypsin in serum-free medium.

activity has been seen when small concentrations of trypsin or chymotrypsin have been added to the cytotoxicity assay. It should be noted that although such data point rather strongly toward some involvement of proteases in NK activity, they do not indicate whether these enzymes are themselves the lytic molecules, or whether they lead to activation of some other processes that are more directly associated with lysis.

CONCLUSIONS

It clearly is not possible as yet to draw any conclusions as to the actual mechanism of lysis by NK cells. However, this can also be said for the mechanisms of cytotoxicity by each of the other effector cells under consideration in this volume. In fact, many of the current issues and even lines of evidence are rather similar for each of the effector cell types. Hopefully, some common aspects of the mechanisms will be found so that progress with one cell type can be rapidly translated to progress with others. It is appealing to think that the main distinctions among the effector mechanisms are related to the means for the effector cells to recognize their targets, with the subsequent metabolic effects being the same or similar. This possibility is particularly attractive for considerations of the mechanisms of lysis by NK and K cells, since both effectors are in the same small population of LGL (4) and at least the majority of such cells may be able to mediate both functions (56). However, it should be noted that some differences in post-binding inhibition of these two cytotoxic activities have been detected. Ortaldo et al. (42) have found that the phosphorylated sugars that inhibit human NK activity have had no inhibitory effect on ADCC against tumor target cells. Similarly, some conditions of treatment with DZA and homocysteine (53) or with monomeric IgG (A. Sulica and R.B. Herberman, unpublished observations) have shown preferential inhibition of NK activity relative to ADCC activity. Such observations again emphasize the complexity of the problems under study.

Although clear answers are not yet available, it would appear that progress in our understanding of the mechanism of lysis of NK cells has been rather rapid. Hopefully, such progress will continue and real understanding will soon be at hand. It seems likely that major advances will come from biochemical characterization of the enzymes and other factors that have been incriminated, rather than from further studies with inhibitory or augmenting agents for NK activity.

REFERENCES

1. Key, M.E., et al. See this volume.
2. Herberman, R.B. (Ed.). In "Natural Cell-Mediated Immunity Against Tumors." Academic Press, New York, 1321 pp. (1980).
3. Goldfarb, R.H., Timonen, T., and R.B. Herberman. Mechanisms of tumor cell lysis by natural killer cells. See this volume.
4. Timonen, T., Ortaldo, J.R., and R.B. Herberman. Characteristics of human large granular lymphocytes and relationship to natural killer and K cells. J. Exp. Med. 153:569 (1981).
5. Reynolds, C.W., Timonen, T., and R.B. Herberman. Natural killer (NK) cell activity in the rat. I. Isolation and characterization of the effector cells. J. Immunol. 127:282 (1981).
6. Luini, W., Boraschi, D., Alberti, S., Aleotti A., and A. Tagliabue. Morphological characterization of a cell population responsible for natural killer activity. Immunol., in press.
7. Timonen, T., and E. Saksela. Isolation of human natural killer cells by discontinuous gradient centrifugation. J. Immunol. Methods 36:285 (1980).
8. Ferrarini, M., Cadoni, A., Franzi, T., Ghigliotti, C., Leprini, A., Zicca, A., and C.E. Grossi. Ultrastructural and cytochemical markers of human lymphocytes. In "Thymus, Thymic Hormones and T Lymphocytes." Edited by F. Aiuti. Academic Press, New York, p. 39 (1980).
9. Reinherz, E.L., Moretta, L., Roper, M., Breard, J.M., Mingari, M.C., Cooper, M.D., and S.F. Schlossman. Human T lymphocyte subpopulations defined by Fc receptors and monoclonal antibodies. A comparison. J. Exp. Med. 151:969 (1980).
10. Ortaldo J.R., Sharrow, S.O., Timonen, T., and R.B. Herberman. Determination of surface antigens on highly purified human NK cells by flow cytometry with monoclonal antibodies. J. Immunol., in press.
11. Reinherz, E.L., Kung, P.C., Goldstein, G., Levey, R.H., and S.F. Schlossman. Discrete stages of human intrathymic differentiation: analysis of normal thymocytes and leukemic lymphoblasts of T-cell lineage. Proc. Natl. Acad. Sci. USA 77:1588 (1980).
12. Glimcher, L., Shen, F.W., and H. Cantor. Identification of a cell-surface antigen selectively expessed on the natural killer cell. J. Exp. Med. 145:1 (1977).

13. Cantor, H., Kasai, M., Shen, H.W., Leclerc, J.C., and L. Glimcher. Immunogenetic analysis of natural killer activity in the mouse. Immunol. Rev. 44:1 (1979).
14. Kasai, M., Iwamori, M., Nagai, Y., Okumura, K., and T. Tada. A glycolipid on the surface of mouse natural killer cells. Eur. J. Immunol. 10:174 (1980).
15. Young, W.W. Jr., Hakomori, S-I., Durdik, J.M., and C.S. Henney. Identification of ganglio-N-tetrasylceramide as a new cell surface marker for murine natural killer (NK) cells. J. Immunol. 124:199 (1980).
16. Tai, A., and N.L. Warner. Biophysical and serological characterization of murine NK cells. In "Natural Cell-Mediated Immunity Against Tumors." Edited by R.B. Herberman. Academic Press, New York, p. 241 (1980).
17. de Landazuri, M.O., Lopez-Botet, M., Timonen, T., Ortaldo, J.R., and R.B. Herberman. Human large granular lymphocytes: Spontaneous and interferon-boosted NK activity against adherent and nonadherent tumor cell lines. J. Immunol. 127:1380 (1981).
18. Stutman, O., Figarella, E.F., Paige, C.J., and E.C. Lattime. Natural cytotoxic (NC) cells against solid tumors in mice: general characteristics and comparison to natural killer (NK) cells. In "Natural Cell-Mediated Immunity Against Tumors." Edited by R.B. Herberman. Academic Press, New York, p. 187 (1980).
19. Burton, R.B. Alloantisera selectively reactive with NK cells: characterization and use in defining NK cell classes. In "Natural Cell-Mediated Immunity Against Tumors." Edited by R.B. Herberman. Academic Press, New York, p. 19 (1980).
20. Dennert, G. Cloned lines of natural killer cells. Nature 287:47 (1980).
21. Nabel, G., Bucalo, L.R., Allard, J., Wigzell, H., and H. Cantor. Multiple activities of a cloned cell line mediating natural killer cell function. J. Exp. Med. 153:1582 (1981).
22. Kedar, E., Herberman, R.B., Gorelik, E., Sredni, B., Bonnard, G.D., and N. Navarro. Antitumor reactivity in vitro and in vivo of mouse and human lymphoid cells cultured with T cell growth factor. In "The Potential Role of T Cell Subpopulations in Cancer Therapy." Edited by A. Fefer. Raven Press, New York, in press.
23. Ortaldo, J.R., Timonen, T.T., Vose, B.M., and J.A. Alvarez. Human natural killer cells as well as T cells maintained in continuous cultures with IL-2. In "The Potential Role of T Cell Subpopulations in Cancer Therapy." Edited by A. Fefer. Raven Press, New York, in press.
24. Henney, C. See this volume.
25. Kiessling, R. See this volume.
26. Ullberg, M., and M. Jondal. Recycling and target binding capacity of human natural killer cells. J. Exp. Med. 153:615 (1981).
27. Timonen, T., Ortaldo, J.R., and R.B. Herberman. Analysis by

a single cell cytotoxicity assay of natural kill (NK) cell frequencies among human large granular lymphocytes and of the effects of interferon on their activity. Submitted for publication.

28. Grimm, E., and B. Bonavida. Mechanism of cell-mediated cytotoxicity at the single cell level. I. Estimation of cytotoxic T lymphocyte frequency and relative lytic efficiency. J. Immunol 123:2861 (1979).
29. Bonavida, B. See this volume.
30. Reynolds, C.W., Timonen, T., Holden, H.T., Hansen, C.T., and R.B. Herberman. Natural killer (NK) cell activity in the rat. III. Analysis of activity in the athymic (nude) rat. Submitted for publication.
31. Silva, A., Bonavida, B., and S. Targan. Mode of action of interferon-mediated modulation of natural killer cytotoxic activity: recruitment of pre-NK cells and enhanced kinetics of lysis. J. Immunol. 125:479 (1980).
32. Kuribayashi, K., Gillis, S., Kern, D.E., and C.S. Henney. Murine NK cell cultures: effects of interleukin-2 and interferon on cell growth and cytotoxic reactivity. J. Immunol. 126:2321 (1981).
33. Riccardi, C., Vose, B., and R.B. Herberman. Limiting dilution frequency analysis of mouse NK cells growing in mitogen-free IL-2: regulation by T cells and interferon. In "Proceedings of the 9th International RES congress, in press.
34. Saxena, R.K., Adler, W.H., and A.A. Nordin. Modulation of natural cytotoxicity by alloantibodies. IV. A comparative study of the activation of mouse spleen cell cytotoxicity by anti-H2 antisera, interferon, and mitogens. Cell. Immunol. 63:28 (1981).
35. Brunda, M.J., Herberman, R.B., and H.T. Holden. Interferon-independent activation of murine natural killer cell activity. In "Natural Cell-Mediated Immunity Against Tumors." Edited by R.B. Herberman. Academic Press, New York, p. 525 (1980).
36. Brunda, M.J., Herberman, R.B., and H.T. Holden. Antibody-induced augmentation of murine natural killer cell activity. Int. J. Cancer 27:205 (1981).
37. Blalock, J.E. Inhibition of interferon production by RA (vitamin A acid). Tex. Rep. Biol. Med. 35:69 (1977).
38. Goldfarb, R.H., and R.B. Herberman. Natural killer cell reactivity: Regulatory interactions among phorbol ester, interferon, cholera toxin, and retinoic acid. J. Immunol. 126:2129 (1981).
39. Domzig, W., Timonen, T.T., and B.M. Stadler. Human natural killer (NK) cells produce interleukin-2 (IL-2). Proc. Amer. Assoc. Cancer Res. 22:309 (1981).
40. Roder, J.C., Argov, S., Klein, N.M., Petersson, C., Kiessling, R., Anderson, R., Anderson, K., and M. Hansson. Target-effector interaction in the natural killer cell system. V. Energy requirement, membrane integrity, and the possible involvement of lysosomal enzymes. Immunol. 40:108 (1980).

41. Stutman, O., Dien, P., Wisun, R., Percoraro, G., and E.C. Lattime. Natural cytotoxic (NC) cells against solid tumors in mice: some target cell characteristics and blocking of cytotoxicity by D-mannose. In "Natural Cell-Mediated Immunity Against Tumors." Edited by R.B. Herberman. Academic Press, New York, p. 949 (1980).
42. Ortaldo, J.R., Timonen, T.T., Goldfarb, R.H., and R.B. Herberman. Mechanisms of lysis by natural killer cells: Discrimination between binding and post-binding events. Submitted for publication.
43. Fischer, H.D., Gonzalez-Noriega, A., Sly, S.W., and D.J. Morre. Phosphomannosyl-enzyme receptors in rat liver. Subcellular distribution and role in intracellular transport of lysosomal enzymes. J. Biol. Chem. 255:9608 (1980).
44. Wright, S.C., and B. Bonavida. Selective lysis of NK-sensitive target cells by a soluble mediator released from murine spleen cells and human peripheral blood lymphocytes. J. Immunol. 126:1516 (1981).
45. Roder, J., and A. Duwe. The beige mutation in the mouse selectively impairs natural killer cell function. Nature 278: 451 (1979).
46. Roder, J.C., Haliotis, T., Klein, M., Korec, S., Jett, J.R., Ortaldo, J., Herberman, R.B., Katz, P., and A.S. Fauci. A new immunodeficiency disorder in humans involving NK cells. Nature 184:553 (1980).
47. Henkart, M. and P. Henkart. See this volume.
48. Goto, T., Maluish, A., Strong, D.M., and R.B. Herberman. Cyclic AMP as a mediator of protaglandin E-induced suppression of human natural killer cell activity. Submitted for publication.
49. Sulica, A., Gherman, M., Galatiuc, C., Manciulea, M., and R.B. Herberman. Inhibition of human natural killer cell activity by cytophilic immunogloculin G. J. Immunol., in press.
50. Schmidt, A., Ortaldo, J.R., and R.B. Herberman. Inhibition of human natural killer cell reactivity by exogenous adenosine 5'-triphosphate. Fed. Proc., in press.
51. Dicker, P., Heppel, L.A., and E. Rozengurt. Control of membrane permeability by external and internal ATP in 3T6 cells grown in serum-free medium. Proc. Natl. Acad. Sci. USA 77: 2103 (1980).
52. Goldfarb, R.H., Timonen, T., Pick, E., and R.B. Herberman. Evaluation of ability of human large granular lymphocytes and monocytes to display an oxidative burst. Submitted for publication.
53. Hoffman, T., Hirata, F., Bougnoux, P., Fraser, B.A., Goldfarb, R.H., Herberman, R.B., and J. Axelrod. Phospholipid methylation and phospholipase A_2 activation in cytotoxicity by human natural killer cells. Proc Natl. Acad. Sci. 78:3839 (1981).
54. Hudig, D., Haverty, T., Fucher, C., Redelman, D., and J. Mendelsohn. Inhibition of human natural cytotoxicity by macro-

molecular antiproteases. J. Immunol. 126:1569 (1981).
55. Lavie G., Weiss, H., Pick, A., and E.C. Franklin. The role of surface associated proteases in lymphocyte spontaneous cytolytic activity. Fourth Congr. Immunol. Abstracts 11.4.30 (1980).
56. Landazuri, M.O., Silva, A., Alvarez, J., and R.B. Herberman. Evidence that natural cytotoxicity and antibody dependent cellular cytotoxicity are mediated in humans by the same effector cell populations. J. Immunol. 123:252 (1979).

DISTINCTIONS BETWEEN NK CELLS AND CTL

Christopher S. Henney

Program in Basic Immunology
Fred Hutchinson Cancer Research Center
Seattle, Washington 98104

By way of introduction to this session on NK cells and their targets, I thought it might be useful to define some of the differences between NK cells and CTL. Table 1 gives a partial listing of some of these differences. There are, I believe, four criteria which potentially can be used.

(i) cell surface markers
(ii) inhibition of cytotoxicity by antibodies (in the absence of complement) directed at selective cell-surface markers
(iii) target cell susceptibility
(iv) potentiation by lymphokines

With respect to cell-surface markers, (of endogenous murine NK cells; that is, those cells that are present in lymphoid tissues prior to exogenous stimulation), there are several macromolecules which are selectively displayed on NK cells and are either not present, or present to a much lesser degree, on CTL. These include the alloantigens NK-1 and NK-2 described by Glimcher et al (1) and by Burton (2), respectively, and the neutral glycolipid asialo GM1 (3). I think it important to point out, because there is a gathering confusion in the literature, that asialo GM1 is exhibited on the surface of many cell types, including most T lymphocytes and activated macrophages. The important point is that it is not present on CTL populations. Thus, its presence on NK cells provides a useful focus for distinguishing between lytic events mediated by NK cells and by CTL.

On the other hand, CTL clearly bear cell-surface markers which are missing (or represented to a lesser extent) on NK cells. Most notable among these are the alloantigens Lyt 2 and 3.

TABLE I

Some Characteristics Which Distinguish Natural Killer Cells from Cytotoxic T Cells

	NK cells	T cells
Distinguishing cell-surface markers	NK 1 NK 2 Asialo GM1	Lyt 2 Lyt 3 Lack asialo GM1
Inhibitory Antisera	Anti-Lyt 5 not Anti-Lyt 2	Anti-Lyt 2 not Anti-Lyt 5
Target cell specificity	Kill across strain and species barriers. Lymphoma variants described which differ in susceptibility.	Exquisite specificity; MHC restricted. Do not distinguish NK susceptibility variants.
Lymphokine augmentation	Interferon and IL-2	Interferon but not IL-2

One note of caution should be exercised with respect to cell-surface markers on cytotoxic cells cultured for prolonged periods in supernatants of Con A stimulated lymphocytes: there is accumulating evidence that interleukin-2 (IL-2), and probably other lymphokines, can induce the display of markers not detectable prior to culture. For example, we have shown that NK cell populations grown from spleens depleted of Thy 1 bearing cells, invariably bear this alloantigen (4).

Of considerable interest is the finding that antiserum against some surface markers of cytotoxic cells can inhibit lysis in the absence of complement components. Here, too, CTL and NK cells can be distinguished. CTL are inhibited by antisera directed against either the Lyt 2 or Lyt 3 alloantigens, but not by anti-Lyt 5. In contrast, NK cell activity is inhibited by anti-Lyt 5, but not by anti-Lyt 2 or anti-Lyt 3 alloantisera. An example of this distinction, taken from the work of Brooks et al. (4) is shown in Fig. 1.

One of the major foci of the following papers and discussion centers on the specificity of NK cells, and particularly those shared characteristics of cells which are susceptible to NK cell attack. It is apparent that the two families of effector cells (NK and CTL) are readily distinguished by the spectrum of target cells

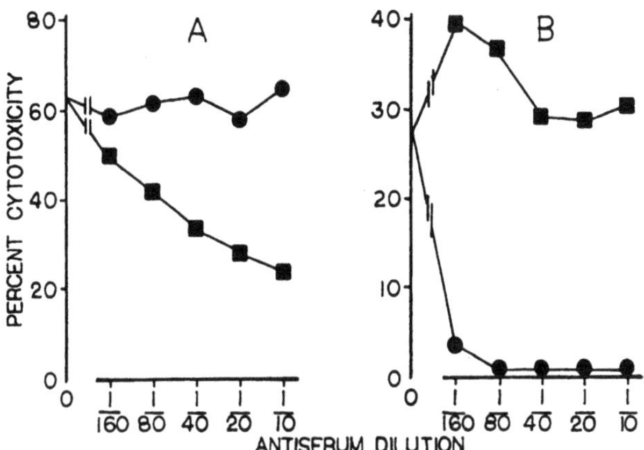

Fig. 1. Specificity of blocking of cytotoxicity by anti-Lyt-2 (●) and anti-Ly-5 (■) antibodies. Lysis of YAC-1 by normal spleen cells at E:T ratio 100:1 (A) and of EL4 by MLR-generated CBA anti-C57BL/6 effectors at E:T ratio 10:1 (B) in presence of various concentrations of antiserum.

which they lyse. NK cells kill a very wide variety of target cells across both strain and species barriers. Lymphomas in particular are susceptible. CTL, in contrast, lyse with exquisite immunological specificity. Furthermore, unlike NK cells, CTL are often restricted in their action by products of the MHC gene complex.

As one approach towards defining some characteristics of NK susceptible target cells, we have derived lymphoma cell variants which vary enormously in their susceptibility to NK cells, but which cannot be distinguished by other cytotoxic cells, including CTL. I will relate some further characteristics of these cells in a subsequent paper in this section, but in the context of this introduction let me simply say that such target cell populations provide a further useful tool for distinguishing NK and CTL effector cells.

Finally, a well known feature of NK cells is that they are activated by lymphokines. The capacity of interferon to boost NK cells is known to the readers of "Time" and "Newsweek" and is the platform from which the clinical trials of interferon as an anti-neoplastic agent have been launched. Interferon, however, also boosts CTL activity and thus this does not serve to distinguish NK and CTL. On the other hand, we have recently shown that interleukin -2 also boosts NK activity (5) but does not raise the cytotoxic activity of CTL, giving yet one more handle by which to identify NK cells from CTL.

REFERENCES

1. Glimcher, L.F., Shen, F.W., and H. Cantor. Identification of a cell-surface antigen selectively expressed on the "Natural Killer" cell. J. Exp. Med. 145:1 (1977).
2. Burton, R.C. Alloantisera selectively reactive with NK cells: characterization and use in defining NK cell classes. In "Natural cell-mediated immunity against tumors," R.B. Herberman (ed.), p. 19 (1980).
3. Young, W.W., Hakomori, S.-I., Durdik, J.M., and C.S. Henney. Identification of ganglio-N-tetrasylceramide as a new cell surface marker for murine natural killer (NK) cells. J. Immunol. 124:199 (1980).
4. Brooks, C.G., Kuribayashi, K., Sale, G., and C.S. Henney. Characterization of five cloned murine cell lines showing high cytotoxic activity against YAC-1 cells. Submitted for publication (1981).
5. Henney, C.S., Kuribayashi, K., Kern, D.E., and S. Gillis. Interleukin-2 augments Natural Killer-cell activity. Nature 291:335 (1981).

A SEARCH FOR TARGET CELL STRUCTURES ASSOCIATED WITH SUSCEPTIBILITY TO NK CELLS

Christopher S. Henney

Basic Immunology Program
Fred Hutchinson Cancer Research Program
1124 Columbia Street
Seattle, Washington 98104

INTRODUCTION

Natural killer (NK) cells, regardless of the species from which they are derived, are characterized by their ability to lyse a wide variety of cell types, most notably lymphomas and other tumor cell lines. Normal tissues, including fibroblasts, thymocytes and a portion of bone marrow cells are also lysed, but, in general, normal cells are much less susceptible than tumor cells to NK cell mediated lysis (1,2).

There are two principle hypotheses which could account for the unusually wide range of target cells which are susceptible to NK cell attack. These are: (i) NK cell "specificities" could be clonally distributed. The broad spectrum of target cells lysed would then represent the sum of activities of individual NK cell clones, each of which would have a limited specificity. (ii) Cells susceptible to the action of NK cells could share a common feature, which, for the sake of simplicity, one might define as a common target "antigen."

Using a number of experimental approaches, we found no evidence to support the concept that NK cell specificity was clonally distributed. On the other hand, several bodies of evidence suggest that NK cells "recognize" a limited number of cell surface macromolecules on susceptible cells. Preliminary evidence employing lymphoma cell variants suggest that target cell surface glycoconjugates might dictate NK cell susceptibility.

RESULTS

Three sets of related experiments were designed to seek evidence for the possibility that NK cells are clonally distributed. In the first, we asked whether NK cell populations could be adsorbed onto monolayers of susceptible cells, and whether such interactions removed NK reactivity against other susceptible target cells. In one experiment typical of this approach, murine NK cell populations were incubated on a monolayer of susceptible L5178Y lymphoma cells. Cells non-adherent to the monolayer were harvested and their activity against a panel of susceptible target cells then assessed. Incubation on L5178Y cells largely removed cytotoxic activity, not only against this cell, but against all NK susceptible target cells tested. In contrast, parallel absorption of NK cell populations on insusceptible cell monolayers (e.g., on normal DBA/2 spleen cells), did not remove NK reactivity (3).

Thus, experiments of this nature established: (a) That NK cells bind to monolayers of NK-susceptible, but not to monolayers of NK-insusceptible cells, and (b) that adsorption on susceptible cell monolayers removed NK reactivity not only to cells of the monolayer phenotype, but also against other NK-susceptible targets.

A similar approach used target cells which had been fluoresceinated by exposure to dicholotriazinyl amino-fluorescein. Such labeled cells were then incubated in suspension with effector cells. The resulting mixture was fractionated using a fluorescence-activated cell sorter into fluorescent and non-fluorescent populations. The NK reactivity of the non-fluorescent population was then assessed, both against the target cell with which it had been incubated and also against a series of other target cells.

It was argued that NK cell interaction with a fluorescent target cell which was susceptible to lysis would result in a cell-cell complex which would fractionate with the fluorescent compartment. Conversely, the non-fluorescent population would be selectively depleted of effector cells capable of binding to the target cell in question. Results of these studies were unequivocal: incubation with susceptible target cells, followed by removal of such cell-cell complexes, was associated with a decline in lytic reactivity against all susceptible target cells tested. In contrast, incubation with a fluorescent but insusceptible target cell was not associated with a decline in NK reactivity.

A third set of experimental results compatible with these binding experiments was obtained using "cold" target inhibition experiments. In this approach, the lysis of ^{51}Cr-labeled susceptible cells was inhibited by the addition of unlabeled competitor cells. NK susceptible target cells were all effective inhibitors of lysis. In contrast, a series of NK insusceptible target cells were very poor inhibitors of the lysis of susceptible cells. A clear positive correlation was seen to exist between the susceptibility of cells to NK attack and their ability to inhibit NK cell-mediated lysis.

Collectively considered, the above results are incompatible with the concept that distinct subpopulations ("clones") of NK cells lyse different target cells. We have thus found no evidence to support the contention that NK "specificities" are clonally distributed. Indeed, recent studies on individual NK cell clones by Colin Brooks in this laboratory (4) have supported these conclusions. In some 20 NK clones examined to date for "specificity," we have never seen indications that clones kill a restricted number of targets. Indeed the spectrum of target cells lysed by NK cell clones directly mimicked that of the parent spleen cell populations from which the clones were derived. Our findings therefore are consistent with the proposition that suceptibility of target cells to NK attack reflects a shared membrane characteristic.

In light of these observations, we have begun to look for the potential molecular basis for NK cell mediated lysis of target cells. We have done so, by seeking variants from a given tumor cell which differ in their susceptibility to NK cell-mediated lysis (5).

To this end, L5178Y lymphoma cells were cloned by limiting dilutions in RPMI 1640 containing 10% fetal calf serum. Samples from each of the resulting clones, approximately 50 in number, were internally labeled by incubation with sodium ^{51}chromate and then tested for sensitivity to NK cell reactivity. As a result of this initial screening, one clone, (cl 27v), was selected as a population particularly susceptible to NK cell mediated lysis. This cell population has been now maintained _in vitro_ for a period exceeding 4 years and has retained its susceptibility phenotype throughout this period. Recloning the cl 27v cell population on several occasions has never revealed evidence of heterogeneity.

After _in vitro_ cloning, a portion of cl 27v cells was transferred to syngeneic, DBA/2 mice and passaged as ascites. In contrast to the _in vitro_ line, the ascites cells were very poorly lysed by NK cells. The ascites cells were then readapted _in vitro_ and have been termed clone 27av. These cells have been cultured for approximately 3 years and have maintained the insusceptible phenotype of the ascites throughout that period.

Clone 27v and cl 27av were equivalently susceptible to alloimmune cytotoxic T cells and were indistinguishable in their ability competitively to inhibit T cell-mediated lysis. Additionally, both cell lines were lysed to an equivalent extent by cytotoxic macrophages and by K cells.

Despite identity as targets for other cytotoxic cells there was a large and striking difference in the abilities of the two cell lines to serve as targets for NK cell-mediated lysis. This distinction was seen with NK cell populations from a variety of sources. These included NK cells derived from a number of lymphoid organelles, a variety of mouse strains, and even NK cell populations from human and subhuman primate sources. The cl 27av cell line was not lysed, even when interferon activated NK cell populations were employed as effector cells.

Not only were the cl 27av cell lines not susceptible to NK cell-mediated lysis, but these cells did not inhibit the lysis of cl 27v cells by NK effector populations. These findings suggest that the susceptible variant binds to NK cells, but that the insusceptible line does not.

These results led us to suggest that cl 27av cells might lack a membrane macromolecule present on cl 27v cells which dictates, or is associated with, susceptibility to NK cells. Thus, we surmised that the variants of L5178Y might serve as useful tools in the search for a molecular basis for NK susceptibility. In collaboration with Drs. D. Urdal, W. Young and S-I. Hakomori of the Biochemical Oncology Program at the Fred Hutchinson Cancer Research Center, we have begun an extensive and systematic biochemical analysis of membrane extracts from the cl 27v and cl 27av cells (6).

Following a number of observations that implicated glycoconjugates as cell surface receptor molecules (7,8), we examined the glycolipids of cl 27v and cl 27av cells.

The L5178Y variants were found to contain completely different glycolipids (6). Clone 27v cells, which were highly susceptible to NK cell attack contained a triplet of orcinol-positive bands that migrated on thin-layer chromatography in the area of the neutral glycolipid standards gangliotriosylceramide and globotetraosylceramide.

All three bands were shown conclusively to be gangliotriosylceramide (Gg_3cer). That is, each band contained the GalNacβ1-4Galβ1-4Glc trisaccraride present on this molecule. The resolution of Gg_3cer into three bands by thin-layer chromatography resulted from differences in the ceramide portion of this glycolipid. In contrast, clone 27av cells, which are resistant to NK mediated lysis, displayed a much simpler glycolipid profile. No glycolipids more complex than ceramide dihexoside and GM_3 were chemically detected. Cell sorter analysis indicated that 100% of the clone 27v cells stained brightly with the antiserum specific for asialo GM_2, whereas the clone 27av cells were uniformly negative. Furthermore, clone 27av cells were completely resistant to lysis by BALB/c monoclonal

IgM anti-asialo GM_2 antibody in the presence of complement, whereas cl 27v cells were effectively lysed by such treatment.

There was then, a positive correlation between the display of asialo GM_2 on the two L5178Y variants and their susceptibility to NK attack. Because of this correlation, we have directly addressed the possibility that asialo GM_2 might be the substrate, or "trigger," for NK cell-mediated lysis of L5178Y cells. This hypothesis was tested by attempting to inhibit NK cell-mediated lysis with anti-asialo GM_2 antibodies. This did not prove possible. Similarly, antiserum directed against MHC products on clone 27v cells also failed to inhibit the NK cell mediated lysis of these cells, although the same antiserum readily inhibited the T cell mediated lysis of the same target cells. Thus, although there was a marked concordance between asialo GM_2 display and susceptibility to NK cells, we have not yet been able to find any direct evidence for a causal relationship between such display and NK susceptibility.

Our current plans involve attempts to fuse asialo GM_2 onto cl 27av cells in order to see whether the NK susceptibility phenotype of these cells is altered. Prospectively, we will also examine other cell surface "markers" of cl 27v cells with a focus on unique glycoproteins.

DISCUSSION

The studies presented here do not support the concept that the "specificity" of NK cells is clonally distributed. Indeed, NK susceptible target cells effectively inhibit the lysis of other susceptible cells and the binding of NK cells to one susceptible target is associated with the removal of activity against all other target cells tested. These observations are, in general, concordant with results obtained from similar experiments by others (2,9), although some investigators, using "cold" target inhibition, have interpreted their results to support the hypothesis of restricted specificity (10).

Our findings, and those of several others, are most compatible with the proposition that susceptibility of target cells to NK attack may reflect a shared membrane characteristic which, for want of a better term, we might call an "antigen." (The structure shared would not necessarily have to be antigenic.) Others have argued, from essentially the same premises, that there are several (but a limited number of) subsets of NK cells, each of which is directed against a different "specificity" (10). It is interesting to note that recent studies involving NK cell clones (4,11) also failed to reveal evidence for a clonal expression of specificity.

It was initially proposed that NK cell activity was directed against either M-MuLV (12) or some type of endogenous MuLV (9,13), but later studies showed that susceptibility or resistance to NK cells did not correlate with the expression of either serologically defined MuLV antigen sor with group-specific antigenic determinants of MuLV (14).

In a recent study using an alternative approach, Roder et al (15) claim to have isolated target cell structures from NK susceptible cell lines which interact with NK cells. The approach was, however, indirect; detergent-solubilized cell surface proteins of YAC-1 lymphoma cells were assessed for their ability to inhibit the binding of mouse spleen cells to YAC targets (a binding assay which the same authors had found to correlate with NK cell activity). Roder et al found that NK susceptible target cells (but not NK insusceptible targets) possessed glycoproteins of 130,000, 160,000, and 240,000 molecular weight which were capable of preventing NK cell binding to susceptible target cells. No mention was made of the ability of these proteins to inhibit NK mediated lysis, and it remains unclear as to whether the cells measured in the binding assay, while they correlate with the cytotoxic activity of the population, are indeed the killer cells. Nevertheless, the findings are intriguing. They are among the most convincing data to date in support of the hypothesis that there are common cell surface macromolecules on NK susceptible target cells, and are the first to indicate that such common features might be membrane-associated glycoconjugates.

Our data presented above, are, in their broadest sense, compatible with Roder's observations, for we have observed a marked difference in the glycolipid profiles of two cell lines which are variants with respect to their susceptibility to the lytic action of NK cells. Thus, among approximately 20 clones of L5178Y which we have studied, only those bearing asialo GM_2 were susceptible to NK cell-mediated lysis (16). It should be added, however, that we have no direct evidence that causally links asialo GM_2 display with NK cell susceptibility and we have, thus far, been unable to inhibit lysis with anti-asialo GM_2 antibodies.

Finally, one other body of evidence suggests that glycoconjugate display may be related to the susceptibility of target tissues to natural cell-mediated cytotoxicity. This is the observation of Stutman et al (16) that NK cell mediated lysis is inhibited by a variety of simple sugars, most notably mannose. Two aspects of these observations are noteworthy: (a) inhibition with mannose was observed over a concentration range of 10 mM to 100 mM, and thus could not be attributed to toxic effects, and (b) the activity of cytotoxic T cells towards the same target cells was not affected by the presence of mannose, so that the inhibitory effects were selective for NK cell mediated lysis.

In sum, three pieces of evidence collectively suggest that recognition of cell surface carbohydrates is a salient feature of the action of NK cells: (a) the ability of glycoproteins found exclusively on NK susceptible target cells to inhibit NK cell binding, (b) inhibition of NK mediated lysis by simple sugars, and (c) the display of aberrant glycolipid forms on at least some NK susceptible target cells. It must be acknowledged, however, that to date the evidence is circumstantial, and more definitive evidence causally linking carbohydrate display with NK cell susceptibility is still awaited.

ACKNOWLEDGEMENTS

I thank the following colleagues who contributed significantly to various aspects of the work presented here: Barbara North Beck, Jeannine M. Durdik, Sen-Itiroh Hakomori, David L. Urdal, and William W. Young.

REFERENCES

1. Henney, C.S., Tracey, D., Durdik, J.M., and G. Klimpel. Am. J. Path. 93:459-468 (1978).
2. Kiessling, R., and H. Wigzell. Immunol. Rev. 44:165-208 (1979).
3. Durdik, J.M., Beck, B.N., Clark, E.A., and C.S. Henney. In "Natural Cell-Mediated Immunity Against Tumors," Herberman, R.B., ED., New York. Academic Press, pp. 805-817 (1980[a]).
4. Brooks, C.G., Kuribayashi, K., Sale, G.E., and C.S. Henney. J. Immunol., submitted for publication (1981).
5. Durdik, J.M., Beck, B.N., Clark, E.A., and C.S. Henney. J. Immunol. 125:683-688 (1980[b]).
6. Young, W.W., Durdik, J.M., Urdal, D., Hakomori, S., and C.S. Henney. J. Immunol. 126:1-6 (1981).
7. Fishman, P.H., and O. Brady. Science 194:906-915 (1976).
8. Hakomori, S., and W.W. young. Scand. J. Immunol. 6:97-117 (1978).
9. Sendo, F., Aoki T., Boyse, E.A., and C.K. Buafo. J. Natl. Cancer Inst. 55:603-609 (1975).
10. Nunn, M.E., and R.B. Herberman. J. Natl. Cancer Inst. 62: 765-771 (1979).
11. Dennert, G. Nature 287:47-49 (1980).
12. Kiessling, R., Klein, E., and H. Wigzell. Eur. J. Immunol. 5:112-117 (1975).
13. Zarling, J.M., Nowinski, R.C., and F.H. Bach. Proc. Natl. Acad. Sci. 72:2780-2784 (1975).
14. Becker S., Fenyo, E.M., and E. Klein. Eur. J. Immunol. 6:882-885 (1976).
15. Roder, J.D., Rosen, A., Fenyo, E.M., and F.A. Troy. Proc. Natl. Acad. Sci. 76:1405-1409 (1979).

16. Stutman, O., Dien, P., Wisun, R.E., and E.C. Lattime. Proc. Natl. Acad. Sci. 77:2895-2898 (1980).

Discussion

R. Herberman

I'd like to take issue with a number of points that you mentioned. In fact, I'd like to take issue on all of your main points. I'm aware of the data from your lab on the first two points in the mouse system in which you've not seen heterogeneity in the specificity of NK cells, either by cold-target inhibition or by monolayer absorption. But there are also some quite well documented examples, from my lab, and Noel Warner's lab, and from others in which by cold-target inhibition one doesn't see reciprocal inhibition.

C. Henney

I don't take exception to that. The point of trying to make this kind of synthesis is if one compares the two general cases, clonally distributed reactivities versus not, one finds a very restricted number of reactivities that cannot account for the vast array of target cells that are killed. Whether in fact there is "one specificity" which all NK cells see, or a limited number, I think for the purpose of this discussion doesn't concern me largely. Whether it's one, two, three, four, it's not the same sort of array that one might see, for example, with the T cell receptor.

R. Herberman

I'll certainly buy that. But I think it is important to distinguish between one versus five specificities and I would submit that the data are more compatible with an oligoclonal than a monoclonal specificity.

C. Henney

I'll accept five. That's fine.

P. Golstein

Perhaps we could have Ron's opinion on the NK clone problem. I mean, you were taking issue against a narrow range of target specificities.

R. Herberman

Yes. I might just briefly summarize some information about the clones. It's true that with most of the published information about NK clones, there is very little indication of heterogeneity. But I think this is partly related to the way the clones were selected. They were selected for anti-YAC activity in the mouse, for example, which tends to restrict the amount of difference. We have seen both with some clones from the human and the mouse limited heterogeneity among the clones. We have some human clones, for example, which will kill K562 very well and not other targets, and some others which kill other targets and not K562. We also have some mouse clones which will kill some monolayer targets but not YAC and vice versa.

C. Henney

Polly Brooks has just finished looking at 21 mouse NK clones against 42 targets. We have never found a clone which kills one target exclusively. There may be quantitative differences between the activity against this panel of targets between one clone and the next, but the major point is that you do not find an anti-K562 clone which kills K562 and doesn't kill other cells.

R. Herberman

We've seen otherwise. We've seen qualitative differences among clones.

C. Henney

You've seen clones that kill one target and kill no other target?

R. Herberman

No. I wouldn't argue for that kind of fine restriction...

C. Henney

OK. I don't know whether this is going to get us very far either. I think we can beg to differ and clearly we do.

CELL SURFACE PROPERTIES INFLUENCING TARGET CELL SENSITIVITY FOR NK LYSIS

Rolf Kiessling and Alvar Grönberg

Department of Tumor Biology
Karolinska Institutet
S 104 01 Stockholm, Sweden

INTRODUCTION

NK cells are defined by the ability of lymphoid cells from non-immunized or non-primed donors to lyse sensitive targets in short term cytotoxicity assays. Since any known "immunogen" is lacking in this system, this raises obvious difficulties in discussing the nature of the NK target structure. We will here make a brief summary of different cell surface properties which have been suggested to be of importance in conferring NK susceptibility to a target cell, focusing on some recent work from our laboratory.

Examples of "Non-specific" and "Specific" Cell Membrane Properties With a Reported Influence on Rendering a Target Cell Susceptible to NK Lysis

Most reports have demonstrated at least a certain "selectivity" in the lytic activity of mouse NK cells, as measured both in direct cytolytic assays or by cold target competition tests. Thus, certain in vitro passaged leukemia lines are generally found to be the most sensitive targets, although sensitivity has also been observed with some solid tumors (1) and even with primary normal tissues (2). Syngeneic as well as allogeneic tumors are susceptible to lysis (3,4) and even xenogeneic targets can be lysed, indicating some specificities conserved across the species barrier (5), although the most efficient lysis generally occurs with target cells and effectors from the same species. One point to be stressed is that the classification of a given target as sensitive or resistant depends on the degree of activation of the NK effector. Thus, with highly activated NK cells lysis can be seen against cells normally resistant to "endogenous" NK cells. The common interpretation of this is that activated cells lower the "threshold" for the NK cells to recognize their targets. Only scarce evidence exists that activated NK cells recognize "new" or qualitatively different specificities than endogenous ones (6), although this point deserves further investigation.

There are several questions to be asked about the "specificity" of NK cells. First, it could indeed be questioned whether the binding of an NK cell to a target involves at all a recognition event of a "receptor-antigen" type. Thus several entirely non-specific properties of a tumor target cell are known to influence the sensitivity to lysis (see Table 1). Becker et al. demonstrated that the liability to hydrophobic interaction of mouse lymphoma cells, as measured by aqueous biphasic partitioning, could be related to their susceptibility to lysis by NK cells (3). Since cell surface sialic acid would influence hydrophobicity, this finding is in line with recent results from our laboratory. Using a panel of NK insensitive and sensitive variants derived from the YAC lymphoma we found an inverse correlation between the levels of neuraminidase-releasable surface sialic acid and sensitivity to NK cells (7). Interferon (IFN) has

TABLE 1. Examples of "non-specific" and "specific" cell membrane properties reported to influence NK killing

Non-specific	Ref.	Specific	Ref.
Cell surface hydrophobicity	Becker et al., 1979 (3)	Virally induced antigens	Herberman et al., 1975 (4); Hatzfeld et al., 1981 (26)
Sialic acid composition	Yogeeswaran et al., 1981 (7)	Differentiation antigens	Gidlund et al., 1981 (22)
Glycolipid composition	Young et al., 1981 (10); Yogeeswaran et al., 1981 (7)	MHC antigens	Vanky et al., 1980 (30)
Cell membrane repair mechanisms	Kunkel and Welsh, 1981 (12)	Carbohydrate composition	Stutman et al., 1980 (29)
Ability to activate NK cells in vitro	Timonen et al., 1980 (13)	Specific glycoproteins	Roder et al., 1979 (28)

been shown to have a dual role in the NK system; while augmenting the effector cell lytic activity it seems to confer protection to the target cell (8,9). Further supporting the influence of sialic acid on the NK system we have recently found an increase in lipid-associated cell surface sialic acid as a result of IFN treatment of the target cell (Yogeeswaran et al., unpublished results) suggesting that this molecule may play a protective role from NK lysis in IFN treated cells. This would then suggest that cell surface sialic acid may reduce NK sensitivity either directly by masking the target antigen or indirectly by negative charge repulsion. However, we have failed to fully restore the sensitivity of the NK resistant or IFN protected targets by removal of terminal sialic acid residues from cell surface glycoproteins and glycolipids with neuraminidase (7). Thus, the reduction in sensitivity in NK-resistant variant cell lines may not be simply due to high negative charge or antigen masking, but may also involve a secondary recognition event.

Young et al. (10) have characterized clones of the L5178Y lymphoma with respect to glycolipid expression correlating to their NK susceptibility. They found that clones lacking asialo G_{M2} were NK resistant, although they failed to see any simple relationship between the quantity of asialo G_{M2} and NK sensitivity when investigating a larger number of individual subclones of the same lymphoma. We have recently confirmed their finding in a study of cell surface glycolipid composition of NK sensitive and insensitive variants of the YAC lymphoma (7). Only one neutral glycolipid, with the chromatographic migration of asialo G_{M2}, showed a positive correlation with sensitivity of target cells to NK lysis. From these two studies it could be concluded that in mouse lymphomas asialo G_{M2} probably must be displayed on the cell surface in order to confer susceptibility to NK cells, but that increased amounts of this glycolipid do not correlate with increased susceptibility to attack. This conclusion has been further substantiated by failure to inhibit NK cell mediated lysis by anti-asialo G_{M2} serum, and to increase NK sensitivity in resistant cell lines by enrichment with asialo G_{M2} (10, and our unpublished results).

These observations suggest that asialo G_{M2} alone may not be the target structure for NK cells. In addition, in the present study we observed that the concentrations of higher ganglioside homologues with migration of G_{M1}, G_{D1a}, G_{D1b} and G_T correlated positively with sensitivity of target cells to NK cell mediated lysis. These observations of the presence of asialo G_{M2}, G_{M2}, G_{D1a}, G_{D1b} in NK-sensitive target cells suggest the involvement of the alternate pathway for ganglioside biosynthesis (CM $\longrightarrow$ CD $\longrightarrow$ asialo G_{M2} $\longrightarrow$ G_{M1} $\longrightarrow$ G_{D1a} $\longrightarrow$ G_{D1b} $\longrightarrow$ G_T)(11). In contrast, NK-insensitive targets lack asialo G_{M2} suggesting that the classical pathway for ganglioside biosynthesis (CM $\longrightarrow$ CD $\longrightarrow$ G_{M3} $\longrightarrow$ G_{M2} $\longrightarrow$ G_{M1} $\longrightarrow$ G_{D1a} $\longrightarrow$ G_{D1b} $\longrightarrow$ G_T) may be operative in these cell lines. Further work is necessary to document the metabolic basis of the differences between the variant cells and their relationship to susceptibility to NK cell mediated lysis. Assay of the critical enzyme asialo G_{M2} : sialyl transferase, which converts asialo G_{M2} to G_{M2}, should help resolve questions on these apparent differences in glycolipid metabolism. It should be added that the observed requirement for asialo G_{M2} to be expressed on NK sensitive cell lines does not seem to be valid in human NK systems, where several NK sensitive cell lines do not express this molecule (Yogeeswaran and Grönberg, unpublished observation).

One point to be stressed when discussing target susceptibility to NK lysis, is that this may not just reflect the availability of the target structure. Other phenomena, such as the ability of target cells to repair their membranes (12) or to activate NK cells in vitro (13), may play a role in determining their sensitivity.

A wide variety of more specific cell surface molecules have been suggested as "antigens" for NK cells (see Table 1). One can ask whether this indeed indicates that NK cells can recognize several different types of cell surface molecules, and if they may express individually specific, clonally distributed receptors of varying specificity. In our own studies in the murine lymphoma system, we have failed to find any evidence for such a clonal variability in the specificity of NK cells (for discussion on this point see Kiessling and Wigzell (14)) but reports on such a heterogeneity pattern have been coming forth in studies on mouse as well as human NK cells (4,15). Arguments on NK cell specificity in relation to clonally distributed receptors for diverse target structures will only be settled in a conclusive manner with the availability of cloned NK cells in vitro. Reports on NK cell lines already exist but have so far yielded inconclusive results; while Dennert (16) found that each of a number of long term cell lines established from cloned NK cells exhibited the same rank order of cytolysis against a panel of diverse target cells, Nabel et al. (17) concluded that each clone displayed a specificity of a more restricted nature.

There are several lines of evidence indicating that cells within one lineage are more susceptible to NK lysis in their early stages of differentiation. This has been shown with both normal and malignant cells as NK targets. With regard to normal cells, it is particularly intriguing that human bone marrow contains a fraction of cells susceptible to NK lysis (18). Moreover, we have recently demonstrated that human NK cells, fractionated on Percoll density gradients, can inhibit granulocytic macrophage colony forming cells (GM-CFC) in vitro (18) but do not seem to exert any effect on stem cells of the erythroid lineage (see Figure 1; 19). Although in this system it is not clear whether NK cells are active via a lytic mechanism or via some cytostatic mechanism, such as their ability to produce IFN (13) which may inhibit stem cell matur-

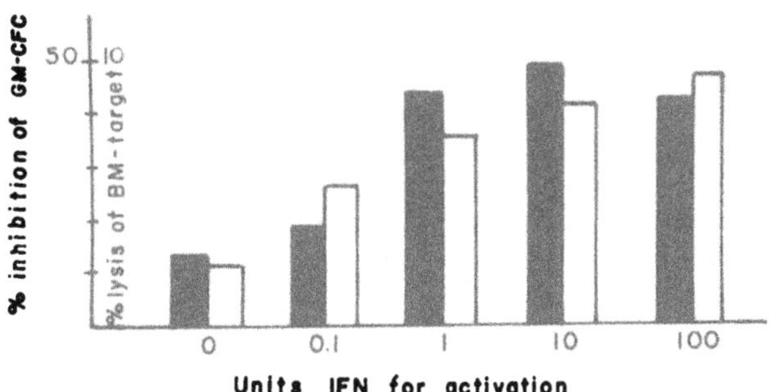

Fig. 1. Inhibition of granulocytic macrophage colony forming cells (GM-CFC)(■) and activation of natural killer cell lysis against bone marrow (BM)(□) by autologous peripheral blood lymphocytes (PBL) preincubated with different amounts of interferon at a PBL:BM ratio of 5:1 and 25:1 respectively.

ation (20), these experiments indicate that NK cells may have important stem cell regulatory functions in vivo.

In agreement with the concept that NK cells may function to lyse cells at a particular stage of their differentiation, Stern et al (21) found that embryonal carcinoma cells representing various stages of differentiation displayed a strikingly different pattern with regard to NK susceptibility. Here, only cell types representing early stages were sensitive to NK-mediated cytolysis in contrast to the more differentiated endodermal cell lines which showed close to complete resistance. This would support the view that, depending on the stage of differentiation, normal as well as malignant cells may be under surveillance by natural killer cells in vivo.

Recently, the same authors addressed the question of differentiation-related NK susceptibility taking advantage of defined cell lines in vitro with known ability to undergo controlled differentiation in the presence of various agents (22). Three different tumor cell lines (a human erythroid leukemia, a human histiocytic lymphoma and a murine Friend-virus leukemia) were explored. They all did demonstrate a striking positive correlation between a decrease in NK susceptibility linked with the induction of differentiation using different inducers. This finding further supported the view that susceptibility to natural killer cell mediated lysis may vary in relation to the stage of diffentiation of the target cell. It was pointed out, however, that NK sensitivity is not always restricted to target cells at an early stage of their respective differentiation lineage. In fact, examples of highly differentiated tumor cells, e.g., myeloma cells being quite susceptible to NK lysis (23), the wide variability of NK sensitivity amongst tumors of the same histogenetic type (24) and the fact that treatment of tumor cells with butyrate in some cases can lead to an increase in NK sensitivity (25), strongly argue against too simplistic a view in this regard. The results do, however, demonstrate that the various differentiation stages expressed by a particular cell type in a defined differentation pathway are important in determining NK susceptibility.

ACKNOWLEDGEMENTS

This investigation was supported by grant CA 26782-02, awarded by the National Cancer Institute, DHEW and the Swedish Cancer Society.

REFERENCES

1. Stutman, O., Paige, C., and E. Figarella. Natural cytotoxicity against solid tumors in mice. I. Strain and age distribution and target cell susceptibility. J. Immunol. 121:1819 (1978).
2. Hansson, M., Kiessling, R., Andersson, B., Kärre, K., and J. Roder. Natural killer (NK) cell sensitive T-cell subpopulation in the thymus: Inverse correlation to NK activity of the host. Nature 278:174 (1979).
3. Becker, S., Stendahl, O., and K.-E. Magnusson. Physicochemical characteristics of tumor cells susceptible to lysis by natural killer (NK) cells. Immunol. Communications 8:73 (1979).
4. Herberman, R.B., Nunn, M.E., and D.H. Lavrin. Natural cytotoxic reactivity of mouse lymphoid cells against syngeneic and allogeneic tumors. I. Distribution of reactivity and specificity. Int. J. Cancer 16:216 (1975).
5. Hansson, M., Kärre, K., Bakacs, T., Kiessling, R., and G. Klein. Intra- and interspecies reactivity of human and mouse natural killer (NK) cells. J. Immunol. 121:6 (1979).
6. Welsh, R.M., Jr., Zinkernagel, R.M., and L.A. Hallenbeck. Cytotoxic cells induced during lymphocytic choriomeningitis virus infection of mice. II. "Specificities" of the natural killer cells. J. Immunol. 122:475 (1979).
7. Yogeeswaran, G., Grönberg, A., Hansson, M., Dalianis, T., Kiessling, R., and R.M. Welsh. Correlation of glycosphingolipids and sialic acid in YAC-1 lymphoma variants with their

sensitivity to natural killer cell mediated lysis. Int. J. Cancer 28:517 (1981).
8. Trinchieri, G., and D. Santoli. Anti-viral activity induced by culturing lymphocytes with tumor-derived or virus-transformed cells. Enhancement of human natural killer cell activity by interferon and antagonistic inhibition of susceptibility of target cells to lysis. J. Exp. Med. 147:1314 (1978).
9. Welsh, R., Kärre, K., Hansson, M., Kunkel, L., and R. Kiessling. Interferon-mediated protection of normal and tumor target cells against lysis by mouse natural killer cells. J. Immunol. 126: 219 (1981).
10. Young, W.H., Durdik, J.M., Urdal, D., Hakamori, S., and C.S. Henney. Lymphoma cell glycolipids and NK cell susceptibility. J. Immunol. 126:1 (1981).
11. Yogeeswaran, G., and B.S. Stein. Glycosphingolipids of metastatic variant RNA virus-transformed nonproducer Balb/3T3 cell lines: altered metabolism and cell surface exposure. J. Natl. Cancer Inst. 65:967 (1980).
12. Kunkel, L.A., and R.M. Welsh. Metabolic inhibitors render "resistant" target cells sensitive to natural killer cell mediated lysis. Int. J. Cancer 27:73 (1981).
13. Timonen, T., Saksela, E., Virtanen, I., and K. Cantell. Natural killer cells are responsible for the interferon production induced in human lymphocytes by tumor cell contact. Eur. J. Immunol. 10:422 (1980).
14. Kiessling, R., and H. Wigzell. An analysis of the murine NK cell as to structure, function and biological relevance. Immunol. Rev. 44:165 (1979).
15. Jensen, P.J., and H.S. Koren. Heterogeneity within the population of NK and K cells. J. Immunol. 124:395 (1980).
16. Dennert, G., Yogeeswaran, G., and S. Yamagata. Cloned lines with natural killer activity: specificity, function, and cell surface markers. J. Exp. Med. 153:545 (1981).
17. Nabel, G., Bucalo, L.R., Allard, J., Wigzell, H., and H. Cantor. Multiple activities of a cloned cell line mediating natural killer cell function. J. Exp. Med. 153:1582 (1981).
18. Hansson, M., Kiessling, R., and B. Andersson. Human fetal thymus and bone marrow contain target cells for natural killer cells. Eur. J. Immunol. 11:8 (1981).
19. Hansson, M., Beran, M. Andersson, B., and R. Kiessling. Inhibition of GM-CFC maturation by autologous and allogeneic human NK cells. Submitted for publication.
20. McNeill, T.A., and I. Gresser. I. Inhibition of haemopoietic colony growth by interferon preparations from different sources. Nature New Biol. 244:173 (1973).
21. Stern, P., Gidlund, M., Örn, A., and H. Wigzell. Natural killer cells mediate lysis of embryonal carcinoma cells lacking MHC. Nature 285:341 (1980).
22. Gidlund, M., Örn, A., Pattengale, P.K., Jansson, M., Wigzell, H., and K. Nilsson. Natural killer (NK) cells kill tumor cells

at a given stage of differentiation. Nature, in press.
23. Pattengale, P.K., Gidlund, M., Nilsson, K., Sundström, C., Örn, A., and H. Wigzell. Lysis of human B lymphocyte-derived lymphoma/leukemia cells of established cell lines by inteferon-activated natural killer (NK) cells. Int. J. Cancer 28:459 (1981).
24. Riesenfeldt, I., Örn, A., Gidlund, M., Axberg, I., Alm, G., and H. Wigzell. Positive correlation between in vitro NK activity and in vivo resistance towards AKR lymphoma cells. Int. J. Cancer 25:399 (1980).
25. Blazar, B., Patarroyo, M., Klein, E., and G. Klein. Increased sensitivity of human lymphoid lines to natural killer cells after induction of the Epstein-Barr viral cycle by superinfection or sodium butyrate. J. Exp. Med. 151:614 (1980).
26. Hatzfeld, A., Pinter, A., Koo, G.C., and Boyse, E.A. Relation of gp70 to spontaneous cytolytic activity of mouse spleen cells. Immunogen. 12:153 (1981).
27. Koren, H.S., Andersson, S.J., and J.W. Larrick. In vitro activation of a human macrophage-like cell line. Nature 279:328 (1979)
28. Roder, J.C., Rosen, A., Fenyö, E.M., and F.A. Troy. Target effector interactions in the natural killer system. Isolation of target structure. Proc. Natl. Acad. Sci. USA 76:1405 (1979).
29. Stutman, O., Dien, P., Wisun, R., Pecoraro, G., and E.C. Lattime. Natural cytotoxic (NC) cells against solid tumors in mice: Some target cell characteristics and blocking of cytotoxicity by D-mannose. In "Natural cell-mediated immunity against tumors." R.B. Herberman, Ed. Academic Press, p. 949 (1980).
30. Vanky, F.T., Argov, S.A., Einhorn, S.A., and E. Klein. Role of allo-antigens in natural killing. Allogeneic but not autologous tumor biopsy cells are sensitive for interferon-induced cytotoxicity of human blood lymphocytes. J. Exp. Med. 151: 1151 (1980).

DISCUSSION

P. Golstein

Have these experiments, showing that NK cells have a tendency to kill allo more than self been done with purified T-deprived populations?

R. Kiessling

No, they have not been done with T-deprived populations. There still remains a possibility that it may represent some kind of in vitro activated T cell. That's a good point, I think. We haven't really excluded that possibility.

P. Golstein

I mean it could also be allo-activated T cells pushing NK cells?

R.Kiessling

Yes. That's a possibility. I think there may very well be some kind of in vitro activation going on in that system, because it's also a long-term incubation assay, where we incubate for 16 to 18 hours and they are not sensitive in the short term cytotoxic assays.

M. Mayer

Let me ask you a couple of questions about the relationship betwen K cells and NK cells. It's not entirely clear to me to what extent separation experiments, by selective depletion of one or the other population, bear on that question? That is, if you attempt to remove the cells that have Fc receptors, does that lead to a relative enrichment of the remaining cells with respect to NK activity?

R. Kiessling

That of course is the clear similarity between K cells and NK cells, that both seem to have Fc receptors. In the human, it's very easily detected. In the mouse somewhat less easily detectable.

M. Mayer

Now what about comparisons of the relative velocities of killing? If one compares the velocity of killing with the same population of targets in the same concentration, but in one case you introduce antibody and the other case you do not, how much does the antibody change the rate of killing?

R. Kiessling

I think the kinetics of the rate of killing are very similar in the two systems. The problem in studying K cell activity is of course that we very often have a background of NK activity in the system, so that you have to choose the target which is resistant to NK cells.

M. Mayer

I mean targets that are susceptible both ways. What is the rate per minute or per hour of how many cells are killed without antibody? And then with antibody? That's what I'm going after.

R. Kiessling

I don't think I can give you any precise figures on that.

C. Henney

If Ron Herberman doesn't have it I suspect that it's not been done.

R. Herberman

As Rolf said, we've avoided doing those experiments because of difficulties of interpretation when using a sensitive target. Our comparisons have been between NK on the one hand versus other targets that are resistant to NK that are coated with antibody. And there I would agree with Rolf that the kinetics are the same. But we've not done the experiment that you're asking about.

P. Perlmann

Many workers do not see the good correlation between binding and killing that you report. Is this due to the fact that your effector cells are purified on a nylon wool column?

R. Kiessling

I think that one of the reasons that we see it is that we limit our studies to rather homogeneous types of tumors. If we look at a wider variety of different tumors, then we may not see this correlation as clearly. Also, as I understand it, if you look at some human suspension tumors the correlation between frequency of target binding and killing is not that clear either. What you have to look for then is more of the frequency of binding cells which go on to kill rather than the frequency of binders totally. I think that the disadvantage with the mouse target binding assays of course is it's difficult to get a pure NK population. One has to go to some other fractionation to get LGL in the mouse system similar to what people are now doing in the human system.

P. Lachmann

I was just going to take minor exception to the general statement that human NK cells have Fc receptors. I have no doubt whatever, that if you look at systems where you're killing measles virus persistently in infected HeLa cells, you can show this activity with no difficulty at all in Fc negative cells.

P. Perlmann

One of the difficulties is that you may have a preparation of purified T cells which have no Fc receptors for IgG. But if you culture these cells under certain conditions, for instance in the presence of some tumor cells or foreign cells, they may rapidly develop Fc receptors.

C. Henney

I think there's general accord that there's considerable heterogeneity within the NK population with respect to a whole number of markers and that the display of those markers in fact can change with culture and isolation procedures.

R. Herberman

It's frequently said that Fc receptor negative populations in various situations can still have NK activity. However, part of that may be the presence of low affinity Fc receptor positive cells. If one separates by rosetting to get a putative Fc receptor negative population there's usually still ADCC activity present in those populations, which is a clear demonstration that there are Fc receptor positive cells there. That is particularly true in the mouse. A very good example of that is with the cultured cells and IL2. It's been virtually impossible to show that most of those cells are Fc receptor positive by rosetting with EA, yet they have good levels of ADCC activity.

SOLUBLE CYTOTOXIC FACTORS AND THE MECHANISM OF NK CELL MEDIATED CYTOTOXICITY[1]

Benjamin Bonavida and Susan C. Wright

Department of Microbiology and Immunology
UCLA School of Medicine
University of California
Los Angeles, California 90024

[1]Supported by Grant CA-13800 awarded by the National Cancer Institute and in part by National Cancer Institute Training Grant CA-09120 to S.C. Wright

INTRODUCTION

The mechanism of lysis by natural killer (NK) cells has been delineated into three discrete steps, namely binding or recognition, programming for lysis or the lethal hit, and target cell disintegration independent of the killer cell. This delineation closely resembles the mechanism of lysis by cytotoxic T lymphocytes (1). However, unlike the T cell system, lysis by NK cells is not antigen restricted and a wide range of target cells is sensitive to the NK lytic attack. These results may be best explained if a common denominator is intimately involved in the mechanism of lysis by NK cells. What is the nature of this common denominator and how can it be verified experimentally? We have proposed a model which could accommodate the known features of the NK cytotoxic system. This model suggests that the initial recognition and interaction between an NK effector cell and a target cell leads to activation of the lytic step. This activation step may result in the release of cytotoxic mediators which can lyse the sensitive NK targets. Data presented in this communication support the proposal that it is the target cell's sensitivity to the lytic activity of the cytotoxic mediators that is the "common denominator" of the NK system.

In this study, we will focus on the possible role of a soluble cytotoxic mediator in NKCMC. Several lymphotoxins have been described in a variety of experimental systems (2-6). Although evidence has been produced which suggests that lymphotoxins play a role in alloimmune T cell-mediated cytotoxicity and in ADCC, they have not been studied in the NK system. Our approach has been to delineate whether soluble cytotoxic mediators are involved in NKCMC and if detected, could they play a role in the mechanism of NKCMC. Our studies show that NKCF can be detected and are selectively cytotoxic for NK sensitive targets. Furthermore, several lines of evidence are presented which establish that there exists a good correlation between lysis by NKCF and lysis in NKCMC.

MATERIALS AND METHODS

These have been described in detail in previous publications (7-9). Briefly, NKCF have been obtained from normal mouse spleen cells or human peripheral blood cells following stimulation with PHA or NK sensitive targets. Cytotoxicity was measured indirectly using a miniaturized Marbrook chamber separated by a nucleopore membrane in which the lower chamber contained the effector cells and stimulatory agent, and the upper chamber contained the target cells. Lysis of target cells was measured by trypan blue dye exclusion. Alternatively, cytotoxicity was measured in a microassay by preparing cell-free supernatants containng NKCF and testing for cytotoxicity on target cells by trypan blue exclusion or ^{51}Cr-release assay. The cytotoxic assays were 16-48 hours long. The production of NKCF in cell-free supernatants and testing NKCF activities in the microassay system have been recently described. Essentially, spleen cells were stimulated by YAC-1 cells in FCS-free medium for 24-48 hours at 37°C. The supernatant was filtered through 0.45 μ filters and stored at -20°C until tested. The supernatant was tested on microtiter plates and lysis was detected by trypan blue uptake or by release of ^{51}Cr from dead targets.

RESULTS AND DISCUSSION

Generation and Detection of NKCF Selectively Lytic to NK-Sensitive Targets

Our initial studies to delineate NKCF have used the same conditions previously used for the detection of lymphotoxins with several modifications. Thus, murine spleen cells were stimulated with PHA-coated L929 fibroblasts, PHA, or Con A in a miniaturized Marbrook chamber. The effector cells were cultured in the top chamber on a 0.2μ nucleopore membrane. Significant target lysis was obtained 24-40 hours following culture as assessed by trypan blue dye uptake. Only murine targets sensitive to NK activity in a 4 hour ^{51}Cr-release assay (YAC-1 and R1♂1) or an 18 hour ^{51}Cr-release assay (FLD-3 and WEHI-164) were lysed by the mediators (Table I)(7). These preliminary findings suggested that the soluble mediators may play a role in NKCMC.

TABLE I. GENERATION AND DETECTION OF NKCF SELECTIVE FOR NK TARGETS

	Percent Cytotoxicity			
	Direct		Indirect	
Target	Marbrook Chambers PHA, Con A	YAC-1	Micro Assay 48 h.	^{51}Cr-release 16 h.
YAC-1	56	30	21	25
RL♂1	35	28	ND	ND
YAC ascites	3	ND	ND	ND
RL♂1 ascites	0	ND	ND	ND
FLD-3	ND	25	15	ND
WEHI-164	ND	14	18	17
P815	0	3	0	0
EL4	0	2	0	0
AKSL2	1	1	0	0
K562	ND	3	0	4
Molt-4	ND	4	0	ND

However, in order to establish a role for a soluble mediator in NKCMC, we were faced with establishing conditions which mimic the NK cytotoxic system. A first requisite was the demonstration that NK targets stimulate release of NKCF selective for NK target killing and that NK effectors release the NKCF. These requirements were experimentally verified. Thus, coculture of murine spleen cells with YAC-1 cells induced release of NKCF active in both the Marbrook culture assay system and in the microassay system. The effector cells which release NKCF were shown to be Thy 1.2 negative and asialo-GM1 positive. Furthermore, lysis was selective for NK target cells. These results, therefore, suggested that lysis of NK targets by NKCF correlated well with lysis in NKCMC (9).

Correlation Between Lysis of NK Targets by NKCF and Lysis in NKCMC

We were encouraged with the above studies since they provided a good system to explore the role of NKCF in NKCMC. We have approached the studies in two directions, namely to verify experi-

TABLE II. CORRELATION BETWEEN LYSYS BY NKCF AND NKCMC

Lysis by NKCF	Lysis in NKCMC
A. Good Correlation	
1. Selective lysis of NK targets (used in short- and long-term assays)	1. Selective lysis of NK target
2. Species specificity of NKCF	2. Species specificity of NKCMC
3. NK targets stimulate production of NKCF	3. NK targets activate NK cytotoxicity
4. NKCF released by NK effector cells	4. Lysis by NK effector cells
5. High NK strains (CBA, nude) release potent NKCF	5. High NK activity by high NK strains
6. NKCF neutralized by certain monosaccharides	6. NKCMC is inhibited by certain monosaccharides.
7. Binding of NKCF by NK targets	7. Binding of NK-sensitive targets by NK effector cells
8. Neutralization of NKCF by RAT*	8. Inhibition of NKCMC by RAT*
9. Lysis of NK_B targets requires 16-24 hours	9. Lysis of NK_B target requires 16-24 hours
10. Release of mediator 16-18 hours	10. Release of mediators for NK_B target may take place in 6-11 hours
B. Poor Correlation	
1. Release of mediator 6-18 hours	1. Release of mediator must be immediate in short-term NKCMC
2. Lysis of NK_A target requires 12-16 hours	2. Lysis is less than 2-4 hours

mentally the role of NKCF in NKCMC and to biochemically characterize the NKCF. In this report, we will only describe the known features of cytotoxicity by NKCF and their relationship to NKCMC. The salient features of these studies are summarized in Table II. Clearly, several requirements have been met in order to implicate a role of NKCF in NKCMC. These include: (1) NK targets are selectively lysed by NKCF in both the short-term and long-term assays (Table I). As in NKCMC, NK targets grown in culture are susceptible to lysis, whereas NK targets grown in vivo are resistant to lysis. (2) There was a remarkable species specificity of NKCF. Thus, murine NKCF lysed only murine NK targets (7). (3) NK-sensitive targets stimulate the production of NKCF, whereas some NK-resistant targets are poor stimulators (9). (4) The production of NKCF is mediated by NK effector cells as shown by elimination of its production following treatment of effector cells with anti-asialo-GM1 and complement, but not with anti-Thy 1.2 (9). These studies indicate that production of NKCF does not require mature T lymphocytes since both Thy 1.2 depleted spleen cell populations and nude spleen cells produce NKCF. (5) There was a good correlation between the potency of NKCF released in different strains of mice and their ability to mediate NKCMC in ^{51}Cr-release assay. Thus, both CBA and BALB/c nu/nu mice release potent NKCF, whereas Bg/Bg mice release NKCF with poor activity (9). (6) There was, to a certain extent, selective absorption of NKCF by NK-sensitive targets, while NK-resistant targets absorbed NKCF poorly (9). (7) The relationship between NKCF and NKCMC was investigated using blocking antibody reagents. Thus, RAT* serum which was shown to inhibit NKCMC also neutralized the cytotoxic activity of NKCF (8). These results, therefore, suggested that there exists a close association between lysis in NKCMC and lysis by NKCF.

Other aspects of lysis by NKCF necessitated further studies and interpretations. For instance, while lysis in NKCMC takes place in a short time (2-4 hours), lysis by NKCF requires 16-28 hours. It may be that NKCF becomes too dilute after diffusing away from the effector cell to mediate lysis within 2-4 hours. Also, it may be that NKCFs lose activity after they are released into the soluble form and are most active when effector cells are in contact with target cells. Alternative possibilities have not been ruled out and are being seriously considered to resolve this issue.

Proposed Model for NKCMC

Based on our studies and the known characteristics of the mechanism of lysis by NK effector cells, we propose a model for NKCMC which takes into account a role for NKCF. According to this model, cell mediated cytotoxicity occurs as a discrete series of events which ultimately lead to lysis of the target cell. The first step is NK-effector cell recognition and binding to the NK-sensitive target. In the second step, the target cells must deliver a signal to the effector cell to activate the lytic machinery. This signal may be delivered through the NK effector cell receptor or through other receptors. The third step involves the binding of or transfer of NKCF from the effector cell to the target cell membrane. The final event is target cell death due to the cytotoxic activity of NKCF and independent of the presence of the effector cell. If any of these steps is interrupted or defective in any given effector-target cell interaction, then target cell lysis will not take place. The proposed model also offers several possible reasons why a target cell may resist NK cytotoxic activity. The target cell may not be recognized by the effector cell or, if it is, it may not be able to signal the effector cell to activate the lytic mechanism. Alternatively, target cells may lack binding sites for NKCF or else may be inherently resistant to the lytic activity of NKCF after they bind to the membrane.

The uniqueness of this model is that several features proposed can be tested and verified experimentally. Our studies at present are pursuing such investigations.

CONCLUDING REMARKS

The studies described above suggest, for the first tme, that a soluble cytotoxic mediator may be involved in the mechanism of NK cytotoxicity. Several lines of evidence have been presented that support the contention that a strong correlation exists between lysis by NKCF and lysis in NKCMC. However, there remain a few logistic problems which need to be resolved before implicating a role of NKCF in NKCMC. These problem, once, resolved, should provide some insight into the lytic stage of NKCMC. Furthermore, biochemical studies to characterize the cytotoxic factors and delineate their mode of action are now feasible. The extension of the NK studies to other cytotoxic systems (e.g., CTL, ADCC, macrophages) awaits direct examination).

SUMMARY

Soluble cytotoxic factors from mouse spleen cells have been shown to selectively lyse NK sensitive target cells. Lysis of target cels is assessed by trypan blue uptake or ^{51}Cr-release assay in a 16-48 hour assay. The possible role of such natural killer cytotoxic factors (NKCF) in the mechanism of natural killer cell-mediated cytotoxicity (NKCMC) has been examined. Several lines of evidence are presented which indicate that there exists a strong correlation between lysis by NKCF and lysis in NKCMC. For instance, (1) NKCF are generated following stimulation of mouse spleen cells with NK sensitive targets; (2) Lysis of NKCF is selective for NK sensitive targets and is species specific; (3) Mice with poor NK activity, such as Bg/Bg mice, produce poor NKCF: (4) There is concomittant inhibition of NKCMC and NKCF activities by blocking

RAT* serum; and (5) Several known characteristics of the mechanism of NKCMC are shown to be shared in the NKCF system. Based on these findings, we propose a model for NKCMC in which lysis by NK effector cells is the result of multiple steps, namely target binding to an NK effector cell, activation of the lytic mechanism, and involvement of NKCF to mediate lysis. Accordingly, for targets to be NK sensitive, they ought to be able to interact and bind with NK effectors, activate the NK cells, bind NKCF, and be sensitive to the NKCF lytic activity.

REFERENCES

1. Martz, E. Contemp. Top. in Immunobiol. 7:301 (1977).
2. Walker, S., and Z.S. Lucas. Transpl. Proc. 5:137 (1973).
3. Hiserodt, J.C., Tiangco, G.T., and G.A. Granger. J. Immunol. 123:332 (1979).
4. Granger, G.A., Hiserodt, J.C., and C. Ware. In "Biology of the Lymphokines," S. Cohen, E. Pick, and J.J. Oppenheim, eds., p. 141. Academic Press, New York (1979).
5. Kondo, L.L. Roseneau, W., and D.W. Wara. J. Immunol. 126: 1131 (1981).
6. Ware, C.F., and G.A. Granger. J. Immunol. 126:1934 (1981).
7. Wright, S.C., and B. Bonavida. J. Immunol. 126:1516 (1981).
8. Wright, S.C., Hiserodt, J.C., and B. Bonavida. Transpl. Proc. 13:770 (1981).
9. Wright, S.C., and B. Bonavida. J. Immunol., in press.

DISCUSSION

L. Simpson

Will your cytotoxic factor kill Con A blasts or LPS blasts?

B. Bonavida

No, it has absolutely no activity on those cells.

P. Henkart

How would you account for lack of innocent bystander effects with this kind of a mechanism?

B. Bonavida

When you do such experiments, using a short-term assay, there must be a threshold concentration for the factor to be detected. There may also be inactivators of the factor. We have some prelimininary information that such inactivators exist.

M. Mayer

I was just going to emphasize what you've said, that the innocent bystander objection would not be applicable if the factor is extensively or essentially removed by binding in the micro-environment of contact.

A. Allison

But how can one do an innocent bystander experiment with NK cells? you have to have an NK sensitive innocent bystander.

G. Berke

Tony, I think one can set up a conjugation between an A and B cell, then allow it to go awhile, and then introduce a C cell which is labeled. If indeed the interaction of A and B leads to the generation of a factor, then that factor should be ready to go when the C cell is introduced.

B. Bonavida

As I mentioned, Gideon, if you stimulate the spleen cells with the YAC cells for about 6 hours, there's enough cytotoxic activity in the supernate, but it requires 12-18 hrs for its activity.

G. Berke

Could you compare your factor to lymphotoxin?

B. Bonavida

There has not been a good comparison as far as I know.

P. Golstein

Your soluble factor made by NK cells - can you absorb it using NK sensitive targets?

B. Bonavida

Yes, we've done a whole series of experiments to test the effectiveness of various NK sensitive and resistant targets to absorb the activity. We find that if you compare YAC cells with EL4 or P815, which are NK resistant, the YAC cells are 10 to 20 times more effective in absorbing the cytotoxic activity on a cell for cell basis. So there seems to be a preferential absorption of the factor on NK sensitive target cells, although more targets need to be studied.

UNDERSTANDING THE NK CYTOLYTIC PROCESS BY STUDYING MECHANISMS OF ACTIVATION

Stephen R. Targan, M.D.
Geriatric Research and Education Center
Medical and Research Services
Wadsworth VA Medical Center

and

Department of Medicine
UCLA Center for the Health Sciences
Los Angeles, California 90024

It has become apparent from recent observations that the definition of the human NK effector cell is more complex then initially suspected. The effector cell which is a lymphocyte has been most accurately defined functionally by its ability to lyse particular "sensitive" target cells (1-4); however, the active NK cell appears to be Fc receptor positive and possibly of T-cell lineage (5). In addition, a large granular lymphocyte has been isolated which has many of these aforementioned characteristics and also possesses most of the NK and activated NK lytic activity (6). Recent observations have shown that NK activity can be augmented by various *in vitro* modalities. These stimuli appear to be divided into those that can augment NK activity within minutes to 24 hours of culture (Interferon (IF), Poly-IC, viruses) and those that require 48-72 hours of incubation before detectable augmentation (B-cell lines (MLC), pokeweed mitogen, and fetal calf serum) (2, 5, 7-10). The variable length of exposure required for each of these classes of agents to augment NK activity suggest that there may be multiple stages of differentiation and responsiveness of NK cells. Pre-NK cells have been defined as effector cells possessing NK receptors and therefore able to bind target cells, but needing further activation in order to express their lytic capabilities (11). In addition, agents such as interferon can also enhance the lytic abilities of the pre-NK and NK cells to become functionally more efficient killer cells (activated NK cells) (11).

Hence, there could possibly be three distinct lytic mechanism with the NK cell type.

The endogneous NK cell appears to be able to recognize and lyse tumor cells, virally infected fibroblasts, fetal fibroblasts and thymus cells (12-15). Interestingly, Zarling et al (8) and Masucci et al (16) showed that following interferon activation, heretofore NK resistant, freshly isolated leukemia cells as well as tissue culture target cells (Daudi), could be lysed by these "new" effector cells (8,16). Morever, these endogenous as well as interferon activated NK cells may be involved in autoregulation of at least thymocytes, bone marrow stem cells and epithelial cells (17; Targan, Unpublished Results). It is yet undetermined what aspect of interferon activation allows these cytotxic cells to extend their specificity to include these types of target cells.

The specific structures on target cells involved in either recognition by NK cells or possibly triggering of their lytic mechanisms, has not been elucidated. Previous studies suggest that human NK cells recognize multiple target antigens (18-21). This suggests that there may be subsets of NK cells each capable of recognizing different specific antigens as well as common antigens on all NK targets. Moreover, Durdik et al (22), and Roder (23) suggest that in the mouse NK system it may be the presence of a specific macromolecule on the membrane surface that renders resistant target cells susceptible to NK lysis. Furthermore, Roder and Kiessling have demonstrated in back cross experiments that target binding by NK cells may well be H2 linked in the mouse (24). Nonetheless, the actual role of any target surface proteins in the NK binding and lytic process has not been delineated.

Few studies have addressed the question of the cytolytic mechanism of endogenous NK cells. The division of the NK lytic process into recognition and binding, and post-binding events has recently ben demonstrated by Roder (25). The structure of this NK cell lysis has been studied by several other groups using pharmacologic and enzyme perturbation of NK cells (25). Various attempts using pharmacologic manipulation have partially or completely inhibited natural killer cellular cytotoxicity (NKCC), with target binding and lysis affected in a differential manner (26). Removal of the surface structure of effector cells by enzymes has resulted in the loss of lytic potential, probably due to the removal of binding capability (27, 28). Clearly, the binding and lytic process can be affected by different agents. This suggests that they represent distinct steps along the pathway of NK lysis of target cells. However, even though these studies show differences in inhibition of target binding and lysis, no specific or defineable structure has been implicated in any phase of the actual lytic process of these cells.

Based on our studies, the mechanisms of NK activation occur by both induction of cytolytically inactive pre-NK cells to lytically active NK cells, as well as enhancement of multiple target lytic capabilities of active NK cells. We have used the former model to ascertain what types of manipulations would prevent and/or enhance expression of lysis. In this manner a better understanding of what facets of the post-recognition binding stages of the NK lytic mechanism are present on pre-NK cells and what alterations are required for the completion and/or linkage of the components of this system so that lysis occurs may be obtained. Several possibilities are pictured in the figure (Fig. 1). Since pre-NK cells can bind to targets in this system the intial mechanism of neoexpression of target receptors is unlikely. One must consider, however, that when monolayer targets are used, interferon increases both the number and binding of lytically active cells (Targan, Unpublished Results). Nonetheless, the latter three mechanisms in the figure are all consistent with three recent observations that give insight into the requirements for this lytic expression.

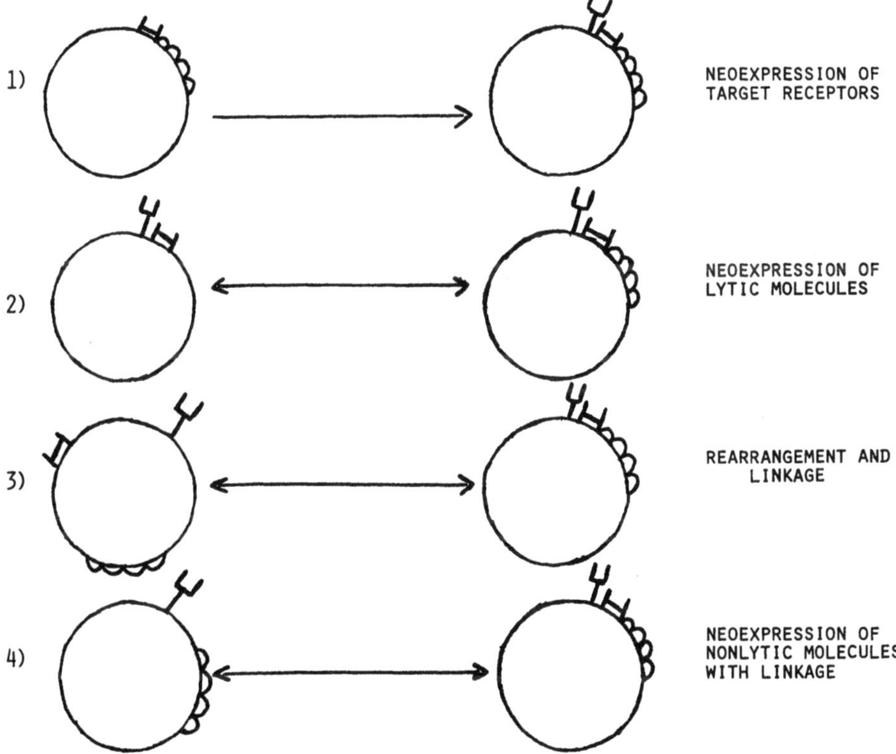

Fig. 1. Induction of single hit lysis.

NK cells and pre-NK cells can be exposed to interferon for brief periods (5 minutes) without being activated. If free interferon is removed by washing and the cells allowed to further incubate at 37 C for 30 minutes to 2 hours, NK cells are activated. Therefore, it is during this time that the cellular processing required for pre-NK cells to express their lytic potential occurs. Various perturbations (pharmacologic, enzymatic, immunologic, or physical) of NK and pre-NK cells can be performed during these 2 hours and their effect on the activation of the lytic potential of pre-NK cells can be ascertained.

Pre-NK activation is inhibited if these cells are bound to target cells prior to expression of their lytic potential (29). It seems that after binding, the effector cells become commited to either kill or not to kill and are no longer inducible by interferon. The mechanism of this block is not clear. It may be that the binding of the effector cell to targets neutralizes adenylcyclase activity or perturbs the membrane in such a fashion so that the exogenous signals are not transmitted into this cell, or induces the aggregation of interferon receptors to the cellular pole. Consistent with these observations was Santoli and Kaprowski's findings that pre-incubation of effector cells with interferon gave a greater augmentation of NK cytotoxicity than if interferon was added directly to a 4 hour ^{51}Cr release cytotoxicity assay (2). This suggested that the augmentation could be muted, even in this assay system in which both recycling of effector cells can occur, and where time of interferon exposure does not alter the targets ability to be lysed.

We have recently demonstrated that the activation of NK lysis can be both enhanced as well as blocked by the interaction of two distinct activators, prostaglandin and interferon. The enhancement of activation appears not to be due to recruitment of separate subsets of pre-NK cells but rather the synergistic enhancement of the recycling capabilities of the same set of NK cells. Furthermore, by first priming NK cells with IFN or PGE_2 and allowing expression of enhanced lytic potential to occur over a 3 hour time span, this activation can be prevented by subsequent exposure of these cells to the other modulator prior to completed activation. This appears to occur by blockage of recruitment of pre-NK cells into the lytic pool. There is a temporal relationship as to which of these above modulations is operative. That is, if PGE_2 is added during the cellular processing required for full expression of NK activation induced by IFN, pre-NK lytic potential is inhibited. If on the other hand, PGE_2 is added after completion of full expression of the IFN induced activated lytic process, there is enhancement of the number of lytic target interactions that each NK cell can perform.

This dual interaction of these two potential biologic modulators may give some insight into the similarities and differences in cellular mechanisms involved in expression of the lytic process by the cytotoxically inactive pre-NK cells and in the ability for NK cells to recycle. There is a temporal relationshop between priming of the NK cell by one agent and whether inhibition or synergism of activation occurs after pulsing with the second agent. This suggests that the sequential IFN-PGE_2 enhancement of recycling may be generated by different cellular mechanisms than the initiation of the lytic potential produced by each agent alone. Prior studies habe demonstrated that IFN alone may enhance this recycling (30,31), but clearly, the interaction of two different modulators can further increase the number of target cells which can be lysed by an individual NK cell (31).

The actual cellular changes responsible for these potential lytic alterations cannot be answered by the data of this study. However, one explanation could be that some NK cellular changes induced by the first agent must occur before the second agent can potentiate recycling. Therefore, the expression of the synergistic modulation by the second agent could be dependent upon a cellular product induced by the first. One possibility for this could be that the initial activation maximally increases the availability of lytic molecules that are incorporated into the cellular membrane. Once this has occured, a second modulation could not add further to the production of lytic molecules, but instead, it could operate by altering the membrane structure so as to facilitate their incorporation and/or stability. Thus, after contact and lysis of a target cell by such modulated NK cells, they would still have the necessary machinery to bind and lyse further susceptible targets. Nonetheless, the lack of such synergistic activation by sequential IFN treatment of NK cells certainly suggests that an additional interdependent mechanism is responsible for PGE_2 and IFN enhancement of recycling.

In addition to synergistic activation, PGE_2 can inhibit expression of pre-NK lytic potential. This occurs only during pre-activation cellular processing. This suggests that lack of expression of activation may be due to competition of each of these for some essential substrate. Thus, with simultaneous activation neither pathway would have enough of this molecule available to complete the processes needed for full expression of activation.

One level of experession for these above modulations could involve cellular membrane changes. Thus, after completion of membrane changes induced by IFN, further PGE_2 modulation could result in synergism. On the other hand, if these membrane alterations occur simultaneously before final expression, they would cancel each other's effect. This idea of the role for the cellular membrane in this lytic activation is consistent with prior observations made on IFN's modulation of the cytoskeleton (32) , as well as its ability to enhance expression of Fc receptors and MHC transmembrane proteins (33,34). In addition, the ability to prevent pulsed IFN activation by subsequent target binding further implicates the mobility of the cellular membrane in such lytic activation (29).

In a different context, prior work has shown that DNA synthesis was not required for IFN activation of NK cytotoxicity (5,35). However, de novo RNA as well as protein synthesis was required (5,35). Although the need for these cellular pro cesses have not been demonstrated for PGE_2 activation, this suggests several potential regulatory points of interaction of these two modulators. Thus, PGE_2's synergism of IFN activation (enhanced recycling) could be dependent upon IFN's induction of RNA, their translation into peptides, or the changes these molecules induced at the membrane level. In contrast, PGE_2 could inhibit IFN induced pre-NK lysis by competing for molecules involved in mRNA transcription, peptide translation or post-translational events. Thus, it remains to be shown at what level the enhancement of NK recycling produced by PGE_2 and IFN interactions is also dependent on RNA or protein synthesis. Thorough understanding of which of these subcelluar events are operative will give a better insight into how the cellular mechanisms responsible for the actual lytic process relate to those involved with NK cells recycling capabilities.

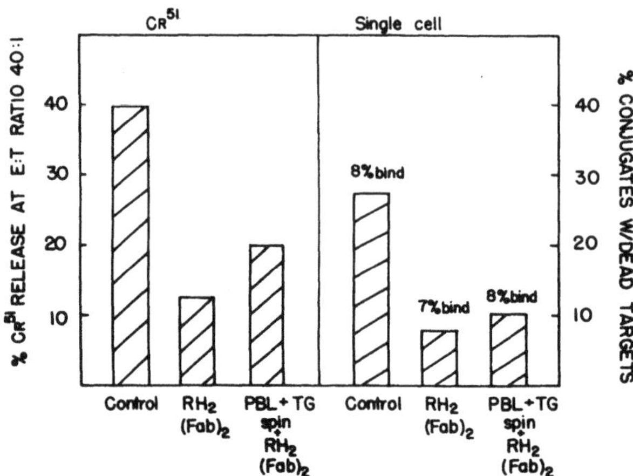

Fig. 2. Inhibition of Cr^{51} Releast and Single Cell by RH_2 $(Fab)_2$

$(Fab)_2$ produced from RH_2 antisera was added to the cytolytic assay either before or following conjugation formation. Its effect on overall NK lysis was measured in a 3 hour Cr^{51} release assay and its effect on target binding and/or single hit lysis was measured in a 3 hour single cell cytotoxic assay.

TABLE 1

DONOR	CONTROL K562 (TI)	MOLT (%I)	17.2 K562 (TI)	MOLT (%I)
1	59	-	12 (80)	-
2	50	38	21 (58)	21 (45)
3	50	-	-	-
4	65	-	-	-

TABLE 1a
BINDING ASSAY DONOR 1

	# Binding
Control	24/400
17.2 Preconjugation	24/400
17.2 Postconjugation	21/400

To analyze at what phase of NK lysis monoclonal 17.2 inhibited, we used a ^{51}Cr release assay and a single cell assay. By adding 17.2 prior to forming conjugates in a single cell assay, we could establish where there was no inhibition of the initial effector-target interaction.

TABLE 2. INHIBITION OF IFN ACTIVATION BY PRETREATMENT WITH 17.2

GROUP	E/T RATIO* 40	20	10
Control	31	25	18
IFN	63	52	35
17.2**	37	27	11
17.2 + IFN+	41	40	16

*^{51}Cr E/T Ratios

**PBL pretreated with monoclonal antibody 17.2 for 30 minutes at 37°C and washed x2 with PBS.

+17.2 treated cells exposed to 50 units of IFN for 1 hour at 37°C.

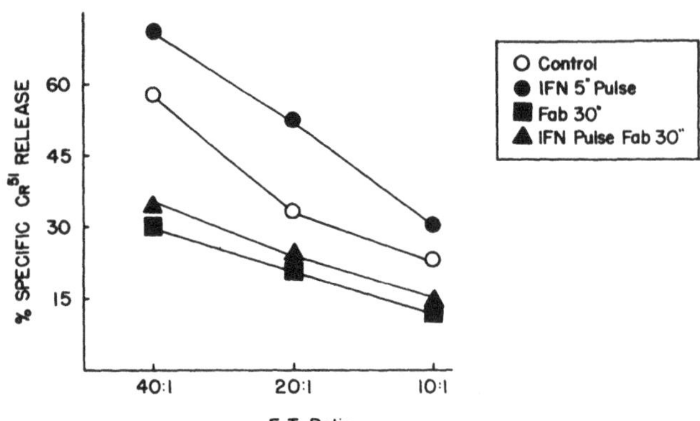

Fig. 3. RH_2 Fab_1 blockage of IFN activation after IFN pulse. PBL were treated with 20 units of interferon for 5 minutes. The cells were then washed and followed by addition of RH_2 and then allowed to incubate at 37°C for two hours prior to testing in a Cr^{51} release assay. These manipulations were done to demonstrate that inhibition of interferon activation was not due to the prevention of binding of interferon to these cells.

Finally, we have produced a heterologous antiserum and monoclonal antibody to lymphocyte populations containing alloimmune periodate activated NK and cytotoxic T cells (36). Both the antiserum RH_2 and the monoclonal antibody 17.2 block 50% to 100% of NK lysis if present during the cytotoxic reaction. These antisera have been absorbed on target cells and thus, most likely do not effect directly the blockage of target cell molecules. RH_2 blocks NK killing both at the level of target recognition and post recognition events (Fig. 2). The monoclonal (17.2) blocks at post binding events (Table 1 and 1a). If NK cells are pulsed with these reagents directly following interferon priming, the usual activation of NK lysis is inhibited (Fig. 3, Table 2). This suggests that whatever molecules these agents react with are important in the production/ linkage of postbinding pre-NK lytic components. Furthermore, neoexpression of these molecules at the end of in vitro activation is unlikely since RH_2 or 17.2 is washed out of the system and not present for the entire 2 hour incubation. This does not preclude, however, the possibility that more of these molecules are produced intracellularly and that the antibody blocks their inclusion or linkage into the proper lytic sequence in the membrane.

Initial target cell recognition by cells of NK lineage does not necessarily lead to lysis. It is clear from these data that cellular processing requiring some membrane modulation is required for completing the cellular machinery that leads to lysis. How much of this machinery is lacking from pre-NK cells and how many alterations must occur before lysis proceeds is unknown. This differentiation is not terminal, however, in that six hours after activation under proper conditions pre-NK cells return to their baseline recognition nonlytic state. This suggests that lytic activation of these pre-NK cells most probably results from rearrangement and linkage of existing structures into a functional unit.

A second mechanism by which interferon activates NK cells is to enhance each individual cell's lytic capacity. A population of NK cells kill in a random fashion over three hours with all lytic events being complete by 3 hours (11,37). After interferon treatment these cells now kill by 10 to 15 minutes of the assay; as if all lytic machinery had been enhanced so that they kill in a synchronous fashion, i.e. more rapidly. This observation at the single cell level probably correlates well with interferon enhancement of the NK cell's ability to recycle and kill multiple targets. Killing more rapidly represents a "loaded NK" cell. Once the NK cell has killed it is capable of immediately binding and killing another target. In contrast, it appears that in the endogenous state there is a relative refractory period before this second event can occur. It is not clear what the fate of the lytic unit on the NK cell is following initiation of lysis, i.e., are they cleaved and transferred from the membrane or do they remain intact? If by addition of interferon to cultures of NK cells more molecules are made available or their stability or ability to be replaced in the NK membrane are enhanced, then the already active cells become more efficient killer cells. Thus, more lytic machinery would be available after an individual lytic event for the cell to rapidly proceed on to a second lytic event.

In conclusion, there are multiple facets of the NK cell lytic mechanism that can be studied by using these activation models. What is clear is that it is important to not only investigate the components of single hit non-augmented NK lysis but also what is involved in enhancing an individual effector cell's lytic efficiency, i.e., the rate of single target lysis and the number of targets lysed per NK effector cell. Therefore, equal amounts of chromium release in two populations of NK cells as measured by the total lytic units per lymphocyte population may very well be measuring activity of individual effector cells with vastly different lytic capabilities. It remains for the specific cellular and molecular components responsible for these cytotoxic functions and/or alterations in the lytic mechanism to be defined.

REFERENCES

1. Pross, H.F., and M.G. Baines. Spontaneous human lymphocyte-mediated cytotoxicity against tumor target cells. VI. A brief review. Cancer Immunol. Immunother. 3:74 (1978).

2. Santoli, D., and H. Kaprowski. Mechanisms of activation of human killer cells against tumor and virus infected cells. Immunol. Rev. 44:125. (1979).
3. Jondal, M., Spina C., and S. Targan. Human Spontaneous killer cells: selective for tumor-derved target cells. Nature 272:62 (1978).
4. Bonnard, G.D., and H.W. West. Cell mediated cytotoxicity in humans. A criticial review of experimental models and clinically oriented studies. In: Immunodiagnosis of Cancer. Edited by R.B. Herberman and K.R. McIntire. Marcel Dekker Publishers, New York. (1978).
5. Herberman, R., Djeu, H., Kay, D., Ortaldo, J.R., Ricardi, C., Bonnard, G.D., Holden, H.T., Fagnani, R., Santoni, A., and P. Puccetti. Natural killer cells: characteristics and regulation of activity. Immunol. Rev. 44:43 (1979).
6. Timonen, T., Ortaldo, J.R., and R.B. Herberman. Characteristics of human large granular lymphoctyes and relationship to natural killer and K cells. J.Exp. Med. 153:569. (1981).
7. Jondal, M. and S.R. Targan. In vitro induction of cytotoxic effector cells with spontaneous killer (SK) cell specificity. J. Exp. Med. 147:1621 (1978).
8. Zarling, J.M., Eskra, L., Borden, E.C., Horoszcwicz, J., and W.A. Cantar. Activation of human natural killer cells cytotoxic for human leukemia cells by purified interferon. J. Immunol. 123:63 (1979).
9. Kasai, M., Leclerc, J.C., McVay-Boudreau, L., Sheni, F.W., and H. Cantor. Direct evidence that natural killer cells in non-immune spleen cell populations prevent tumor growth in vivo. J. Exp. Med. 149:1260 (1979).
10. Seeley, J.K., and S.H. Golub. Studies on cytotoxicity generated in human mixed lymphocyte cultures. I. Time course and target spectrum of several distinct concomitant cytotoxic activities. J. Immunol. 120:1415 (1978).
11. Targan, S. and F. Dorey. Interferon activation of "prespontaneous killer" (pre-SK) cells and alteration kinetics of lysis of both "pre-SK" and active SK cells. J. Immunol 124:2157 (1980).
12. Welsh, R.M. Jr. Mouse natural killer cells: induction, specificity, and function. J. Immunol. 122:1631 (1978).
13. Hansson, M., Kiessling, R., Anderson, B., Karre, K., and J. Roder. NK cell-sensitive T-cell subpopulation in thymus: inverse correlation to host NK activity. Nature 278:174. (1979).
14. Ono, A., Amos, D.B., and H.S. Koren. Selective cellular natural killing against human leukaemic T cells and thymus. Nature 266:546 (1977).
15. Kiessling R., Hochman, P.S., Haller, O., Shearer, G.M., and G. Cudkowicz. Evidence for a similar or common mechanism for natural killer cell activity and resistance to hemopoietic grafts. Eur. J. Immunol. 79:655 (1977).

16. Masucci, M.G., Masucci, G., Klein, E., and W. Berthold. Target selectivity of interferon-induced human killer lymphocytes related to theri Fc receptor expression. (1980).
17. Hansson M., Kiessling, R., and R. Welsh. Interaction between NK cells and normal tissue: definition of a NK-sensitive thymocyte population. In: Natural Cell-Mediated Immunity Against Tumors. Edited by R.B. Herberman. Academic Press, New York, p 855 (1980).
18. Ortaldo, J.R., Oldham, R.K., Cannon, G.C., and R.B. Herberman. Specificity of natural cytotoxic reactivity or normal human lymphocytes against a myeloid leukemia cell line. J. Natl. Cancer Inst. 59:77 (1977).
19. Callewaert, D.J., Lightbody, J.J., Kaplan, J., Jaroszewski, J., Peterson, W.D., and J.C. Rosenberg. Spontaneous cytotoxicity of cultured human cell lines by normal PBL. II. Specificity for target antigens. Cell Immunol. 42:103 (1979).
20. Takasugi, M., Akira, D., Takasugi, J., and M. Mickey. Specificities of human cell-mediated cytotoxicity. J. Natl. Cancer Inst. 59:69 (1977).
21. Phillips, W.H., Ortaldo, J.R., and R.B. Herberman. Selective depletion of human natural killer cells on monolayers of target cells. J. Immunol. 125:2322 (1980).
22. Durdik, J.M., Beck, B.N., Clark, W.A., and C.S. Henney. Characterization of a lymphoma cell variant selectively resistant to natural killer cells. J. Immunol 125:683 (1980).
23. Roder, J.C., Rosen, A., Fenyo, E.M., and F.A. Troy. Target-effector interaction in the natural killer cell system: Isolation of target structures. Proc. Natl. Acad. Sci. USA 76:1405 (1979).
24. Roder, J.C., and R. Kiessling. A model of target cell recognition and lysis by natural killer cells. Adv. Exp. Med. Biol. 114:745 (1979).
25. Roder, J.C., and T. Haliotis. A comparative analysis of the NK cytolytic mechanism and regulatory genes. In "Natural Cell-Mediated Immunity Against Tumors." Edited by R.B. Herberman. Academic Press, New York, P379. (1980).
26. Roder, J.C., and M. Klein. Target-effector interaction in the natural killer cell system. IV. Modulation by cyclic nucleotides. J. Immunol. 123:2785. (1979).
27. Kiuchi, M., and M. Takasugi. The nonselective cytotoxic cell (N cell). J. Natl. Cancer Inst. 56:575. (1976).
28. Perussia, B., Trinchieri, G., and J.C. Cerottini. Functional studies of Fc receptor-bearing human lymphocytes: effect of treatment with proteolytic enzymes. J. Immunol 123:681 (1979).
29. Lilve, A., Bonavida, B., and S. Targan. Mode of action of interferon-mediated modulation of natural killer cytotoxic activity: Recruitment of pre-NK cells and enhanced kinetics of lysis. J. Immunol. 125:479. (1980).
30. Ullberg, M., and M. Jondal. Recycling and target-binding capacity of human natural killer cells. J. Exp. Med. 153:615. (1981).

31. Targan, S., Britvan, L. and F. Dorey. Activation of human NKCC by moderate exercise: increased frequency of NK cells with enhanced capability of effector-target lytic interactions. J. Clin. Exp. Immunol. 45:352 (1981).
32. Chany, Rousset, C.S., Bourgeade, M.F., Mathieu, D., and A. Gregoire. In " Regulatory Functions on Interferons." Edited by J. Vilcek, Gresser I., and T.C. Merigan. New York Academy of Sciences, New York, p 254. (1980).
33. Fridman, W.H., Gresser, I., Bandu, M.T., Aguet, M., and C. Neauport-Sautes. Interferon enhances the expression of Fc receptors. J. Immunol. 124:2436. (1980).
34. Itoh, K., Inoue, M., Kataoka, S., and K. Kumagi. Differential effect of interferon expression of IgG- and IgM-Fc receptors on human lympohocytes. J. Immunol. 124:2589. (1980).
35. Ortaldo, J.R., Herberman, R.B., and J.Y. Djeu. Characteristics of augmentation of interferon of cell-mediated cytotoxicity. In " Natural Cell-Mediated Immunity Against Tumors." Edited by R.B. Herberman. Academic Press, New York, P 593. (1980).
36. Hiserodt, J., Britvan, L., and S. Targan. Blockage of natural killer cytotoxicity by heterologous and monoclonal antibodies (In Submission). (1981).
37. Targan S., Grimm, E., and B. Bonavida. A single cell marker of active NK cytotoxicity: Only a fraction of target binding lymphocytes are killer cells. J. Clin. Lab. Immunol. 4:165. (1980).

DISCUSSION

E. Martz

When you say these antibodies block post-binding, have you checked to see if they weaken or detach ET conjugates?

S. Targan

The number of conjugates is not altered after these antisera are added. We have done some kinetic experiments adding these antisera following initiation, and at no time does there appear to be a difference.

V. Hu

Can lectins induce NK binding to and lysis of insusceptible targets?

S. Targan

I would defer to Ben if he wants to say anything about that.

B. Bonavida

The findings so far show very clearly that in humans they are mediated by different cells. The NK cell does not mediate LDCC and vice versa. This was done by looking at double target cells bound to one lymphocyte; one of the targets was the NK sensitive K562, and the other target was a Con A pre-treated NK-resistant Raji cell.

R. Herberman

Some studies on that point have been performed by Michael Brunda in my lab. He used spleen cells from nude mice to avoid a possible contribution by polyclonal activation of CTL. Certain lectins clearly increased the amount of killing of K562 or some other resistant targets, but did not increase the killing of YAC-1 or some other sensitive targets.

S. Targan

Was there binding changes on those? Or was it merely an activation of the cells? Do you know?

R. Herberman

There was clearly binding, as part of the mechanism, but I'm not sure that was the whole explanation.

P. Golstein

I wanted to follow up on Eric's point about inhibition by your monoclonal, which blocks post-binding. How was the experiment actually done? I mean, did you add your monoclonal before looking at conjugates? Or did you first get conjugates and then add your monoclonal?

S. Targan

We did it both ways. And the results were the same either way. That is, if we pre-added them and allowed the antisera to be in during the time of the assay, without washing it out, we got inhibition but no change of conjugates and the other way, the same thing.

P. Golstein

This doesn't block T kill?

S. Targan

We haven't looked at T kill. We have looked at ADCC and it inhibits ADCC. Post-binding also.

MECHANISMS OF TUMOR CELL LYSIS BY NATURAL KILLER CELLS

Ronald H. Goldfarb*, Tuomo Timonen+, and Ronald B. Herberman+

*Cancer Metastasis Research Group, Department of Immunology and Infectious Disease, Pfizer Central Research, Groton, Connecticut 06340

+Laboratory of Immunodiagnosis, National Cancer Institute, National Institutes of Health, Bethesda, Maryland 20205

INTRODUCTION

Immune reactivity against malignant cells is well-documented for a number of lymphoid cell types (1). The foremost features of anti-tumor immune effector cells appears to be their capacity to recognize and subsequently kill tumor cells. Nevertheless, the mechanism(s) by which effector cells of the immune response mediate tumor cell lysis is largely unknown. The lack of precise knowledge concerning lytic pathways is evident for well studied immune killer cells, such as cytotoxic T lymphocytes, as well as for effector cells that have only recently received intense experimental scrutiny, such as natural killer (NK) cells.

This article will focus on possible mechanisms of tumor cell cytolysis mediated by NK cells, a relatively small subpopulation of lymphoid cells that may play an important role in natural host defense against cancer and infectious diseases (2). Special emphasis will be placed on the potential contributions of neutral serine proteases and phospholipases in NK cell-mediated destruction of tumor cells. Aspects of our recent experimenal findings will be discussed in detail. In addition, what is known concerning the mechanism of NK lysis will be compared to the events that appear to be involved in target cell lysis triggered by other immune effector cells, particularly cytotoxic T lymphocytes and activated macrophages. Furthermore, NK cells and K cells, that mediate antibody-dependent cell-mediated cytotoxicity (ADCC), may be in the same effector cell population, and therefore, investigations concerning the mechanism of ADCC may be directly relevant to the mechanism of NK cell killing.

MECHANISMS OF IMMUNE LYSIS: OVERVIEW

In considering the possible mechanism of cytolysis mediated by NK cells, it is useful to review highlights concerning the mechanism of target killing by other immune effector cells. Although the mechanism of T cell-mediated tumor cell lysis is not fully understood, a great deal of investigative effort has been made in this area; T cell killing is, therefore, the best available model for comparison with the discrete steps that may contribute to tumor cell lysis by NK cells.

The process of T cell-mediated cytolysis appears to consist of distinct and complex stages that have been well studied at both the molecular and cellular levels (3, 4, 5, 6). It has been documented that cytotoxic T lymphocytes bind to target molecules through cell surface receptors, program target cells for subsequent killer-cell independent lysis, and then detach and can then repeat the same type of interactions with additional target cells. These events have been determined by use of: a myriad number of drugs with various modes of action as probes; temperature effects; kinetic analysis; and the investigation of individual effector cell-target cell conjugates (3).

The first step in NK cell-mediated lysis of tumor cells also appears to involve binding to target cells, and subsequent conjugate formation. The succeeding steps involved in the process leading to target cell lysis are, however, not well understood. Several possible mechanisms have been suggested for NK lysis and will be considered below. These mechanisms include: activation of cell surface proteases or local secretion of proteases in the effector cell-target cell conjugate micro-environment; activation of phospholipase A_2 with concommitant generation of lytically active lysolecithin; production of reactive oxygen species such as superoxide; release of soluble factors including lymphotoxins or activation of membrane-bound lymphotoxins; and colloid osmotic lysis of target cells as a consequence of cell surface damage to target cells due to physicochemical alterations triggered by conjugate formation.

REQUIREMENTS FOR EFFECTOR CELL-TARGET CELL CONTACT FOR NK MEDIATED KILLING

Evidence has recently been reviewed for the requirement of effector cell-target cell contact in lysis by cytolytic T cells, macrophages, and for ADCC (7). It has also been suggested that the binding of NK cells to target tumor cells is required for target cell cytolysis. An assay for the binding of natural killer cell-containing spleen cells to target cells has been reported (8), and target cell binding was detected five to ten minutes before measurable cell damage was observed (8). Trypsinization of the effector cell population led to inhibition of both conjugate formation and lysis; in addition, both functions were reported to be regenerated with coincident kinetics (8). These results suggest that binding needs to take place prior to a lytic event. In contrast to cytotoxic T cells, which are completely prevented from binding and killing target cells in the presence of metabolic inhibitors, or at low temperature, mouse NK cells have been reported to still bind to targets, albeit with decreased stability, but not kill under these conditions (8).

The isolation of target molecules from several NK-sensitive target cells has been reported (9). Preincubation of mouse lymphoid cells with detergent-solubilized, cell surface molecules of NK-susceptible mouse target cells, such as YAC-1 lymphoma cells, prevented subsequent binding of NK-containing cells to intact target cells; this solubilized cell surface preparation, however, failed to inhibit cytolysis (9). These inhibitory molecules were shown to be glycosylated proteins with molecular weights of 130,000, 160,000 and 240,000 daltons (9). These molecules were not observed in NK insensitive target cells, and their expression appeared to vary directly among target cells with their sensitivity to lysis (9).

The binding of effector cells to tumor cell targets has also served as an assay for the examination of NK cell specificity. Both mouse and human NK cells have been shown to bind in a selective fashion to monolayers of NK-susceptible target cells. As of yet, this method has not been used for the examination of target structural molecules. However, this technology has been used to determine whether reactivity against some targets remains following depletion of effector cells on targets attached to monolayers (reviewed in reference 7).

The actual frequency of contacts between human large granular lymphocytes (LGL), that account for human NK activity (10, 11), and tumor target cells has been enumerated. LGL were isolated by adsorption-elution of the effector cells from K562 target cells. NK activity and LGL mrophology were enriched in the target cell-adherent populations and in normal human donors; the number of LGL that bound to K562 targets correlated with the levels of NK activity (10).

Recent results with highly purified LGL have confirmed that the binding of target cells is an initial step required in NK cell-mediated cytolysis (Ortaldo, Timonen, Goldfarb, and Herberman, manuscript in preparation). For example, EDTA inhibited the binding of human LGL to targets and also inhibited lysis. Various inhibitors of human NK activity, such as cholera toxin or phorbol-12-myristate-13-acetate (12), were found to have different effects in this assay; the former agent inhibited the lytic reaction but had no effect on binding, whereas the latter agent inhibited the binding of NK cells to target cells (Ortaldo, Timonen, Goldfarb, and Herberman, unpublished observations). It therefore appears that binding is an important step in NK killing, and that different agents can affect binding in various ways. Nevertheless, it should be noted that a recent report (13) has suggested that a soluble, cytotoxic factor, released from mouse spleen cells and human peripheral blood lymphocytes, may be selectively lytic for NK-sensitive target cells. This factor was generated in a Marbrook chamber with effector cells separated from target cells, suggesting an exception to the requirement for effector-target contact described above. More detailed biochemical studies with material derived from pure NK populations will be required to probe the significance of this observation.

THE ROLE OF NEUTRAL SERINE PROTEASES IN KILLER CELL LYSIS OF TARGET CELLS

A role for serine proteases in tumor cell lysis by immune effector cells has been examined by a number of investigators in several experimental systems. Proteases play a role in degradative alteration of cellular components and have the ability to modify both cellular and extracellular protein components (14). It is possible that proteases with invasive potential can contribute to cell killing either indirectly or directly through well-regulated limited proteolysis of cell surface or other cellular components.

Specific inhibitors of neutral serine proteases have been used as probes to determine the role of these enzymes in killer cell function. Diisopropylfluorophosphate (DFP), for example, serves as an active site inhibitor and titrant of neutral serine proteolytic enzymes. DFP has been shown to inhibit target cell killing by cytolytic T cells (15). In addiiton, it has been reported that target cell lysis by cytotoxic T lymphocytes is dependent upon cell-surface activated proteases (16). A cytotoxic protease has indeed been isolated from human peripheral blood lymphocytes, and could cause lysis of pre-labeled tumor cell targets (17). Lymphocyte plasma membranes, with the potential for tumor cell cytotoxicity, may have a membrane-associated proteolytic enzyme (18), and it has also been suggested that intact lymphocytes display cell-surface associated protease activity (19). Further support for a role of neutral proteases in target cell lysis has come from observations that low levels of exogenously added enzymes caused enhanced T cell cytolysis as well as ADCC (20). However, one study concluded that protease action is not likely to be the mechanism of T cell mediated cytolysis (21); although inhibition of T cell killing was observed upon treatment with protease inhibitors, it was concluded that such activity was due to toxic side effects rather than to specific inhibition of protease action.

Neutral serine proteases may also play an active role in the mechanism of tumor cell lysis mediated by activated macrophages (22, 23, 24). One protease, isolated from macrophages, was shown to be cytolytic for target cells and it has been suggested that tumor cell cytolysis by activated macrophages is mediated, at least to some extent, by the neutral serine proteases secreted by macrophages. As with T cells and NK cells, macrophages bind to target cells; it has been shown that the ability of macrophages to bind to tumor cells and to secrete a cytolytic protease are independent functions. Nevertheless, expression of both functions is required for macrophage mediated target cell lysis (25). With regard to the role of proteases in macrophage killing, it is of interest that macrophages produce neutral serine proteases, particularly plasminogen activator (26). Furthermore, it has been reported that a cascade of regulatory, DFP-sensitive proteases appears to play a role in the functional regulation of activated macrophages (27).

Inhibitors of serine proteases, such as DFP and tosyl-lysyl-chloro-methyl-ketone (TLCK), have also been shown to suppress ADCC by human peripheral blood mononuclear cells (28); an established human lymphoblastoid line was used as a target cell, and was sensitized with an alloantiserum. This work is of particular interest with respect to NK killing since NK cells are closely related to K cells mediating ADCC and may, in fact, be the same cells. It is, therefore, intriguing to speculate that earlier reports, which document inhibition of ADCC activity by protease inhbiitors (28), may also be of direct relevance to the mechanism of NK lysis. Although it seems likely that NK activity is dependent on cell surface receptors which are distinct from the receptors for the Fc portion of IgG that are directly involved in ADCC (29), the subsequent mechanism of lysis of bound target cells may be identical for both ADCC and NK cell-mediated cytolysis.

THE ROLE OF NEUTRAL SERINE PROTEASES IN NK CELL-MEDIATED CYTOLYSIS

It has been suggested that proteases may also play a role in the mechanism of tumor cell cytolysis by NK cells. An inhibitor of serine proteases was reported to have no effect on binding of NK cells to target cells, but rather to inhibit their subsequent lysis (8). it was suggested that following binding, and subsequent to effector cell-target cell conjugate formation, a "lytic unit" on the NK cells is triggered, and that this unit involves a proteolytic activity (8). Since inhibitors of glycolysis also inhibited NK activity, it was speculated that energy was required for either exposing the active site of the enzyme on the exterior of the effector cell or for the creation of a degradative interaction with the target (8). Interestingly, various immunological factors (e.g., anti-Ig) can indeed activate membrane-bound tryptic-like serine proteases, and thereby cause signal transmission. This has been reported to be the case for Ig receptor-mediated signals for activation of B cell precursor proteins (30). It was found that the binding of anti-Ig to Ig molecules on the surface of B lymphocytes activated a membrane-bound, tryptic-like neutral serine enzyme. This enzyme split precursor proteins present in the cytoplasm of resting B lymphocytes (M.W. 150,000 daltons) to an active cytoplasmic factor (M.W. 45,000 daltons), which, in turn, induced a protein kinase activity in the nucleus.

Several recent reports have described further evidence for a role of proteases in NK reactivity against tumor cells. Human NK activity was inhibited by protease inhibitors of either low or high molecular weight (31) or by proteinase substrates (32); the latter report suggested that human NK activity is inhibited by substrates for chymotrypsin and plasmin but not by substrates for elastase and collagenase. Another preliminary report suggested an important role for surface-associated chymotryptic and tryptic proteases in the spontaneous lysis of tumor cells (33). In addition, it was suggested that elastase activity might play some role in NK mediated tumoricidal activity.

Although these interesting reports suggest that serine proteases contribute to NK lysis, direct evidence for a role of proteolytic activity in lysis of tumor cells by NK cells has not been provided. In addition, these preliminary studies were not performed on pure populations of effector cells and the protease inhibitors might have indirectly exerted their inhibitory effects on NK reactivity by affecting other, regulatory cells. Therefore, in order to unambiguously evaluate the role of proteases in the mechanism of NK lysis, it is imperative to study pure cell populations. With proteases this is indeed a critical point, since even a small number of contaminating cells could contribute potent proteases which might be active at picogram or nanogram levels. Conversely, it is possible that a protease produced by a contaminating cell type might degrade a proteolytic enzyme produced by NK cells and, thereby, interfere with the detection and isolation of relevant molecules.

Another suggestive piece of evidence for a role of protease activity in the NK cell lytic mechanism has been provided by recent findings that beige mice and humans with Chediak-Higashi syndrome have diminished NK activity (34, 35). Neutral proteases are low or undetectable in the leukocytes of individuals with these diseases (36), and these two observations may be related in a direct fashion. It is of interest that the proteases which are altered in expression may be localized to azurophilic granules in the cytoplasm. Such granules appear to be particularly characteristic of human and rat NK cells (i.e., LGL). In support of this possible link, it has been noted (T. Timonen, unpublished observation) and confirmed (R. H. Goldfarb, unpublished observation) that patients with Chediak-Higashi syndrome have only unusually large azurophilic granule(s) in the cytoplasm of their LGL.

In order to elucidate further the exact role of proteolytic enzymes in NK activity, we have examined highly enriched populations of human NK cells (7, 11). Our efforts were directed at both the examination of extracellular and cell-associated proteases produced by LGL, and the use of specific, non-toxic protease inhibitors on these pure populations.

Our experimental results have suggested that neutral serine proteases are indeed produced by NK cells, and that such enzymes may play a role in the mechanism of tumor cell lysis. Human cell subpopulations with 75-95% LGL were found to have neutral serine protease activity. Neutral serine proteolytic activity was monitored on iodinated fibrin, a well characterized substrate for protease assay, as previously described (37). This activity was also found in LGL preparations enriched to greater than 99% purity, by

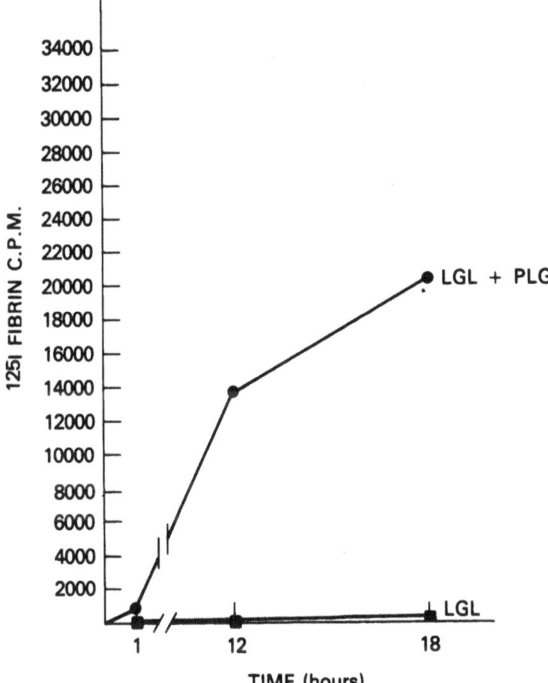

Fig. 1 Production of plasminogen activator by human NK cells. 5×10^6 human large granular lymphocytes, in the presence or absence of pure human plasminogen (6 μgm) were incubated on ^{125}I-fibrin coated tissue culture wells in serum-free medium supplemented with crystalline bovine serum albumin (6 mg/ml). At the indicated time points supernatants were harvested and directly counted in a gamma counter to determine ^{125}I-fibrin degradation products as an index of plasminogen-dependent or independent proteolytic activity.

an additional purification step of rosetting with sheep erythrocytes at 29°C. The proteolytic activity was detected in intact LGL following overnight culture on iodinated fibrin, and also in extracellular culture fluids. In addition, proteolytic activity in homogenates of LGL was found to be associated with subcellular fractions enriched for cell surface membranes. Figure 1 demonstrates that the proteolytic activity associated with LGL appears to have the capacity to generate plasmin from plasminogen, as detected by well established methods for the assay of plasminogen activators (37). It therefore appears that NK cells, as well as macrophages, produce plasminogen activator. Previously, the production of plasminogen activator by lymphocytes was not documented (E. Reich, personal communication) and the finding with NK cells was unexpected. However, there are recent indications that plasminogen activator may perhaps be associated with lymphocytes. Lymph node lymphocytes, putatively devoid of contaminating macrophages, were reported to produce plasminogen activator (38); in addition, plasminogen activator production was associated with B lymphocytes, and reported to be associated with the cell membrane (39). Furthermore, it has been claimed that thymocytes were able to produce plasminogen activator (40, 41). One might argue that the protease activity described above for NK cells might be attributable to small numbers of monocytes that may be found in the LGL population. However, we have observed that our LGL-enriched populations, following rosetting with sheep erythrocytes at 29°C, contained no detectable cells that were able to ingest fluorescently labeled latex beads, thereby indicating little or no residual monocytes among the LGL (Goldfarb, Timonen, and Herberman, unpublished observations). In addition, upon morphological analysis of Giemsa-steroid cytocentrifuge preparations, all of the cells appeared to be LGL (>99%) whereas no cells with the morphology of monocytes was observed. Subsequent work has demonstrated that cultures of LGL, grown in the presence of T cell growth factor, also produce plasminogen activator (Goldfarb, Timonen, and Herberman, unpublished observations). Preliminary biochemical characterization of the plasminogen activator associated with human LGL has been initiated by well documented methodology (42) and will be reported in detail elsewhere (Goldfarb, Timonen, and Herberman, manuscript in preparation).

In order to determine whether the apparent association of proteases with NK cells was of physiological significance, we examined the effect of selective protease inhibitors on NK activity. We have employed highly selective proteinase inhibitors of microbial origin (43) which display little or no toxicity and are, therefore, superior to inhibitors such as TLCK which are potentially toxic.

We have also investigated the effects of exogenously added proteases on the NK activity of LGL. In order to critically examine this issue, we established a ^{51}chromium release assay in serum-free conditions, to eliminate serum-containing protease inhibitors, and in which cell viability was high (Goldfarb and Herberman, unpublished observations). The entire chromium release assay was, therefore, performed with washed target cells and effector cells, under serum-free conditions in which both effectors and targets remained highly viable, with the background release comparable to normal serum-containing chromium release tests. The serum-free medium was supplemented with highly purified human or bovine serum albumin which was tested and determined to be free of contaminating proteases or inhibitors. Our results indicate that exogenous trypsin and chymotrypsin, added in nanogram amounts to these serum-free conditions, enhanced the LGL-mediated natural killing of K562 cells as shown in Figure 2. These findings are reminiscent of the

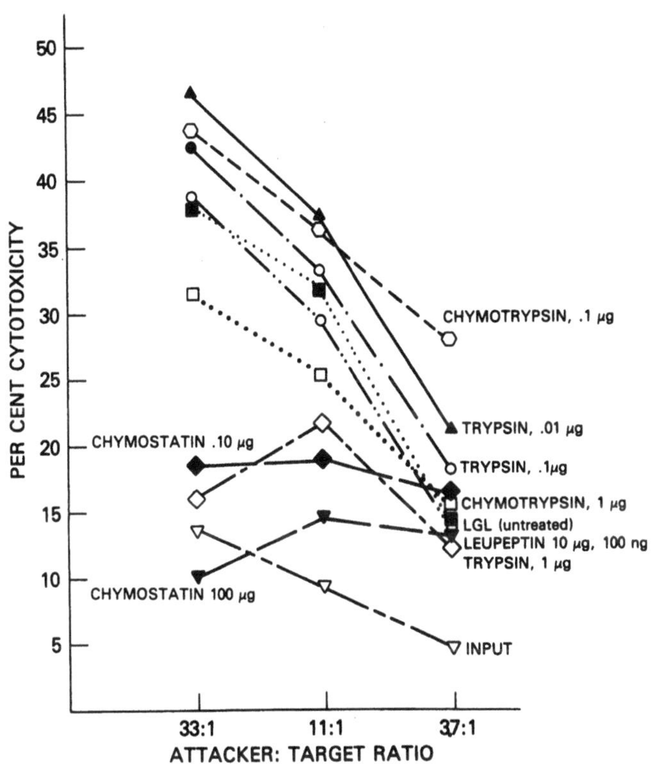

Fig. 2 Effect of proteases and inhibitors on human NK activity. The entire assay was performed in serum-free medium supplemented with crystalline bovine serum albumin (6 mg/ml). All samples were preincubated for 60 minutes at 37°C. The cells were not washed after treatments. The assay for cell-mediated cytotoxicity was as previously described (12), except all steps were done in serum-free conditions.

results of other investigators that have employed low levels of proteases in cytolysis experiments with immune T cells (20). We have also found that the specific inhibitor of chymotrypsin, chymostatin, profoundly inhibited NK mediated cytolysis (Figure 2). Leupeptin, an agent with inhibitory potential for tryptic enzymes, including plasminogen activator (44), also inhibited NK activity, as shown in Figure 2. The specificity of the proteases and the inhibitors employed, as well as the enzymatic activity of the proteases, were confirmed by established methods (37).

The results described above suggest a major role for proteolytic activity in NK killing. This activity may be directly mediated by molecules on the surface of NK cells; alternatively, extracellular and/or cell-associated protease activity may be triggered in either target cells or killer cells subsequent to killer cell-target cell interaction. A recent report has shown that chymostatin can inhibit the aggregation of activated human peripheral blood lymphocytes (45) and it has been suggested that chymotryptic-like activity may be involved in the aggregation of human peripheral blood lymphocytes stimulated by PHA. It has been suggested that surface membrane-bound lymphocyte proteases may be important in altering the cell surface membrane, and result in discharge of biochemical signals that in turn lead to cell proliferation and aggregation. Therefore, it is possible that inhibition of NK activity by chymostatin may be due to inhibition of an NK cell protease that is involved indirectly, rather than directly, in target cell killing.

PHOSPHOLIPASES IN NK MEDIATED CYTOLYSIS

Other physiologic enzymes that may play a role in NK activity are the phospholipases. Phospholipase A_2 has the capacity to convert lecithin to the membrane-reactive, degradative detergent, lysolecithin. Although it has been demonstrated that phospholipases may not play a role in T cell killing of target cells (3,46) this enzyme might still be of importance in cytolysis of tumor cells by other types of effector cells. It was shown that inhibition of phospholipase activity by Rosenthal's inhibitor (dimethyl DL-2,3-distearoyloxypropyl-2'-hydroxyethyl ammonium acetate) diminished ADCC activity (47). However, the ADCC system involved mouse spleen cells and chicken erythrocytes as targets, and macrophages rather than K cells appear to be responsible for the reported reactivity. We have observed that Rosenthal's inhibitor can also inhibit human LGL-mediated killing of tumor cells, as shown in Figure 3. Furthermore, exogenous phospholipase A_2 led to enhanced cytolysis by LGL (Figure 3). A detailed study of the effects of phospholipase inhibitors on NK activity by human PBL has also implied a role for both phospholipase A_2 activity and phospholipid transmethylation in cytolysis (48); LGL were also shown to develop increased phospholipase A_2 activity upon incubation with NK-susceptible target cells.

TREATMENT	PERCENT CYTOTOXICITY***	PERCENT INHIBITION	PERCENT AUGMENTATION
LGL-NON-TREATED	59.5	–	–
ROSENTHALS' INHIBITOR			
10^{-3}M	−3.5	100	–
10^{-4}M	46.8	21.3	–
PHOSPHOLIPASE A2 6.5 U	78.3	–	31.6%
LYSOLECITHIN*	12.4	21.0	–
LYSOLECITHIN**	52.1	12.4	–

$$\text{LECITHIN} \xrightarrow[\text{A2}]{\text{PHOSPHOLIPASE}} \text{LYSOLECITHIN + FATTY ACID (lytic agent)}$$

*LYSOLECITHIN CONCENTRATIONS TOXIC FOR LGL
**LYSOLECITHIN CONCENTRATIONS NON-TOXIC FOR LGL
***A:T RATIO ≡100:1

Fig. 3 The effect of phospholipase A_2 on human NK activity. The assay for cell-mediated cytotoxicity was as previously described (12).

POSSIBLE ROLE OF SUPEROXIDE OR OTHER REACTIVE OXYGEN SPECIES IN LYSIS BY NK CELLS

Much attention has been focused on the production of superoxide or other reactive oxygen species as possible mechanism(s) for cell mediated cytotoxicity. In the presence of myeloperoxidase and a halide, granulocyte-derived hydrogen peroxidase appears to mediate the destruction of eukaryotic cells (49, 50). Activated mouse peritoneal macrophages, upon triggering, release hydrogen peroxide and superoxide anions. Some evidence has been obtained for a role of hydrogen peroxide as the molecule that mediates extracellular cytolysis of lymphoma cell lines by activated macrophages and granulocytes (51, 52). A role for such a mechanism has also been suggested for ADCC by activated macrophages, with the binding of IgG antibodies to the Fc receptors on activated macrophages triggering an oxidative, extracellular response (53). However, the role of oxidative mechamisms in ADCC appears to be controversial, perhaps due to use of different target cells which may vary in their susceptibility to either oxidative or non-oxidative pathways (53, 54, 55).

Recently we have examined the possible role of superoxide or other reactive oxygen species in the mechanism of NK cell-mediated lysis of tumor cells. We have found that LGL do not display any oxidative burst in response to challenge with a number of well-characterized inducers, including PMA, A23187, Concanavalin A, NaF, FMLP, and phopholipase C I; in contrast, monocytes tested in parallel were stimulated as expected (Goldfarb, Timonen, Pick, and Herberman, manuscript in preparation).

POSSIBLE ROLE OF LYMPHOTOXINS IN NK CELL-MEDIATED CYTOLYSIS

Lymphotoxins have been suggested to play a central role in cell-mediated lysis of target cells (56); there has, however, been no clear documentation that production of cytolysis by any type of effector cells is due to liberation of this mediator into culture supernatants (6). If lymphotoxins are involved in cell-mediated cytolysis, it would appear to be a localized event occurring at the site of surface membrane contacts between effector cells and their targets. Evidence for a role of lymphotoxin in the lytic action of mouse NK cells has not been reported, but several investigators have suggested the possibility that NK activity may be mediated by secretion of lymphotoxin (57, 58, 59). It has been reported that guinea pig lymphotoxin, cytostatic to guinea pig cells, might increase the susceptibility of target cells to natural cell-mediated cytolysis (60). It should be pointed out that, at this time, it is not known whether the soluble factor described for NK activity is a conventional lymphotoxin (13).

POSSIBLE INTER-RELATIONSHIPS AMONG LYTIC MECHANISMS

The evidence suggesting a role of various enzymes or metabolic processes in the mechanism of NK activity need not be mutually exclusive. It is possible that interactions take place between various processes involved in cell mediated lysis of tumor cells, with lysis resulting from a sequence involving several interrelated events.

Phospholipases may be of major importance in effecting target cell destruction as described above. However, phospholipase action may reflect interactions with other metabolic processes. For example, an endogenous protease might lead to the activation of a latent precursor form of phospholipase (61, 62), or lead to the activation of some as yet undefined regulatory cascade that is controlled through limited proteolysis. Proteases produced by NK cells may therefore play a role in phospholipase activation through limited proteolysis of precursor molecules and, therefore, regulate the lytic potential of phospholipases through zymogen activation. Alternatively, both phospholipases and proteases may cooperatively function, either simultaneously or in temporal sequence, to degrade lipids and/or protein components of tumor target cells. These activities may in turn contribute to a common cascade of events controlled by other regulatory molecules (e.g., interferon) or may regulate other effector mechanism (e.g., superoxide formation). It is also possible that a protease might lead to the generation of an amphipathic "plug" which might be introduced into target cells and thereby disrupt the target cell membrane phospholipid bilayer (see M. Mayer and P. J. Lachman, this volume) with subsequent cytolysis.

As discussed above, reactive oxygen species such as superoxide have been implicated in the mechanism of cell-mediated cytotoxicity by various effector cell types. It is of interest that reports suggest that serine proteases, possibly cell surface membrane-associated, are involved in oxide production by human polymorpho-nuclear leukocytes (63, 64, 65). It was therefore suggested that serine proteases might be essential for the initiation and maintenance of superoxide production in response to triggering stimuli. This superoxide production and proteolytic activity may interact in the mechanism(s) of tumor cell cytolysis.

The possible role of proteolytic enzymes in the mechanisms of cell-mediated tumor cell cytolysis has also been examined relative to lymphotoxin. It has been reported that an enzyme on tumor target cells, which can be inactivated by inhibitors of proteolytic enzymes, is required for lymphotoxin-mediated target cell cytolysis (66). It has been suggested that alpha lymphotoxin, present on effector cells in an inactive form, requires esterase or protease-mediated activation for subsequent tumor cell lysis. Therefore, the alpha subunits of lymphotoxin may be considered as lytically inactive target cell precursor-zymogens that require proteolytic activation (66). It appears in this case that a target cell protease functions as a regulatory molecule, converting by limited proteolysis a normally dormant effector cell molecule into a potently lytic molecule. Interestingly, it has been reported that guinea pig lymphotoxin can activate membrane phospholipase A (67). In this system the activation of phospholipase A followed immediately after binding of lymphotoxin, suggesting that this may be a prerequisite for the cytotoxic activity of lymphotoxin. Therefore, a role for lymphotoxin in NK activity may be interrelated with either or both proteases and phospholipases. It would be of interest to determine whether other reported soluble mediators (13) also display protease or phospholipase activity.

The examples listed above illustrate how apparently distinct mechanisms may be, in fact, closely linked, with more than one event being required in the mechanism leading to the eventual lysis of target cells. Other essential inter-relationships also may exist. It has been demonstrated, for example, that fibroblasts and tumor cells may be lysed by C3a (68). This may be related to the ability of a protease (e.g., plasmin or plasminogen activator) to initiate the complement cascade by converting C1 to $\overline{C1}$ and by cleaving C3 to C3a and C3b. In addition, it has recently been observed that cytotoxic, activated macrophages lead to impairment of mitochondrial respiration in tumor cells (69); protease or superoxide production might be envisioned as the events required to produce this inhibition.

In summary, precise definition of the mechanisms involved in lysis by NK cells will probably be difficult and elusive. More definitive evidence for a role of a particular biochemical event in cytotoxicity by NK cells will not necessarily indicate that this mechanism is the primary, final, or sole event. It will also be necessary to determine the exact number and order of discrete steps and biochemical processes that take place between the initial contact of effector cells with target cell and the subsequent cytolysis. Ultimate resolution of the mechanism of NK killing will require molecular and biochemical examination of homogeneously pure molecules derived from highly purified cell populations.

REFERENCES

(1) Herberman, R.B. Immunologic defenses against cancer. In, The pathophysiology of human immunologic disorders, ed. J. J. Twomey, Urban & Schwarzenberg. In Press.
(2) Herberman, R.B. Possible roles of natural killer (NK) cells. In, Immunobiology of transplantation, cancer, and pregnancy, ed. P. K. Ray, Plenum Press. In Press.
(3) Berke G. Interaction of cytotoxic T lymphocytes and target cells. Prog. Allergy 27:69-133, 1981.
(4) Golstein, P., and Smith, E.T. 1977. Mechanism of T-cell mediated cytolysis: the lethal hit stage. Contemp. Top. Immunobiol. 7:273-300.
(5) Henney, C.S. 1977. T-cell mediated cytolysis: an overview of some current issues. Contemp. Top. Immunobiol. 7:245-272.
(6) Martz, E. 1977. Mechanism of specific tumor-cell lysis by alloimmune T lymphocytes. Resolution and characterization of discrete steps in the cellular interaction. Contemp. Top. Immunobiol. 7:301-361.
(7) Goldfarb, R.H., and Herberman R.B. Characteristics of natural killer cells and possible mechansims for their cytotoxic activity. In Advan. Inflamm. Res., ed. G. Weissman, Raven Press. In Press.
(8) Roder, J.C., Kiessling, R., Bibberfeld, P., and Andersson, B. 1978. Traget-effector interaction in the natural killer (NK) cell system. II. The isolation of NK cells and studies on the mechanism of killing. J. Immunol. 121:2509-2517.
(9) Roder, J.C., Rosen, A., Fenyo, E.M., and Troy, F.A. 1979. Target-effector interaction in the natural killer cell system: isolation of target structures. Proc. Natl. Acad. Sci. USA,

76:1405-1409.
(10) Timonen, T., Saksela, E., Ranki, A., and Hayry, P. 1979. Fractionation, morphological and functional characterization of effector cells responsible for human natural killer activity against cell-line targets. Cell. Immunol. 48:133-148.
(11) Timonen, T., Ortaldo, J.R., and Herberman, R.B. 1981. Characteristics of human large granular lymphocytes and relationship to natural killer and K cells. J. Exp. Med., 153:569-582.
(12) Goldfarb, R.H., and Herberman, R.B. 1981. Natural killer cell reactivity: Regulatory interactions among phorbol ester, interferon, cholera toxin, and retinoic acid. J. Immunol. 126:2129-2135.
(13) Wright, S.C., and Bonavida, B. 1981. Selective lysis of NK-sensitive target cells by a soluble mediator released from murine spleen cells and human peripheral blood lymphocytes. J. Immunol., 126:1516-1521.
(14) Goldfarb, R.H. Proteases in tumor invasion and metastasis. In The biology of metastatis., ed. L. A. Liotta and I. R. Hart. In Press.
(15) Ferluga, J., Asherson, G.L., and Becker, E.L. 1972. The effect of organophosphorous inhibitors, p-nitrophenol, and cytochalasin B on cytotoxic killing of tumor cells by immune spleen cells and the effects of shaking. Immunol. 23:577-590.
(16) Redelman, D., and Hudig, D. 1980. The mechanism of cell mediated cytotoxicity. I. Killing of murine cytotoxic T lymphocytes requires cell surface thiols and activated proteases. J. Immunol., 124:870-878.
(17) Hatcher, V.B., Oberman, M.S., Lazarus, G.S., and Grayzel, A.I. 1978. A cytotoxic proteinase isolated from human lymphocytes. J. Immunol. 120:665-670.
(18) Ferluga, J., and Allison, A.C. 1974. On the mechanism by which T lymphocytes exert cytotoxic effects. Nature, 250: 673-675.
(19) Tokes, Z.A. 1976. Estimation of cell surface associated protease activity and its application to lymphocytes. J. Supramolec. Struc., 4:507-513.
(20) Kedar, E., Ortiz de Landazuri, M., and Fahey, J.L. 1974. Enzymatic enhancement of cell-mediated cytotoxicity and antibody-dependent cell cytotoxicity. J. Immunol., 112: 26-36.
(21) Matter, A. 1975. A study of proteolysis as a possible mechanism for T cell mediated target cell lysis. Scand. J. Immunol., 4:349-356.
(22) Adams, D.O. 1980. Effector mechanisms of cytolytically activated macrophages: I. Secretion of neutral serine proteases and effect of protease inhibitors. J. Immunol., 124: 286-292.
(23) Adams, D.O., Kuo-Jang, J., Farb, R., and Pizzo, S.V. 1980. Effector mechanisms of cytolytically activated macrophages.

II. Secretion of a cytolytic factor by activated macrophages and its relationship to secreted neutral proteases. J. Immunol., 124:293-300.

(24) Piessens, W.F., and Sharma, S.D. 1980. Tumor cell killing by macrophages activated in vitro with lymphocyte mediators. 5. Role of proteases, inhibitors, and substrates. Cellular Immunol., 56:286-291.

(25) Adams, D.O., and Marino, P.A. 1981. Evidence for a multistep mechanism of cytolysis by BCG-activated macrophages: The interrelationship between the capacity for cytolysis, target binding, and secretion of a cytolytic factor. J. Immunol., 126: 981-987.

(26) Unkeless, J.C., Gordon, S., and Reich, E. 1974. Secretion of plasminogen activator by stimulated macrophages. J. Exp. Med., 139:834-850.

(27) Chapman, H.A., Vavrin, Z., and Hibbs, J.B. 1979. Modulation of plasminogen activator secretion by activated macrophages: Influence of serum factors and correlation with tumoricidal potential. Proc. Natl. Acad. Sci. USA, 76:3899-3903.

(28) Trinchieri, G., and DeMarchi, M. 1976. Antibody dependent cell mediated cytotoxicity in humans. III. Effect of protease inhibitors and shaking. J. Immunol., 116:885-891.

(29) Herberman, R.B., editor. 1980. natural cell mediated immunity against tumors. Academic Press, New York.

(30) Kishimoto, T., Kikutani, H., Nishizawa, Y., Sakaguchi, N., and Yamamura, Y. 1979. Involvement of anti Ig-activated serine protease in the generation of cytoplasmic factors that are responsible for the transmission of Ig-receptor mediated signals. J. Immunol., 123:1504-1510.

(31) Hudig, D., Haverty, T., Fucher, C., Redelman, D., and Mendelsohn, J. 1981. Inhibition of human natural cytotoxicity by macromolecular antiproteases. J. Immunol., 126:1569-1574.

(32) Hudig, D., Redelman, D., and Mendelsohn, J. 1980. Inhibition of human natural cytotoxicity by proteinase substrates. Fed. Proc., 469.

(33) Lavie, G., Weiss, H., Pick, A.I., and Franklin, E.C. 1980. The role of surface associated proteases in lymphocyte spontaneous cytolytic activity. Fourth Cong. Immunol. Abstracts, 11, 4. 30.

(34) Haliotis, R., Roder, J., Klein, M., Ortaldo, J., Fauci, A., and Herberman, R.B. 1980. Chediak-Higashi gene in humans. I. Impairment of natural-killer function. J. Exp. Med., 151:1039-1048.

(35) Roder, J.C., and Duwe, A.K. 1979. The beige mutation in the mouse selectively impairs natural killer cell function. Nature, 278:451-453.

(36) Vassali, J., Granelli-Piperno, A., Griscelli, C., and Reich, E. 1978. Specific protease deficiency in polymorphonuclear leukocytes of Chediak-Higashi syndrome and beige mice. J. Exp. Med., 147:1285-1290.

(37) Goldfarb, R.H., and Quigley, J.P. 1978. Production of plasminogen activator by chick embryo fibroblasts: synergistic effect of Rous sarcoma virus transformation and treatment with the tumor promoter phorbol-myristate-acetate. Cancer Res., 38:4601-4608.

(38) Maillard, J., Toullet, F., Favreau, C., and Chadenier, F. 1978. Stimulated lymph node lymphocytes release a plasminogen activator. Ann. Immunol. Inst. Pasteur., 129:499-502.

(39) Maillard, J.L., and Favreau, C. 1981. Plasminogen activation by normal B lymphocytes, a function associated with the cell membrane. J. Immunol., 126:1126-1130.

(40) Fulton, R.J., and Hart, D.A. 1980. Detection and partial characterization of lymphoid cell surface proteases. Cell. Immunol., 55:394-405.

(41) Fulton, R.J., and Hart, D.A. 1981. Characterization of a plasma-membrane associated plasminogen activator on thymocytes. Biochim. Biophys. Acta, 642:345-364.

(42) Goldfarb, R.H., and Quigley, J.P. 1980. Purification of plasminogen activator from Rous sarcoma virus transformed chick embryo fibroblasts treated with the tumor promoter phorbol-12-myristate-13-acetate. Biochem., 19:5463-5471.

(43) Umezawa, H., and Ayogi, T. 1977. Activities of proteinase inhibitors of microbial origin. In, Proteinases in mammalian cells and tissues, ed. A. Barrett, pp. 637-662, North Holland Biomedical Press.

(44) Zimmerman, M., Quigley, J.P., Ashe, B., Dorn, C., Goldfarb, R.H., and Troll, W. 1978. Direct fluorescent assay of urokinase and plasminogen activators of normal and malignant cells: kinetics and inhibitor profiles. Proc. Natl. Acad. Sci. USA, 75:750-753.

(45) Lane, J.T., Lo, F., and Prasad, C. 1980. Chymostatin inhibits cellular aggregation of activated human peripheral blood lymphocytes. Life Sci., 27:451-456.

(46) Berke, G. 1977. Recent advances and questions in lymphocytotoxicity. In, Regulatory mechanisms in lymphocyte activation, ed. D. O. Lucas, pp. 812-816, Academic Press, New York.

(47) Frye, L.D., and Friou, G.J. 1975. Inhibition of mammalian cytotoxic cells by phosphatidylcholine and its analogue. Nature, 258:333-335.

(48) Hoffman, T., Hirata, F., Bougnoux, P., Fraser, B.A., Goldfarb, R.H., Herberman, R.B., and Axelrod, J. 1981. Phospholipid methylation and phospholipase A_2 activation in cytotoxicity by human natural killer cells. Proc. Natl. Acad. Sci. USA, 78:3839-3843.

(49) Clark, R.A., and Klebanoff, S.J. 1975. Neutrophil-mediated tumor cell cytotoxicity: role of the peroxidase system. J. Exp. Med., 141:1442-1447.

(50) Clark, R.A., Klebanoff, S.J., Einstein, A.B., and Fefer, A. 1978. Peroxidase-H_2O_2-halide system cytotoxic effect on

mammalian tumor cells. Blood, 45:161-170.
(51) Nathan, C.F., Bruckner, L.H., Silverstein, S.C., and Cohn, Z.A. 1979. Extracellular cytolysis by activated macrophages and granulocytes. I. Pharmacologic triggering of effector cells and the release of hydrogen peroxide. J. Exp. Med., 149:84-99.
(52) Nathan, C.F., Bruckner, L.H., Silverstein, S.C., and Cohn, Z. 1979. Extracellular cytolysis by activated macrophages and granulocytes. II. Hydrogen peroxide as a mediator of cytotoxicity. J. Exp. Med., 149:100-113.
(53) Nathan, C., and Cohn, Z. 1980. Role of oxygen dependent mechanisms in antibody-induced lysis of tumor cells by activated macrophages. J. Exp. Med., 152:198-208.
(54) Nathan, C., Bruckner, L., Kaplan, G., Unkeless, J.C., and Cohn, Z. 1980. Role of activated macrophages in antibody-dependent lysis of tumor cells. J. Exp. Med., 152:183-197.
(55) Nathan, C.F., Murray, H.W., and Cohn, Z. 1980. The Macrophage as an effector cell. N. Eng. J. Med., 303:662-626.
(56) Granger, G.A., Hiserodt, J.C., and Ware, C.F. 1979. Cytotoxic and growth inhibitory lymphokines, ed. S. Cohn, E. Pick, and J. P. Oppenheim, pp. 141-163, Academic Press, New York.
(57) Ballas, Z.K., and Henney, C.S. 1979. The relationship between lymphokines and cell-mediated cytotoxicity. In, Biology of the lymphokines, ed. S. Cohen, E. Pick, and J. Oppenheim, pp. 165-180, Academic Press, New York.
(58) Bonnard, G., and West, W. 1979. Cell mediated cytotoxicity in humans. A critical review of experimental models and clinically oriented studies. In, Immunodiagnosis of Cancer, Part 2, ed. R. B. Herberman and K. R. McIntire, pp. 1032-1105. Marcel Dekker, Inc., New York.
(59) Peter, H.H., Eife, R.E., and Kalden, J.R. 1976. Spontaneous cytotoxicity (SCMC) of normal human lymphocytes against a human melanoma cell line: a phenomenon due to a lymphotoxin-like mediator. J. Immunol., 116:342-348.
(60) Evans, C.H. 1981. The role of lymphotoxin in natural cell-mediated cytotoxicity. Cell Immunol., 63:1-15.
(61) Van Den Bosch, H. 1980. Intracellular phospholipases A. Biochim. Biophys. Acta, 604:191-246.
(62) Rittenhouse-Simmons, S. 1981. Differential activation of platelet phospholipases by thrombin and ionophore A23187. J. Biol. Chem., 256:4153-4155.
(63) Goldstein, B.D., Witz, G., Amoruso, M., and Troll, W. 1979. Protease inhibitors antagonize the activation of polymorphonuclear leukocyte oxygen consumption. Biochem. Biophy. Res. Comm., 88:854-860.
(64) Kitagawa, S., Takaku, F., and Sakamoto, S. 1979. Serine protease inhibitors inhibit superoxide production by human polymorphonuclear leukocytes and monocytes stimulated by various surface active agents. FEBS Letters, 107:331-334.
(65) Kitagawa, S., Takaku, F., and Sakamoto, S. 1980. Evidence

that proteases are involved in superoxide producion by human polymorphonuclear leukocytes and monocytes. J. Clin. Invest., 65:74-81.

(66) Weitzen, M., and Granger, G.A. 1980. The human L.T. system. VIII. A target cell dependent enzymatic activation step required for the expression of the cytotoxic activity of human lymphotoxin. J. Immunol., 125:719-724.

(67) Kobayashi, Y., Sawada, J., and Osawa, T. 1979. Activation of membrane phospholipase A by guinea pig lymphotoxin (GLT). J. Immunol., 122:791-794.

(68) Temple, A., and Allison, A.C. 1980. Cytolysis of fibroblasts by C3a. Brit. J. Cancer, 42:21-25.

(69) Granger, D.L., Taintor, R.R., Cook, J.L., and Hibbs, J.B. 1980. Injury of neoplastic cells by murine macrophages leads to inhibition of mitochondrial respiration. J. Clin. Invest., 65:357-370.

DISCUSSION

J. Hibbs

Ron, did you say that the plasminogen activator activity was membrane-associated. It wasn't secreted?

R. Goldfarb

It exists in both forms, but we don't have a firm feeling for which form of the enzyme, if either, is critically involved. Although the enzyme appears to play some role, we're not yet sure whether it is a direct effect or an indirect effect. I should also note that this effect is not seen with all proteases that we've tried. For instance, alphathrombin, in the system that I described, had no positive stimulatory effect, nor did specific inhibitors of alphathrombin abrogate activity. In addition, other enzymes which are not neutral proteases, such as metalloproteases or type 4 collagenase have no effect on the system as well. We believe that at least there is some restricted specificity in terms of a neutral serine protease of tryptic and/or chymotryptic specificity.

P. Henkart

In view of the possible role of sialic acid on the target cell, what about the possibility that what the proteases are doing is just knocking sialic acid off glycoproteins?

R. Goldfarb

It's possible that some sialic acid could be degraded as an indirect result of these or other proteases, but I haven't pursued those studies. It's a possibility.

SECTION III. THE USE OF ANTISERA, MONOCLONAL ANTIBODIES, AND CLONED EFFECTOR CELLS N THE STUDY OF CELL-MEDIATED CYTOLYSIS

INTRODUCTION

The development of cloned lines of cytotoxic effector cells (Nabholz, Kaufmann) together with monoclonal antibody (mAb) technology, has introduced a much needed level of precision and reproducibility into an old problem: the serological identification of effector cell surface molecules possibly involved in the cytolytic process. The past history of the search for such molecules is summarized in the first part of Eric Martz's paper. The recent tremendous ferment in this area is reflected by the large number of papers on this topic in this volume.

To date, attention has been focused almost exclusively on CTL surface molecules, although some of the antibodies have beeen tested in other cytotoxic systems (See Golstein et al). One theme that seemed to emerge from various sessions is the need to use some of the well-defined CTL antibodies to look for the presence of and possible role for cross-reacting antigens on effectors in ADCC, NKCC and LDCC. Perhaps investigators with well-defined lytic systems could share antisera or mAb in an attempt to address one of the major questions of this workshop; namely, whether similar or different mechanisms are involved in the various lytic systems.

Identification of such molecules is made operationally through the ability of various antisera or mAb to block cytolysis. To date, three major types of surface components have been detected through this approach: Lyt-2, the LFA-1 antigen, and the component reactive with the "RAT-STAR" antibody. The development of further mAb of these types and characterization of the target antigens detected may lead to a better understanding of the cytolytic process.

The number of CTL-blocking antibodies is manageable at present, but will probably increase dramatically over the next year or so since this is such a promising general approach to studying the mechanism of CMC. However, the number of different membrane molecules recognized by these blocking antibodies is relatively limited, and may remain so.

In this section Martz et al. update their studies of Lyt2 and LFA-1 antibodies, both of which they feel block at the recognition-binding stage. However, it seems unlikely that at least Lyt2 antibodies bind directly to the CTL receptor; Fitch has described CTL clones that have no Lyt2, and Kaufmann's CTL hybridoma bears no detectable Lyt2. As pointed out by MacDonald and others, PEL are fairly insensitive to blocking by Lyt2 antibodies. Hayot et al. describe an Lyt-2^+ CTL clone specific for I region determinants that is inhibited neither by Lyt-2 or Lyt-2 antibodies.

Fitch's group (Dialynas et al.; Lancki et al.) describe a variety of CTL-blocking mAb. Most of them appear to recognize LFA-1-like molecules, although one precipitates a MHC class I-like molecule. One mAb (FP 384.5; Lancki et al.) is unique of all the antibodies described so far in that it blocks only a single CTL clone.

MacDonald et al. use one of their Ly2,3 mAb to ask whether blocking of CTL lysis correlates with the effect of the same antibody on other T cell functions. They find that the same degree of inhibition is observed with lysis, proliferation and lymphokine secretion. They also put forward the interesting postulate that CTL Ly23 molecules may be involved in stabilization of T cell-partner cell interactions. Schmitt-Verhulst et al., however, looked at the effect of two different mAb (one α-Lyt2 and the other α-LFA-1) on the proliferation and cytotoxicity of two different CTL clones. They found that the effect of the antibodies on proliferation depends on the antibody itself, and on how proliferation is induced. Golstein et al. report on a mAb that inhibits both proliferation and killing in some CTL lines, but only killing in others. Hayot et al also suggest that the precise effect of a given mAb on CTL function can be affected by the target cell used in the lytic assay. It may thus be a bit too soon to generalize on the relatedness of T cell functions on the basis of sensitivity to particular antibodies.

Bonavida also finds that Lyt2 antibodies block at the binding stage. He shows that selective removal of Lyt2 antigens with further trypsin inhibits binding. Further evidence on the action of the RAT* antibody at a post-binding stage is presented in his paper, together with a preliminary description of the molecule precipitated by the RAT* antibody.

Malissen et al. describe seven murine mAb inhibiting the cytolytic activity of human alloimmune cloned CTL. These antibodies precipitate a 30K dalton membrane protein. Somewhat like α-Lyt2 in mice, these mAb block different CTL clones with differing degrees of efficiency.

SOMATIC CELL GENETICS OF CYTOLYTIC T LYMPHOCYTES

M. Nabholz

Swiss Institute for Experimental Cancer Research
CH-1006 Epalinges
Lausanne, Switzerland

I would like to make some general comments about the use of cell genetics in the analysis of cytolytic mechanisms. To start you might well ask why somatic cell genetics, what is the importance of somatic cell genetics? I would answer that if you want to prove to me that you have identified a molecule on a CTL which is important for, say, its cytolytic activity, you can do it in one of two ways: You can either put this molecule into a vesicle or liposome of completely defined composition and show that this liposome has cytolytic activity; and I think it is quite clear that we are far from being able to do that type of experiment. Or you can use a cytolytic T-cell line which expresses the molecule and derive from this cell line variants which lack this molecule and show that they are no longer able to kill target cells. If such variants are the result of gene mutations then their further analysis should lead to testable hypotheses concerning the genetic control and the mechanism of cytolysis, as well as the differentiation of CTL. Now, let me outline briefly what the prerequisites for a somatic cell genetic analysis of a differentiated function are. The first one is that you have cell lines, i.e. cloned established cell populations, which stably express the function that you want to study. The second one is that you have to be able to derive variants from such cell lines that are affected in the specific function. Preferably such variants should be mutants and I will make a few comments about that in a minute. The third prerequisite is that there must be systems for a genetic analysis of such variants, systems for complementation tests and for recombination and segregation analysis. That is, you have to have a substitute for sex. And of course the most commonly used system today is somatic cell hybridization.

Now, let me make a few comments about the use of CTL lines for somatic cell genetics: simplifying things a bit there are two ways in which CTL lines have been derived. The first one was originally described by Gillis and Smith (for a recent review on the use of CTL-lines for somatic cell genetics, see ref. 1) and has been used by many investigators: you transfer and culture a population of lymphocytes that is enriched for CTL of a particular specificity by in vitro stimulation in medium supplemented only with a TCGF-containing supernatant. The cells will grow quite well for awhile, but if you try to clone them it doesn't work very well, and only after such populations have undergone some sort of "crisis" you obtain a cell line which is clonable with good effeciency and is reasonably stable. This process usually lasts several months. We have called such lines, operationally, CTL-B lines. The other way was first described by Glasebrook and Fitch who took MLC populations and cloned them right away in microcultures in the presence of stimulator cells and TCGF. They established clones which also seem to be able to grow for indefinite periods of time. We have called such lines CTL-A lines. What are the differences between these two types of lines? Both are dependent on TCGF, but CTL-A lines depend on the addition of filler cells (irradiated spleen cells). I don't want to go into the question of whether these have to be allogeneic or not. CTL-B lines have been selected for being able to grow in the absence of filler cells because they have been maintained in TCGF-containing medium without the addition of any irradiated spleen cells. Morphologically CTL-A lines look normal, like those killer cells that we saw in Sanderson's film. They are of normal size. Also their karyotype is more or less normal. CTL-B lines, on the other hand, are clearly not normal cells anymore. They are larger and heterogeneous in their morphology - you can distinguish different lines from each other simply by looking through the microscope - some adhere more, some adhere less to plastic, some are bigger, some are smaller, etc. Their karyotype is highly abnormal and differs from line to line. Their stability with regard to CTL-function and specificity is variable. Some clones are more stable than others. In general one has the impression that CTL-B clones tend to be less stable than CTL-A clones, although that is still a bit anecdotal. Clearly, the use of lines with karyotypes containing too many unrecognizable chromosomes, or that do not express CTL-funtions stably enough, for somatic cell genetic purposes become problematical.

Now, as I pointed out before, for somatic cell genetics, you should have, on the one hand, stable CTL-lines and, on the other, a source of genetic variants, i.e., mutants, because the whole approach is based on the comparison of such variants with the active lines. It is clear both from CTL-A and from CTL-B lines, though from the latter probably more easily, that you can get spontaneous variants which do not kill anymore. These are quite rare, but you can easily isolate variants which kill much less efficiently than the parental line. Such spontaneous variants are of unknown origin and you usually have no clue what the variation is due to. It may be epigenetic or genetic; multiple small variations may have finally abolished the cytolytic activity of these cells; you may have no idea where to start analyzing them. If people start to work with such variants, I predict that they will have a lot of trouble with conclusive interpretations for their findings. I therefore think that it is very important to work with well characterized genetic variants, i.e., mutants. Now if you look at the relevant literature, you will discover that it is by no means easy to make sure that any particular variant is a mutant and not something else (for discussion see ref. 2), and that you have to live with. But there are, I think, some criteria which one can apply to distinguish probable mutants from other types of variants. The first one is that the frequency of the variants is increased by treatment with mutagens. That is very important but not always easy to show, because to measure mutation frequencies is not a trivial proposition even in the simplest type of situation. It becomes much more complicated and a big project when you have to apply repeated cycles of selection with antibody and complement to obtain variants, which is almost always the case in the isolation of antigen-loss variants. The second criterion is stability - that is, if you remove the selective agent your variants should not - either rapidly or slowly - revert to the wild type phenotype. (Slow reversion has been observed, for instance, in H2-loss variants of a Balb/c myeloma (3).) The third criterion is further genetic and, possibly, biochemical characterization: if you can show that a variant has an alteration in the gene the product of which you have been selecting against, then you're OK, of course. Now, just to stress one point concerning the use of mutants: I think if you want to evaluate the functional significance of a particular trait, for instance the expression of an antigen, you have to analyze several independently derived mutants. It is not enough to look at one or two. And you have to characterize to some extent the nature of the lesions in the mutants, to investigate whether they affect regulatory or structural genes. Only when you have reasonably consistent answers to all these questions can you really make definitive statements about why variants no longer express the characteristic function of the parental cells.

I think that's all I want to say about mutants, except to point out that up to now all we can say is: "Well, that antigen might be important or that other, so let's select antigen loss variants." The real thing would be to be able to select for loss of cytolytic activity, and I propose that this meeting set up a prize for anybody who designs such a selection systems. Whoever wants to have a go at it should remember that systems for the selection of mutations affecting autosomal dominant genes have to be powerful because such mutations are expected to be very rare.

Let me end with a few comments about somatic cell hybrids. Somatic cell hybridization (for a review see ref. 4) can obviously be used to determine whether mutations are recessive or dominant. Complementation analysis determines, by crossing phenotypically identical mutants with each other, the number of loci controlling the expression of the affected trait. And co-segregation analysis may allow one to assign genes to particular chromosomes, or parts of chromosomes.

This technique has also been applied to the study of differentiation. By crossing cell lines belonging to different histiotypes one hopes to identify the genes which control the expression of the differentiated functions of these cells, and to determine their mode of action.

On the whole, the yield of conclusions from such experiments has been rather meager, but some of them have provided information on the nature of the commitment of a differentiated cell. It appears that, at least in some cases, the capacity of a gene to be expressed is "imprinted" on the chromosome carrying the gene, and maybe on the gene itself. To give an example: there are data which indicate that in hybrids between mouse Friend virus leukemia infected cells and human cells, which contain only the human chromosome carrying the α- globin genes, the capacity of these genes to be expressed depends on the tissue of origin of the chromosome. They can only be induced if the human parental cells belong to the erythroid lineage (5). This implies that the homologous genes of two parental cells with different functions may remain "imprinted" differently in a hybrid derived from them: the two cell types behave as if they were genetic variants with regard to such genes, and if there are not too many differences then crosses between such cell lines can be used to identify the differently imprinted genes.

From some of our recent work it appears, indeed, that (thymoma x CTL) hybrids may help us to identify some of the genes controlling the CTL-phenotype. In the immediate post-Köhler-Milstein era it was, of course, very fashionable to try to "immortalize" CTL by crossing them with T lymphomas. Apart from Kaufmann and her collaborators everybody was unsuccessful. That sort of situation can have three types of explanations: the first one is that the surviving hybrids are derived from inactive cells contaminating the CTL-population or CTL line. (Even in a cloned CTL-line it is hard to rule out the existence of one inactive variant per 10^4 cells, which is about the highest frequency of hybrids you can easily achieve). The second possibility is that in the hybrids the CTL-function is extinguished by some gene product(s) contributed by the lymphoma parent. To prove that, one has to find segregants which re-express the function because they have lost the lymphoma chromosomes carrying such repressing genes. The third alternative is that the hybrids always lose some CTL-chromosomes carrying genes which are essential for the CTL-function and not expressed in the lymphoma parent.

Our more recent findings (6) suggest that it is this last explanation which applies to the earlier failures to obtain cytolytically active hybrids. From crosses of AKR-thymomas with normal CTL or CTL-lines, cytolytic hybrids can easily be isolated if selection is carried out in the presence of TCGF. The active hybirds are dependent on TCGF but independent variants can be derived from them. These are almost always cytolytically inactive. These observations are consistent with the hypothesis that in CTL but not in thymomas one or several linked genes are active which make these cells TCGF dependent and cytolytically competent. In hybrids with thymoma cells these CTL-genes but not their thymoma homologues remain expressed, and TCGF-independent variants are the result of the loss of the CTL-chromosome carrying them.

If our hypothesis turns out to be correct then "imprinting" of these genes may be one of the crucial steps in the maturation of T cells.

REFERENCES

1. Nabholz, M. The somatic cell genetic analysis of cytolytic T-lymphocyte functions. In "Isolation, Characterization and Utilization of T Lymphocyte Clones." G. Fathman and F.W. Fitch, eds., Academic Press, in press.
2. Siminovitch, L. On the Nature of Hereditable Variation in Cultured Somatic Cells. Cell 7:1 (1976).
3. Rajan, T.V., Nathenson, S.G., and M.D. Scharff. Regulatory Variants for the Expression of H-2 Antigens. I. Isolation and Characterization. J. of the National Cancer Inst. 56: 1221 (1976).
4. Ringertz, N.R., and R.E. Savage. Cells Hybrids. Academic Press (1976).
5. Deisseroth, A., Bode, U., Fontana, J., and D. Hendrick. Expession of human α-globin genes in hybrid mouse erythroleukaemia cells depends on differentiated state of human donor cell. Nature 285:36 (1980).
6. Conzelmann, A., Corthesy, P., and M. Nabholz. Correlation between cytolytic activity, growth factor dependence and lectin resistance in cytolytic T-cell hybrids. In "Isolation, Characterization and Utilization of T Lymphocyte Clones." G. Fathman and F.W. Fitch, Eds., Academic Press, in press.

DISCUSSION

E. Martz

I wondered if you could comment on what would be the mutagen of choice to produce the kinds of mutations that you would like to get. I was at a Gordon Conference this summer, in which someone led me to believe that ethylmethane sulfonate tends to produce very large deletions in those systems where the genetic effect can be characterized, and therefore it may not usually produce a point mutation.

M. Nabholz

I don't think EMS produces large deletions, but I'm not completely sure. There is a tendency to take mutagens which work in bacteria and where the effect is known, and apply them to eucaryotic cells. I think there are very few mutagens where the effect is very clear, except for things like x-ray where it is known that you produce deletions. I think EMS in general works often as a point mutagen.

(UK)

Have you some information about the size in kb of structures affected by EMS?

E. Martz

No, I'm afraid I really can't remember the details, but it was not a mammalian system.

LYT-2 NEGATIVE AND T CELL GROWTH FACTOR INDEPENDENT CYTOTOXIC T LYMPHOCYTE HYBRIDOMAS

Yael Kaufmann

Department of Cell Biology
The Weizmann Institute of Science
Rehovot 76100, Israel

INTRODUCTION

Homogeneous populations of cytotoxic T lymphocytes (CTL) are essential for studying the CTL receptor and killing mechanism. Such populations are obtained mainly through continuous CTL lines. However, the limiting amounts of cells thus produced, the months required to establish these lines and the need for repeated stimuli to maintain CTL growth and activity represent major drawbacks. To circumvent these problems we developed functional CTL-hybridomas which proliferate autonomously both in culture and *in vivo* (1-3). Previous attempts to generate T cell growth factor (TCGF)-independent CTL-hybridomas were unsuccessful (4,5), possibly due to CTL-induced nonspecific lysis of the fusion partner during hybridization. Our approach was based on the assumption that nonspecific lysis during hybridization may be prevented by a transient inactivation of CTL with trypsin prior to fusion and cytotoxicity regenerated in the hybrid cells after fusion, as is the case with trypsin-inactivated parental CTL (1). Using this approach, we have generated functional CTL-hybridomas which constitutively express their killing potential.

The growth characteristics and killing activity of the autonomous CTL-hybridomas have been described previously (1-3). Here we demonstrate the independence of the cytotoxicity of these CTL-hybridomas from TCGF, by the failure to detect any secreted TCGF in the hybrid growth media and by the inability of added TCGF to further stimulate cytotoxicity.

The lytic specificity of the CTL-hybrid clones, which was previously found to be restricted to allogeneic leukemic target cells

(TC;2), was further examined by addition of phytohemagglutinin (PHA) to the lysis assay. Since PHA induces nonspecific lysis of TC by CTL (6), it was expected that the CTL-hybridomas would likewise lyse nonspecific, otherwise resistant, TC. This expectation was based on the assumption that the lytic specificity demonstrated for the CTL-hybridomas was due to the presence of suitable antigenic determinants on the sensitive TC and not to their exceptional fragility. Indeed, in the presence of PHA the CTL-hybridomas induced nonspecific TC lysis, similar to the parental CTL. This result indicated that the cytotoxicity of the hybridomas can be expressed specifically presumably through TC antigens, or nonspecifically, via the lectin.

Lyt-2 alloantigen has been detected on most murine CTL and was implicated in TC recognition or cytolytic process (7-9). The relevance of Lyt-2 to the lytic capacity of CTL was examined here using the CTL-hybridomas. The Lyt-2 antigen was not exposed on two independent CTL-hybrid clones, one derived from a mixed lymphocyte culture (MLC) and the other from peritoneal exudate lymphocytes (PEL). Furthermore, the hybridomas' specific cytotoxicity was not inhibited by monoclonal antibodies directed against Lyt-2. These data suggested that exposure of Lyt-2 antigen on CTL is not essential for the expression of specific lytic activity.

THE SPECIFICITY OF TC KILLING BY THE CTL-HYBRIDOMAS CAN BE BYPASSED WITH PHA

The CTL-hybridomas were generated by fusion of BALB/c anti EL4 CTL ($H-2^d$ anti $H-2^b$) with AKR thymoma cells BW5147. The CTL populations used for fusion were obtained from BALB/c mice primed with leukemia EL4 of C57BL/6 and restimulated either _in vivo_ (PEL) or _in vitro_ (MLC). Cytolytically active cultures obtained from the two sources were cloned and subcloned (1,2). Both types of CTL-hybridomas lysed several $H-2^b$ leukemic target cells and did not lyse non-$H-2^b$ tumors, similar to the parental CTL. However, unlike parental CTL populations, the hybridomas did not lyse normal lymphoblasts stimulated with either Concanavalin A (Con A) or lipopolysaccharide (2). To determine whether this pattern did not simply reflect a differential resistance to lysis of some normal TC versus tumor cells, the assays were done in the presence of PHA which promotes nonspecific CTL mediated lysis (6). The CTL-hybridomas which specifically lysed EL4 but not $H-2^b$ lymphoblasts or YAC ($H-2^a$) tumor cells did lyse both resistant TC when PHA was present (Fig. 1). The promotion of hybrid-mediated lysis of these TC by PHA suggests that their resistance to specific lysis is not due to refractoriness to lysis but can be attributed to the lack of certain TC determinants specifically recognized by the hybridomas. This result and previous findngs about the killing of $H-2^b$ leukemic TC (EL4, RBL5, ALC5 and ALB.B2) by the CTL-hybridomas (2), are consistent with the hypothesis that the hybridoma-mediated lysis is specific for a viral or tumor antigen and is restricted by $H-2^b$.

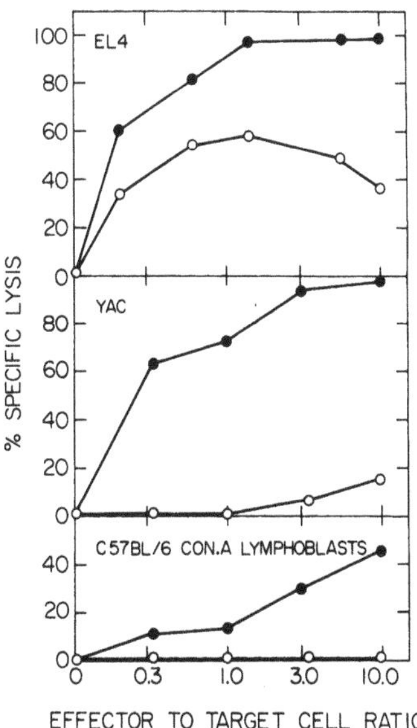

Fig. 1. PHA promotes nonspecific lysis of target cells by CTL-hybridomas.

CTL-hybrid clone P.47 was tested at various effector-to-TC ratios for lysis of the following ^{51}Cr-labeled and neuraminidase-treated (2) TC: EL4 (C57BL/6 H-2^b leukemia), YAC (A/SN, H-2^a leukemia, highly sensitive to natural killer-mediated lysis) and Con A lymphoblasts generated by incubation of C57BL/6 spleen cells in the presence of 2 μg/ml Con A for 3 days. The Con A lymphoblasts were pretreated with 20 mg/ml methyl-alpha-D-mannopyranoside to remove residual Con A. Incubation was for 4 hours with EL4 and for 5 hours with YAC or Con A lymphoblasts. Spontaneous release values from EL4, YAC and Con A blasts were 15%, 12% and 40%, respectively.

(o) No PHA in the assay; (•) lysis in the presence of 10 μg/ml PHA.

THE CTL-HYBRIDOMAS EXPRESS THEIR KILLING POTENTIAL INDEPENDENTLY OF TCGF

Nabholz et al. (10) suggested that the expression of cytolytic competence is restricted to TCGF-dependent clones. This suggestion was based on the behavior of TCGF-dependent continuous CTL clones and hybridomas derived from these lines (11). Yet, the CTL-hybridomas generated by us express efficient and specific cytotoxicity while growing for months in standard tissue culture medium without the addition of any known stimulus. It was still possible that the apparent autonomous expression of cytotoxicity depends on growth factors secreted by the CTL-hybridomas themselves. To test this possibility, hybrid growth media were examined for TCGF activity. MLC memory cells, which respond to TCGF by increased proliferation and cytotoxicity, were used as indicators in the search for TCGF in CTL-hybridomas' conditioned media. As can be seen in Table I, growth media from both hybridomas could not replace TCGF in either promoting DNA synthesis or restimulating killing activity of the indicator cells. In a complementary assay, the effect of an externally added TCGF on the activity of the hybridomas was tested. In this experiment (Table 1), CTL-hybridomas were grown for 3 days in TCGF containing medium before their proliferation and cytotoxicity was examined. The externally added TCGF did not affect the activities of the MLC-derived CTL-hybridomas while it partially inhibited the PEL-derived hybridomas. The absence of detectable TCGF in the hybridomas' growth media and the inability of TCGF-containing fractions to further stimulate the CTL-hybridomas show that their killing potential is expressed autonomously. It may be that constitutive cytotoxic clones (TCGF independent) which had existed in the original, heterogeneous parental CTL populations were immortalized by hybridization. Alternatively, the tumorigenic fusion partner released the CTL-hybrid progeny cells from the dependence of parental CTL on growth stimuli without interfering with cytotoxicity.

THE FUNCTIONAL CTL-HYBRIDOMAS DO NOT EXPRESS SURFACE LYT-2 ANTIGEN

Recent studies from several laboratories have indicated that T cell-mediated cytolysis of allogeneic or syngeneic tumor cells can be inhibited by either conventional alloantisera or monoclonal antibodies directed against Lyt-2 (7-9, 12). Antibodies reactive with H-2, Thy-1 or other antigens of the effector cells do not inhibit cytolysis under the same conditions. These findings sugested a relation between Lyt-2 and the T cell receptor (7-9). To investigate the possible involvement of Lyt-2 in the lytic process, the effect of anti-Lyt-2 on the lytic activity as well as the expression of Lyt-2 on parental CTL populations and CTL-hybrid clones were examined. Monoclonal antibodies directed against constant determinants of mouse Lyt-2 (13) were used in these experiments. Supernatants of the culture media of hybridoma subclone 53-6.72 was concentrated to generate high antibody titer. The cytotoxicity of the two CTL-hybrid clones was not affected even at 30-fold the concentration which caused 50% inhibition with the control primary MLC (Fig. 2). In contrast to anti-Lyt-2, several other antibodies such as rat monoclonal antibodies directed against CTL (P. Golstein et al., submitted) and the serum of a rabbit which had been immunized against the CTL-hybridomas (unpublished results) proved inhibitory

TABLE I

TCGF is not detected in the CTL-hybridomas' growth media and added TCGF does not stimulate their activities

Effector cells*	Conditioned medium**	DNA synthesis*** (^{3}H TdR incorporation)	Cytotoxicity**** (^{51}Cr release)
		(cpm x 10^{-2})	(Percent lysis)
MLC 2° memory cells	---	3	18
	TCGF	157	100
	Md. hybridoma culture sup.	1	20
	P. hybridoma culture sup.	2	20
Md. hybridoma	---	1087	39
	TCGF	992	37
P. hybridoma	---	694	47
	TCGF	528	22

*MLC 2° memory cells (CBA anti C57BL/6) were used as indicator cells, 16 days following secondary stimulation. CTL-hybrid clones Md.26/15 and P.47/21 were examined.

**TCGF conditioned medium was from BALB/c splenocytes incubated for 48 hours with 2 μg/ml Con A. Hybridoma culture supernatants were taken from hybrid cutures grown to $1x10^6$ cells/ml. Before use the conditioned media were diluted 1:2 in fresh Dulbecco-modified Eagle's medium containing 10% fetal calf serum, $5x10^{-5}$ M 2-mercaptoethanol and 4 mg/ml methyl-α-D-mannopyranoside. MLC indicator cells were incubated in conditioned media for 5 days and hybridomas for 3 days.

***Thymidine uptake was determined at the end of the preincubation period, after a 4-h pulse of ^{3}H TdR (10 μCi/ml).

****Cytotoxicity was tested in a 4-h assay under standard conditions (2) with $1x10^4$ effector cells and $1x10^4$ ^{51}Cr-labeled EL4 target cells. Spontaneous release was 15%.

to the CTL-hybridoma mediated lysis. In agreement with several reports (7-9,12), CTL activity generated in primary MLC (BALB/c anti C57BL/6) was inhibited by the anti-Lyt-2 antibodies, while cytotoxicity of PEL, generated in the same strain combination, was only slightly affected over a wide range of anti-Lyt-2 concentrations (Fig. 2). This result confirms a recent study by MacDonald et al. (14) who demonstrated that the majority of PEL-derived clones, although exposing high levels of Lyt-2 antigen, are not inhibited by anti-Lyt-2 antibodies.

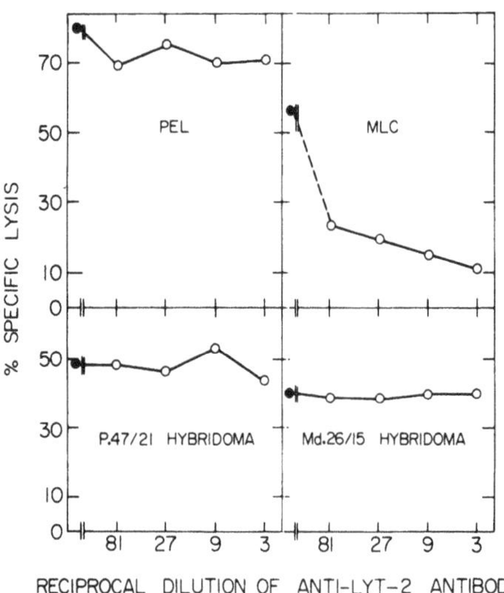

Fig. 2. Effect of anti-Lyt-2 on the lytic activity of CTL and CTL-hybridomas.

The anti-Lyt-2 antibody used was the rat monoclonal antibody 53-6.72 prepared by Ledbetter and Herzenberg (13) and supplied by the cell distribution center of the Salk Institute. Hybrid growth medium was precipitated with 50% ammonium sulfate and reconstituted in one-tenth of the original volume.

Aliquots of $1x10^4$ effector cells: BALB/c anti-EL4 PEL 1° (15); BALB/c anti-C57BL/6 MLC 1° (15); P.47/21 hybridoma and Md.26/15 hybridoma, were preincubated for 20 minutes at 37°C with various dilutions of the anti-Lyt-2. Cytotoxicity was then tested against $1x10^4$ ^{51}Cr-labeled, neuraminidase-treated (2) EL4 target cells in a 3-hour assay (PEL) or in a 4-hour assay (MLC and hybridomas). The filled-in symbols correspond to the lytic activity of each effector preparation in the absence of antibody.

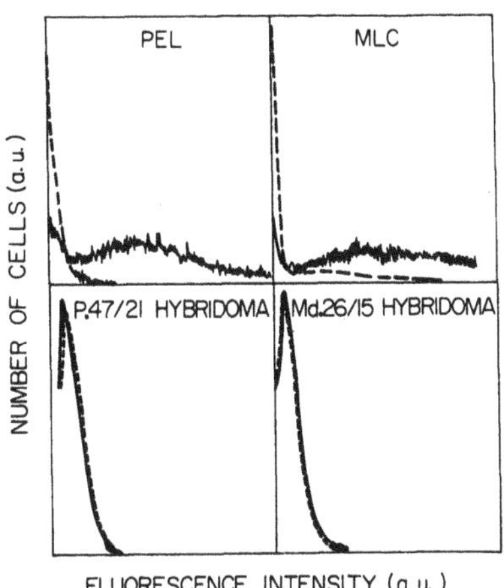

Fig. 3. Cytofluorometric analysis of Lyt-2 expression on CTL and CTL-hybridomas.

Aliquots of $2x10^6$ BALB/c anti-EL4 CTL: PEL 1° (15) or MLC 2° (1) or $1x10^6$ CTL-hybridomas; clones P.47/21 or Md/26/15 were incubated for 30 minutes at 4°C in 1:3 dilution of anti-Lyt-2 described in Fig. 2, washed and stained with fluoresceinated rabbit anti-rat Ig. Samples were analyzed by the FACS II. For each cell preparation, anti-Lyt-2 staining (solid lines) was compared to control staining in the presence of the fluoresceinated reagent alone (dashed lines).

The expression of Lyt-2 on parental CTL and on CTL-hybrid clones was examined by flow cytofluorometric analysis using the same monoclonal anti-Lyt-2 antibodies. Aliquots of cells were incubated at 1:3 dilution of the concentrated Lyt-2 supernatant, washed and stained with fluorescent rabbit anti-rat immunoglobulin reagent. Control aliquots were incubated with only the fluorescent reagent. Figure 3 depicts the Lyt-2 fluorescence distributions of PEL, MLC and the CTL-hybridomas that were assessed for cytotoxicity in Fig. 2. As shown, both parental CTL populations expressed considerable amounts of Lyt-2 while the CTL-hybridomas exhibited only background fluorescence and were thus considered Lyt-2 negative.

The absence of Lyt-2 from CTL-hybridoma surfaces and the inability of anti-Lyt-2 to inhibit their specific killing activity distinguishes them from several CTL populations and clones which have been reported to expose Lyt-2 and, in some cases, to be inhibited by anti-Lyt-2 antibodies (7-9,12,14). This discrepancy could be taken to indicate that the CTL-hybridomas utilize a different cytotoxic mechanism, or alternatively, that Lyt-2 is unrelated to cytotoxicity. The first interpretaiton seems less likely, because of the great similarity in the requirements of hybridoma- and parental CTL-mediated killing of their target cells. Thus, both reactions occur at 37°C and not at 21°C; and both are inhibited by EDTA, cytochalasin B (2) and anti-CTL monoclonal antibodies (Golstein et al., submitted). In addition, the cytotoxicity of the hybridoma can be abolished by preincubation with trypsin or with the trypsin inhibitor TLCK (2), as in the case with CTL (1,16). These similarities and the finding that the hybridomas do not induce antibody-dependent cytotoxicity (2), support the view that the CTL-hybridomas utilize the parental CTL mechanisms for recognition and killing during TC lysis.

Although Lyt-2 positive cells were found to be responsible for cytotoxicity in most allogeneic and syngeneic situations reported so far (7-9,12,17), exceptions to this "rule" are the Lyt-2 negative, long-term allospecific CTL-line (18) and primary MLC (19) directed against I-A molecules. These, as well as our observations with CTL-hybridomas (Figs. 2 & 3), indicate that Lyt-2 molecules are not obligatory in TC lysis. Hence, views holding Lyt-2 as a common characterizing marker for all CTL and involving it in the killing mechanism need to be reexamined. It is interesting to note that the Lyt-2 negative CTL line (18) resembles the CTL-hybridomas in that its growth and cytotoxicity are not dependent on added TCGF, in contrast to most continuous CTL-lines.

CONCLUDING REMARKS

CTL-hybridomas provide an efficient tool for studying T lymphocyte cytotoxicity, with clear technical and scientific advantages when compared to CTL populations and lines. Previous analyses of the killing activity and growth characteristics of several CTL-hybrid clones revealed that they specifically lyse TC *in vitro* in a reaction similar to that mediated by parental CTL (2). They grow rapidly in culture without addition of stimulus and can also proliferate efficiently *in vivo* in F1 mice (3), thus providing an unlimited supply of homogeneous cells for the study of unique killer structures and functions. Another advantage, resulting from the hybridomas' tendencies to lose chromosomes and suppress additional genes of the nontumorigenic partner, is the potential of separating dispensable CTL components from those essential to specific cytotoxicity. This may have occurred in the active CTL-hybridomas which did not express the parental Lyt-2 surface antigen and yet expressed cytotoxicity, although selective fusion of Lyt-2 negative CTL cannot be ruled out. Likewise, cytotoxic capacity was separated from TCGF dependency, implying that the two properties are not directly linked as previously suggested (10). TCGF may support cell proliferation and maintenance of CTL lines, functions that are provided in the hybridoma by the tumorigenic fusion partner. A promising future approach will be the comparative biochemical analysis of nonfunctional hybrid variants. Such nonfunctional variants were recently derived in our laboratory from active clones.

ACKNOWLEDGEMENTS

The author wishes to thank Dr. Z. Eshhar and Dr. G. Berke for helpful discusisons. The skilled assistance of Mrs. T. Oren and Ms. T. Waks is gratefully acknowledged. This research was supported in part by the United States-Israel Binational Science Foundation (Grant #2642-81).

REFERENCES

1. Kaufmann, Y., Berke, G., and Z. Eshhar. Functional cytotoxic T lymphocyte hybridomas. Transpl. Proc. 13:1171 (1981).
2. Kaufmann, Y., Berke, G., and Z. Eshhar. Cytotoic T lymphocyte hybridomas which mediate specific tumor cell lysis in vitro. Proc. Natl. Acad. Sci. USA 78:2502 (1981).
3. Kaufmann, Y., Berke, B., and Z. Eshhar. Cytolytic T cell hybridomas. In "Lymphokines, a Forum for Immunoregulatory Cell Products," ed. M. Feldmann (Academic Press, New York), Vol. 5, in press.
4. Kohler, G., Lefkovits, I., Elliot, B., and A. Coutinho. Derivation of hybrids between a thymoma line and spleen cells activated in a mixed leukocyte reaction. Eur. J. Immunol. 7:758 (1977).
5. Grutzmann, R., and G. Hammerling. Characterization and functional analysis of T cell hybrids. Curr. Top. Microbiol. Immunol. 81:188 (1978).
6. Forman, J., and G. Möller. Generation of cytotoxic lymphocytes in mixed lymphocyte reactions. I. Specificity of the effector cells. J. Exp. Med. 138:672 (1973).
7. Nakayama, E., Shiku, H., Stockert, E., Oettgen, H.F., and L.J. Old. Cytotoxic T cells: Lyt phenotype and blocking of killing activity by Lyt antisra. Proc. Natl. Acad. Sci. USA 76:1977 (1979).
8. Sarmiento, A., Glasebrook A.L., and F.W. Fitch. Monoclonal antibodies block cytolysis by T cells. J. Immunol. 125:2665 (1980).
9. Hollander, N., Pillemer, E., and I. Weissman. Blocking effect of Lyt-2 antibodies on T cell functions. J. Exp. Med. 152:674 (1980).
10. Nabholz, M., Conzelman, A., Acuto, O., North, M., Haas, W., Pohlit, W., Boehmer, H.W., Hengartner, H., Mach, J.P., Engers, H., and J.P. Johnson. Established murine cytotoxic T cell lines as tools for a somatic cell genetic analysis of T cell functions. Immunol. Rev. 51:125 (1980).
11. Nabholz, M., Cianfriglia, M., Acuto, O., Conzelmann, A., Haas,

W., Boehmer, H.V., MacDonald, H.R., and J.P. Johnson. Cytolytically active murine T cell hybrids. Nature (London) 287: 437 (1980).
12. Shinahara, N., and D.H. Sachs. Mouse alloantibodies capable of blocking cytotoxic T cell function. I. Relationship between the antigen reactive with blocking antibodies and the Lyt-2 locus. J. Exp. Med. 150:432 (1979).
13. Ledbetter, J.A., and L.A. Herzenberg. Xenogeneic monoclonal antibodies to mouse lymphoid differentiation antigens. Immunol. Rev. 47:362 (1979).
14. MacDonald H.R., Thiernesse, N., and J.-C. Cerottini. Inhibition of T cell-mediated cytolysis by monoclonal antibodies directed against Lyt-2: Heterogeneity of inhibition at the clonal level. J. Immunol. 126:1671 (1981).
15. Kaufmann, Y., and G. Berke. Cell surface glycoproteins of cytotoxic T lymphocytes induced in vivo and in vitro. J. Immunol. 126:1443 (1981).
16. Chang, T., and H.N. Eisen. Effects of N^{α}-tosyl-l-lysyl-chloromethylketone on the activity of cytotoxic T lymphocytes. J. Immunol. 124:1028 (1980).
17. Dialynas, D.P., Loken, M.R., Glasebrook A.L., and F.W. Fitch. $Lyt\text{-}2^{-}/Lyt\text{-}3^{-}$ variants of a cloned cytotoxic T cell line lack an antigen receptor functional in cytolysis. J. Exp. Med. 153:595 (1981).
18. Swain S.L., Dennert, G., Wormsley, S., and R.W. Dutton. The Lyt phenotype of a long-term allospecific T cell line. Both helper and killer activities to IA are mediated by Ly-1 cells. Eur. J. Immunol. 11:175 (1981).
19. Vidovic, A., Juretic, A., Nagy, Z.A., and J. Klein. Lyt phenotype of primary cytotoxic T cells generated across the A and E regions of the H-2 complex. Eur. J. Immunol. 11:499 (1981).

DISCUSSION

A. Glasebrook

If you stimulate with mitogens do you get any IL2 production? You'd have to change your test system, of course. You couldn't use the MLC hybridoma, but you could use a clone at least.

Y. Kaufmann

I am doing these experiments now. I cannot give you a definite answer yet.

P. Golstein

I'd like to know if Marcus' hybrids show a lag period as well, or if this is peculiar to these hybridomas.

M. Nabholz

We haven't tested that carefully.

R. MacDonald

I was under the impression from the early publications I saw that you used neuraminidase or enzyme-modified target cells. Is that true in the results you have been showing or are these unmodified target cells?

Y. Kaufmann

Yes. These target cells were all pre-treated with neuraminidase, which enhances only the specific killing, and never affects non-specific killing.

C. Henney

Is it necessary to do that?

Y. Kaufmann

No. It's only a question of assay time. You have to wait a little bit longer to see the same level of killing without pre-treatment. The reason I use this pre-treatment with neuraminidase is that I am convinced that normal spleen cells do not kill following neuraminidase treatment of target cells. Because of the long lag period, spontaneous release can be quite high. Enzyme treatment shortens the total assay time and lowers spontaneous release.

B. Bonavida

Will your hybrid grow in vivo?

Y. Kaufmann

Yes. Several hybrids grow in ascites form in vivo in F1 mice. They proliferate very well.

THE MOLECULAR BASIS FOR CYTOLYTIC T LYMPHOCYTE FUNCTION: ANALYSIS WITH BLOCKING MONOCLONAL ANTIBODIES

Eric Martz[a], Denise Davignon[b], Konrad Kürzinger[b], and Timothy A. Springer[b]

[a]The Department of Microbiology, University of Massachusetts, Amherst MA 01003

[b]The Laboratory of Membrane Immunochemistry, Sidney Farber Cancer Institute, Harvard Medical School, Boston MA 02115

INTRODUCTION

Cytolytic T lymphocytes (CTL) were identified during the late 1960's (1,2) and are thought to be important effector cells in immunity to viruses (3) and in allograft rejection (4). Despite considerable effort during the past decade, little has been learned about the biochemical basis for the killing event. Not only do the presumed molecular mediators remain unidentified, but fundamental physiological questions remain unanswered.

The primary target cell site damaged by the CTL has not been identified. While electrolyte fluxes have been observed at the time of programming for lysis (5), the sodium influx or depolarization of membrane potential expected to ensue if membrane "holes" have been created (similar to those produced by complement) have not been documented.

It is often supposed that the primary lesions are in the target cell membrane, and that these lead to colloid osmotic lysis of the sort documented for complement-mediated lysis of erythrocytes. However, a colloid osmotic lytic phenomenon has not been substantiated for viable nucleated cells, such as tumor cells, even in the case of complement (a view also held by Sanderson, 6). Such cells are capable of considerably more complicated responses to damage than are red cells (7,8). Experiments employing macromolecular "osmotic protectants" to estimate the size of the membrane lesions

(?) induced by CTLs are open to alternative interpretations (6; section VI.C in 9).

What, then, have we learned about the mechanism of CTL-mediated killing during the past decade?

1. The CTL is not only antigenically specific, but, once it recognizes a target, remains exquisitely selective in sparing antigenically "innocent" bystander cells (4). This excludes release of a stable, non-specific toxin. A labile and/or specific toxin remains possible (Cf. 10).
2. The CTL remains unharmed during killing, and can kill multiple target cells sequentially in time (11,12).
3. Nevertheless, CTLs can be killed by other CTLs (13,14), although this leaves open the possibility of spatially or temporally limited resistance to their own toxin.
4. The target cell probably plays no active role in its own demise, since target cells whose metabolism has been irreversibly poisoned by glutaraldehyde are killed efficiently (15).
5. Once differentiated, the CTL needs no protein synthesis during killing, probably even to kill repeatedly (16).
6. Some lectins induce CTLs to kill nonspecifically (17) by a mechanism very similar to that employed in specific killing (18). Nevertheless, mere adhesion with a CTL is not sufficient for killing (19), suggesting that the lytic mechanism requires triggering by the antigen receptors. This conclusion is also consistent with the outcome of elegant unidirectional recognition experiments involving two CTL populations (20).
7. Individual CTL cells can vary in killing efficiency. Secondary CTL form conjugates in half the time required by primary CTL (89), and in individual binary conjugates, secondary CTL kill their targets in half the time required by primary CTL (21).
8. Assays have been developed which resolve the killing process into three steps: recognition-adhesion (probably two events but not yet clearly resolved), programming for lysis (the lethal hit), and killer cell-independent lysis (9,22).
9. Completion of programming for lysis can occur within minutes after contact with the target (23,24).
10. The recogniton-adhesion step requires Mg^{++}; Ca^{++} is unnecessary and insufficient (25). Programming for lysis is calcium (or strontium) dependent (22,26,27); killer cell independent lysis requires neither divalent cation (9).
11. Cytochalasins inhibit primarily or solely the recognition-adhesion step (28,29), while other pharmacologic inhibitors appear to act both on recognition-adhesion and on programming for lysis (29,30).
12. It seems likely that the primary lesion produced by CTLs

in the target cell is functionally different from that produced by complement, based on studies with mast cell targets (31,32, and Martz, Parker, Gately, and Tsoukas, this volume) and on morphologic observations of lysis (6).

REASONS FOR LACK OF MOLECULAR UNDERSTANDING OF CTL FUNCTION

Molecular understanding of the mechanism of CTL-mediated killing has been slow to develop. With the exception of Hiserodt's tantalizing but unconfirmed report of a labile antigen-specific lysis produced by CTL-rich T lymphocytes (10), attempts to detect lytic effector molecules in CTL extracts or supernatants have been unrewarding (9,33). No T cell antigen-receptor is well understood in molecular terms at the present time, including the CTL receptor (Cf. 34). Even attempts to isolate target H-2 antigens in a form which will bind specifically to CTL, much less competitively block killing, have been largely unsuccessful (35-39). Finally, it has not been feasible to simplify the target cell, for example, to an erythrocyte (there are no reports of specific CTL-mediated killing of erythrocytes) or a liposome (Cf. 40).

SEARCH FOR PROTEINS UNIQUE TO CTL

A more general approach to a molecular understanding of CTL-mediated killing is to search for unusual or unique CTL proteins. Kimura (41) reported that Lyt-2^+ (but not Lyt-2^-) T lymphoblasts express an external membrane glycoprotein of 145,000 M_r (T145) only after activation. A subsequent study, however, found this SDS-PAGE band lacking on peritoneal exudate lymphocytes with high cytolytic activity (42).

Gately (43) found an intensely-labeled band of 11,000 M_r (T11) on SDS-PAGE of purified plasma membranes of [^{35}S]methionine internally-labeled CTL-rich lymphocytes. The band was present at lower specific activity in the endoplasmic reticulum fraction, and was virtually absent from the cytosol or nuclei-mitochondria fractions, indicating that it is located primarily in the plasma membrane.

T11 was prominent on the T cells in primary or secondary allo-specific CTL-containing lymphocyte populations generated _in vitro_ and on Concanavalin A-induced lymphoblasts, but absent or nearly absent from normal splenocytes, LPS-induced B lymphoblasts, or tumor cells such as P815 mastocytoma or the T lymphoma EL4 (Table I). Most interestingly, T11 was absent or nearly absent from PHA-induced lymphoblasts. This latter population contained 30% T lymphoblasts (the same proportion as the allo-specific CTL populations) but lacked lectin-dependent cytolytic activity. Thus, T11 expression appears to be restricted to a subpopulation of activated T lymphocytes, quite possibly CTL.

TABLE I. T11 Distribution

Cell Type	Thy-1+	T cell Blasts	T11	Lytic Activity
1° MLC CTL	80%	30%	++++	++
2° MLC CTL	80	30	++++	++
Con A Blasts	90	80	++	+
PHA Blasts	90	30	±	-
Normal Spleen	60	0	-	-
LPS Blasts[b]	0	0	-	-
1° MLC[b]	0	0	-	-
P815	0	0	-	-
EL4	100	100	-	-
RDM4			±	-

[a]From Gately and Martz (43).

[b]Thy-1+ cells removed with Ab+C.

The functions of T145 and T11 are unknown. Unless an antibody to such a molecule were to block killing, there appears to be no general approach to ascertaining the function of such a molecule. Consider, for example, our ignorance about the function of Thy-1, which was discovered seventeen years ago (44).

TABLE II. Monoclonal antibodies that block murine CTL-mediated killing in the absence of complement by binding to the CTL

Antigen on CTL	M_r(s) of reduced antigen x 10^{-3}	References
Lyt-2,3	30, 35	45, 59-61, 64, 65, 73-75
LFA-1	95, 180	45, 63, 68, 69, 76, 77

TABLE III. Monoclonal antibodies which do not block murine CTL-mediated killing when directed towards the CTL

Antigen on CTL	M_r(s) of reduced antigen x 10^{-3}	References
B2-microglobulin	12	46, 78
Thy-1	25	45, 46, 59, 74, 79
Ia	28, 35	45, 46
H-2	45	59, 80, 81, reviewed in 9
TL	50	59
Lyt-1	70	45, 59
Lgp-100	100	45
Common leucocyte antigen (T200, Ly 5)	200	45
9 misc. antigens defined by monoclonal xenoantibodies	46, 60, 115 140, 250	45
Immunoglobulins		reviewed in 9
Ly-6		45
Misc. murine leukemia virus glycoproteins		59
Numerous misc. alloantisera		60
Misc. xenoantisera against mouse CTL		82, 83 as elaborated on page 216 in 46
Anti-idiotypic antisera*		84-87, page 140 in 88

*All had demonstrated activity on other T cell functions.

MONOCLONAL ANTI-CTL ANTIBODIES WHICH BLOCK KILLING

Recently, it has been demonstrated that CTL-mediated killing can be blocked with monoclonal antibodies (MAbs) against either of two molecular species on the CTL membrane in the absence of complement (Table II). This represents the first breakthrough in identifying molecules likely to play an essential role in CTL function. Screening for MAbs which block CTL-mediated killing now provides a systematic approach towards linking specific molecules with CTL functions.

The fact that certain antibodies block killing by binding to the CTL is remarkable in light of past failures to find such antibodies, summarized in Table III. Antibodies to more than a dozen distinct molecules expressed on CTLs fail to block killing (45 and Table III). This comparison is what distinguishes Lyt-2,3 and LFA-1 as being uniquely involved in CTL function.

Previously, six papers have reported blocking of murine CTL-mediated killing with conventional antisera thought to act on the CTL. In three cases, however, action on the target cell was not rigorously excluded (46-48). In the remaining three cases (49-51), action via the target cell was excluded but the xenoantisera employed recognized multiple specificities, making identification of the crucial molecules impractical. Blocking monoclonal antibodies avoid this problem since they usually bind to a single molecular species.

Human CTLs have been most consistently blocked with OKT3 MAb (52-54, but see 55). The murine homolog of the human molecule recognized by OKT3 is not clear. Blocking has also been found with anti-Leu-2a MAb (56), which appears to recognize the human homolog of Lyt-2,3 (57). The OKT5 and OKT8 MAbs, which may recognize the same molecule, have produced weaker blocking (52) but not consistently (52-54).

Some caution should be used in categorizing CTL molecules, or the MAbs which recognize them, as "blocking" or "non-blocking." We have seen that the 53.6 anti-Lyt-2 MAb of Ledbetter and Herzenberg (58) is a potent blocker of CTL-mediated killing, while the M5/24 anti-Lyt-2,3 MAb we developed (45) is a relatively poor blocker. The reason for this difference has not yet been resolved; possibilities include differences in avidity or in the exact position of the determinant recognized on the Lyt-2,3 molecule. A similar situation exists for the anti-Leu-2a and anti-leu-2b MAbs in the human CTL system (56). Clearly, the fact that one or more MAbs to a given molecule fail to block CTL-mediated killing does not preclude later discovery of a MAb to the same molecule which blocks well, or vice versa. Moreover, it is conceivable that certain pairs or trios of pooled MAbs may block while no individual member of the group is able to block by itself.

MECHANISM OF BLOCKING WITH ANTI-LYT-2,3 AND THE ROLE OF THE LYT-2,3 MOLECULE

In 1979, two groups independently discovered that antibodies to Lyt-2,3 block killing (59,60). Action via the CTL was established by using target cells genetically incapable of expressing the relevant alloantigen. Such antibodies block the formation of shear-resistant CTL-target conjugates (61), and thus act on the recognition-adhesion step. Moreover, Fan, Ahmed and Bonavida (61) obtained two kinds of direct evidence suggesting that the 53.6 anti-Lyt-2 MAb of Ledbetter and Herzenberg (58) does not act on the lethal hit. First, they showed that the number of target cells which are killed, as a percentage of those bound to CTLs in isolated binary conjugates, is not reduced by anti-Lyt-2 MAb (although the MAb reduced the number of conjugates which formed). Second, addition of MAb after formation of conjugates (and their dispersion in dextran-containing medium to prevent recycling) such that the lethal hit occurred in the presence of MAb did not reduce subsequent ^{51}Cr-release.

In a more recent study, Shinohara and coworkers (62), using a calcium pulse analysis, have confirmed that mouse allo-anti-Lyt-2 blocks the recognition-adhesion step. Moreover, they provide evidence that anti-Lyt-2 reverses already completed recognition-adhesion events within 5 minutes. The same study (62) also noted that for effective blocking, the antibody must be present during CTL-target interaction. CTL which were pretreated and rinsed were not blocked. (We have made similar observations with M7/14, but the story is apparently more complicated, see 63.)

MacDonald and coworkers (64) have shown that H-2^b anti-H-2^d CTL clones differ considerably in their susceptibility to blocking by anti-Lyt-2 (MAb 53.6). These differences are not accounted for by differences in density of Lyt-2 expression on the CTLs. It seems likely that high avidity clones are less inhibited than low avidity clones.

Ledbetter and coworkers have presented evidence that the Lyt-2 and Lyt-3 antigenic determinants are carried on separate disulfide-bonded polypeptides (65). They found that selective removal of Lyt-3 with trypsin, which left over 60% of Lyt-2 intact, affected the killer activity of various CTL populations differently. In one case where removal of Lyt-3 left substantial killing activity, killing was less inhibited by anti-Lyt-3 and more inhibited by anti-Lyt-2 antibodies.

Fan and Bonavida (66) treated CTLs more extensively with trypsin until Lyt-2 was removed. Under these conditions, H-2, Thy-1, and some Lyt-1 remained. Nevertheless, the trypsinized CTL lost specific killing ability and specific conjugate-forming ability. Incubation of the trypsinized CTLs at 37°C for 3 hours allowed about 50% recovery of Lyt-2 expression, killing, and conjugate-forming ability.

Dialynas, Glasebrook and Fitch (67) treated CTL clones with the mutagen ethyl methane sulfonate and selected for antigen-loss variants. A clone which no longer expressed a monoclonal Thy-1.2 determinant retained specific killing activity. However, a clone which no longer expressed several monoclonally defined Lyt-2,3 determinants lost the ability to kill specifically. Non-specific Con A-dependent killing ability was retained, however, showing that the Lyt-2,3 antigens were not essential for lethal hit delivery. The question of whether the variant clones lost the entire molecule or only lost certain antigenic determinants while continuing to express the molecule remains open.

These data (66,67) suggest that the Lyt-2,3 molecule may be essential for specific recognition.

IDENTIFICATION OF LYMPHOCYTE FUNCTION-ASSOCIATED ANTIGEN ONE (LFA-1)

In 1979, we began screening for monoclonal blocking antibodies. We immunized rats with mouse CTLs. We hoped that xenoimmunization would increase the number of immunogenic CTL molecules; this may have been the case since no alloantibodies to LFA-1 have been reported. Secondly, we wanted to avoid antibodies to the target cell. For this purpose, we used mouse anti-rat CTLs as immunogen in the rat (a "doubly xenogeneic" protocol), and then studied the blocking of the

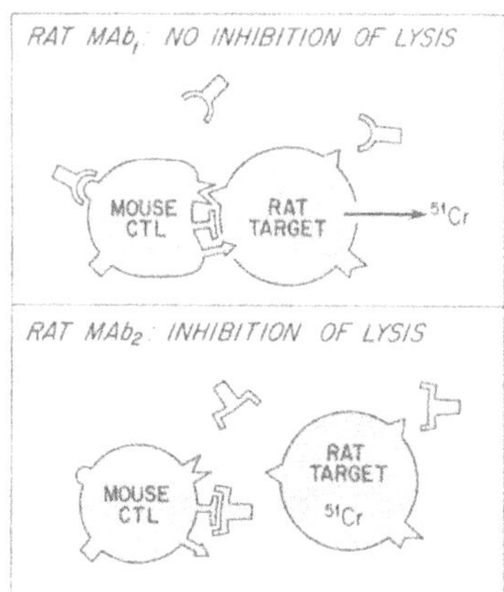

Fig. 1. Doubly xenogeneic rationale for development of blocking monoclonal antibodies. Rat MAbs are tested for blocking on a mouse CTL anti-rat lymphoma target cell system. Antibodies which might block by binding to the target are avoided since the target cell is syngeneic with the rat antibody donor.

mouse anti-rat killing by the resulting rat anti-mouse antibodies (Fig. 1). Both the donor of the antibody and the ^{51}Cr-labeled assay target were thus of inbred Lewis rat genotype (45). The hybridomas were rat-mouse fusions made with the non-secreting mouse myeloma derivative NSI.

Screening was also conducted for T lymphocyte-specific binding, and this was actually the basis for the decision to clone a group of hybridomas which turned out to include one producing antibody with potent CTL-blocking activity. This antibody, designated M7/14, was unique among 24 monoclonal antibodies tested for blocking. These antibodies distinguished at least 14 different molecules on the CTL membrane; only M7/14 and two anti-Lyt-2,3 antibodies blocked killing (45 and Table II).

M7/14 produced an $IgG2_a$ which immunoprecipitates two non-covalently linked polypeptide chains of 95,000 and 180,000 M_r (45,68; Kürzinger, Ho, and Springer, submitted for publication). The molecule recognized by M7/14 was designated lymphocyte function-associated antigen one (LFA-1, 45) and was shown to be distinct from previously described lymphocyte membrane molecules. The molecular weights of LFA-1 clearly distinguish it from T11 (43) and T145 (41), and direct comparison on SDS-PAGE (68) shows it to be distinct from Thy-1, H-2, Lyt-1, Lyt-2,3 and T200 (also known as the common leucocyte antigen of Ly-5). In biosynthetic labeling, both chains of LFA-1 incorporate [^{3}H]-glucosamine, suggesting that both are glycoproteins (unpublished). Pierres, Goridis, and Golstein and Fitch and coworkers have developed MAbs which block CTL-mediated killing and appear to recognize the same LFA-1 molecule (63 and articles in this volume).

The xenoantibody M7/14 recognizes lymphocytes from all 9 inbred strains of mice tested, and blocks various xenogeneic, allogeneic, and syngeneic CTL-target systems (69). Thus, the specificity of M7/14 is neither idiotypic nor allotypic.

TISSUE DISTRIBUTION AND DENSITY OF LFA-1

LFA-1 expression is not restricted to CTL or even to T cells (68). It was found by quantitative flow cytofluorometry (FACS analysis) on 100% of thymocytes, peripheral T lymphocytes, and B lymphocytes. It is present on 80% of bone marrow leucocytes, suggesting that myeloid cells express LFA-1. Thioglycollate-induced macrophages were largely negative, erythrocytes were negative, and tissue homogenates of lung, liver, brain, and kidney did not absorb M7/14 antibody (68).

Based on fluorescence (FACS) analysis of LFA-1 density, normal splenic C57BL/6J T lymphocytes are two-thirds dim and one-third bright. The two subpopulations differ by 4-fold in LFA-1 density (68). The dim T cells are 1.7-fold brighter than B cells, and the bright T cells, about 7-fold. The average density for pooled T lymphocytes is 3.5-fold greater than that for B cells.

Activation of T lymphocytes by allogeneic secondary MLC (to produce a population with high CTL activity) or by Con A increased the LFA-1 per cell by 5-fold compared to normal splenocytes, whereas H-2 per cell increased only 2-fold (68). The increase in LFA-1 was similar to that in Thy-1, and greater than that of Lyt-2,3 (Thy-1 and Lyt-2,3 densities were calculated for the positive subpopulations only).

Activation of B cells by LPS increased LFA-1/cell by 2.3-fold, but this increase was less than the corresponding 3.2-fold increase in H-2/cell.

In side-by-side SDS-PAGE analysis, the polypeptides immunoprecipitated by M7/14 from LPS activated B lymphocytes, Con A-activated T lymphocytes, or thymocytes were indistinguishable.

EFFECTS OF M7/14 ANTIBODY ON NON-CTL FUNCTIONS

Experiments to determine the effects of M7/14 in various systems (69) have led us to the working hypothesis that LFA-1 is crucial in the interactions of T cells with other cells. In addition to blocking CTL-mediated killing, M7/14 MAb inhibits allogeneic and xenogeneic mixed lymphocyte culture proliferative responses, the macrophage-dependent, antigen-specific proliferation of primed T lymphocytes *in vitro*, and T cell dependent primary antibody (plaque-forming cell) responses to sheep red blood cells. On the other hand, responses of LFA-1-bearing cells (B lymphocytes) which do not involve known cellular interactions are not inhibited, showing that M7/14 is not generally inhibitory for proliferation: LPS-induced proliferation of B cells and the T cell-independent primary antibody (PFC) response to haptenated-Ficoll are not inhibited. Furthermore, addition of M7/14 to mixed lymphocyte cultures at one day or later is not inhibitory, showing that M7/14 does not block T cell proliferation *per se*.

MECHANISM OF INHIBITION OF CTL-MEDIATED KILLING BY ANTIBODY TO LFA-1

The unlikely possibility that M7/14 is an autoreacive antibody which could bind to the rat lymphoma target cells used in the ^{51}Cr-release assay was excluded by quantitative flow cytofluorometry (45).

The density of LFA-1 on lymphocyte populations high in CTL activity is 2.5-fold less than the density of H-2, and 10-fold less than Thy-1 (all based on quantitation with $IgG2_a$ MAbs, 68). Since MAbs to H-2 and Thy-1 do not block killing, blocking by anti-LFA-1 cannot be accounted for by a non-specific blanketing effect resulting from high antigen density. Also, the density of Lyt-2,3 is slightly greater than that of LFA-1.

Blocking of xenogeneic C57BL/6J anti BN-lymphoma killing averaged 90% in 17 experiments (45). Inhibition was not diminished even when highly active CTLs or high effector/target ratios were employed: 94% inhibition was found in 6 experiments in which corrected ^{51}Cr-release was 88-99% in the absence of M7/14 (45). Inhibition of allogeneic killing was somewhat less (50-80%, 69). The purified immunoglobulin inhibited as well as the dialyzed hybridoma culture supernatant. Half maximal inhibition in the xenogeneic system occurred at 600 ng IgG/ml (69). M7/14 was not toxic to the effector cell (69).

The possibility that the inhibition might be a result of CTL agglutination, preventing intermixing with target cells, was ruled out by microscopic observation. Whereas M7/14 gave profound inhibition of killing with little or no agglutination, anti-Thy-2 (M5/49) agglutinated half of the lymphocytes but produced little or no inhibition of killing (69).

The formation of shear-resistant, microscopically counted CTL-target conjugates was inhibited by M7/14 (69).

ROLE OF THE LFA-1 MOLECULE IN CTL FUNCTION

It is not excluded that M7/14 recognizes the specific antigen receptor on CTL, but this is rendered highly unlikely by the expression of LFA-1 not only on B lymphocytes and 80% of bonemarrow cells (68), but on the macrophage-like cell line P388D1 and on the mastocytoma P815 (unpublished data).

It appears unlikely that M7/14 interferes directly with the mechanism of programming for lysis, since it inhibits conjugate formation (strong adhesion formation) and this seems sufficient to account for the inhibition of killing. Although CTL-target contact in the absence of strong adhesion may permit limited killing under certain circumstances (70,71), it seems clear that the strong adhesion triggered by antigen recognition (25) greatly increases the efficiency of killing (9,70).

The most likely role for LFA-1 would thus appear to be a role in adhesion formation between T cells and other cells (target cells, and macrophages and/or B lymphocytes). This is currently under investigation. It is interesting to note that while macrophages appear to lack LFA-1 (68), they express the Mac-1 molecule (72) which may be homologous to LFA-1. Not only are the molecular weights of the polypeptide chains quite similar between Mac-1 and LFA-1, but the smaller polypeptides in each case appear closely related or identical on the basis of recent peptide mapping (Kürzinger, Ho and Springer, submitted for publication).

SUMMARY

During the past decade the mechanism of CTL-mediated killing has been resolved into 3 steps, and its cation requirements, and general nature have been well defined. However, biochemical understanding of the CTL-target interaction has made little progress. Recently, we have developed a monoclonal antibody (MAb) which blocks killing by binding to a previously undescribed molecule on the CTL membrane, a molecule which we therefore have termed lymphocyte function-associated antigen one (LFA-1). LFA-1 and Lyt-2,3 are the only presently identified sites for such blocking; antibodies to over a dozen other molecules expressed on the CTL do not block killing. Present evidence suggests that LFA-1 is crucial in the adhesive interaction of T cells with other cells (e.g., targets, macrophages, perhaps B cells). The continuing search for blocking MAbs provides a systematic way to link specific molecules with CTL function.

ACKNOWLEDGEMENTS

Supported by NIH grants CA-14723, CA-31798, CA-31799, AI-00458, AI-18003, by an American Cancer Society Faculty Award (to T.A.S.), and by postdoctoral fellowships from the Massachusetts Division of the American Cancer Society (D.D.) and the Deutsche Forschungsgemeinschaft (K.K.).

ABBREVIATIONS USED IN THIS PAPER

CTL, cytolytic T lymphocyte; LFA-1, lymphocyte function-associated antigen one; M7/14, the blocking monoclonal antibody (or more properly the hybridoma which secretes it) which recognizes and defines LFA-1; MAb, monoclonal antibody; M_r, relative molecular mass.

REFERENCES

1. Brunner, K.T., J. Mauel, J.-C. Cerottini, H. Rudolf, and B. Chapuis. In vitro studies of cellular and humoral immunity induced by tumor allografts. In "Mechanisms of Inflammation Induced by Immune Reactions," P.A. Miescher and P. Grabar, eds., pp. 342-357 (1967).
2. Berke G., G. Yagil, H. Ginsburg, and M. Feldman. Kinetic analysis of a graft reaction induced in cell culture. Immunol. 17:723-740 (1969).
3. Doherty, P.C., and R.M. Zinkernagel. T-cell-mediated immunopathology in viral infections. Transplant. Rev. 19:89-120 (1974).
4. Cerottini, J.-C., and K.T. Brunner. Cell-mediated cytotoxicity, allograft rejection, and tumor immunity. Adv. Immunol. 18:67-132 (1974).
5. Martz, E. Early steps in specific tumor cell lysis by sensitized mouse T lymphocytes. II. Electrolyte permeability increase in the target cell membrane concomitant with programming for lysis. J. Immunol. 117:1023-1027 (1976).
6. Sanderson, C.J. The mechanism of lymphocyte-mediated cytotoxicity. Biol Rev. 56:153-197 (1981).
7. Boyle, M.D.P., S.H. Ohaninan, and T. Borsos. Studies on the terminal stages of antibody-complement-mediated killing of a tumor cell. II. Inhibition of transformation of T* to dead cells by 3'5'cAMP. J. Immunol. 116:1276-1279 (1976).
8. Burakoff, S.J., E. Martz, and B. Benacerraf. Is the primary complement lesion insufficient for lysis? Failure of cells damaged under osmotic protection to lyse in EDTA or at low temperature after removal of osmotic protection. Clin. Immunol. and Immunopathol. 4:108-126 (1975).
9. Martz, E. Mechanism of specific tumor cell lysis by alloimmune T-lymphocytes: Resolution and characterization of discrete steps in the cellular interaction. Contemp. Top. Immunobiol. 7:301-361 (1977).
10. Hiserodt, J.C., G.J. Tiangco, and G.A. Granger. The LT system in experimental animals. IV. Rapid specific lysis of ^{51}Cr-labeled allogeneic target cells by highly unstable high MW lymphotoxin-receptor complex(es) released in vitro by activated alloimmune murine T lymphocytes. J. Immunol. 123:332-341 (1979).
11. Martz, E., and B. Benacerraf. Multiple target cell killing by the cytolytic T-lymphocyte and the mechanism of cytotoxicity. Transplantation 21:5-11 (1976).
12. Zagury, D., J. Bernard, N. Thierness, M. Feldman, and G. Berke. Isolation and characterization of individual functionally reactive cytotoxic T lymphocytes: conjugation, killing and recycling at the single cell level. Eur. J. Immunol. 5:818-822 (1975).
13. Golstein, P. Sensitivity of cytotoxic T cells to T-cell mediated

cytotoxicity. Nature 252:81-83 (1974).
14. Kuppers, R.C., and C.S. Henney. Evidence for direct linkage between antigen recogntion and lytic expression in effector T cells. J. Exp. Med. 143:684-689 (1976).
15. Bubbers, J.E., and C.S. Henney. Studies on the synthetic capacity and antigenic expression of glutaraldehyde-fixed target cells. J. Immunol. 114:1126-1131 (1975).
16. Thorn R.M., and C.S. Henney. Studies on the mechanism of lymphocyte-mediated cytolysis. VI. A reappraisal of the requirement for protein synthesis during T cell-mediated lysis. J. Immunol. 116:146-149 (1976).
17. Bevan, M.J., and M. Cohn. Cytotoxic effects of antigen- and mitogen-induced T cells on various targets. J. Immunol. 114:559-565 (1975).
18. Gately, M.., and E. Martz. Comparative studies on the mechanisms of nonspecific, Con A-dependent cytolysis and specific T cell-mediated cytolysis. J. Immunol. 119:1711-1722 (1977).
19. Parker, W.L., and E. Martz. Lectin-induced nonlethal adhesions between cytolytic T lymphocytes and antigenically unrecognizable tumor cells, and nonspecific "triggering" of cytolysis. J. Immunol. 124:25-35 (1980).
20. Kuppers, R.C., and C.S. Henney. Studies on the mechanism of lymphocyte-mediated cytolysis. IX. Relationships between antigen recognition and lytic expression in killer T cells. J. Immunol. 118:71-76 (1977).
21. Grimm, E., and B. Bonavida. Mechanism of cell-mediated cytotoxicity at the single cell level. I. Estimation of cytotoxic T lymphocyte frequency and relative lytic efficiency. J. Immunol. 123:2861-2869 (1979).
22. Golstein, P., and E.T. Smith. The lethal hit stage of mouse T and non-T cell-mediated cytolysis. Differences in cation requirements and characterization of an analytical "cation pulse" method. Eur. J. Immunol. 6:31-37 (1976).
23. Wagner, H., and M. Rollinghoff. T cell-mediated cytotoxicity: Discrimination between antigen recognition, lethal hit and cytolysis phase. Eur. J. Immunol. 4:745-750 (1974).
24. Martz, E. Early steps in specific tumor cell lysis by sensitized mouse T-lymphocytes. I. Resolution and characterization. J. Immunol. 115:261-267 (1975).
25. Martz, E. Immune lymphocyte to tumor cell adhesion: magnesium sufficient, calcium insufficient. J. Cell Biol. 84:584-598 (1980).
26. Gately, M.K., and E. Martz. Early steps in specific tumor cell lysis by sensitized mouse T lymphocytes. III. Resolution of two distinct roles for calcium in the cytolytic process. J. Immunol. 122:482-489 (1979).
27. Plaut, M., J.E., Bubbers, and C.S. Henney. Studies on the mechanism of lymphocyte-mediated cytolysis. VII. Two stages in the T cell-mediated lytic cycle with distinct cation requirements. J. Immunol. 116:150-155 (1976).

28. Golstein, P., C. Foa, and I.C.M. MacLennan. Mechanism of T-cell-mediated cytolysis: The differential impact of cytochalasins at the recognition and lethal hit stages. Eur. J. Immunol. 8:302-309 (1978).
29. Gately, M.K., and E. Martz. Inhibition of the lethal hit phase of T cell-mediated cytolysis by pharmacologic agents. Fed. Proc. 38:1166 (Abs. #4960) (1979).
30. Golstein, P. and E.T. Smith. Mechanism of T cell-mediated cytolysis: The lethal hit stage. Contemp. Top. Immunobiol. 7:273-300 (1977).
31. Martz E., C.D. Tsoukas, and W.J. Wechter. Evidence against Ca^{++} poisoning by killer cells: Mast cells killed by T lymphocytes do not secrete prelytically. J. Supramol. Struct. Suppl. 3:311 (Abstract 818) (1979).
32. Ko, L., and D. Lagunoff. Depletion of mast cell ATP inhibits complement-dependent cytotoxic histamine release. Exp. Cell Res. 100:313-321 (1976).
33. Henney, C.S. T cell mediated cytolysis: Consideration of the role of a soluble mediator. J. Reticuloendothelial Soc. 17:231-235 (1975).
34. Todd, R.F., and G. Berke. Functional characterization of membrane components of cytotoxic peritoneal exudate T lymphocytes. I. Search for T cell receptor activity in lymphocyte membrane fractions. Immunochemistry 11:313-320 (1974).
35. Whisnant, C.C., K.H. Singer, and D.B. Amos. Interaction of cytotoxic T lymphocytes with target cells. I. Specific inhibition by detergent-solubilized, partially purified mouse histocompatibility anitgens. J. Immunol. 121:2253 (1978).
36. Todd, R.F. III, R.D. Stulting, and D.B. Amos. Lymphocyte-mediated cytolysis of allogeneic tumor cells in vitro. I. Search for target antigens in subcellular fractions. Cellular Immunol. 18:304-323 (1975).
37. Nagy, Z.A., and B.E. Elliott. The receptor specificity of alloreactive T cells. Distinction between stimulator K, I, and D region products and degeneracy of third-party H-2 recognition by low-affinity T cells. J. Exp. Med. 150:1520-1537 (1979).
38. Linna, T.J., H.D. Engers, J.-C. Cerottini, and K.T. Brunner. Inhibition of cytolytic T lymphocyte activity with subcellular alloantigen preparations and with unlabeled allogenic target cells. J. Immunol. 120:1544-1549 (1978).
39. Gilmer, P.J., H.O. McDevitt, and H.M. McConnell. Inhibition of specific T cell-target cell conjugates by target cell plasma membranes. J. Immunol. 120:774 (1978).
40. Ozato, K., H.K. Ziegler, and C.S. Henney. Liposomes as model membrane systems for immune attack. I. Transfer of antigenic determinants to lymphocyte membranes after interactions with hapten-bearing liposomes. J. Immunol. 121:1376 (1978).
41. Kimura, A.K., and H. Wigzell. Cell surface glycoproteins of murine cytotoxic T lymphocytes. I. T 145, a new surface

glycoprotein selectively expressed on Ly 1^-2^+ cytotoxic T lymphocytes. J. Exp. Med. 147:1418-1434 (1978).

42. Berke, G., Y. Kaufmann, and D. Gabison. Cell surface determinants of cytotoxic T lymphocytes: possible role in lymphocyte-target cell interaction. Fed. Proc. 39:1198 (Abstract #4891) (1980).
43. Gately, M.K., and E. Martz. T11: A new protein marker on activated murine T lymphocytes. J. Immunol. 126:709-714 (1981).
44. Reif, A.E., and J.M. Allen. The AKR thymic antigen and its distribution in leukemias and nervous tissues. J. Exp. Med. 120:413 (1964).
45. Davignon, D., E. Martz, T. Reynolds, K. Kurzinger, and T.A. Springer. Lymphocyte function-associated antigen one (LFA-1): a surface antigen distinct from Lyt-2/3 that participates in T lymphocyte-mediated killing. Proc. Natl. Acad. Sci. USA 78:4535-4539 (1981).
46. Kimura, A.K., and H. Wigzell. Cytotoxic T lymphocyte membrane components: An analysis of structures related to function. Cont. Top. Mol. Immunol. 6:209-244 (1977).
47. Redelman, D., and P.E. Trefts. In vitro studies of the rabbit immune system. VIII. Rabbit anti-mouse cytotoxic T-effector cells are inhibited by anti-rabbit T-cell serum in the absence of complement. J. Immunol. 121:1532-1539 (1978).
48. Rabinowitz, R., and M. Schlesinger. Inhibition of the activity of cytotoxic murine T lymphocytes by antibodies to idiotypic determinants. Immunol. 39:93-99 (1980).
49. Kimura, A.K. Inhibition of specific cell-mediated cytotoxicity by anti-T-cell receptor antibody. J. Exp. Med. 139:888-901 (1974).
50. Rabinowitz, R., R. Laskov, and M. Schlesinger. Inhibition of cell-mediated lysis by xenoantibodies reactive with effector T lymphocytes. Eur. J. Immunol. 10:219-223 (1980).
51. Hiserodt, J.C., and B. Bonavida. Studies on the induction and expression of T cell-mediated immunity. XI. Inhibition of the "Lethal Hit" in T cell-mediated cytotoxicity by heterologous rat antiserum made against alloimmune cytotoxic T lymphocytes. J. Immunol. 126:256-262 (1981).
52. Platsoucas, C.D., and R.A. Good. Inhibition of specific cell-mediated cytotoxicity by monoclonal antibodies to human T cell antigens. Proc. Natl. Acad. Sci. USA 78:4500-4504 (1981).
53. Chang, T.W., P.C. Kung, S.P. Gingras, and G. Goldstein. Does OKT3 monoclonal antibody react with an antigen-recognition structure on human T cells? Proc. Natl. Acad. Sci. USA 78: 1805-1808 (1981).
54. Tsoukas, C.D., R.I. Fox, D.A. Carson, S. Fong, and J.H. Vaughan. Monoclonal antibody OKT3 blocks the function of human cytotoxic T-lymphocytes against autologous EBV-transformed target cells. Submitted for publication.
55. Reinherz, E.L., R.E. Hussey, and S.F. Schlossman. A monoclonal antibody blocking human T cell function. Eur. J. Immunol. 10:

758-762 (1980).
56. Evans, R.L., D.W. Wall, C.D. Platsoucas, F.P. Siegal, S.M. Fikrig, C.M. Testa, and R.A. Good. Thymus-dependent membrane antigens in man: inhibition of cell-mediated lympholysis by monoclonal antibodies to T_{H2} antigen. Proc. Natl. Acad. Sci. USA 78:544-548 (1981).
57. Ledbetter, J.A., R.L. Evans, M. Lipinski, C. Cunningham-Rundles, R.A. Good, and L.A. Herzenberg. Evolutionary conservation of surface molecules that distinguish T lymphocyte helper/inducer and cytotoxic/suppressor subpopulations in mouse and man. J. Exp. Med. 153:310-323 (1981).
58. Ledbetter, J.A., and L.A. Herzenberg. Xenogeneic monoclonal antibodies to mouse lymphoid differentiation antigens. Immunological Rev. 47:63-89 (1979).
59. Nakayama, E., H. Shiku, E. Stockert, H.F. Oettgen, and L.J. Old. Cytotoxic T cells: Lyt phenotype and blocking of killing activity by Lyt antisera. Proc. Natl. Acad. Sci. USA 76:1977-1981 (1979).
60. Shinohara, N., and D.H. Sachs. Mouse alloantibodies capable of blocking cytotoxic T-cell function. I. Relationship between the antigen reactive with blocking antibodies and the Lyt-2 locus. J. Exp. Med. 150:432-444 (1979).
61. Fan, J., A. Ahmed, and B. Bonavida. Studies on the induction and expression of T cell-mediated immunity. X. Inhibition by Lyt-2,3 antisera of cytotoxic T lymphocyte-mediated antigen-specific and nonspecific cytotoxicity: Evidence for the blocking of the binding between T lymphocytes and target cells and not the post-binding cytolytic steps. J. Immunol. 125: 2444-2453 (1980).
62. Shinohara, N., M. Taniguchi, and M. Kojima. Mouse alloantibodies capable of blocking cytotoxic T cell function. III. Studies of the mechanism of blocking of CML by anti-Lyt-2 antibodies. J. Immunol. 127:1575-1578 (1981).
63. Pierres, P., C. Goridis, and P. Golstein. Inhibition of murine T cell-mediated cytolysis and T cell proliferation by a rat monoclonal antibody immunoprecipitating two lymphoid cell surface polypeptides of 94,000 and 180,000 molecular weight. Eur. J. Immunol., in press (1981).
64. MacDonald, H.R., N. Thiernesse, and J.-C. Cerottini. Inhibition of T cell-mediated cytolysis by monoclonal antibodies directed against Lyt-2: heterogeneity of inhibition at the clonal level. J. Immunol. 126:1671-1675 (1981).
65. Ledbetter, J.A., W.E. Seaman, T.T. Tsu, and L.A. Herzenberg. Lyt-2 and Lyt-3 antigens are on two different polypeptide subunits linked by disulfide bonds. Relationship of subunits to T cell cytolytic activity. J. Exp. Med. 153:1503-1516 (1981).
66. Fan, J., and B. Bonavida. Studies on the induction and expression of T cell-mediated immunity. XII. The concomitant loss and recovery of membrane-associated Lyt-2 antigens, lymphocyte-target cell binding, and the antigen-specific and -nonspecific

cytotoxic activity of alloimmune T lymphocytes after treatment with trypsin. J. Immunol. 127:1856-1864 (1981).
67. Dialynas, D.P., M.R. Loken, A.L. Glasebrook, and F.W. Fitch. Lyt-2⁻/Lyt-3⁻ variants of a cloned cytolytic T cell line lack an antigen receptor functional in cytolysis. J. Exp. Med. 153:595-604 (1981).
68. Kurzinger, K., T. Reynolds, R.N. Germain, D. Davignon, E. Martz., and T.A. Spjringer. A novel lymphocyte function-associated antigen (LFA-1): cellular distribution, quantitative expression, and structure. J. Immunol. 127:596-602 (1981).
69. Davignon, D., E. Martz, T. Reynolds, K. Kurzinger, and T.A. Springer. Monoclonal antibody to a novel lymphocyte function-associated antigen (LFA-1). Mechanism of blockade of T lymphocyte-mediated killing and effects on other T and B lymphocyte functions. J. Immunol. 127:590-595 (1981).
70. Shortman, K., and P. Golstein. Target cell recognition by cytolytic T cells: Different requirements for the formation of strong conjugates or for proceeding to lysis. J. Immunol. 123: 833-839 (1979).
71. Martz, E. Inability of EDTA to prevent damage mediated by cytolytic T-lymphocytes. Cellular Immunol. 20:304-314 (1975).
72. Springer, T.A. Mac-1,2,3, and 4: Murine macrophage differentiation antigens identified by monoclonal antibodies. In: "Heterogeneity of mononuclear phagocytes," O. Forster, ed., Academic Press, New York. In press (1980).
73. Shinohara, N., U. Hammerling, and D.H. Sachs. Mouse alloantibodies capable of blocking cytotoxic T cell function. II. Further study on the relationship between the blocking antibodies and the products of the Lyt-2 locus. Eur. J. Immunol. 10:589-594 (1980).
74. Hollander, N., E. Pillemer, and I.L. Weissman. The blocking effect of Lyt-2 antibodies on T cell functions. J. Exp. Med. 152:674-687 (1980).
75. Sarmiento, M., A.L. Glasebrook, and F.W. Fitch. IgG or IgM monoclonal antibodies reactive with different determinants on the molecular complex bearing Lyt-2 antigen block T cell-mediated cytolysis in the absence of complement. J. Immunol. 125:2665-2672 (1980).
76. Springer, T.A., K. Kurzinger, T. Reynolds, R.N. Germain, D. Davignon, and E. Martz. Monoclonal antibodies as probes of surface structures participating in T lymphocyte function. In: "Monoclonal Antibodies and T Cell Hybridomas," U. Hammerling, G. Hammerling, and J. Kearney, eds., Elsevier. In press (1981).
77. Golstein, P., and M. Pierres. Monoclonal antibodies as probes to study the mechanism of T cell-mediated cytolysis. Proc. 14th Leukocyte Cult. Conf., in press (1981).
78. Lightbody, J.J., L. Urbani, and M.D. Poulik. Effect of beta-2 microglobulin antibody on effector function of T-cell mediated cytotoxicity. Nature 250:227-228 (1974).

79. Golstein, P. H. Wigzell, H. Blomgren, and E.A.J. Svedmyr. Cells mediating specific in vitro cytotoxicity. II. Probable autonomy of thymus-processed lymphocytes (T cells) for the killing of allogeneic target cells. J. Exp. Med. 135:890-906 (1972).
80. Lindah., K.F., and H. Lemke. Inhibition of killer-target cell interaction by monoclonal anti-H-2 antibodies. Eur. J. Immunol. 9:526-536 (1979).
81. Epstein, S.L., K. Ozato, and D.H. Sachs. Blocking of allogeneic cell-mediated lympholysis by monoclonal antibodies to H-2 antigens. J. Immunol. 125:129-135 (1980).
82. Rothstein, T.L., M.G. Mage, J. Mond, and L.L. McHugh. Guinea pig antiserum to mouse cytotoxic T lymhocytes and their precursors. J. Immunol. 120:209 (1978).
83. Sullivan, K.A., G. Berke, and D.B. Amos. An antigenic determinant of cytotoxic lymphocytes. Transplantation 16:388-391 (1973).
84. Braun, M. and F. Saal. The T-cell receptor and cytotoxicity. An anti-idiotype antiserum that inhibits a graft-versus-host reaction does not inhibit cell-mediated cytotoxicity. Cellular Immunol. 30:254-260 (1977).
85. Lindahl, K.F. Antisera against recognition sites: lack of effect on the mixed leucocyte culture interaction. Eur. J. Immunol. 2:501-504 (1972).
86. Sherman, L.A., S.J. Burakoff, and B. Benacerraf. The induction of cytolytic T lymphocytes with specificity for p-azophenylarsonate coupled syngeneic cells. J. Immunol. 121:1432 (1978).
87. Rubin, B., P. Golstein, O. Nordfang, and B. Hertel-Wulff. Generation of H-2-reactive T cell lines that bear the 5936 idiotype(s). J. Immunol. 124:161-167 (1980).
88. Binz, H., and H. Wigzell. Antigen-binding, idiotypic T-lymphocyte receptors. In: "Contemporary topics in immunobiology volume 7: T cells," O. Stutman, Ed., Plenum Press, New York, pp. 113-177 (1977).
89. Glasebrook, A.L. Conjugate formation by primary and secondary populations of murine immune T lymphocytes. J. Immunol. 121:1870-1877 (1978).

DISCUSSION

C. Henney

Following Rob's observation that CTL from various sources behave differently with respect to blocking with anti-Ly2, I wonder if you've made analogous studies with LFA1?

E. Martz

I'm glad you asked that. In fact, we had observations very similar to MacDonald's with Lyt2; namely, that while we could block a xenogeneic system quite well (90%), we could not block the same C57BL/6 killing against P815 very well at all. But LFA1 antibodies in our hands block every system we've tested to a very high degree and much more consistently.

C. Henney

How about cytotoxic effector cells which are not CTL? NK for example, or K cell lysis?

E. Martz

We have not studied K cell mediated lysis. We have looked at normal mouse NK against YAC, and what we found is that among this panel of antibodies, M7/14 was the best blocker. It was not, however, as good a blocker as it was on T cell mediated killing. The blocking was around 50% instead of 90%. The problem with that is that the YAC target cell possesses a high density of LFA1, as does the CTL. Therefore, I don't think we can interpret whether the antibodies are acting on the target or the killer.

C. Henney

Are you saying it can block at the target level?

E. Martz

I'm simply saying that in the NK system both cells possess the antigen and therefore the blocking that we see is difficult to interpet.

R. MacDonald

Can you pretreat CTL and get the blocking effect?

E. Martz

In the T cell system, yes. I don't believe we tried it in the NK cell system. In the T cell system, if we pretreat the CTL, we do get some blocking, but it's about only 30% blocking. If we pre-treat the target we get no blocking, but given the variability of the system, it's really difficult to use the modest inhibition you get as the basis for saying the antigen is not on the target. But, in essence, pretreatment does not work very well if you wash before you do the assay. The antibody must be present during the assay to give 90% inhibition.

P. Lachmann

Does inhibition work with Fab or $(Fab)_2$?

E. Martz

We haven't done that.

L. Simpson

You've presumably looked for H2 and immunoglobulin determinants on these two chain structures?

E. Martz

We have multiple monoclonal antibodies against H2. We have not done immunoglobulin. But none of the H2 antibodies we have bind.

(UK)

You said that your antigen was absent from activated macrophages. I think only BCG activated macrophages are fully cytotoxic. Did you look for this antigen on BCG treated macrophages?

E. Martz

No, we have not really concerned ourselved with the question of whether cytotoxic macrophages possess the antigen. Tim Springer is quite interested in macrophage antigens, and I think papers on that will be forthcoming in the near future.

MECHANISM OF T CELL-MEDIATED CYTOLYSIS: AN INVESTIGATION OF CELLS AND STAGES AFFECTED BY CYTOLYSIS-INHIBITING MONOCLONAL ANTIBODIES

Brigitte Hayot, Michel Pierres and Pierre Golstein

From the Centre d'Immunologie INSERM-CNRS de
Marseille-Luminy Case 906
13288 Marseille Cedex 9, France

INTRODUCTION

A key question when studying the mechanism of T cell-mediated cytolysis (1-4) is whether specialized molecules are at play at the surface of effector cells, not only at the recognition stage but also at the post-recognition lethal hit stage (2) of cytolysis. Detection of such molecules could greatly benefit from the availability of monoclonal antibodies (mAb) interfering with the cytolytic mechanism. With this in mind, we developed a range of rat anti-mouse mAb selected for their ability to inhibit cytolysis (5,6). Six of them were used i nthis work; some of their characteristics are given below.

This paper focuses on the following two points, essential for an assessment of the potential usefulness of these mAb. First, was inhibition of cytolysis achieved via interaction of these mAb with the effector or the target cells? Although the answer was that interaction of each of these mAb with the effector cells was sufficient to bring about inhibition, the extent of inhibition seemed, at least in some cases to be a function of the target cells as well. Second, on which stage(s) of the cytolytic process (i.e., recognition, lethal hit or target disintegration, ref. 2) were these mAb acting? We found that none acted at the last stage; methodological limitations made it difficult to ascertain whether inhibition was at recognition and/or lethal hit.

CYTOLYSIS-INHIBITING mAb

These were prepared as described in detail (5) by fusing spleen

TABLE I

Monoclonal antibodies used in this study

Full Designation	Short Designation	Inhibition of			Recognized antigen: Molecular Weight
		Specific Cytolysis	Con A-mediated Cytolysis	Con A-mediated Proliferation	
H35-17.2	17.2	+	-	-	70K (30K, 35K)
H35-27.9	27.9	+	-	-	70K (3K, 35K)
H35-89.9	89.9	+	+	+	180K and 94K
H49-57.1	57.1	+	ND[b]	ND	70K (30K, 35K)
K58.55.3	55.3	+	ND	ND	70K (30K, 35K)
H59-101.7	101.7	+	ND	ND	70K (30K, 35K)

[a] From ref. 5 and unpublished data with C. goridis.

[n][b] ND = not done.

cells (from rats immunized with b anti-d MLC cells) and Y3-Ag1.2.3 myeloma cells, selecting positive fusion wells for the ability of the corresponding supernatants to inhibit cytolysis by b anti-d cells of L1210 target cells and further cloning. Antibodies were partially purified from culture supernatants using $(NH_4)_2SO_4$ salt fractionation at 50% saturation. Precipitates were resuspended to one tenth of the original volume. These preparations, referred to as mAb, were used after dialysis in the experiments described below. Six mAb from 4 individual fusions were investigated. While 3 mAb have not yet been extensively analyzed, some results are available for the 3 others (summarized in Table I, from ref. 5 and unpublished data with C. Goridis). 17.2 mAb recognizes an antigen which is probably Lyt-2 according to its molecular weight and tissue distribution; formal demonstration of identity with Lyt-2 is in progress using sequential immunoprecipitation. 27.9 Ag seems different from 17.2 Ag by its tissue distribution, although a relationship between both antigens exists and is under investigation. 89.9 mAb was studied in detail before (5), immunoprecipitates two polypeptide chains and is peculiar in its ability to inhibit, not only specific cytolysis, but also Concanavalin A (Con A)-mediated cytolysis and proliferation. 57.1, 55.3 and 101.7 mAb have not yet been studied in detail; they could be similar to 17.2 or 27.9 mAb on the basis of molecular weight of the corresponding antigens and functional behavior (see below).

CYTOLYSIS-INHIBITING mAb EXERT THEIR EFFECT BY ACTING ON EFFECTOR RATHER THAN TARGET CELLS

Effector and/or target cells were preincubated with medium or mAb, washed and used in a cytolytic test. For all six mAb tested, preincubation of target cells did not lead to less cytolysis, while preincubation of effector cells with mAb consistently did (Table II). Similar results were obtained using 10^2 dilutions of mAb (not shown). The date presented in Table II generalized a result previously obtained with 89.9 mAb (5) and strongly suggested that these mAb exerted their inhibitory effect by acting on the effector cells.

Another approach was to use in standard cytolysis tests target cells which could not be recognized by the inhibitory mAb. For instance, 17.2 mAb inhibited cytolysis by b anti-k cells of $LMTK^-$ target cells (Fig. 1, _right_); $LMTK^-$ are fibroblasts which do not bear the 17.2 antigen and have no detectable Fc receptors for 17.2 mAb (not shown). Also, 17.2 and 89.9 mAb inhibited cytolysis by b anti-rat cells of Y3.Ag1.2.3 target cells (Fig. 1, _left_); these target cells are unlikely to be recognized by these mAb, since they were used as tumor "parents" for the constitution of the hybridomas making these mAb. These experiments showed that at least 17.2 and 89.9 mAb need not interfere with the target cells to exert their inhibitory effect on cytolysis.

TABLE II

Effect on cytolysis of preincubating effector or target cells or both with each of 6 cytolysis-inhibiting mAb

mAb	Exp	Preincubated cells[a]						Spont. Rel.[c]
		Effectors		Targets		Effectors and Targets		
		mAb	med	mAb	med	mAb	med	
17.2	1	40[b]	56	60	64	20	69	15
	2	29	45	44	40	31	59	8
27.9	1	39	56	56	64	28	69	15
	2	27	45	43	40	34	59	8
89.9	3	33	44	53	51	18	52	17
57.1	4	21	34	37	39	24	53	17
	5	16	42	43	43	21	56	7
55.3	6	17	35	41	39	11	51	8
101.7	5	23	42	47	43	28	56	7
	7	20	29	34	34	24	37	15

[a] Effector b anti-d cells and/or ^{51}Cr-labeled L1210 target cells were preincubated in tubes at a 20:1 ratio with (mAb) or without (med) 10^{-1} dilutions of the indicated mAb in Ca^{++} free medium. Cells were then washed and distributed in microplate wells for cytolysis test, with addition of complementary cells and or an excess of Ca^{++}. Incubation ws then for 4 h, with addition of an excess of EDTA after 30 min.

[b] Cytolysis, expressed as % ^{51}Cr-release; spontaneous release not subtracted.

[c] Spontaneous release of target cells alone.

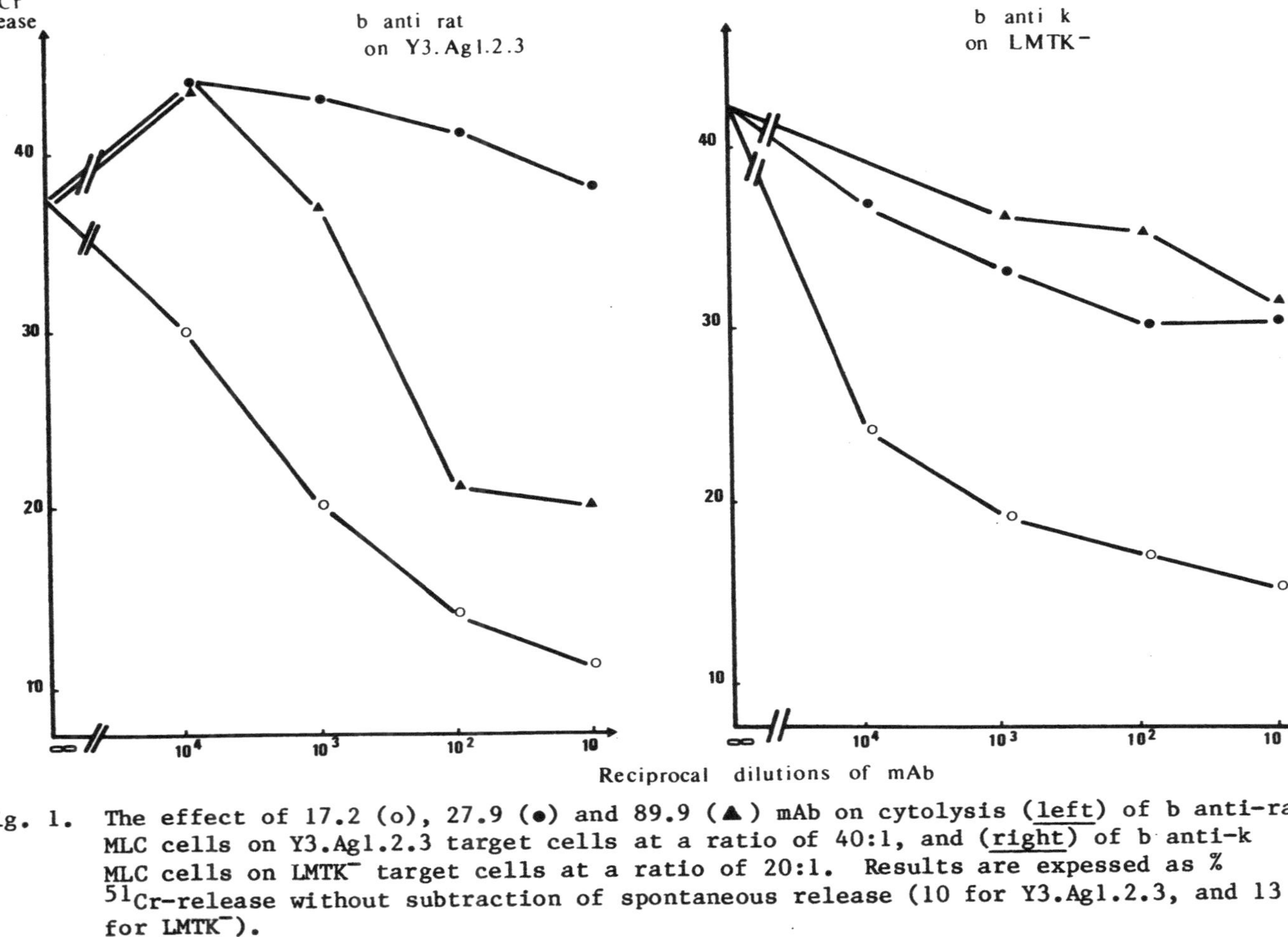

Fig. 1. The effect of 17.2 (o), 27.9 (●) and 89.9 (▲) mAb on cytolysis (left) of b anti-rat MLC cells on Y3.Ag1.2.3 target cells at a ratio of 40:1, and (right) of b anti-k MLC cells on LMTK⁻ target cells at a ratio of 20:1. Results are expessed as % ^{51}Cr-release without subtraction of spontaneous release (10 for Y3.Ag1.2.3, and 13 for LMTK⁻).

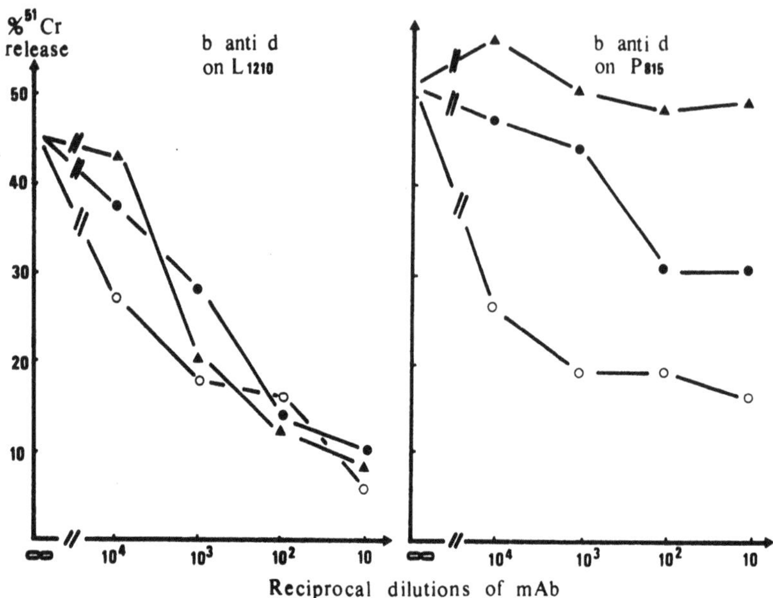

Fig. 2. The effect of 17.2 (o), 27.9 (●) and 89.9 (▲) mAb on cytolysis of b anti-d MLC cells (left) on L1210 target cells and (right) on P815 target cells. Effector:target cell ratios were 20:1. Results are expressed as % ^{51}Cr-release without subtraction of spontaneous release (6 for L1210, 10 for :815).

TARGET CELLS INFLUENCE THE INHIBITION OF CYTOLYSIS BY mAb

Although, as shown in the previous section, the effect of these cytolysis-inhibiting mAb was primarily on the effector cells, target cells were found to influence the inhibitory effect in two different ways (which may or may not be related). First, preincubation with mAb of a mixture of effector and target cells often led to more inhibition than preincubation of effector cells alone (Table II). These preincubations were done in the absence of Ca^{++}. This showed that interaction of effector and target cells at a pre-lethal hit stage facilitated the inhibitory effect of mAb. Second, the use of different tumor target cells seemed to influence the extent of inhibition by at least some mAb. This was already reflected in Fig. 1, but was studied in numerous experiments in the more appropriate combination b anti-d effector cells tested on either L1210 or P815 target cells. The pattern shown in Fig. 2 was always found, with 17.2, 27.9 and 89.9 mAb equally inhibitory when using L1210 target cells, but less inhibitory in that order when using P815 target cells. This difference in sensitivity to inhibition by mAb was apparently not linked to specificity of cytolysis, since the cytolysis by d anti-B cells in the presence of Con A was more inhibited

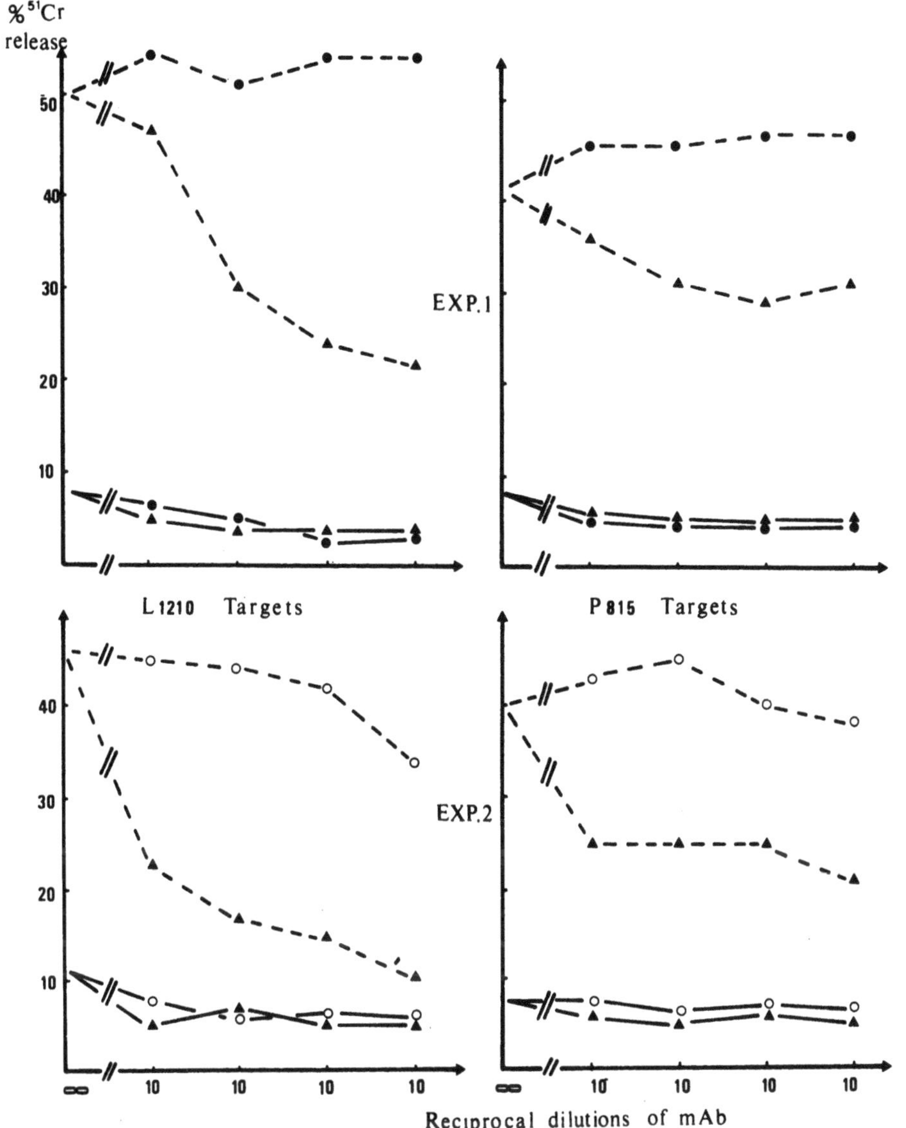

Fig. 3. The effect of 17.2 (o), 27.9 (●) and 89.9(▲) mAb on cytolysis by d anti-b MLC cells (left) on L1210 target cells and (right) on P815 target cells, in the presence of Con A (---) or in its absence (____), in two separate experiments (upper and lower panels). Effector:target cell ratios were (20:1. Results are expressed as % ^{51}Cr-release without subtraction of spontaneous release (4 or 5 in all cases).

by 89.9 mAb when L1210 rather than P815 were used as target cells (Fig. 3). In the experiments shown in Fig. 3, only 89.9 mAb but neither 17.2 nor 27.9 mAb inhibited to a large extent Con A-mediated cytolysis, confirming earlier results (5). The fact that differences in inhibition by 89.9 mAb of lysis of L1210 or P815 cells were also found with "irrelevant" effector cells in the presence of Con A strongly suggested that it was the very nature of the target cells that modulated the extent of inhibition of cytolysis by mAb.

THE TARGET CELL DISINTEGRATION STAGE OF CYTOLYSIS IS NOT AFFECTED BY THESE mAb

A Ca^{++} pulse experiment aiming at locating the stage of cytolysis (2,9) inhibited by 27.9 mAb is shown in Fig. 4. Addition of 27.9 mAb initially or just before addition of Ca^{++} almost completely inhbited cytolysis, while addition of 27.9 mAb just after addition

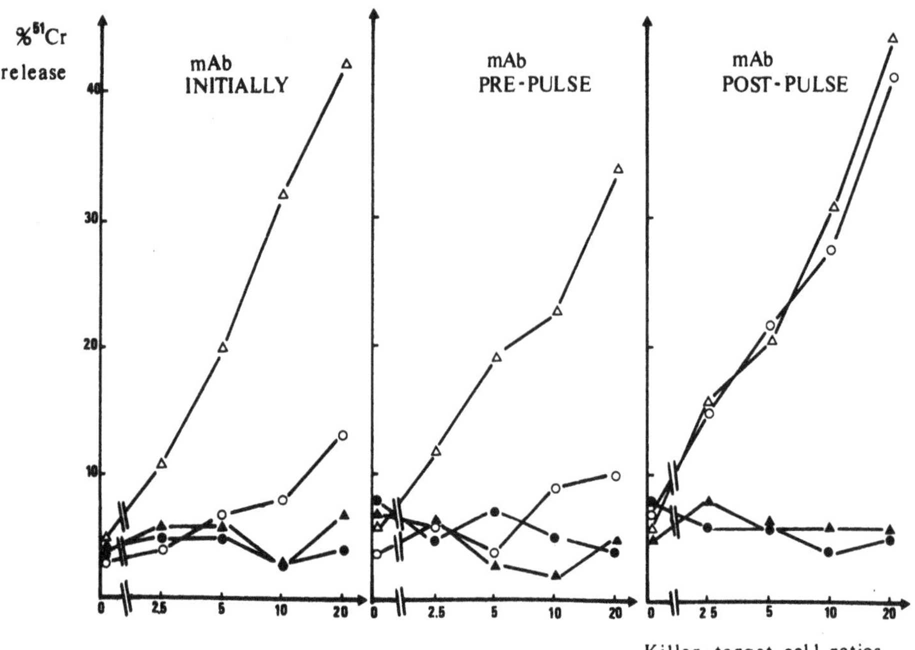

Fig. 4. The effect of the addition of 27.9 mAb in a Ca^{++} pulse experiment at various stages of cytolysis by b anti-d MLC cells (open symbols) or d anti-b MLC cells (full symbols) on L1210 target cells at varius killer:target cell ratios. Circles are with addition of 27.9 mAb, triangles are medium controls. Results are expressed as % ^{51}Cr-release without subtraction of spontaneous release.

TABLE III

Stage-locating Ca^{++} pulse experiments with each of 6 cytolysis-inhibiting mAb

mAb	Exp	Effector cells[a]	Addition of mAb or medium						Spt. release
			Initially[b]		prepulse		post-pulse		
			mAb	med	mAb	med	mAb	med	
17.2	1	b anti d	6[c]	22	7	23	25	26	8[d]
		d anti b	8	6	7	9	8	8	
27.9	2	b anti d	13	42	10	34	41	44	6
		d anti b	4	7	4	5	5	6	
89.9	3	b anti d	13	40	18	37	34	36	8
		d anti b	9	8	10	11	8	8	
57.1	4	b anti d	16	59	18	50	62	62	9
		d anti b	10	14	11	14	15	15	
55.3	4	b anti d	21	59	39	50	62	62	9
		d anti b	10	14	13	14	15	15	
101.7	5	b anti d	9	23	9	20	19	22	8
		d anti b	7	8	9	9	9	9	

[a] Effector cells were b anti-d or d anti-b MLC cells, target cells were L1210 cells, at a ratio of 20:1.

[b] mAb or medium were added to the mixtures of effector and target cells either initially, or prepulse (10 min. before addition of Ca^{++}) or post-pulse (just after addition of EDTA).

[c] Cytolysis expressed as % ^{51}Cr-release; spontaneous release not subtracted.

[d] Spontaneous release of target cells alone.

of EDTA did not inhibit cytolysis at all (Fig. 4). An experiment with similar results was previously shown using 89.9 mAb (5). Indeed, all 6 mAb showed the same pattern of inhibition when adding the mAb initially or pre-pulse but not post-pulse (Table III). Thus, none of these mAb inhibited cytolysis at the target cell disintegration stage. This conclusion is consistent with the above-mentioned findings that these mAb acted at the effector cell level, since the target cell disintegration stage is effector cell-independent (see 2 for review).

WHICH OF THE RECOGNITION OR LETHAL HIT STAGES IS INHIBITED BY THESE mAb

The results of the Ca^{++} pulse experiments above did not allow us to locate the effect of the cytolysis-inhibiting mAb at recognition or at lethal hit. An independent way to investigate recognition was therefore used, namely specific conjugate formation between effector and target cells (11,12). However, it was previously shown (10) that conjugate formation required events in excess of specific recognition. Inhibition of conjugate formation by mAb may reflect impairment of these events rather than impairment of specific recognition *per se*. Therefore, the only conclusive experimental result would be the *lack* of inhibition by mAb of conjugate formation, which would allow us to locate inhibition at the lethal hit stage.

Table IV gives a summary of all the conjugation experiments done under our standard experimental conditions. While some of the

TABLE IV

Conjugate formation. We followed, with only slight modifications, the method described and discussed in detail before (10). Briefly, a suspension of 2 x 10^5 effector cells (iron-plus-magnet purified MLC cells) with or without mAb as incubated for 30 min. at 37°C in a U-shaped well of a Cooke microtiter plate. Neutral red-labeld or more often unlabeled L1210 cells (of DBA/2 origin, $H\text{-}2^d$; 2 x 10^5 per well) were then added, the plate was briefly centrifuged and left for 10 min. at room temperature. A volume (40 µl) of Trypan Blue solution was added to each well, the contents of which in a total volume of 240 µl was then resuspended by 10 rapid in-and-out passages through the yellow disposable plastic tip of an automatic pipette (Gilson Pipetman, set at 200 µl). A sample was introduced into a hemocytometer chamber for counting under phase contrast optics. Results are expressed as the number per chamber of target cells with at least one bound lymphocyte. A figure of 100 corresponds to at least 100 bound lymphocytes, thus at least 15% of the total number of lymphocytes present in the chamber. Counting of conjugates was always done on coded preparations, i.e., without knowledge of the experimental groups at play.

TABLE IV

The effect of each of 6 cytolysis-inhibiting mAb on conjugate formation under standard conditions

		Effector Cells:											
		b anti-d						d anti-b					
		Reciprocal Ab dilution:						Reciprocal Ab dilution:					
mAb	Exp	10	10^2	10^3	10^4	10^5	med	10	10^2	10^3	10^4	10^5	med
17.2	1	25	12	12	19	ND	30	4	1	2	5	ND	4
	2	40	13	20	20	ND	39	15	14	14	12	ND	14
	3	123	63	33	62	70	105	27	20	30	24	26	17
	4	34	59	27	51	88	47	32	28	17	17	21	11
27.9	5	148	137	184	112	151	188	66	75	79	57	49	75
	6	59	62	68	60	67	64	32	28	26	26	24	13
	7	126	105	113	92	137	121	20	16	24	16	23	9
	8	60	50	40	47	ND	65	24	21	18	14	ND	7
89.9	9	7	5	6	34	83	102	1	12	15	8	21	31
	10	4	3	8	36	197	103	8	4	9	4	23	32
57.1	11	58	40	48	43	41	43	22	22	21	16	13	15
	12	54	68	53	68	52	55	19	22	17	17	16	13
55.3	13	25	50	71	89	87	98	30	35	19	33	48	38
	14	27	16	15	31	49	41	17	6	6	11	12	4
101.7	15	14	26	41	49	57	36	23	21	17	12	12	6
	16	51	62	77	50	66	54	32	32	31	16	11	21

mAb gave variable results (for instance, 17.2 mAb had a tendency to inhibit conjugate formation with a concentration "prozone" effect), two mAb gave a clearcut pattern. First, 89.9 mAb inhibited both specific and non-specific conjugate formation. This is in line with the cell disagglutinating action of this mAb reported before (5). This did not occur when conjugates were made with peritoneal exudate lymphocytes instead of MLC cells; however, cytolysis by peritoneal exudate lymphocytes was only poorly inhibited by 89.9 mAb (not shown). Second, 27.9 mAb and perhaps also 57.1 mAb did not inhibit conjugate formation under these experimental conditions (Table IV). However, when we tried to confirm this lack of inhibition using slightly different experimental conditions (i.e., incubation of cells and mAb at 37°C instead of room temperature, N. Hollander, personal communication), 27.9 mAb was found to inhibit conjugate formation (Table V).

We then resorted to a somewhat different approach, reasoning that the inhibition of cytolysis observed when 27.9 mAb was added pre-pulse (Fig. 4) could be due either to an "upstream" effect (reversal of recognition) or to a "downstream" effect (inhibition of lethal hit). To investigate this, effector and target cells were mixed, in the absence of mAb, under Ca^{++} pulse conditions (i.e., in medium B, which allows recognition and conjugate formation). After incubation for 30 min. at 37°C, 27.9 mAb was added, incubation at 37°C proceeded for variable lengths of time, Ca^{++} was added, and both the number of conjugates and ^{51}Cr-release were checked. Table VI shows that such addition of 27.9 mAb post-recognition, pre-pulse, did not revert preformed conjugates while it inhibited ^{51}Cr-release. Another experiment of this sort gave similar results (not shown). This suggested that 27.9 mAb added pre-pulse acted downstream by inhibiting lethal hit (but see below).

TABLE V

The effect of 27.9 mAb on conjugate formation at 37°C°

		Effector Cells:											
		b anti d						d anti b					
		Reciprocal Ab dilutions:						Reciprocal Ab dilution:					
mAb	Exp	10	10^2	10^3	10^4	10^5	med	10	10^2	10^3	10^4	10^5	med
27.9	1	15	28	52	19	22	72	2	4	6	3	4	3
	2	13	19	26	40	40	60	4	10	10	4	10	3

Legends as for Table IV, except that incubation of the effector-L1210 target cell mixture in the presence of 27.9 mAb was at 37°C instead of at room temperature.

TABLE VI

Comparison of the effect of 27.9 mAb added post-recognition pre-pulse on number of conjugates and ^{51}Cr-release

Incubation with 27.9 mAb (min.)	Conjugates				Incubation with 27.9 mAb (min.)	^{51}Cr-release			
	b anti d		d anti b			b anti-d		d anti-b	
	mAb	med	mAb	med		mAb	med	mAb	med
10	33	45	5	5	10	32	ND	9	ND
15	47	43	7	7	12	33	ND	7	ND
25	43	39	9	7	17	33	ND	7	ND
					25	33	60	7	7

Iron-plus-magnet treated b anti-d or d anti-b MLC cells were mixed with ^{51}Cr-labeled L1210 cells in medium B, in cytolysis test or conjugate formation conditions, in wells of microplates. The microplates were centrifuged and incubated for 30 min. at 37°C. 27.9 mAb at a 10^{-1} final dilution or medium was then added. Incubation at 37°C was resumed for 10 to 25 min., then Ca^{++} was added in all wells. Conjugates were counted 2 min. after addition of Ca^{++}, and results are expressed as indicated in the legend of Table IV. For cytolysis, EDTA was added 20 min. after addition of Ca^{++}, and incubation proceeded for a further 3 h before sampling of supernates; results are expressed as % ^{51}Cr-release. ND = not done.

DISCUSSION

Monoclonal antibodies may be valuable tools to identify molecules involved in T cell-mediated cytolysis. Monoclonal antibodies putatively directed against such molecules can be detected via their inhibitory effect on cytolysis. We selected 6 xenogeneic rat anti-mouse mAb for their inhibitory effect on T cell-mediated cytolysis (5,6). One of these mAb, 17.2 mAb, was very probably directed against Lyt-2. Inhibition of cytolysis by anti-Lyt-2 mAb has already been extensively studies (13-18). Another one, 89.9 mAb, which we analyzed in detail before (5,6) was similar to the M7/14 mAb described by others (19,20).

Cytolysis-inhibiting mAb were found to fall into two categories. First some mAb inhibit cytolysis by acting on the target cells, most likely by masking target molecules (see for instance 21; M. Pierres, in preparation). Second, some mAb inhibit cytolysis by acting on the effector cells. This seems to be the case for anti-Lyt-2 mAb and M7/14 mAb (see references above) and also for the 6 mAb we studied. To demonstrate this, we used preincubation experiments and, for some of these mAb, target cells devoid of the corresponding antigens and Fc receptors. A possibly related observation is that the nature of the effector cells often conditions the extent of inhibition. For instance, 89.9 mAb inhibited cytolysis by MLC cells much more than cytolysis by sensitized peritoneal cells (unpublished results), which was also found using anti-Lyt-2 mAb (18). However, we found tht the nature of the target cells also seemed to play a role in the extent of inhibiton by these effector cell-acting mAb. We are not aware of any previous report on this point, which we cannot readily explain and which remains to be clarified using, for instance, Fab'_2 of each of these mAb.

The 6 mAb used here were also investigated as to the stage of cytolysis (recognition, lethal hit or target cell disintegration) they inhibited. Ca^{++} pulse experiments demonstrated that none of these mAb inhibited the post-pulse target cell disintegration stage (while one report suggested that a rat anti-mouse antiserum could inhibit cytolysis at this stage, 22). To investigate whether inhibition occurred at recognition or lethal hit, we resorted to a study of inhibition of conjugate formation by these mAb. We found that all 6 mAb inhibited conjugate formation, even 27.9 mAb, when the temperature of incubation was raised to 37°C. We do not believe this to be very conclusive in itself, since conjugate formation involves events other than specific recognition (10) which may be the ones inhibited by mAb. The same objection, that inhibition of conjugate formation does not necessarily mean inhibition of specific recognition _per se_, may apply to published work using anti-Lyt-2 mAb (16).

In our studies using conjugates, two mAb, however, stood out. First, 89.9 mAb was unique in its ability to inhibit both specific and non-specific conjugates, which is in line with the general cell disagglutinating effect of this mAb reported before (5) and may or may not be related to its cytolysis-inhibiting effect. The similar antibody M7/14 was reported to inhibit specific conjugate formation, but non-specific conjugates were not investigated (20). Second, 27.9 mAb when added post-recognition, pre-Ca^{++} pulse inhibited cytolysis without reversing preformed conjugates. While this does not mean that when added initially 27.9 mAb cannot affect recognition, it might suggest that 27.9 mAb affects, only or also, the lethal hit stage of cytolysis. A reservation to this conclusion would be the possibility that 27.9 mAb added post-recognition pre-pulse reverses recognition in some subtle, presently undetectable way, i.e., without affecting preformed conjugates. Another possibility would be that 27.9 antigens are somehow involved in both recognition and lethal hit, with for each a different threshold of inhibition by 27.9 mAb.

At another level of discussion, each of the antigens detected by these cytolysis-inhibiting mAb may be (a) either crucially necessary for the mechanism of T cell-mediated cytolysis, or (b) not necessary, but the binding of the corresponding mAb sterically interferes with the action of other, necessary structures, or (c) not necessary, but the binding of the corresponding mAb provides an "off" signal to some of the metabolic pathways of the killer cells. The first of these hypotheses may be abandoned if cells could be found which would be "antigen-negative", but still cytolytic.

ACKNOWLEDGEMENTS

We thank M.-F. Luciani for providing excellent technical help. This work was supported by CNRS, INSERM and DGRST.

REFERENCES

1. Henney, C.S. T-cell-mediated cytolysis: an overview of some current issues. Contemp. Top. Immunobiol. 7:245 (1977).
2. Golstein, P., and E.T. Smith. Mechanism of T-cell-mediated cytolysis: the lethal hit stage. Contemp. Top. Immunobiol. 7:273 (1977).
3. Martz, E. Mechanism of specific tumor-cell lysis by alloimmune lymphocytes: resolution and characterizations of discrete steps in the cellular interaction. Contemp. Top. Immunobiol. 7:301 (1977).
4. Berke, G. Interaction of cytotoxic T lymphocytes and target cells. Progress in Allergy 27:69 (1979).
5. Pierres, M., Goridis, C., and P. Golstein. Inhibition of murine T cell-mediated cytolysis and T cell proliferation by a rat monoclonal antibody immunoprecipitating two lymphoid cell surface polypeptides of 94,000 and 180,000 molecular weight. Eur. J. Immunol., in press (1981).
6. Golstein, P., and M. Pierres. Monoclonal antibodies as probes to study the mechanism of T cell-mediated cytolysis. Proc. 14th Leuc. cult. Conf., in press (1981).
7. Golstein, P., Foa, C., and I.C.M. MacLennan. Mechanism of T cell-mediated cytolysis: the differential impact of cytochalasins at the recognition and lethal hit stages. Eur. J. Immunol. 8:302 (1978).
8. Galfre, G., Milstain, C., and B. Wright. Rat x Rat hybrid myelomas and a monoclonal anti-Fd portion of mouse IgG. Nature 277:131 (1979).
9. Golstein, P., and E.T. Smith. The lethal hit stage of mouse T and non-T cell-mediated cytolysis: differences in cation requirements and characterization of an analytical "cation pulse" method. Eur. J. Immunol. 6:31 (1976).
10. Shortman, K., and P. Golstein. Target cell recognition by

cytolytic T cells: different requirements for the formation of strong conjugates or for proceeding to lysis. J. Immunol. 123:833 (1979).
11. Berke, G., Gabison, D., and M. Feldman. The frequency of effector cells in populations containing T lymphocytes. Eur. J. Immunol. 5:813 (1975).
12. Martz, E. Early steps in specific tumor cell lysis by sensitized mouse T-lymphocytes. I. Resolution and characterization. J. Immunol. 115:261 (1975).
13. Shinohara, N., Hammerling, U., and D.H. Sachs. Mouse alloantibodies capable of blocking cytotoxic T cell function. II. Further study on the relationship between the blocking antibodies and the products of the Lyt-2 locus. Eur. J. Immunol. 10:589 (180).
14. Nakayama, E., Dippold, W., Shiku, H., Oettgen, H.F., and L.J. Old. Alloantigen-induced T-cell proliferation: Lyt phenotype of responding cells and blocking of proliferation by Lyt antisera. Proc. Natl. Acad. Sci. USA 77:2890 (1980).
15. Hollander, N., Pillemer, E., and I.L. Weissman. Blocking effect of Lyt-2 antibodies on T cell function. J. Exp. Med. 152:674 (1980).
16. Fan, J., Ahmed, A., and B. Bonavida. Studies on the induction and expession of T cell-mediated immunity. X. Inhibition by Lyt 2,3 antisera of cytotoxic T lymphocyte-mediated antigen-specific and non-specific cytotoxicity: evidence for the blocking of the binding between T lymphocytes and target cells and not the post-binding cytolytic steps. J. Immunol. 125: 2444 (1980).
17. Sarmiento, M., Glasebrook, A.L., and F.W. Fitch. IgG or IgM monoclonal antibodies reactive with different determinants on the molecular complex bearing Lyt 2 antigen block T cell-mediated cytolysis in the absence of complement. J. Immunol. 125:2665 (1980).
18. MacDonald H.R., Thiernesse, N., and J.-C. Cerottini. Inhibition of T cell-mediated cytolysis by monoclonal antibodies directed against Lyt-2: heterogeneity of inhibition at the clonal level. J. Immunol. 126:1671 (1981).
19. Kurzinger, K., Reynbolds, T., Germain, R.N., Davignon, D., Martz, E., and T.A. Springer. A novel lymphocyte function-associated antigen (LFA-1): cellular distribution, quantitative expression and structure. J. Immunol. 127:596 (1981).
20. Davignon, D., Martz, E., Reynolds, T., Kurzinger, K., and T.A. Springer. Monoclonal antibody to a novel lymphocyte function-associated antigen (LFA-1). Mechanism of blockade of T lymphocyte-mediated killing and effects on other T and B lymphocyte functions. J. Immunol. 127:590 (1981).
21. Lindahl, K.F., and H. Lemke. Inhibition of killer-target cell interaction by monoclonal anti-H-2 antibodies. Eur. J. Immunol. 9:526 (1979).
22. Hiserodt, J.C., and B. Bonavida. Studies on the induction and

expression of T cell-mediated immunity. XI. Inhibition of the "lethal hit" in T cell-mediated cytotoxicity by heterologous rat antiserum made against alloimmune cytotoxic T lymphocytes. J. Immunol. 126:256 (1981).

FUNCTIONAL RELATIONSHIPS OF LYMPHOCYTE MEMBRANE STRUCTURES PROBED WITH CYTOLYSIS AND/OR PROLIFERATION-INHIBITING H35-27.9 AND H35-89.9 MONOCLONAL ANTIBODIES

Pierre Golstein, Michel Pierres, Anne-Marie Schmitt-Verhulst, Marie-Francoise Luciani, Michel Buferne, Zelig Eshhar and Yael Kaufmann

From the Centre d'Immunologie INSERM-CNRS de Marseille-Luminy, Case 906, 13288 Marseille Cedex 9, France, and the Departments of Cell Biology and Chemical Immunology, The Weizmann Institute of Sciences, Rehovot, Israel

INTRODUCTION

The mechanism(s) of T lymphocyte "functions" such as cytolysis (1-4) or proliferation involve those cell surface structures that insure specific recognition and may involve other cell surface structures as well. Detection of these may be via the use of monoclonal antibodies (mAb) selected for their ability to inhibit lymphocyte functions. Indeed, anti-Lyt-2 mAb have been extensively studied as to their inhibitory effect on mouse T cell-mediated cytolysis, with repeated suggestions that Lyt-2 itself may be related to the T cell specific receptor (5-10). We have developed a range of xenogeneic rat anti-mouse mAb selected for their ability to inhibit T cell-mediated cycolysis (11,12). Three of them will be used in the present report: H35-17.2 mAb, which is most probably an anti-Lyt-2 mAb, as an experimental counterpoint to the two other mAb; H35-27.9 mAb, which differs from an anti-Lyt-2 mAb at least by the tissue distribution of the structures it recognizes; and H35-89.9 mAb, which immunoprecipitates from lymphoid cell surfaces two polypeptides of 180K and 94K molecular weight.

Using these mAb, we made a series of observations on the relationships between lymphocyte cell surface structures and functions (in this report, the relationships between a lymphoid cell structure and a lymphoid cell function are defined by the ability of a mAb directed against this structure to inhibit this function). First, H35-89.9 mAb inhibited T but not B cell proliferation, and H35-27.9 mAb inhibited T but not NK cell-mediated cytolysis, while in both cases the corresponding antigens were present on both inhibited and non-inhibited cells. Second, in some cloned cytolytic T cell lines or hybridomas, H35-89.9 mAb inhibited both cytolysis and proliferation, while in others it inhibited cytolysis but not proliferation. Third, the determinant recognized by the cytolysis-inhibiting H35-27.9 mAb was not found on a given cytolytic T cell hybridoma. These findings suggested that the functional relationships of a lymphoid cell surface structure may not be the same from one cell type to another, and for a given type from one function to another; and that a cell surface structure involved, when bound by the corresponding mAb, in the inhibition of a function may not be necessary for this function.

CYTOLYSIS-INHIBITING RAT mAb

These were prepared as described in detail before (11). Antibodies were partially purified from culture supernatants or ascitic fluid using $(NH_4)_2SO_4$ at 50% saturation. Precipitates were resuspended to one tenth of the original volume. These preparations, dialyzed, are referred to as mAb. The three mAb studied, H35-17.2, H35-27.9 and H35-89.9 (often abbreviated below to 17.2, 27.9 and 89.9 mAb) had been investigated before (11; this volume; and unpublished data with C. Goridis). These mAb all inhibited T cell-mediated cytolysis irrespective or its specificity (11), by acting on the effector cells. 17.2 mAb recognized an antigen which was probably Lyt-2 according to its molecular weight and tissue distribution. 27.9 mAb recognized an antigen which was different from Lyt-2 by its tissue distribution (see below, Fig. 6 and 7) although on thymocytes Lyt-2 and 27.9 determinants seem to be present on structurally similar molecules (in preparation). 89.9 mAb immunoprecipitated two membrane structures of 180K and 94K molecular weight and was peculiar in its ability to inhibit, not only specific cytolysis, but also Con A-mediated cytolysis and proliferation (11). Other mAb used were directed against Thy-1.2 (clone J1J, kindly provided by J. Sprent, Philadelphia, PA, USA or clones kindly provided by A. Marshak-Rothstein et al. from MIT, Cambridge, MA, USA).

Cytolytic T cell clones BD4-2 and BD4-13 were derived by limiting dilution from C57BL/6 anti-DBA/2 MLC cells in the presence of irradiated BALB/c spleen cells in RPMI 1640 containing 5% FCS, 25% supernatant from Con A-stimulated rat spleen cells and 10 mg/ml α-methylmannoside. The clones were expanded in the same supplemented medium. Their characteristics will be described elsewhere (A.M. Schmitt-Verhulst et al., in preparation). Cytolytic T cell hybridomas, the preparation (by fusion of cytolytic T cells and AKR tumor cells BW5147), characteristics and anti-EL4 cytolytic activity of which were described before (13,14) were either Md26 derived from MLC cells or P47 derived from sensitized peritoneal exudate cells. Tumor target cells were L1210 (T lymphoma of DBA/2

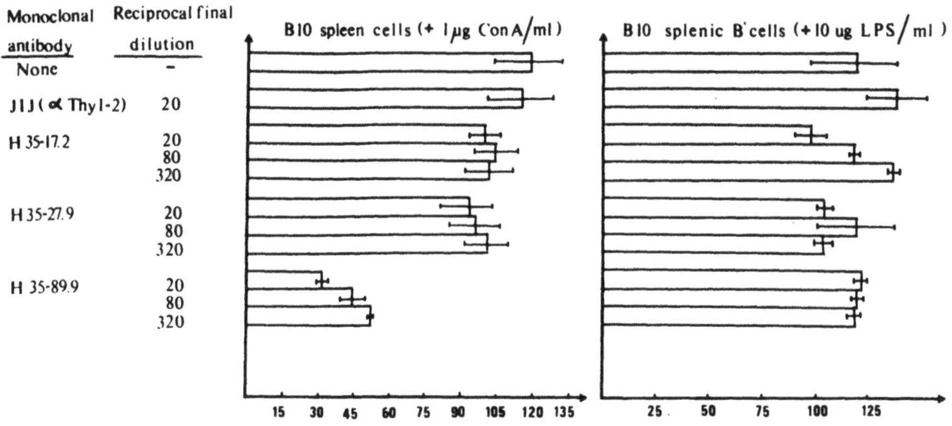

Fig. 1. The inhibitory effect of H35-89.9 mAb on lectin-induced proliferation of T (left) but not B (right) spleen cells. C57BL/10 spleen cells, either unseparated or depleted of T cells by treatment with an anti-Thy-1.2 mAb (JIJ) and complement, were cultured in Click's medium with 5% fetal calf serum in flat-bottomed wells of microtiter plates (2×10^5 cells/well) in the presence of either 1 μg/ml Con A or 10 μg/ml LPS. Various amounts of mAb were added at initiation of cultures to the indicated final dilutions. Thymidine uptake was determined after a 12 h pulse of ^3H TdR (1 μCi/well) on day 2 (left) or 3 (right). Each bar represents mean ± standard deviation of triplicate assays.

origin, H-2^d), YAC (T lymphoma of A/Sn origin, H-2^a) and EL4 (T lymphoma of C57BL/6 origin, H-2^b). Two different sublines of EL4 cells were used, carried in vitro at the Centre d'Immunologie or passaged in vivo at the Weizmann Institute respectively.

INHIBITION OF LYMPHOID CELL FUNCTIONS BY 89.9 mAb

Two sets of unexpected observations were made as to the inhibition of lymphoid cell functions by 89.9 mAb. First, lectin-mediated T but not B cell proliferation (11 and Fig. 1) could be inhibited by 89.9 mAb. In striking contrast, by quantitative immunoadsorption the same amount of 89.9 antigen (Ag) was found on both T and B cells (11). Similar results were obtained with M7/14 mAb (16,17). Moreover, 89.9 Ag appeared similar on T and B cells not only quantitatively, but also qualitatively, since the same 180K and 94K structures could be immunoprecipitated with 89.9 mAb from both T (11) and B cells (unpublished results with C. Goridis). This indicated that the relationships of 89.9 Ag with proliferation were different in T and B cells.

Second, both T cell-mediated cytolysis and proliferation were inhibited by 89.9 mAb at the T cell population level (11) and for some T cell clones (11 and unpublished). However, in some cases there was a dissociation between inhibition of proliferation and cytolysis. This was first found using T cell hybridomas, the cytolytic activity of which was inhibited by 89.9 mAb, while their proliferation was not (Fig. 2, left panels). In these experiments, the effect of 89.9 mAb on Con A-stimulated spleen cells served as a positive control for inhibition proliferation. The inability of 89.9 mAb to inhibit proliferation of these hybridoma cells was not linked to the constitutive character of the growth of these cells, since the same phenomenon of inhibition of cytolysis but not of proliferation was also found with some TCGF-dependent long term lymphoid cell clones. In Fig. 2, right panels, both clone BD4-2

Fig. 2. The effect of H35-89.9 mAb on cytolytic T cell hybridomas (left) and TCGF-dependent clones (right). Cytolytic T cell hybridomas were either Md26 (——) or P47 (---). Their cytolytic activity was tested (lower left) in a 5 h ^{51}Cr-release test on in vivo-carried neuraminidase-treated EL4 cells at effector:target cell ratios of 0.5:1 and 2:1 respectively. Proliferation of hybridoma cells was tested (upper left) in flat-bottomed wells of microtiter plates. Each well received 2 x 10^3 hybridoma cells plus the indicated final concentration of mAb in a total volume of 200 μl. After either 1 h (▲) or 45 h (▼) of incubation, ^{3}H-thymidine (2 μCi/well) was added to triplicate cultures for a further 4 h period of incubation. BALB/c spleen cells (4 x 10^4/well) incubated for 45 h with Con A (0.5 μg/ml) served as control (●). Results are expressed as % of cpm without mAb, which were, for Md26, 27,800 (1 h) and 440,000 (45 h), for P47 28,000 (1 h) and 280,000 (45 h), for spleen cells 9,100. Cytolytic T cell clones were either BD4-2 (——) or BD4-13 (---). This cytolytic activity was tested (lower right), one day after passage, in a 4 h ^{51}Cr-release test on L1210 cells at effector:target cell ratios of 5:1 and 1:1 respectively. Less than 5% cytolysis of control EL4 target cells was observed (not shown). Proliferation of T cell clones was tested (upper right) in flat-bottomed wells of microtiter plates. Each well received, in a total volume of 200 μl, 1 x 10^4 cloned cells, 5 x 10^5 irradiated (2500 R) BALB/c spleen cells, Con A supernatant (25% final, α-methylmannoside (2.5 mg/ml) and the indicated final concentration of mAb. After 40 h of incubation ^{3}Hthymidine was added as indicated above for a further 6 h period of incubation. Results are expressed as % of cpm without mAb, which were 4730 for BD4-2 and 12,670 for BD4-13.

% OF CONTROL 3H TdR INCORPORATION
% 51Cr RELEASE
RECIPROCAL DILUTIONS OF H35-89.9 MONOCLONAL ANTIBODY
none

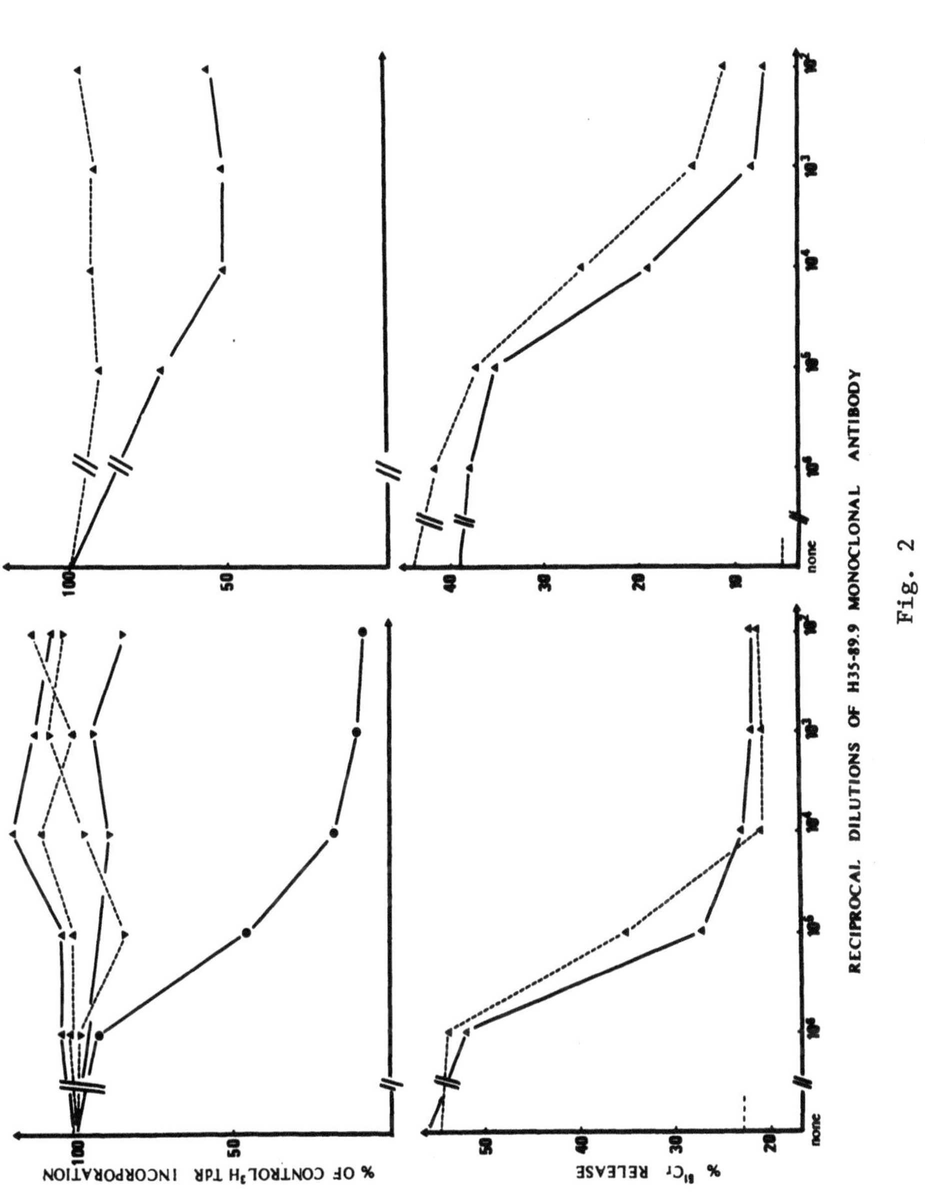

Fig. 2

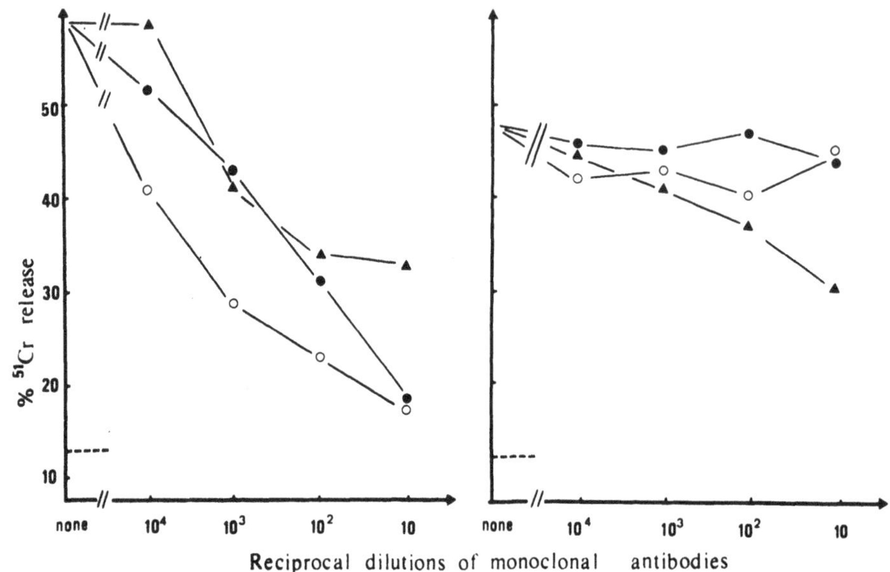

Fig. 3. The effect of three monoclonal antibodies on T and NK cell-mediated cytolysis. Effector cells, either MLC-generated b anti-A cells at a ratio of 10:1 ("T", left) or nylon wool column-passed normal CBA spleen cells at a ratio of 50:1 ("NK", right) were incubated for 4 h with ^{51}Cr-labeled YAC (H-2^a) target cells in the presence of various dilutions of H35-17.2 (O), H35-27.9 (●) and H35-89.9 (▲) mAb. Similar results were obtained using CBA nu/nu spleen cells as NK cells. C57BL/6 anti-B10.A MLC cells did not lyse control EL4 target cells. Control bg/bg normal spleen cells, devoid of detectable T, NK and K cytolytic activity lysed neither EL4 nor YAC target cells (not shown). Horizontal dotted lines indicate spontaneous ^{51}Cr-release of target cells incubated alone.

and clone BD4-13 were inhibited by 89.9 mAb in terms of cytolysis, but only clone BD4-2 was partially inhibited in terms of proliferation. Similar results were obtained with two subclones of BD4-2 and two subclones of BD4-13 (not shown). In all these experiments, the inhibition by 89.9 mAb of cytolytic activity of cloned cells demonstrated the presence of 89.9 Ag at their surface. The proliferation of some of these cells was nevertheless not inhibited by 89.9 mAb. This indicated that within a given T cell, 89.9 Ag could be related to one function (cytolysis) and related <u>or not</u> to another (proliferation).

INHIBITION BY 27.9 mAb OF T BUT NOT NK CELL-MEDIATED CYTOLYSIS

We wondered whether mAb that inhibit T cell-mediated cytolysis would inhibit NK cell-mediated cytolysis as well. To avoid differences in inhibition by mAb due to target cell effects, we used for both types of cytolysis the same YAC target cells (Fig. 3). T cell-mediated cytolysis by b anti-a MLC effector cells was significantly inhibited by each of the three mAb used (17.2, 27.9 and 89.9 mAb). In contrast, NK cell-mediated cytolysis by nylon wool column-passed normal spleen cells was inhibited neither by 17.2 nor by 27.9 mAb, while 89.9 mAb still gave some inhibition (Fig. 3). Similar results were obtained using nu/nu spleen cells as NK cells (not shown).

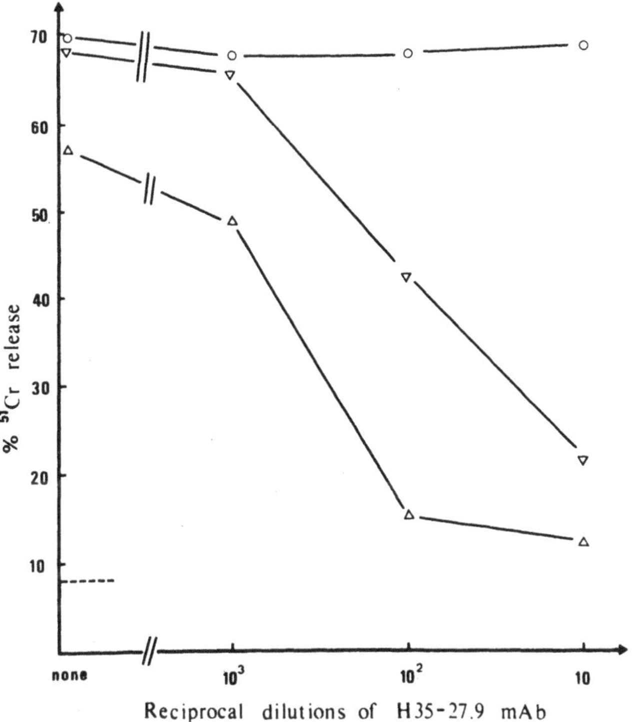

Fig. 4. The effect of H35-27.9 mAb and complement on NK effector cells. Spleen cells from CBA nu/nu mice were incubated with various dilutions of H35-27.9 mAb and medium (O) or normal rabbit serum as a source of complement at a dilution of 1/20 (▽) or 1/5 (△). The spleen cells were then washed and tested for cytolysis of YAC target cells, in a 4h ^{51}Cr-release assay, at a ratio, not corrected for complement-mediated cell death, of 20:1. Dotted line indicates spontaneous ^{51}Cr-release by YAC cells alone. NK lysis was high in this experiment; its decrease by pretreatment with H35-27.9 mAb and complement was also observed in experiments with lower levels of lysis (not shown).

The lack of inhibition of NK cell-mediated cytolysis by 17.2 and 27.9 mAb may be due to the absence of the corresponding antigens on the effector cells. Both mAb had previously been shown to be cytolytic in the presence of complement. While pre-treatment of effector cells with 17.2 mAb and complement led to little alteration of subsequent NK lysis (not shown), pre-treatment with 27.9 mAb and complement drastically decreased NK lysis (Fig. 4). This demonstrated the presence of 27.9 Ag at the surface of NK cells. Their presence at the surface of cytolytic T cells was shown by inhibition of cytolysis by 27.9 mAb, and also by complement-mediated lysis of cytolytic T cell clones (not shown). Thus, although differences in 27.9 Ag density between NK and mixed leucocyte culture-derived cytolytic T cells could not be excluded, clearly both T and NK effector cells bore 27.9 Ag, and 27.9 mAb inhibited cytolysis by the former but not by the latter. This suggested that the relationships of 27.9 Ag with the cytolytic mechanism were different in T and NK cells.

Md26, A CYTOLYTIC T CELL HYBRIDOMA, BEARS NO DETECTABLE 27.9 Ag

The Ags we investigated (17.2, 27.9 and 89.9 Ag) were functionally connected with cytolysis, either because they were a necessary part of the mechanism of cytolysis, or because they could interfee with this mechanism without being part of it. The former possibility would be excluded if a given cytolytic cell could be shown not to bear one of these Ag. We screened a small range of cloned cytolytic T cell lines and hybridomas for inhibition of cytolysis by mAb. When comparing hybridomas Md26 and P47, we found that their respective cytolytic activity could be inhibited to the same extent by the same dilutions of 89.9 mAb, but that Md26 contrarily to P47 was hardly inhibited at all by 27.9 mAb (Fig. 5).

Md26 could either bear no 27.9 Ag, or bear functionally unconnected 27.9 Ag. This point was investigated using two approaches. First, ^{51}Cr-labeled Md26 and P47 were treated with anti-Thy-1.2 mAb, 17.2 mAb or 27.9 mAb in the presence of complement. Fig. 6 shows that Md26 and P47 hybridoma cells could be lysed to the same extent, either by high dilutions of anti-Thy-1.2 mAb or by relatively low dilutions of 17.2 mAb; this gave some indications as to the relative amounts of both Ag, and more important here suggested that the "lysability" of both hybridomas by mAb and complement was similar. In sharp contrast, P47 cells were lysed at a 10^{-4} dilution of 27.9 mAb and Md26 cells were not lysed at a 10^{-1} dilution of this mAb (Fig. 6). This suggested a difference of at least 1000 fold in the amount of 27.9 Ag present on these hybridomas. Also, cytofluorometry (Fig. 7) showed similar relative values for both hybridomas with 17.2 mAb on the one hand and 89.9 mAb on the other hand; however, with 27.9 mAb, Md26 cells were at background level and P47 cells significantly above it.

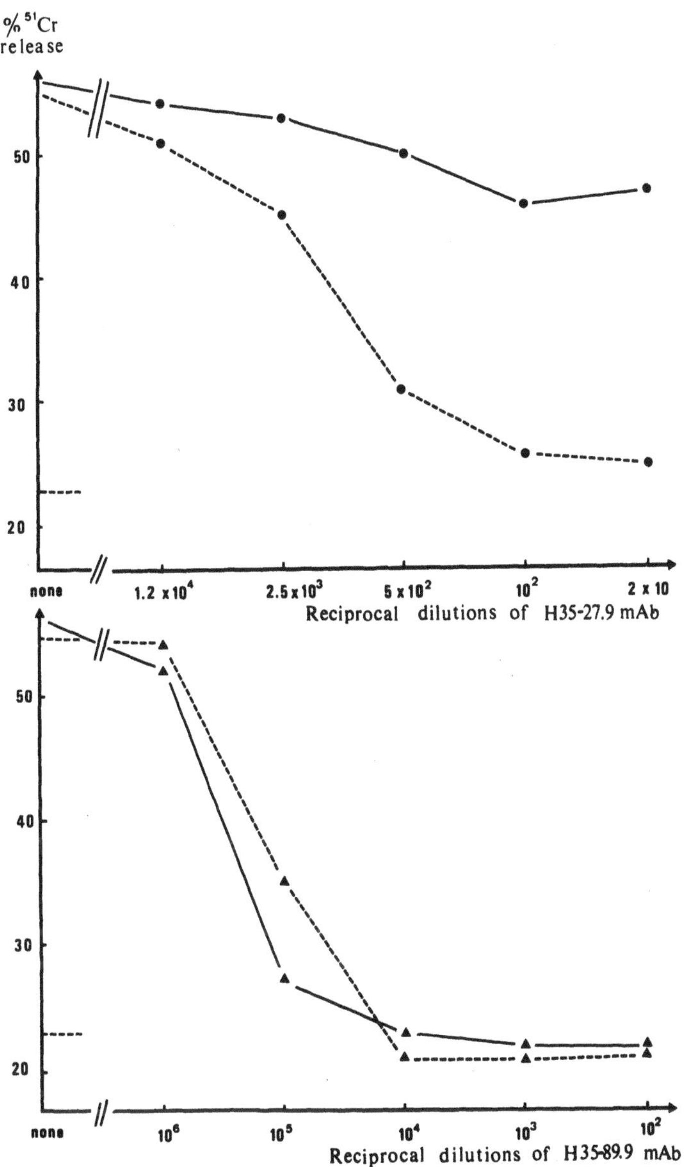

Fig. 5. The effect of H35-27.9 mAb (top) or H36-89.9 mAb (bottom) on the cytolysis of ^{51}Cr-labeled target cells by hybridomas Md26 (———) or P47 (----) at effector:target cell ratios of 0.5:1 and 2:1 respectively. Horizontal dotted lines indicate spontaneous ^{51}Cr-release of target cells incubated alone.

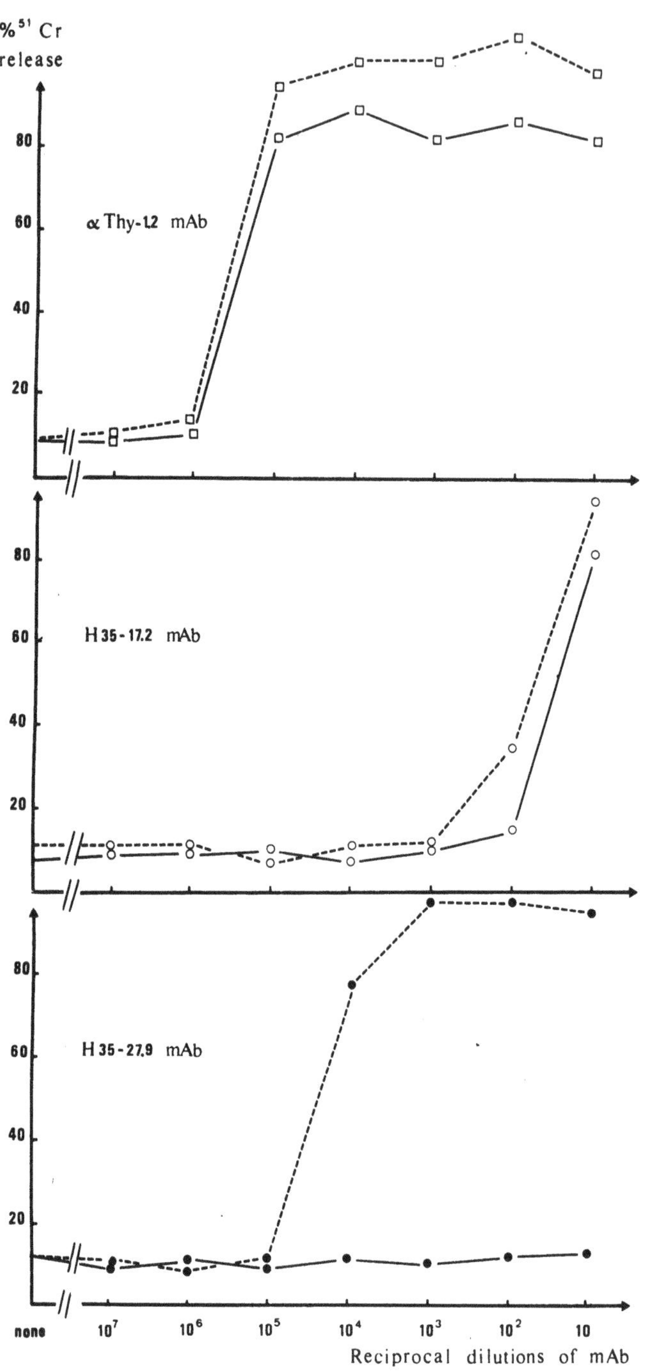

% 51 Cr release
80
60
40
20
α Thy-1.2 mAb
H 35-17.2 mAb
H 35-27.9 mAb
none
10^7
10^6
10^5
10^4
10^3
10^2
10
Reciprocal dilutions of mAb

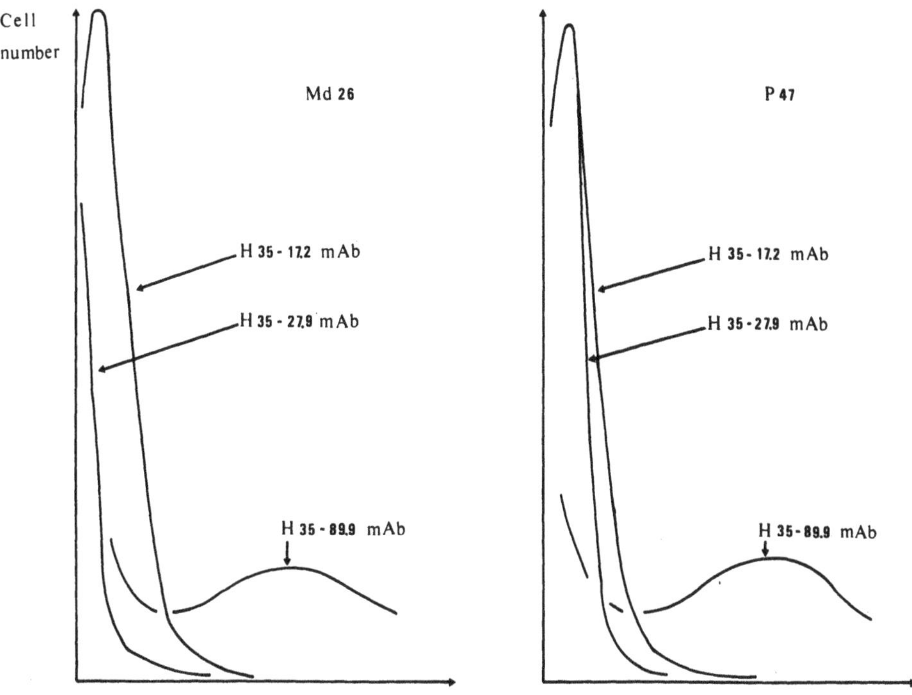

Fig. 7. Cytofluorometric analysis of cells from hybridomas Md26 (left) or P47 (right) incubated with the indicated mAb and stained with fluoresceinated rabbit anti-rat Ig. Fluorescence intensity is in arbitrary units. In a control group with an irrelevant mAb, the staining was similar to that of Md26 cells plus H35-27.9 mAb (not shown).

These results showed that 27.9 Ag was not detectable at the surface of Md26 hybridoma cells. This accounted for the lack of inhibition by 27.9 mAb cytolysis by these cells. More important, this showed that detectable amounts of 27.9 Ag were not necessary for the mechanism of cytolysis by Md26 hybridoma cells. It could be argued that these hybridoma cells may have inherited from their AKR tumor "parent" a functional molecule allelic to the 27.9 Ag-bearing structure and not recognized by 27.9 mAb. However, the results

Fig. 6. The effect on ^{51}Cr-labeled Md26 (——) or P47 (----) hybridoma cells of anti-Thy-1.2 (top), H35-17.2 (middle) or H35-27.9 (bottom) mAb in the presence of complement. Spontaneous ^{51}Cr-release of Md26 and P47 was 9% and 10% respectively.

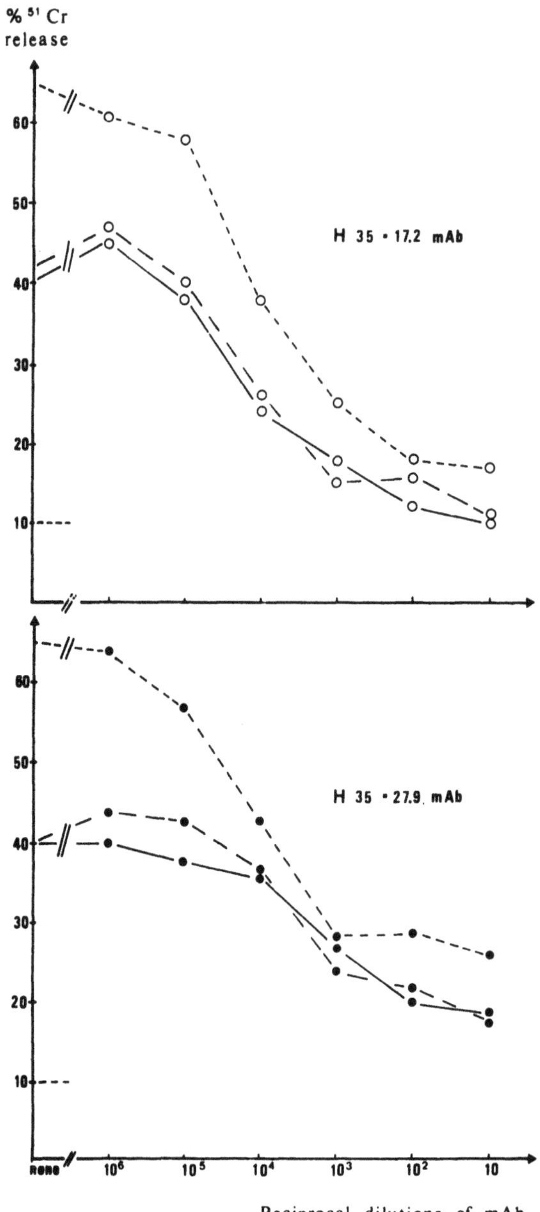

Fig. 8. The effect of H35-17.2 mAb (top) or H35-27.9 mAb (bottom) on the cytolysis of ^{51}Cr-labeled L1210 target cells by C57BL/6 anti-BALB/c (——), CBA anti-BALB/c (---) or AKR anti-BALB/c (----) MLC effector cells at effector:target cell ratios of 1:1, 1:1 and 5:1 respectively. Horizontal dotted lines indicate spontaneous ^{51}Cr-release of L1210 target cells incubated alone.

shown in Fig. 8 demonstrated that cytolytic AKR cells could be inhibited by 27.9 mAb to the same extent as CBA or B6 cytolytic cells, and thus bore 27.9 Ag. In summary, Md26 hybridoma cells lacked detectable 27.9 Ag and should bear no allelic form of the 27.9 Ag. This did not prevent these cells from being cytolytic.

DISCUSSION

We investigated the relationships between the lymphoid cell surface structures recognized by some mAb, and the functions these mAb inhibited. We used three mAb, of which two (27.9 and 89.9 mAb) were not identical with Lyt-2, the third mAb (17.2 mAb) probably directed against Lyt-2 being used here as an experimental counterpoint.

We found that 27.9 mAb inhibited T but not NK cell-mediated cytolysis (a situation of possible practical interest, reciprocal to that found with anti-Lyt-5 antibodies; ref. 18 and C. Henney, personal communication) and that 89.9 mAb inhibited T but not B cell proliferation (confirming previous findings with 89.9 mAb, ref. 11; and the comparable M7/14 mAb, ref. 16,17). In both cases, the corresponding antigens were present on inhibited as well as non-inhibited cells. Thus, the functional relationships of 89.9 Ag were different in T and B cells, and the functional relationships of 27.9 Ag were different in T and NK cells. This showed that cell surface structures related to a given function in one cell type may not be related to it in another cell type, without necessarily implying that the mechanism of the function differs from one cell type to the other. A similar observation was recently reported for anti-Lyt-2 mAb, which inhibited cytolysis by only some of a range of Lyt-2 bearing clones (10) and was also made with 17.2 and 27.9 mAb on distinct cytolytic T cell clones (this volume).

A "split coupling" between structures and functions was observed with 89.9 mAb, which inhibited cytolysis and proliferation in some cells, and cytolysis but not proliferation in other cells. This showed that some T cells (and B cells) escape a proliferation control which can be mediated on most T cells via 89.9 surface structures. This also strongly suggested that the inhibition by 89.9 mAb of cytolysis and proliferation was not due to the alteration of a step common to both processes contrary to the simplest interpretation previously raised (11).

We do not know yet what relationships there may be between proliferation, cytolysis and the 180K and 94K polypeptides immunoprecipitated by 89.9 mAb. More generally, we do not know by which pathway(s) the interaction of a given mAb with the corresponding surface structure leads to inhibition of a function. The results discussed above may provide, for further investigation of this problem, cells apparently identical as to the surface structures they bear, but different as to the functional relationships of these structures.

Another approach to the same problem is as follows. Interaction of a cell surface structure with the corresponding mAb may lead to inhibition of a function, either because the structure itself is necessary for this function, or because the mAb-structure interaction provides a "shut-off" signal, or because the interaction affects an antigenically unrelated, functionally important neighboring structure. The first of these possibilities would be ruled out by the demonstration of the existence of "structure-negative, function-positive" cells. We indeed found one T cell hybridoma, Md26, with no demonstrable surface 27.9 Ag and with cytolytic activity. The conclusion that 27.9 Ag-bearing structures are not necessary for cytolysis, however, meets with at least three reservations. First, 27.9 Ag may exist at the Md26 cell surfaces in amounts undetectable by the techniques used. Second, the 27.9 Ag may not be detected, but the 27.9 Ag-bearing structure may still be present on these cells. Third, hybridomas may exert cytolysis by pathways different from those used by conventional cytolytic T cells. If these reservations do not hold, it may indeed turn out that the 27.9 Ag-bearing structure is not necessary for T cell-mediated cytolysis. We did not expect this, considering the preoccupation of this structure with T rather than NK cell-mediated cytolysis (this report), moreover, possibly at the lethal hit stage (accompanying report).

Whether the cell surface structures recognized by 27.9 or 89.9 mAb are necessary for cytolysis could also be investigated by immunoselection on cytolytic T cell lines using these mAb in the presence of complement. A dissociation of function and surface structure in the surviving cells would be informative. The results, however, may not be unambiguous, since in the case of Lyt-2 some Lyt-2-negative T cell lines or clones were reported to lyse in a specific way (19), or in a non-specific way (20) or to lyse only in the presence of lectins (21). This sort of information, however, will be essential in order to focus further research on molecules directly involved in the mechanism of T cell-mediated cytolysis.

ACKNOWLEDGEMENTS

This work was supported by INSERM, CNRS, DGRST and the United States-Israel Binational Science Foundation. Part of this work was done during a stay of P. Golstein in G. Berke's laboratory at the Weizmann Institute within a French INSERM-Israeli CNRD agreement.

REFERENCES

1. Henney, C.S. T-cell-mediated cytolysis: an overview of some current issues. Contemp. Top. Immunobiol. 7:245 (1977).
2. Golstein, P., and E.T. Smith. Mechanism of T cell-mediated cytolysis: the lethal hit stage. Contemp. Top. Immunobiol. 7:273 (1977).
3. Martz, E. Mechanism of specific tumor-cell lysis by alloimmune lymphocytes: resolution and characterization of discrete steps in the cellular interaction. Contemp. Top. Immunobiol. 7:301 (1977).
4. Berke, G. Interaction of cytotoxic T lymphocytes and target cells. Progress in Allergy 27:69 (1979).
5. Shinohara, N., Hämmerling, U., and D.H. Sachs. Mouse alloantibodies capable of blocking cytotoxic T cell function. II. Further study on the relationship between the blocking antibodies and the products of the Lyt-2 locus. Eur. J. Immunol. 10:589 (1980).
6. Nakayama, E., Dippold., W., Shiku, H., Oettgen, H.F., and L.J. Old. Alloantigen-induced T-cell proliferation: Lyt phenotype of responding cells and blocking of proliferation by Lyt antisera. Proc. Natl. Acad. Sci. USA 77:2890 (1980).
7. Hollander, N., Pillemer, E., and I.L. Weissman. Blocking effect of Lyt-2 antibodies on T cell functions. J. Exp. Med. 152:674 (1980).
8. Fan, J., Ahmed, A., and B. Bonavida. Studies on the induction and expression of T cell-mediated immunity. X. Inhibition by Lyt-2,3 antisera of cytotoxic T lymphocyte-mediated antigen-specific and non-specific cytoxicity: evidence for the blocking of the binding between T lymphocytes and target cells and not the post-binding cytolytic steps. J. Immunol. 125: 2444 (1980).
9. Sarmiento, M., Glasebrook A.L., and F.W. Fitch. IgG or IgM monoclonal antibodies reactive with different determinants on the molecular complex bearing Lyt-2 antigen block T cell-mediated cytolysis in the absence of complement. J. Immunol. 125:2665 (1980).
10. MacDonald, H.R., Thiernesse, N., and J.-C. Cerottini. Inhibition of T cell-mediated cytolysis by monoclonal antibodies directed against Lyt-2: heterogeneity of inhibition at the clonal level. J. Immunol. 126:1671 (1981).
11. Pierres, M., C. Goridis, and P. Golstein. Inhibition of murine T cell-mediated cytolysis and T cell proliferation by a rat monoclonal antibody immunoprecipitating two lymphoid cell surface polypeptides of 94,000 and 180,000 molecular weight. Eur. J. Immunol., in press (1981).
12. Golstein, P., and M. Pierres. Monoclonal antibodies as probes to study the mechansim of T cell-mediated cytolysis. Proc. 14th Leuc. Cult. Conf., in press (1981).
13. Kaufmann, Y., Berke, G., and Z. Eshhar. Functional cytotoxic

T lymphocyte hybridomas. Transplantation Proc. 13:1171 (1981).
14. Kaufmann, Y., Berke, G., and Z. Eshhar. Cytotoxic T lymphocyte hybridomas which mediate specific tumor cell lysis in vitro. Proc. Natl. Acad. Sci. USA 78:2502 (1981).
15. Golstein, P., Foa, C., and I.C.M. MacLennan. Mechanism of T cell-mediated cytolysis: the differential impact of cytochalasins at the recognition and lethal hit stage. Eur. J. Immunol. 8:302 (1978).
16. Kürzinger, K., Reynolds, T., Germain, R.N., Davignon, D., Martz, E., and T.A. Springer. A novel lymphocyte function-associated antigen (LFA-1): cellular distribution, quantitative expression and structure. J. Immunol. 127:596 (1981).
17. Davignon, D., Martz E., Reynolds, T., Kürzinger, K., and T.A. Springer. Monoclonal antibody to a novel lymphocyte function-associated antigen (LFA-1). Mechanism of blockade of T lymphocyte-mediated killing and effects on other T and B lymphocyte functions. J. Immunol. 127:590 (1981).
18. Cantor, H., Kasai, M., Shen, F.W., Leclerc, J.C., and L. Glimcher. Immunogenetic analysis of "natural killer" activity in the mouse. Immunological Rev. 44:3 (1979).
19. Swain, S.L., Dennert, G., Wormsley, S., and R.W. Dutton. The Lyt phenotype of a long-term allospecific T cell line. Both helper and killer activities to Ia are mediated by Ly-1 cells. Eur. J. Immunol. 11:175 (1981).
20. Nabholz, M., Conzelmann, A., Acuto, O., North, M., Haas, W., Pohlit, H., Von Boemer, H., Hengartner, H., Mach, J.-P., Engers, H., and J.P. Johnson. Established murine cytolytic T cell lines as tools for a somatic cell genetic analysis of T cell functions. Immunological Rev. 51:125 (1980).
21. Dialynas, D.P., Loke, M.R., Glasebrook A.L., and F.W. Fitch. Lyt-2$^-$/Lyt-3$^-$ variants of a cloned cytolytic T cell line lack an antigen receptor functional in cytolysis. J. Exp. Med. 153:595 (1981).

DISCUSSION

(UK)

Have you some information on the $F(ab)_2$ blocking effect of your monoclonal antibodies?

P. Golstein

This was done with H35-89.9 mAb twice, using an $F(ab)_2$ preparation that blocked only at a titer which was ten times less than the whole antibody and we cannot be sure what it means exactly.

R. Herberman

Have you done the blocking with $F(ab)_2$ in NKCC?

P. Golstein

No. H35-89.9 mAb blocks partially NK kill as indicated by Eric Martz, but we could not go further in analysis because this antibody is non-cytolytic in the presence of complement. H35-27.9 was much more informative because it did not block NK kill, but we could lyse NK effector cells in the presence of complement.

M. Mayer

I wanted to ask a technical question. Do you wash out excess antibody after the pre-treatment?

P. Golstein

The standard experiments were done by pre-incubating effectors for 30 minutes in the presence of antibody, then adding the targets, not washing, letting everything remain together. When pre-treating the effector cells and washing we have only perhaps 50% inhibition.

CYTOLYTIC T CELL CLONES AGAINST H-2I REGION PRODUCTS: AN ANALYSIS USING MONOCLONAL ANTIBODIES AGAINST Ia, Lyt-2 AND P94,180 CELL SURFACE ANTIGENS

Anne Pierres, Anne-Marie Schmitt-Verhulst,
Christian Devaux, Pierre Golstein, Daniel Birnbaum,
Christo Goridis, and Michel Pierres

From the Centre d'Immunologie INSERM-CNRS de Marseille-Luminy, Case 906
13288 Marseille cédex 9, France

INTRODUCTION

Interactions between mouse lymphoid cell populations across major histocompatibility complex (MHC) differences activate a variety of alloreactive T cells differing in their functional characteristics, cell surface phenotype and molecular specificity. Early studies indicated that class I (i.e., H-2K/D) or class II (i.e., Ia) MHC antigens could stimulate Lyt-1^-, 2^+ cytolytic or Lyt-1^+2^- helper/amplifier allospecific T cell populations, respectively (1). However, in recent years such an absolute functional dichotomy of the H-2 complex has been challenged by several lines of evidence. First, class I antigens could in some instances cause strong T cell proliferation, and second, generation of effector cytolytic T cell (CTL) was documented during allogeneic interactions across I-region disparities (2). Class II antigens - besides their crucial role in immunoregulation - may thus function as transplantation antigens controlling skin graft rejection *in vivo* and cell mediated lympholysis *in vitro* (3-7). Studies based on genetic evidence, cold target inhibition and blocking of cytolysis by anti-Ia alloantisera have demonstrated that both I-A and I-E can serve as targets for class II specific CTL populations (8-10). In addition, the latter were shown to differ from class I specific CTL by their Lyt-$1^+2^{-\text{or low}}$ cell surface phenotype and hence might represent a distinct subset of alloreactive T cells (11).

Analysis of CTL specific for *I* region determinants has been facilitated by recent technological developments such as generation and maintenance of cloned cytolytic T cells (12,13) and the construction of hybridomas producing monoclonal antibodies (mAb) against target (14-16) or effector cell surface antigens. For example, we have characterized in a previous study a series of A.TH anti-A.TL ($\underline{I}^s$ anti-$\underline{I}^k$) derived mAb which defined distinct epitopes arranged in spatially distant clusters on the A^k and E^k molecules (17). Also, in recent investigations from this (18-19) and other (20-22) laboratories, attempts have been made to identify cell surface structures involved in T cell mediated cytolysis. Our approach was to construct monoclonal antibody-producing hybridomas by hybridizing rat myeloma and spleen cells from rats immunized with *in vitro*-generated allospecific T cell populations. A range of rat monoclonal antibodies were selected for their ability to inhibit in the absence of complement T cell mediated cytolysis at the level of the effector cells. These monoclonal antibodies were shown to recognize either the Lyt-2 (or 3) molecule(s) or a cell surface structure composed of two non-covalently linked chains with an apparent molecular weight of 94,000 and 180,000 daltons (designated thereafter p94,180). In the present study such monoclonal antibodies directed against target or effector cell surface structures have been used to assess the fine specificity, cell surface phenotype and susceptibility to cytolysis inhibiting monoclonal antibodies of class II specific cytolytic T cell clones.

DERIVATION OF $A^{\underline{k}}$ and $E^{\underline{k}}$ SPECIFIC CTL CLONES

In vivo-primed spleen cells from the A.TH mice alloimmune to A.TL lymphoid cells were restimulated *in vitro* by irradiated (2000 R) A.TL stimulator cells and cloned 48 hours later by limiting dilution in the presence of concanavalin A stimulated rat spleen cell culture supernatants (Rat Con A Sup) as described (23). Some clones were selected for their lytic activity against ^{51}Cr-labeled *E. Coli* lipopolysaccharide (LPS) blasts derived from A.TL spleen cells, and were maintained by weekly restimulation by A.TL irradiated spleen cells in the presence of Rat Con A Sup. The cytolytic activity of two representative clones, named A15.1.17 and A15.1.16 against LPS blasts from various *H-2* recombinant mouse strains is shown in Table I. Both clones lysed B10.BR ($\underline{A}^k$, $\underline{E}^k$) targets. The specificity of clone A15.1.17 for a determinant carried by the A^k molecule was suggested by its ability to lyse B10.A(4R) but not B10.A(5R) or B10.HTT targets. Conversely clone A15.1.16 was apparently specific for a determinant expressed on the $\underline{E}^k$ molecule since it exerted lytic activity against B10.A(5R) and B10.HTT but not B10.A(4R) targets. This was confirmed by blocking effector-target cell interactions with anti-$\underline{A}^k$ or anti-$\underline{E}^k$ monoclonal antibodies. Thus, as shown in Table II, mixtures of anti-$\underline{A}^k$ or of anti-$\underline{E}^k$ mAb strongly inhibited the cytolytic activity of clone A15.1.17 or A15.1.16, respectively. These results were in agreement with earlier data demonstrating that both A and E molecules could serve as potential targets for class II specific cytolytic T cell populations (5,9,10).

TABLE I: Cytolytic Activity of A.TH Anti-A.TL Derived T Cell Clones Against ^{51}Cr Labeled LPS Blast Targets From H-2 Recombinant Mouse Strains

Target Cells	H-2 composition of targets					Cytolytic T cell clones	
	K	A	E	D	H-2T	A15.1.17	A15.1.16
B10.S	s	s	s	s	a	-3.3	0.2
B10.BR	k	k	k	k	a	29.0	47.5
B10.A(4R)	k	k	b	b	.	24.8	0.9
B10.A(5R)	b	b	k	d	d	0.3	50.4
B10.HTT	s	s	k	d	.	0.4	35.8
B10.A(4R)x B10.A(5R) F_1	k/b	k/b	b/k	b/d	./d	32.0	43.8

Cytolytic T cell clones were tested 3 days after restimulation in a 4h standard cytotoxicity assay utilizing $5x10^4$ ^{51}Cr labeled LPS blasts targets and an effector to target ratio of 5:1. Results are expressed as %specific ^{51}Cr release calculated as follows: (E-C) - T X 100. Spontaneous release of of each target ranged between 38 and 48%. Each figure represents the mean of triplicate assays. Standard errors were <5.

The observation that in vivo priming was usually required for optimal development of class II specific CTL (14) contrasted with the high frequency of helper/amplifier T cell activated by I-region disparities during primary mixed lymphocyte cultures. This may suggest differences in the size of the precursor pool of these two I-region specific T cell subsets and/or a differential susceptibility to regulatory T cells. Evaluation of such parameters awaits further studies using, for example, limiting dilution assays.

TOPOLOGICAL MAPPING OF THE ALLODETERMINANT RECOGNIZED BY CYTOLYTIC CLONE A15.1.17

The anti-A^k cytolytic clone A15.1.17 was investigated in more detail. As indicated in Table II, this clone exerted lytic activity against A.TL, CBA and B10.BR LPS blast targets (all I-A^k, I-E^k). In contrast, no cytolysis was observed on targets from strains with the H-2 haplotypes f, u, r, b, q and d (Table III). Hence, clone

TABLE II: Blocking of I-A- and I-E Specific CML With Monoclonal Anti-Ia Antibodies

Target cells (LPS spleen blasts)	Monoclonal antibodies	Clone A15.1.16 (anti-I-E^k)	% Inhibition	Clone A15.1.17 (anti-I-A^k)	% Inhibition
A.TH	None	0.9 ($\pm$0.3)[a]	-	-2 ($\pm$5)	-
A.TL	None	22.3 ($\pm$2)	-	26.5($\pm$3)	-
A.TL	pool anti-A^k (1/40)[b]	25.1 ($\pm$4)	0	-6.5($\pm$1)	100
A.TL	pool anti-E^k (1/40)[c]	4.4 ($\pm$1)	81.3	30.5($\pm$3)	0
A.TL	anti-A^S (1/4)[d])	26.0 ($\pm$2)	0	31.3($\pm$6)	0

a) See footnote of Table I. E:T ratio was 5:1. Spontaneous release of A.TH and A.TL LPS blast targets was 39% and 34% respectively.

b) Pool of 17 anti-A^k mAb (17); all monoclonal antibodies were used as purified antibodies from culture supernatants at a concentration of 1mg/ml.

c) Pool of 18 anti-E^k mAb (17). See b).

d) MKD-S4 : a(B10.D2 x D1.LP) F1 anti-B10.S monoclonal antibody used as saturated culture supernatant.

A15.1.17 recognized a private determinant of the I-A^k molecule (hereinafter referred to as the A^k molecule). Monoclonal anti-A^k antibodies have been shown to define epitopes arranged in spatially distant clusters (16,17). This is illustrated in Fig. 1, left which shows that mAb H39-58.11 and H40-481.3 (anti-Ia.1) exhibited cross-inhibition of binding, thereby identifying A^k determinants either identical or in close proximity one to another. In contrast, mAb H8-138.4 (anti-Ia.2) detected a private determinant presumably located at another site of the A^k molecule since it failed to inhibit the binding of ^{125}I-labeled mAb H39-58.11 or H40-481.3 mAb. Fig. 1, right shows the inhibition of the lytic activity of clone A15.1.17 with these anti-Ia^k mAb. Strong inhibition of effector-target cell interactions was observed with anti-A^k mAb H38-58.1 and H40-481.3 but not with anti-A^k mAb H38-138.4 or anti-E^k mAb H40-394.2. A similar study was carried out using 15 A.TH derived anti-A^k mAb which

TABLE III: Cytolytic Activity of Anti-A^k Clone A15.1.17 Against ^{51}Cr Labeled LPS Blasts From Strains With Standard H-2 Haplotypes

Target cells (LPS) blasts)	H-2 composition				% specific ^{51}Cr release (± SE)[a] at the following E:T ratios:		
	K	A	E	D	8 : 1	2 : 1	0.5 : 1
A.TH	s	s	s	d	-1(±2)	-0.6(±1)	-0.7(±0.5)
A.TL	s	k	k	d	25.8(±4.7)	31.3(±2.6)	23.5(±3.8)
CBA/J	k	k	k	k	35.8(±6.7)	34.8(±5.9)	33.4(±7.9)
B10.BR	k	k	k	k	30.7(±5.2)	29.6(±3.6)	21.3(±2.4)
B10.M	f	f	f	f	-3.8(±0.8)	-3.6(±3.)	-0.9(±2.2)
B10.PL	u	u	u	u	-8.1(±2.7)	-2.4(±3.9)	-4.9(±4.2)
B10.RIII	r	r	r	r	-8.5(±3.3)	-4.7(±2.6)	-3.1(±2.7)
C57BL/10	b	b	b	b	-3.2(±1.7)	-3.2(±5.2)	1.2(±3.7)
DBA/1	q	q	q	q	-4.9(±1.0)	-0.4(2.4)	0.6(3.5)
DBA/2	d	d	d	d	-4.9(±2.6)	-4.6(±2.7)	-3.5(±2.0)

a) See footnote of Table I. Spontaneous release of the different targets was in the range of 37 to 58%.

defined by competition experiments various clusters of allodeterminants (named I through V) on the A^k molecule. As shown in Table IV, 9 anti-A^k mAb inhibited A15.1.17 mediated cytolysis whereas 6 other anti-A^k mAb failed to do so. Interestingly, all inhibitory mAb defined epitopes belonging to either the epitope cluster I or II. The 6 mAb defining cluster I exhibited complete bidirectional competitive inhibition of binding, and detected epitopes in close proximity one to another. The observation that some antibodies defining epitope cluster II could also inhibit the lytic activity of clone A15.1.17 may be explained by a spatial relationship between these two clusters, as shown by partial competitive inhibition of antibody binding. No inhibition was observed with antibodies defining clusters III, IV and V. The above data show (a) that mAb specific for public A^k determinants (i.e., cluster I) inhibit A15.1.17 mediated cytolysis, although the allodeterminant recognized by

TABLE IV: Topological Mapping of the Antigenic Site Recognized by Cytolytic Clone A15.1.17 on the A^k Molecule by Means of Inhibition of Clone Mediated Lympholysis by Anti-A^k Monoclonal Antibodies

mAb[a]	Specificity[c]	Tentative epitope cluster assignment[d]	Percent specific ^{51}Cr release[e]	Percent Inhibition	Kd Constant[f]
None	-	-	23.3		
H39-58.11	A^k(f,u,r;Ia.1)	I	2.1	91	NT
H40-399.4	A^k(f,u,r;Ia.1)	I	-0.4	100	4±1
H40-481.3	A^k(f,u,r,;Ia.1)	I	-0.4	100	6±1
10.2.16[b]	A^k(f,r,s;Ia.17)	I	-1.5	100	0.6±0.1
H40-269.6	A^k(f,u ; -)	I	10.4	56	NT
H40-395.3	A^k(f,u ; -)	I	0.3	99	NT
H39-64.5	A^k(- ;Ia.2)	II	5.4	77	NT
H40-348.10	A^k(- ;Ia.2)	II	7.6	68	2±0.3
H39-487.7	A^k(r ;Ia.19)	II	1.2	95	NT
H39-146.1	A^k(- ;Ia.2)	II	22.8	3	2.5±0.5
H8-15.9	A^k(u,b,d,q,j,p; -)	III	21.1	10	NT
H39-49.5	A^k(f,u,b,d,q,p,v;-)	III	22.6	4	NT
H40-164.3	A^k+E^k(u,b,d,p,v,r;-)	III	20.4	13	4.5±0.5
H8-109.13	A^k(- ;Ia.2)	IV	28.4	0	NT
H8-138.4	A^k(- ;Ia.2)	V	21.1	10	NT
H40-298.3	E^k(p,u,r,j,d;Ia.7)		28.4	0	NT
Pool I-E^k	E^k		23.3	0	NT

a) See Ref. (16,17) for detailed characterization of these anti-Ia^k mAb.
b) See Ref. (36).
c) The known cross-reactions with Ia products of other H-2 haplotypes and the correspondence to serum specificities are indicated in brackets.
d) The topological arrangement of A^k determinants in epitope clusters was operationally defined by bidirectional analysis of competitive inhibition of antibody binding to spleen cells. Antibodies within one cluster exhibited complete cross-inhibition of binding. Partial inhibition of binding was observed between some mAb included within clusters I, II and III. (See Ref. 17 for details.)
e) See legend to Table I. The E:T ratio was 3:1 and the spontaneous ^{51}Cr release of A.TL LPS blasts was 43%. Protein-A purified monoclonal antibodies were tested at the concentration of 83 μg/ml.
f) See Ref. (37) .NT : Not tested.

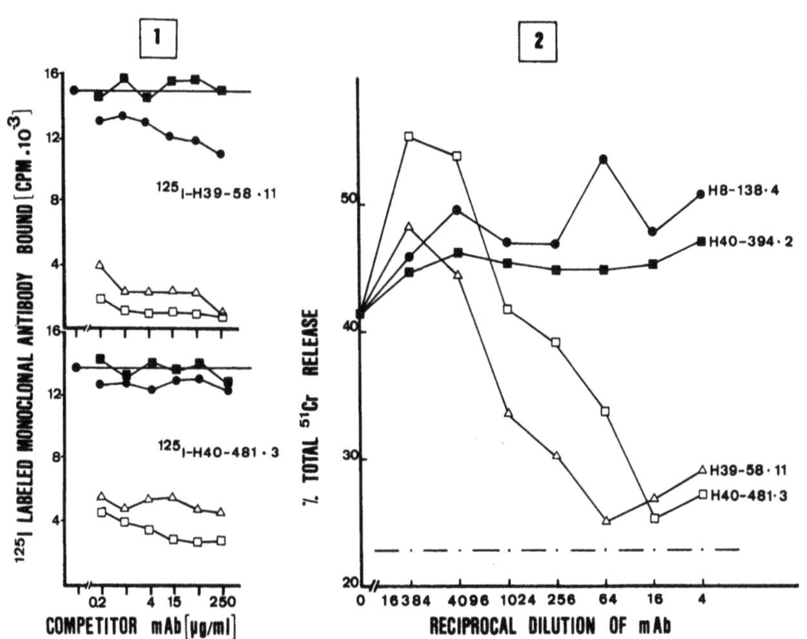

Fig. 1. Pattern of inhibition of clone A15.1.17 (anti-A^k) mediated cytolysis of ^{51}Cr labeled A.TL LPS blasts targets

Right panel: Various dilutions of ascitic fluids from hybridomas producing anti-A^k (H40-481.3 □——□, H39-58.11 △——△ and H8-138.4 ●——●) or anti-E^k (H40-394.2 ■——■) monoclonal antibodies were tested for inhibition of A15.1.17 mediated cytolysis of ^{51}Cr-labeled ATL-LPS blasts in a 4 h standard cytotoxic assay as described in footnote of Table I. The spontaneous ^{51}Cr-release of A.TL targets is indicated by a dotted line. Each figure represents the mean of triplicate assays. Standard erors were ≤ 2.

Left panel: Competitive inhibition of binding of ^{125}I-labeled anti-A^k mAb H39-58.11 (upper part) or H40-481.3 (lower part) to A.TL spleen cells by increasing amounts of the unlabeled competitors H39-58.11 (anti-A^k △——△), H40-481.3 (anti-A^k □——□), H8-138.4 (anti-A^k ●——●) or H40-394.2 (antiE^k ■——■). See reference 17 for details. Each figure represents the mean of duplicate assays. Straight horizontal lines indicate the binding obtained without competitor.

this clone was apparently private; (b) that only two out of 5 anti-Ia.2 mAb directed at private A^k determinant are inhibitory, in agreement with our previous data which demonstrated that such anti-Ia.2 mAb recognized spatially separated A^k determinants; and (c) that the lack of inhibition observed with some anti-A^k mAb is not likely to be related to low affinity binding since mAb H39-146.1 had a dissociation rate constant (Kd) in the same range as that of other anti-A^k mAb capable of inhibiting the lytic activity of clone A15.1.17. Thus, it may be that some anti-A^k mAb (i.e., anti-Ia.2 H39-64.5 and H40-348.10) inhibit cytolysis by masking the antigenic site recognized by this cytolytic clone, whereas others directed at public A^k determinants may act by steric hindrance of effector-target cell interaction or by masking a functionally related zone of the A^k molecule. Analysis of additional alloreactive clones differing in their functional characteristics and molecular specificity (i.e., I-A, I-E or I-A and I-E) with our panel of anti-Ia^k mAb is in progress, and may help to clarify these issues. Anti-H-2 K/D mAb have also recently been used to assess by means of blocking studies the fine recognition of class I-specific CTL populations or clones (25.26). For instance Weyand et al (27) observed that cytolysis exerted by allospecific or TNP-modified $H\text{-}2K^k$-reactive CTL could be selectively inhibited by anti-$H\text{-}2K^k$ mAb defining spatially distant clusters of determinants. This illustrates the potential use of mAb in defining the fine specificity of various alloreactive T cell subsets. Similarly, these reagents could be used at the induction phase of allogeneic interactions where they could interfere with the helper and/or effector T cell activation (28).

CELL SURFACE PHENOTYPE OF ALLOREACTIVE T CELLS SPECIFIC FOR I-REGION CONTROLLED DETERMINANTS

Generally allorecognition of MHC subregion products correlates with the functional characteristics and phenotype of the respective T cell subsets involved. Thus Lyt-2^-, 3^- helper/amplifier cells are class II restricted whereas Lyt-2^+, 3^+ cytotoxic cells are class I restricted 91). Recent compelling evidence from several laboratories led us to reconsider such an absolute rule. First, unrestricted Lyt-2^+ helper T cells may develop during allogeneic recognition of H-2K/D antigens (29). Second, alloreactive CTL populations or long term T cell lines against class II antigens were shown to be Lyt-1^+ (11,30). These results led us to examine the cell surface phenotype of two I-region specific alloreactive clones, differing in their function and molecular specificity. Results shown in Fig. 2 indicate that an anti-E^k proliferative clone named A7-2.16 expressed the phenotype Thy 1.2^+, Lyt-1^+, Lyt-2^-, whereas the anti-A^k cytolytic clone A15.1.17 was Thy 1.2^+, Lyt-1^+, Lyt-2^+. In addition, both clones lacked detectable I-A^s determinants (not shown). How-

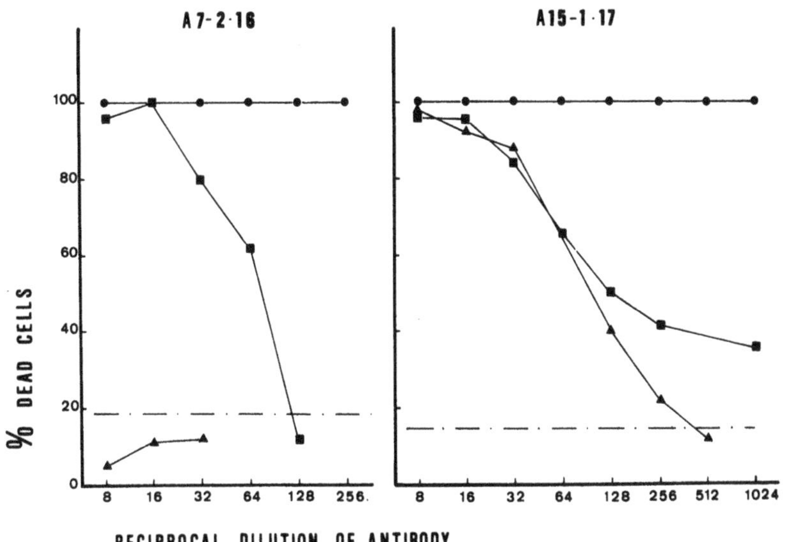

Fig. 2. Cell surface phenotype of cytolytic clone A15.1.17 compared to A7.2.16, an anti-I-E^k proliferative clone.

Various dilutions of antisera J.I.J., a rat anti-Thy-1.2 mAb ●——●; H35-17.2, a rat anti-Lyt-2 Ab▲——▲; and a C3H-CE anti-C3H anti-Lyt-1.2 serum ■——■) were tested for their capacity to lyse A7.2.16 (left panel) and A15.1.17 (right panel) in a standard two stage cytotoxicity assay using absorbed rabbit complement. Monoclonal antibodies were used as culture supernatants. J.I.J. mAb was kindly provided by J. Sprent, Philadelphia, PA, USA and the C3H.CE anti-C3H serum by J. Ray, Jr. NIH, Bethesda, MD, USA. Each figure represents the mean of duplicates. The dotted lines indicate the percentage of dead cells obtained with complement alone.

ever, the cytotoxic titer of the anti-Lyt-2 mAb H35-17.2 was found to be considerably lower on the anti-A^k cytolytic clone A15.1.17 (1/128) than on class I-specific cytolytic clones (>1/1056)(not shown). Furthermore, attempts to immunoprecipitate the Lyt-2 molecule from ^{125}iodinated surface of clone A15.1.17 cells with various rat anti-Lyt 2 mAb have so far failed (C. Goridis, unpublished). These results may therefore suggest either a low expression of the Lyt-2 molecules of A15.1.17 cells, or the recognition of the Lyt-2 molecules of A15.1.17 cells, or the recognition by mAb H35-17.2 of a cross-reactive determinant expressed on a molecule other than Lyt-2 on such cells. This point is of some importance with regard to the failure of various anti-Lyt-2 mAb to inhibit the Lyt-2 function of this clone as will be discussed below.

Although most helper T cell clones have been found Lyt-1$^+$, others may lack this antigen (30,31). In addition, cytolytic T cell clones against various allodeterminants, viral antigens or hapten modified syngeneic cells were shown to express the Lyt-2 and in some instances the Lyt-1 antigens (32). Finally, Dennert et al. have characterized long term cultured T cell lines with cytotoxic and/or proliferative specificity for the A^k molecule which expressed the Lyt-1$^+$, Lyt-2$^-$ cell surface phenotype, a finding in agreement with our data (30). Thus, characterization of alloreactive T cell clones revealed heterogeneity in their cell surface phenotype suggesting different ontogenic pathways. Whether or not such phenotype heterogeneity correlates with distinct functions remains to be examined.

SUSCEPTIBILITY OF ANTI-A^k CLONE A15.1.17 TO INHIBITION OF CYTOLYSIS BY ANTI-LYT-2 AND ANTI-p94,180 RAT mAb

The combined use of alloreactive T cell clones and anti-cell surface mAb should allow exploration of the functional conections of various lymphoid cell surface structures. For example, rat mAb against the Lyt-2, Lyt-3 or p94,180 antigen were found to inhibit the function of cytolytic T cells (18-22).

Since I-region specific cytolytic T cells were characterized by a distinct cell surface phenotype it was of interest to determine the impact of various rat mAb against Lyt-2 or p94,180 antigen on the lytic function of the anti-A^k clone A15.1.17. As shown in Table V the latter was affected neither by the anti-Lyt-1 mAb 53.3.7 nor by a panel of anti-Lyt-2 mAb. In contrast, strong inhibition of cytolysis was obtained with two mAb (H35-89.9 and H68-96.22) which immunoprecipitated from surface iodinated A15.1.17 cells two polypeptides of 94,000 and 180,000 daltons m.w. corresponding to the p94,180 antigen. This sharply contrasted with the ability of anti-lyt-2 and anti-p94,180 mAb to inhibit cytolysis of A.AL (K^k I^k D^d) LPS blasts by C57BL/10 anti-DBA/2 (H-2^b anti-H-2^d) CTL. It is not clear whether the lack of inhibition of A15.1.17-mediated cytolysis by

TABLE V. Effect of Rat Monoclonal Antibodies Against Lyt-1, Lyt-2 or p94,180 Antigens on Anti-A^k Clone A15.1.17 and C57BL/10 Anti-DBA/2 CTL Mediated Cytolysis of A.AL ^{51}Cr Labeled LPS Blasts

Rat monoclonal antibody[b]	Specificity	Clone A15.1.17[a]			C57 BL/10 anti-DBA/2 CTL		
	Dilution of mAb :	None	10^{-1}	10^{-2}	None	10^{-1}	10^{-2}
None	-	21.0			24.9		
53.3.7[c]	Lyt-1		27.1	24.0		26.6	29.9
53.6.7[c]	Lyt-2		26.0	18.7		14.6	18.6
H35-17.2	Lyt-2		27.6	27.3		6.2	17.1
H49-57.4	Lyt-2		23.4	24.1		11.0	17.1
H59-101.7	Lyt-2		23.3	24.8		13.2	19.3
H58-55.3	Lyt-2		26.5	28.2		15.6	22.3
Pool anti-Lyt-2[d]	Lyt-2		26.0	22.5		NT	NT
H35-27.9	Lyt-2		23.3	24.6		14.1	18.7
H35-89.9	p 180,94		7.8	10.8		15.4	15.1
H68-96.22	p 180,94		1.2	6.6		7.1	8.5

a) See footnote to Table I. E:T ratio was 5:1 (A15.1.17) and 10:1 (C57BL/10 anti-DBA/2). Spontaneous release of A.AL LPS targets was 30 and 35% respectively.
b) 50 µl of 10x concentrated hybridoma culture supernatants.
c) See Ref. (35).
d) Mixture of monoclonal antibodies H35-17.2, 53.6.72, H49-57.4 and H59-101.7.

anti-Lyt-2 mAb relates to a complete lack or a low expression of Lyt-2 molecules on these cells. Swain et al. also observed that the lytic activity of an anti-A cytolytic T cell line was not inhibited by anti-Lyt-2 alloantisera (quoted in 33). Thus, this may well represent a common feature of I-region specific CTL clones. Such observations strongly argue against a direct involvement of Lyt-2 molecules in I-region specific cytolysis. Possibly not related is the observation by McDonald et al. (34) describing peritoneal exudate cell-derived class I-specific T cell clones, the cytolytic activity of which was not inhibited by anti-Lyt-2 mAb, although they were clearly Lyt-2^+. Altogether, the present data and others support the view that class II specific CTL represent a distinct subset of T cells, the functional role of which in allo- or self-restricted immunity will have to be evaluated.

ACKNOWLEDGEMENTS

This investigation was supported by INSERM (CRL 80.1.034.1 and 79.5.128.1), CNRS (ATP 7071/12) and DGRST (ACC 81.L.0711). A.P. and C.D. were recipients of fellowships from DGRST.

We wish to thank Sylvie Marchetto and Michel Buferne for expert technical assistance and Colette Kourilsky for her help in preparing this manuscript.

REFERENCES

1. Cantor, H., and E.A. Boyse. Functional subclasses of T lymphocytes bearing different Ly antigens. II. Cooperation between subclasses of Ly^+ cells in the generation of killer activity. J. Exp. Med. 141:1390 (1975).
2. Klein, J. The unity of genes in the major histocompatibility complex. Arthr. and Rheum. 21:590 (1978).
3. Wagner, H., Gotze, D., Ptschelinzew, L., and M. Rollinghoff. Induction of cytotoxic T lymphocytes against I-region-coded determinants: in vitro evidence for a third histocompatibility locus in the mouse. J. Exp. Med. 142:1477 (1975).
4. Nabholz, M., Young, H., rynbeek, A., Boccardo, R., David, C.S., Meo, T., Miggiano, V., and D.C. Shreffler. I-region associated determinants expression on mitogen-stimulated lymphocytes and detection by cytotoxic T cells. Eur. J. Immunol. 5:594 (1975).
5. Klein, J., Geib, R., Chiang, C., and V. Hauptfeld. Histocompatibility antigens controlled by the I region of the murine H-2 complex. I. Mapping of H-2A and H-2C loci. J. Exp. Med. 143:1976 (1976).

6. Klein, J., Chiang, C.L., and V. Hauptfeld. Histocompatibility antigens controlled by the I-region of the murine H-2 complex. II. K/D region compatibility is not required for I-region cell-mediated lymphocytotoxocity. J. Exp. Med. 145:450 (1977).
7. Billings, P., Burakoff, S., Dorf, M.E., and B. Benacerraf. Cytotoxic T lymphocytes specific for I-region determinants do not require interactions with H-2K or K gene products. J. Exp. Med. 145:1387 (1977).
8. Klein, J., Chiang, C.L., and E.K. Wakeland. Histocompatibility antigens controlled by the I region of the murine H-2 complex. III. Blocking with antisera of the in vitro response. Immunogenetics 5:445 (1977).
9. Fischer-Lindhal, K., and B. Hausmann. Expression of the I-E target antigen for T cell killing requires two genes. Immunogenetics 11:571 (1980).
10. Juretic A., Nagy, Z.A., and J. Klein. Generation of cytotoxic T lymphocytes by the H-2 encoded E molecules. Immunogenetics 14:73 (1981).
11. Vidovic, D., Juretic, A., Nagy, Z.A., and J. Klein. Lyt phenotypes of primary cytotoxic T cells generated across the A and E region of the H-2 complex. Eur. J. Immunol. 11:499 (1980).
12. Gillis, S., and K.A. Smith. Long-term culture of tumor specific cytotoxic T cells. Nature (London) 268:154 (1977).
13. Moller, G., Editor. Immunol. Rev. Vol. 51 (1980).
14. Lemke, H., Hammerling, G.J., and U. Hammerling. Fine specificity of antigen controlled by the major histocompatibility complex and by the Qa/TL region. Immunol. Rev. 47:175 (1979).
15. Ozato, K., Mayer, N., and D.H. Sachs. Hybridoma cell lines secreting monoclonal antibodies to mouse H-2 and Ia antigens. J. Immunol. 124:533 (1980).
16. Pierres, M., Kourilsky, F.M., Rebouah, J.P., Dosseto, M., and D. Caillol. Distinct epitopes on K^k gene products identified by monoclonal antibodies. Eur. J. Immunol. 10:950 (1980).
17. Pierres, M., Devaux, C., Dosseto, M., and S. Marchetto. Clonal analysis of B and T cell responses to Ia antigens. I. Topology of epitope regions on $I-A^k$ and $I-E^k$ molecules analyzed with 35 monoclonal antibodies. Immunogenetics, in press (1981).
18. Pierres, M., Goridis, C., and P. Golstein. Inhibition of murine T cell cytolysis and T cell proliferation by a rat monoclonal antibody immunoprecipitating two polypeptides of 94,000 and 180,000 molecular weight. Eur. J. Immunol., in press (1981).
19. Golstein, P., and M. Pierres. Monoclonal antibodies as probes to study the mechanisms of T cell mediated cytolysis. In "Mechanisms of Lymphocyte Activation," K. Resch and H. Kirchner, editors, Elsevier/North-Holland, Amsterdam, pp. 442-445 (1981).

20. Sarmiento, M., Glasebrook, A.L., and F.W. Fitch. IgG or IgM monoclonal antibodies reactive with different determinants on the molecular complex bearing Lyt-2 antigen block T cell mediated cytolysis. J. Immunol. 125:2665 (1980).
21. Hollander, N., Pellemer, E., and I.L. Weissman. Blocking effect of Lyt-2 antibodies on T cell functions. J. Exp. Med. 152:674 (1980).
22. Davignon, D., Martz, E., Reynolds, T., Jurzinger, K., and T.A. Springer. Lymphocyte function associated antigen 1 (LFA-1): a surface antigen distinct from Lyt-2, 3 that participates in T lymphocyte mediated killing. Proc. Natl. Acad. USA 78: 4535 (1981).
23. Glasebrook, A.L., and F.W. Fitch. Alloreactive cloned T cell lines. I. Interactions between cloned amplifier and cytolytic T cell lines. J. Exp. Med. 151:876 (1980).
24. Klein, J., and V. Hauptfeld. Ia antigens: their serology, molecular relationships and their role in allograft rejections. Transpl. Rev. 30:83 (1979).
25. Fischer-Lindhal, K., and H. Lemke. Inhibition of killer-target cell interaction by monoclonal anti-H-2 antibodies. Eur. J. Immunol. 9:526 (1979).
26. Epstein, S.L., Ozato, K., and D.H. Sachs. Blocking of allogeneic cell-mediated lympholysis by monoclonal antibodies to H-2 antigens. J. Immunol. 125:129 (1980).
27. Weyland, C., Hammerling, G.J., and J. Goronzy. Recognition of H-2 domains by cytotoxic T lymphocyte. Nature 292:627 (1981).
28. Brenan, M., and M. Mullbacher. Analysis of H-2 determinants recognized during the induction of H-Y-immune cytotoxic T cell by monoclonal antibodies in vitro. J. Exp. Med. 154: 560 (1981).
29. Swain, S.L., Bakke, A., English, M., and R.W. Dutton. Ly phenotypes and MHC recognition: the allohelper that recognizes K or D is a mature Ly 1, 2, 3 cell. J. Immunol. 123:2716 (1979).
30. Swain, S.L., Dennert, G., Wormgley, S., and R.W. Dutton. The Lyt phenotype of a long-term allospecific T cell line. Both helper and killer activities to I-A are mediated by Ly-1 cells. Eur. J. Immunol. 11:175 (1981).
31. Glasebrook, A.L., Sarmiento, M., Loken, M.R., Dialynas, D.P., Guintaus, J., Eisenberg, L., Lutz, C.T., Wilde, D., and F.W. Fitch. Murine T lymphocyte clones with distinct immunological function. Immunol. Rev. 54:225 (1981).
32. Weiss, A., Brunner, K.T., McDonald, H.R., and J.C. Cerrotini. Antigenic specificity of the cytolytic T lymphocyte response to murine sarcoma virus-induced tumors. III. Characterization of cytolytic T lymphocyte clones specific for Moloney leukemia virus associated cell surface antigens. J. Exp. Med. 152:1210 (1980).

33. Swain, S.L., and R.W. Dutton. Mouse T-lymphocyte subpopulations: relationships between function and Lyt-antigen phenotype. Immunol. Today, Sept. 1980, 61 (1980).
34. McDonald, A., Thiernesse, H., and J.C. Cerrotini. Inhibition of T cell-mediated cytolysis by monoclonal antibodies directed against Lyt-2: heterogeneity of inhibition at the clonal level. J. Immunol. 126:1671 (1981).
35. Ledbetter, J.A., and L.A. Herzenberg. Xenogeneic monoclonal monoclonal antibodies to mouse lymphoid differentiation antigens. Immunol. Rev. 47:63 (1979).
36. Oi, V.T., Jones, P.P., Goding, J.W., Herzenberg, L.A., and L.A. Herzenberg. Properties of monoclonal antibodies to mouse Ig allotypes, H-2 and Ia antigens. Curr. Top. Microbiol. and Immunol. 81:115 (1978).
37. Birnbaum, D., and F.M. Kourilsky. Differences in the cell binding affinity of a cross-reactive monoclonal anti-Ia alloantibody in mice of different H-2 haplotype. Eur. J. Immunol., in press (1981).

THE DIFFERENTIAL EFFECTS OF DISTINCT CYTOLYSIS-INHIBITING MONOCLONAL ANTIBODIES ON GROWTH AND ON CYTOLYTIC ACTIVITY OF T CELL CLONES

Anne-Marie Schmitt-Verhulst, Pierre Golstein, Michel Buferne and Michel Pierres

Centre d'Immunologie INSERM-CNRS de Marseille-Luminy
Case 906
13288 Marseille Cedex 9

The analysis of the involvement of cell-surface structures of cytotoxic T lympocytes (CTL) in lytic interactions with target cells has been approached in recent years by the use of antibodies capable of inhibiting cytolysis. Among antibodies found to inhibit cytolysis via their binding to the effector cells, were allogeneic anti-Lyt2 antibodies (2-6) and a xenogeneic rat anti-mouse antiserum (7). Unlike these antibodies which blocked cytolysis in the absence of added complement, antibodies raised in syngeneic mice, directed at T cell blast-specific structures possibly involved in antigen recognition, required additional complement treatment to eliminate the CTL (8,9). More recently, a systematic search has been made for cytolysis-inhibiting monoclonal antibodies (mAb) secreted by hybridoma cells obtained after fusion of rat cells immunized with mouse T cell populations (1,10-14). This has resulted in the production of mAb directed at two types of cell surface structures: (a) the Lyt2 molecule (1,10,11) and its associated Lyt3 molecule (10,11), and (b) a glycoprotein composed of 180 and 95K polypeptides defined independently by mAb LFA-1 (12,13), mAb described by Fitch and colleagues (14), and by mAb H35-89.9 described by Pierres and colleagues (1).

In parallel with the development of monoclonal reagents, the definition of culture conditions allowing continuous growth of T cells (15) has permitted cloning of CTL and their propagation in culture (16-19). Such T cell clones, in turn, constitute monoclonal reagents in terms of their antigen-specificity, as well as providing tools for the study of the relationship between T cell function and cell surface antigen expression.

We here describe two such CTL clones derived from C57BL/6 (B6) anti-DBA/2 mixed lymphocyte cultures (MLC), which were specific for H-2D-end major histocompatibility complex (MHC) products. In the presence of T cell-growth factor (TCGF) and feeder cells not expressing the $H\text{-}2D^d$ allelic form, the CTL proliferated poorly, but the simultaneous presence of TCGF and $H\text{-}2D^d$-expressing stimulating cells induced a vigorous proliferation.

The effects of two cytolysis-inhibiting mAb, one directed at Lyt2 (H35-17.2)(1), the other at the 180-95 K molecule (H35-89.9) (1) were studied on these CTL clones. The anti-Lyt2 antibody inhibited the antigen-specific component of induction of proliferation and the cytolytic activity of both clones. The anti-(180-95 K proteins) antibody inhibited cytolysis by both clones, but the proliferation of only one clone.

DERIVATION OF CTL CLONES FROM B6 ANTI-DBA/2 MLC

Conditions for MLC and cloning were adapted from those described by Glasebrook et al (18) as follows. B6 spleen cells (25×10^6) were cultured in Falcon flasks with 2500 Rad irradiated DBA/2 spleen cells (25×10^6) in 20 ml RPMI-FCS medium (RPMI 1640 supplemented with HEPES (10 mM), 2-mercaptoethanol (5×10^{-5}M), glutamine (2 mM), sodium pyruvate (1 mM) and heat inactivated fetal calf serum (FCS, Flow Laboratories) (5%), antibiotics (100 u/ml penicillin, 100 u/ml streptomycin) and antimycotics (0.1% Fungizone). After 9 days responding cells (2.5×10^6) were restimulated with DBA/2 stimulating cells (20×10^6) and 5 days later were cloned by plating in 96 well flat bottomed microtiter plates an average of 1 responding cell in the presence of 5×10^5 DBA/2 stimulating cells and 25% Con A SUP. (Supernatant from rat spleen cells cultured with Con A for 20-36 H and supplemented with 10 mg α-methyl mannoside (Sigma) per ml as described (19) is referred to as 100% Con A SUP). After weekly feeding with stimulating cells and Con A SUP, growth-positive wells were transferred to the wells of Costar plates containing 2×10^6 BALB/c stimulating cells and 25% Con A SUP in 2 ml final volume. Of the 14 growth positive wells transferred, cells in 7 continued to proliferate and amongst those, 5 had cytolytic activity. These CTL lines were recloned in the same conditions at an average 0.5 cell per well. Two such clones (here called BD4-2 and BD4-13) were used in these studies.

GROWTH CHARACTERISTICS AND SPECIFICITY OF CLONES BD4-2 AND -13

CTL clones BD4-2 and -13, derived from B6 ($H\text{-}2^b$, Mls^b) anti-DBA/2 ($H\text{-}2^d$, Mls^a) MLC were tested for their dependence on stimulating cells and on TCGF-containing medium for proliferation. Figure 1 indicates that in the absence of Con A SUP, clones BD4-2

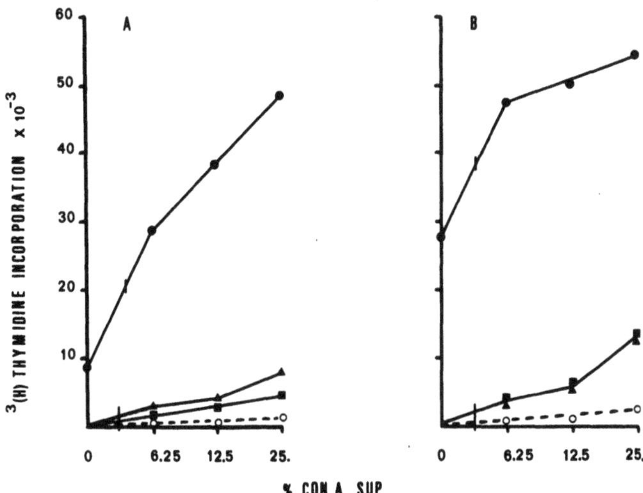

Fig. 1. Proliferative responses of CTL : 1 x 10^4 cells of clones BD4-2 (A) and BD4-13 (B) measured by ^{3}H) thymidine incorporation 48 H after their stimulation without (o) or with 5 x 10^5 feeder cells (2500 Rad) of B/6 (■), DBA/1 (▲), or BALB/c (●) origin and the indicated amounts of Con A SUP.

and BD4-13 were slightly stimulated in the presence of H-2^d stimulating cells (BALB/c, Mls^b), but not in the presence of syngeneic B6 or allogeneic DBA/1 (H-2^q, Mls^a) splenic stimulating cells. The addition of Con A SUP, however, increased the stimulating potential of the H-2^d cells in a dose-dependent fashion and sustained a weak proliferation in the presence of either H-2^b or H-2^q cells. The specificity of the proliferative stimulation of the CTL clones was compared with their lytic specificity in Fig. 2 (See Table I for the information on the allelic forms expressed in the H-2 and at the Mls loci of the mouse strains used as stimulating cell donors). The ability of clones BD4-2 and -13 to lyse B10.A(K^kD^d), but not D2.GD(K^dD^b), nor C3H.OL(K^dD^K) target cells, indicated that the lytic specificity was for the d allelic form of a H-2D mapped product, possibly including the L (20) and/or R (21) molecules. Known Qa, Tla or Qed region products could be excluded as potential target sites (Table I). Similarly an increased stimulation of growth was observed when clones BD4-2 and -13 were stimulated in the presence of Con A SUP with DBA/2 (K^dD^d) or A.AL (K^kD^d) spleen cells, but not with B6 (K^bD^b), D2.GA (K^dD^b), C3H.OL(K^dD^k) or B10.BR (K^kD^k) cells, indicating the requirement for the expression of a H-$2D^d$ product for optimal stimulation of the growth of the clones.

TABLE I

Mouse strain	Alleles at H-2 and Mls[a]											
	K	A	J	E	C	S	D	Qa1	Qa2	Tla	Qed1	Mls
B/6	b	b	b	b	b	b	b	b	a	b	b	b
DBA/w	d	d	d	d	d	d	d	(a)	a	c	b	a
BALB/c	d	d	d	d	d	d	d	b	a	c	b	b
D2.GD	d	d	b	b	b	b	b	.	.	.	(b)	a
B10.A	k	k	k	d	d	d	d	a	a	a	a	b
B10.BR	k	k	k	k	k	k	k	a	b	a	a	b
C3H.OL	d	d	d	d	d	k	k	.	.	b	b	c
A.AL	k	k	k	k	k	k	d	.	.	c	b	c
DBA/a	q	q	q	q	q	q	q	b	.	b	(b)	a

a) Taken from Klein et al. (28), Fischer-Lindhal and Hausmann (29) and Festenstein (30).

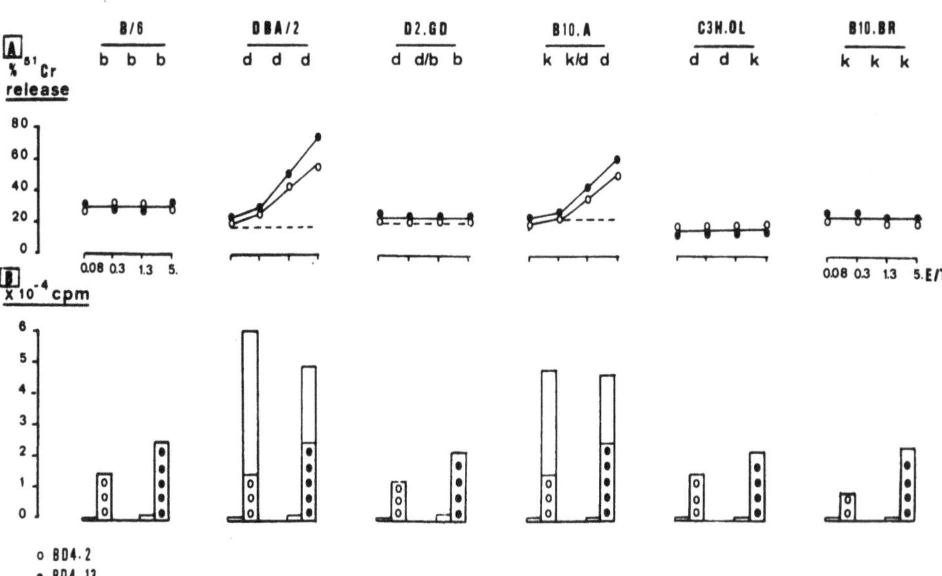

EFFECT OF CYTOLYSIS-INHIBITING mAb ON THE GROWTH OF THE CTL CLONES

Cytolysis-inhibiting rat mAb H35-17.2 (abbreviated 17.2) and H35-89.9 (abbreviated 89.9) prepared as previously described (1), were obtained from culture supernatant precipitated with $(NH_4)_2SO_4$ (50% saturated) and resuspended to one tenth of the original volume. Figure 3 indicates the inhibition pattern of mAb 17.2 and 89.9 on cytolysis by clones BD4-2 (A) and BD4-13 (B) when tested on P815 ($H-2^d$) target cells. A 50% inhibition of cytolysis was obtained in the presence of mAb 17.2 at a dilution of 10^7 and 10^4 for clones BD4-2 and -13 respectively, and in the presence of mAb 89.9 at a dilution of 10^2 regardless of the clone used.

The effects on the proliferation of clones BD4-2 and -13 induced in the presence of Con A SUP and splenic feeder cells presenting (BALB/c) or not (B6) the $H-2D^d$ product were investigated in Figure 4. The $H-2D^d$-dependent stimulation of clone BD4-2 was inhibited by both mAb 17.2 and 89.9 The weaker proliferation of that clone on B6 feeder cells was not affected by the presence of mAb 89.9 (Fig. 4-A). $H-2D^d$-dependent proliferation of clone BD4-13 was strongly inhibited by mAb 17.2, although it was unaffected by the presence of mAb 89.9. The low level of proliferation of clone BD4-13 on B6 feeder cells was again not affected in the presence of mAb 17.2, although it was slightly diminished in the presence of mAb 89.9.

Fig. 2. Mapping of MHC specificity requirements for lysis by CTL clones (A) as measured by ^{51}Cr release from 2 x 10^4 LPD blast target cells from different mouse strains and for stimulation of CTL clone growth (B) as measured by (^3H) thymidine incorporation 48 H after culturing 1 x 10^4 cells in the presence of 5 x 10^5 of the stimulating cells from the mouse strains indicated at the top of the figure and 25% Con A SUP. (A) and (B) data for clone BD4-2 and BD4-13 correspond to open (o) and closed (•) dots respectively. (A) E/T indicates the effector to target cell ratio during the 4 H ^{51}Cr release assay. S.D. of triplicate samples were less than 5%. (---) Background ^{51}Cr release from target cells in the presence of medium. (B) The open bars close to background values on the left side of each dotted bar correspond to (^3H) thymidine incorporation in the presence of the corresponding stimulating cell but in the absence of Con A SUP. For each of the different stimulating cells used the bar representing the proliferative response of clones BD4-2 (o) or BD4-13 (•) is dotted up to the level corresponding to the proliferation in the presence of B6 stimulating cells. S.D. of triplicate cultures were less than 10%.

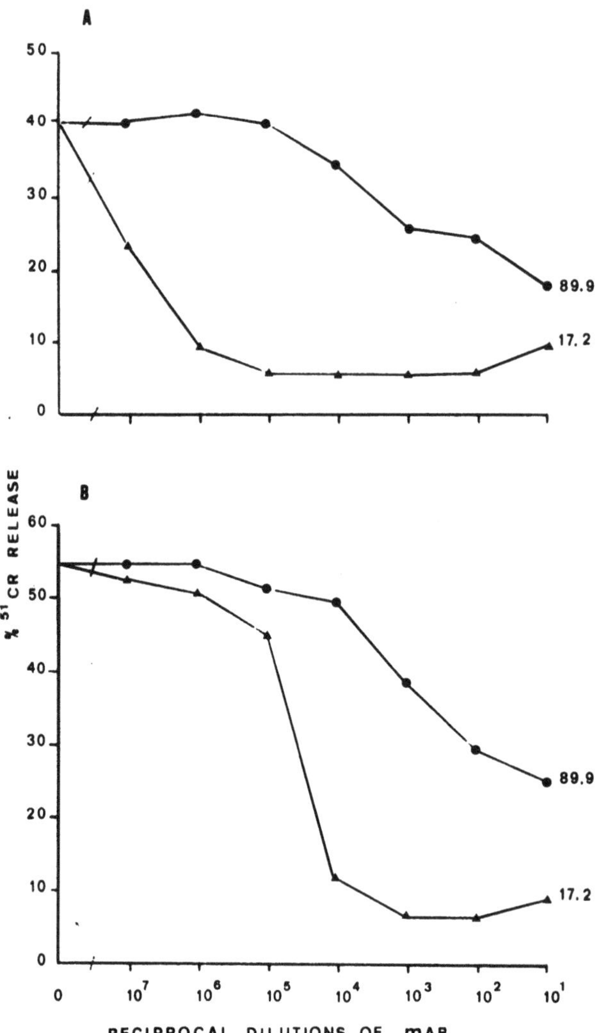

Fig. 3. Inhibition of CTL activity of clone BD4-2 (A) and BD4-13 (B) as measured during a 4 H ^{51}Cr release assay on 1 x 10^4 P815 tumor target cells in the presence of various concentration of mAb 17.2 (▲) or 89.9 (●). E/T was 5/1. Background ^{51}Cr release was 7%.

These results indicate (a) that a single cloned T cell population could be inhibited or not by a mAb depending on whether antigen-dependent or independent, TCGF-dependent proliferation was considered, mAb 17.2 inhibiting the former, but not the latter; (b) that depending on the particular CTL clone, a cytolysis-inhibiting mAb (89.9) will or will not inhibit the proliferation of a clone. This property was a clonal characteristic since subclones

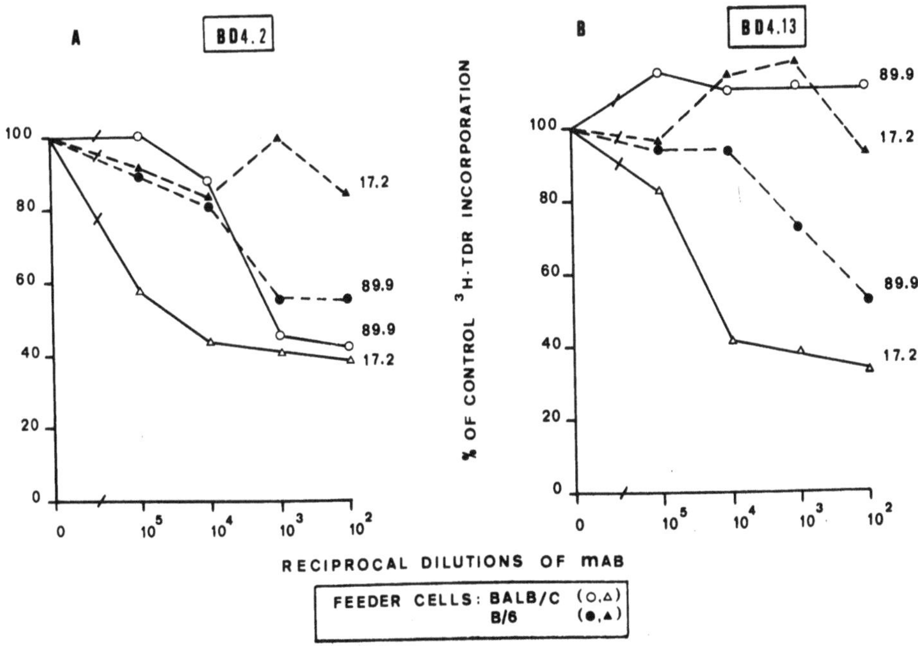

Fig. 4. Inhibition of the proliferative response of CTL clones BD4-2 (A) and BD4-13 (B) in the presence of the indicated amounts of mAb 17.2 (▲,Δ) and 89.9(●, o) when measured in the presence of B/6 (●,▲) or BALB/c (o,Δ) stimulating cells and 25% Con A SUP. Results are expessed as % of ^{3}H-thymidine incorporation in the absence of mAb which was (in cpm for 1 x 10^4 cells) for BD4-2, 2980 $\pm$ 16 on B/6 and 4800 $\pm$ 290 on BALB/c stimulating cells and for BD4-13, 4862 $\pm$ 466 on B/6 and 12700 $\pm$ 2000 on BALB/c stimulating cells.

derived from clones BD4-2 and -13 expressed susceptibility to inhibition by 89.9 (BD4-2-1), or not (BD4-13-10) as indicated in Fig. 5-A and -B respectively.

DISCUSSION

Two types of xenogeneic mAb directed against mouse lymphoid cells and selected for their ability to block anti-allogeneic CTL activity have previously been described (1).

MAb 17.2, probably directed at the Lyt2 antigen on T cells, was found to inhibit direct cytolysis, but not lectin-dependent cytolysis of tumor target cells (1). This mAb did not inhibit any T cell proliferation in the assays previously tested (1) which involved Con A, alloantigen and soluble antigen stimulation of T

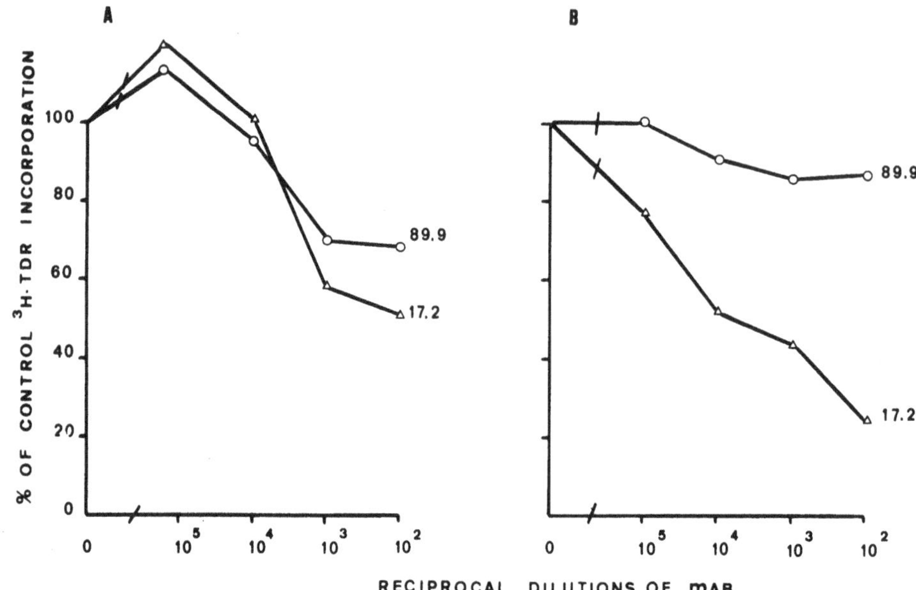

Fig. 5. Inhibition of the proliferative response of CTL sub-clones BD4-2-1 (A) and BD4-13-10 (B) in the presence of the indicated amounts of mAb 17.2 (▲), and 89.9 (o) when measured in the presence of BALB/c stimulating cells and 25% Con A SUP. Results are expressed as % of ^{3}H-thymidine incorporation in the absence of mAb which was (in cpm for 1 x 10^4 cells) 8032 $\pm$ 523 and 19128 $\pm$ 3000.

cells. The results presented here make use of two CTL clones which recognize H-2D^d-mapped products as target antigens and also as stimulating antigens required for optimal TCGF-dependent proliferation (Figures 1 and 2). Clones with similar stimulating properties have recently been described (22), which contrast with initially described CTL clones dependent on TCGF but not on their specific antigen for their growth 16,19). The analysis of the effect of mAb 17.2 on the antigen-dependent and antigen-independent TCGF-dependent proliferation of clones BD4-2 and -13 indicated that the former was inhibited, but not the latter (Fig. 4). These results may explain discrepancies previously reported for the ability of anti-Lyt2 antibodies to block T cell proliferation (1,4-6), thus further subtantiating previous indications on the role of the Lyt2 and/or associated molecules in antigen-CTL interaction, rather than in the lytic event (23) and further suggesting that the same associations of the Lyt2 antigen with the T cell receptor for Class I MHC antigens (6,11) might exist at the stage of the CTL stimulation and at the stage of its lytic interaction with target cells. Such an associaton might not exist for CTL directed at class II alloantigens (24; Pierres, A., Schmitt-Verhulst, A.M., Buferne, M., Golstein, P. and Pierres, M. (this volume).

The second type of cytolysis-inhibiting mAb recognizing a 180 K, 95K antigen (1,12-14) on mouse lymphoid cells, was found to inhibit lectin-induced as well as antigen-induced proliferation of T cells, but not LPD-induced proliferation of B cells (1). The analysis of the effect of this mAb (89.9) on cytolysis (Fig. 3) and proliferation (Fig. 4) of our CTL clones indicated that both clones were equally sensitive to the presence of the mAb when measured for their cytolytic potential but only clone BD4-2 was affected in its antigen-dependent proliferation. Similarly this mAb inhibited cytolysis by, but not proliferation of CTL hybridomas (Golstein, P., Pierres, M., Schmitt-Verhulst, A.M., Luciani, M.F., Buferne, M., Eshhar, Z. and Kaufmann, Y. (this volume). A CTL clone which was totally feeder cell-independent and TCGF-dependent (19) had previously been found to be inhibited by mAb 89.9 for both cytolysis and proliferation (1). It appears tht TCGF-dependency for growth and inhibition of proliferation by mAb 89.9 are not necessarily linked. This does not necessarily preclude the possibility that the mechanism of inhibition of growth by 89.9 might involve a TCGF acceptor site on the cell surface. Indeed, relative avidities for acceptor-TCGF and for acceptor-mAb may vary from clone to clone, as it might be the case for the Lyt2-anti-Lyt2 interaction (25). TCGF-dependency for growth and expression of CTL function are two traits which have been suggested to be linked in certain CTL hybridomas (26), but that correlation does not appear to apply for other CTL hybridomas (27) however.

The mechanism by which the 180-95K surface antigen interferes with either cytolysis by T cells or TCGF-dependent T cell stimulation is as yet unknown. The analysis of the effect of mAb 89.9 on cloned CTL and on CTL hybridomas suggests that its relationship with T cell stimulation might be less stringent than with cytolysis in some individual T cell clones. Such clones thus provide apparent natural "phenotypic variants" in which traits that are associated in the bulk of a T cell population appear to be dissociated.

ACKNOWLEDGEMENTS

We would like to thank C. Kourilsky for secretarial assistance. This work was supported by ACC DGRST 81 L 0711.

REFERENCES

1. Pierres, M., Goridis, C., and P. Golstein. Inhibition of murine T cell-mediated cytolysis and T cell proliferation by a rat monoclonal antibody immunoprecipitating two lymphoid cell surface polypeptides of 94,000 and 180,000 molecular weight. Eur. J. Immunol. (in presss)(1981).
2. Shinohara, N., and D.H. Sachs. mouse alloantibodies capable of blocking cytotoxic T cell function. I. Relationship between the antigen reactive with blocking antibodies and the Lyt-2 locus. J. Exp. Med. 150:432 (1979).
3. Shinohara, N., Hammerling, U., and D.H. Sachs. Mouse allo-antibodies capable of blocking cytotoxic T cell function. II. Further study on the relationship between the blocking antibodies and the products of the Lyt-2 locus. Eur. J. Immunol. 10:589 (1980).
4. Nakayama, E., Dippold, W., Shiku, H., Oettgen, H.F., and L.J. Old. Alloantigen-induced T-cell proliferation: Lyt phenotype of responding cells and blocking of proliferation by Lyt anti-sera. Proc. Natl. Acad. Sci. USA 77:2890 (1980).
5. Fan, J., Ahmed, A., and B. Bonavida. Studies on the induction and expession of T cell-mediated immunity. X. Inhibition by Lyt-2,3 antisera of cytotoxic T lymphocyte-mediated antigen-specific and non-specific cytotoxicity: evidence for the blocking of the binding between T lymphocytes and target cells and not the post-binding cytolytic steps. J. Immunol. 125: 2444 (1980).
6. Hollander, N., Pillemer, E., and I.L. Weissman. Blocking effect of Lyt-2 antibodies on T cell function. J. Exp. Med. 152:674 (1980).
7. Hiserodt, J.C., and B. Bonavida. Studies on the maturation and expression of T cell-mediated immunity. XI. Inhibition of the "lethal hit" in T cell-mediated cytotoxicity by heterologous rat antiserum made against alloimmune T lymphocytes. J. Immunol. 126:256 (1981).
8. Binz, H., Frischknecht, Shen, F.W., and H. Wigzell. Idiotypic determinants on T-cell subpopulations. J. Exp. Med. 149:910 (1979).
9. Krammer, P. The T cell receptor problem. Curr. Top. Micro-biol. and Immunol. (1980).
10. Sarmiento, M., Glasebrook, A.L., and F.W. Fitch. IgG or IgM monoclonal antibodies reactive with different determinants on the molecular complex bearing Lyt-2 antigen block T cell-mediated cytolysis in the absence of complement. J. Immunol. 125:2665 (1980).
11. Ledbetter, J.A., Seaman, W.E., Tse, T.T., and L.A. Herzenberg. Lyt-2 and Lyt-3 antigens are on two different polypeptide sub-units linked by disulfide bonds. Relationship of subunits to T cell cytolytic activity. J. Exp. med. 153:1503 (1981).
12. Kurzinger, K., Reynolds, T., Germain, R.N., Davignon, D., Martz,

E., and T.A. Springer. A novel lymphocyte function-associated antigen (LFA-1): cellular distribution, quantitative expression and structure. J. Immunol. 127:596 (1981).
13. Davignon, D., Martz, E., Reynolds, T., Kurzinger, K., and T.A. Springer. Monoclonal antibody to a novel lymphocyte function-associated antigen (LFA)l). Mechanism of blockade of T lymphocyte mediated killing and effects on other T and B lymphocyte functions. J. Immunol. 127:590 (1981).
14. Fitch, F.W. et al, this volume.
15. Gillis, S., Ferm, M.M., Oe, W., and K.A. Smith. T cell growth factor: parameters of production and a quantitative microassay for activity. J. Immunol. 120:2027 (1978).
16. Nabholz, M., Engers, H.D., Collavo, D., and M. North. Cloned T cell lines with specific cytolytic activity. Curr. Top. Microbiol. and Immunol. 81:176 (1978).
17. von Boehmer, H., and W. Hass. H-2 restricted cytolytic and non-cytolytic T cell clones: isolation specificity and functional analysis. Immunol. Rev. 54:27 (1981).
18. Glasebrook, A.L., Sarmiento, M., Loken, M.R., Dialynas, D.P., Quintans, J., Eisenberg, L., Lutz, C.T., Wilde, D., and F.W. Fitch. Murine T lymphocyte clones with distinct immunological functions. Immunol. Rev. 54:225 (1981).
19. Schmitt-Verhulst, A.M., Albert, F., Guimezanes, A., and M. Buferne. Antigenic and genetic parameters in the stimulation and in the lytic phases of anti-hapten + self cytotoxic T cells and their derived clones: role of the T helper cell. J. Supramol. Structure and Cell. Biochem. (in press)(1981).
20. Lemonnier, F., Neuport-Sautes, C., Korilsky, F.M., and P. Demant. Relationships between private and public H-2 specificities on the cell surface. Immunogenetics 2:517 (1975).
21. Hansen, T.H., Ozato, K., Melino, MR., Coligan, J.E., Kindt, T.J., Jandinsky, J.J., and D.H. Sachs. Immunochemical evidence in two haplotypes for at least three D region-encoded molecules D, L and R. J. Immunol. 126:1713 (1981).
22. Lutz, C.T., Glasebrook, A.L., and F.W. Fitch. Alloreactive cloned T cell lines. IV. Interaction of alloantigen and T cell growth factors (TCGF) to simulate cloned cytolytic T lymphocytes. J. Immunol. 127:391 (1981).
23. Dialynas, D.P., Loden, M.R., Glasebrook, A.L., and F.W. Fitch. Lyt-2$^-$/Lyt-3$^-$ variants of a cloned cytolytic T cell ine lack an antigen receptor functional in cytolysis. J. Exp. Med. 153:595 (1981).
24. Swain, S.L., Dennert, G., Wormsley, S., and R.W. Dutton. The Lyt phenotype of a long-term allospecific T cell line. Both helper and killer activities to I-A are mediated by Lyt-1 cells. Eur. J. Immunol. 11:175 (1981).
25. MacDonald, H.R., Thiernesse, N., and J.C. Cerottini. Inhibition of T cell-mediated cytolysis by monoclonal antibodies directed against Lyt-2: heterogeneity of inhibition at the clonal level. J. Immunol. 126:1671 (1981).

26. Nabholz, M., Cianfriglia, M., Acuto, O., Conzelmann, A., Haas, W., Boehmer, H.V., MacDonald, H.R., Pohlit, H., and J.P. Johnson. Cytolytically active murine T-cell hybrids. Nature 287:437 (1980).
27. Kaufmann, Y., Berke, G., and Z. Eshhar. Cytotoxic T lymphocyte hybridomas which mediate specific tumor cell lysis in vitro. Proc. Natl. Acad. Sci. USA 78:2502 (1981).
28. Klein, J., Flaherty, L., Vandeberg, J.L., and D.C. Schreffler. H-2 haplotypes, genes, regions, and antigens: first lising. Immunogenetics 6:489 (1978).
29. Fisher-Lindhal, K., and B. Hausmann. Qed-1: a target for unrestricted killing by T cells. Eur. J. Immunol. 10:281 (1980).
30. Festenstein, H. Immunogenetic and biological aspects of _in vitro_ lymphocyte allotransformatin (MLR) in the mouse. Transplant. Rev. 15:62 (1973).

HETEROGENEITY OF INHIBITION OF CYTOLYTIC T LYMPHOCYTE CLONES BY MONOCLONAL ANTI-LYT-2/3 ANTIBODIES: PARALLEL EFFECTS ON CYTOLYSIS, PROLIFERATION AND LYMPHOKINE SECRETION

H. R. MacDonald[1], A. L. Glasebrook[2], O. Acuto[3], A. Kelso[2], C. Bron[3] and J.-C. Cerottini[1]

[1]Ludwig Institute for Cancer Research, Lausanne Branch
[2]Dept. of Immunology, Swiss Institute for Experimental Cancer Research
[3]Dept. of Biochemistry, University of Lausanne
1066 Epalinges, Switzerland

INTRODUCTION

The interaction between cytolytic T lymphocytes (CTL) and target cells is presumed to be mediated by antigen-specific receptors on the surface of CTL. One approach to the identification and characterization of such putative receptors is thus to make antisera (or monoclonal antibodies) against CTL and test these reagents for their ability to block cytolytic function. At the present time, only antibodies directed against the Lyt-2/3 antigenic complex (1, 2) or against the LFA-1 surface antigen (3) have been found to consistently inhibit CTL function in the mouse. In both instances, however, the observed inhibition is independent of the immunological specificity of the CTL. Thus, it is unlikely that either of these surface structures correspond to the CTL antigen receptor (although models in which they contribute to a constant portion of such a receptor cannot be excluded).

A major limitation to the interpretation of the inhibitory effects of monoclonal antibodies on CTL has been the fact that only cytolytic activity has been measured. Thus, in cases where positive inhibition is observed, it is difficult to exclude the interpretation that the antibody is reacting with a determinant on a surface molecule which is required for cytolytic function but not for antigen recognition. One means of circumventing this objection would be to investigate other properties of CTL which could potentially depend upon specific antigen recognition. In this regard, CTL clones which proliferate specifically to alloantigens have recently been described by Widmer and Bach (4) and independently by ourselves (1). Furthermore, alloantigen-induced release of lymphokines such as interferon and macrophage-activating factor (MAF) by CTL clones has been reported (5). In the present study, we will demonstrate that 1) the effect of monoclonal anti-Lyt-2/3 antibodies on these various functional activities is heterogeneous when examined at the level of individual CTL clones, and 2) inhibition of proliferation and lymphokine secretion in CTL clones by these antibodies occurs in parallel with inhibition of cytolysis. Based on these findings, a model for the role of the Lyt-2/3 molecular complex in stabilization of antigen receptors on CTL will be proposed.

DIFFERENTIAL EFFECT OF MONOCLONAL ANTI-LYT-2/3 ANTIBODIES ON CYTOLYSIS BY CLONES C10 AND L3

We have previously reported that CTL clones directed against alloantigens may vary considerably in their ability to be inhibited by monoclonal antibodies directed against Lyt-2 (6). In order to investigate this phenomenon in greater detail, we derived a CTL clone (C10) which was particularly insensitive to anti-Lyt-2 inhibition. For this purpose, spleen cells from C56BL/6 mice which had been primed 3 months previously with P-815 (DBA/2) tumor cells were restimulated _in vitro_ with irradiated DBA/2 spleen cells for 5 days. Cells from these cultures were then cloned by limiting dilution (average cell density = 3 cells/well) in the presence of irradiated DBA/2 spleen cells and secondary MLC supernatant as a source of IL-2 (7). Putative clones derived from this procedure were then tested for cytolytic activity in the presence or absence of anti-Lyt-2 antibodies. In one such experiment, 10 of 18 (56%) cytolytic clones tested were only slightly (0-20%) inhibited, in agreement with our previous studies using primed peritoneal exudate cells (6). Several clones from this experiment were then expanded, recloned, and retested for inhibition over a range of concentrations of anti-Lyt-2 antibodies. The data for one such clone (C10), which was selected for detailed analysis, are shown in Fig. 1. It can be seen that lysis of P-815 target cells by clone C10 was not significantly inhibited by doses of anti-Lyt-2 antibody as high as 5 μg per well. In contrast, another C57BL/6 anti-DBA/2 clone (13), which was derived independently from an _in vitro_ primed population (8), and which is readily inhibited by monoclonal anti-Lyt-2 antibodies (9), was completely inhibited at this dose of antibody and significantly inhibited by as little as 5 ng per well. Thus, a quantitative difference of at least 1000-fold in the amount of anti-Lyt-2 antibody required for inhibition of cytolysis was observed between clones L3 and C10.

These differences in inhibition of cytolysis observed between clones L3 and C10 were not restricted to a particular subclass of specificity of anti-Lyt-2 antibody. Thus rat IgM (9) or IgG (9, 10) antibodies against Lyt-2 strongly inhibited lysis of P-815 target

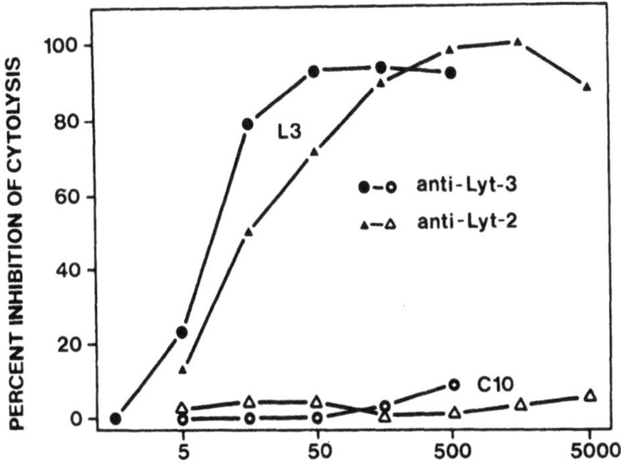

Fig. 1. Differential inhibition of CTL clones L3 and C10 by monoclonal anti-Lyt-2/3 antibodies. Cloned CTL ($6x10^3$) were incubated with the indicated amount of monoclonal anti-Lyt-2 or anti-Lyt-3 antibodies for 15 minutes at 20°C. Then $3x10^3$ ^{51}Cr-labeled P-815 target cells were added for 3 hours and specific lysis was assessed. For purposes of comparison, data are expressed as percent inhibition relative to control lysis in the absence of added inhibitor (59% and 69% for L3 and C10, respectively).

cells but not by C10 (data not shown). In addition, monoclonal antibodies against Lyt-3, a serologically and genetically separable component of the same molecular complex as Lyt-2 (10, 11), likewise inhibited cytolysis by L3 at least 100-fold more efficiently than by C10 (Fig. 1).

EXPRESSION OF LYT-2/3 ANTIGENS BY CLONES C10 AND L3

One trivial explanation for the observed failure of anti-Lyt-2/3 antibodies to inhibit cytolysis by clone C10 would be lack of expression of the corresponding surface antigens. That this is not, in fact, the case is demonstrated by the data in Fig. 2. In this experiment, C10 cells were incubated with monoclonal rat antibodies against Thy-1.2, Lyt-1, Lyt-2 or Lyt-3 followed by fluoresceinated rabbit anti-rat Ig and run on a FACS II flow cytometer. The fluorescence histograms obtained indicated that C10 cells were clearly stained by the Thy-1, Lyt-2 and Lyt-3 reagents (as compared to control staining with the fluorescent anti-Ig along), whereas Lyt-1 staining was undetectable. Similar fluorescence histograms

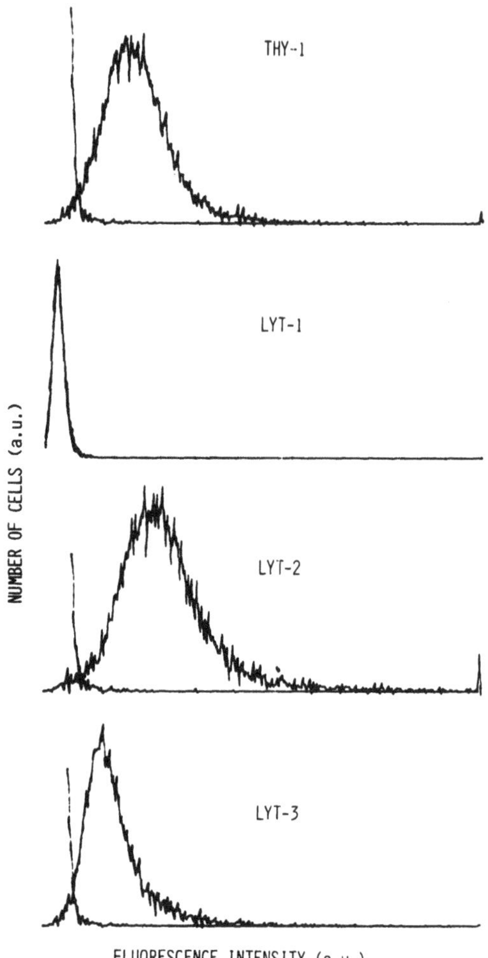

Fig. 2. Expression of surface antigens on CTL clone C10. Aliquots of C10 cells ($3x10^5$) were incubated with rat monoclonal antibodies directed aginst Thy-1.2, Lyt-1, Lyt-2 or Lyt-3 followed by fluoresceinated rabbit anti-rat immunoglobulin. Samples were run on a FACS II and 10,000 viable cells (gated according to forward light scatter) were accumulated for each histogram. The fluorescence for each reagent is compared to the distribution obtained with the fluorescent conjugate alone.

were observed for L3 (data not shown; see also reference 12). Thus, no qualitative or quantitative differences in the expression of Lyt-2/3 antigens on L3 or C10 cells could be detected by flow mirco-fluorometry.

Further immunochemical analysis of Lyt-2 expression on C10 and L3 cells was carrried out by SDS polyacrylamide gel electrophoresis and autoradiography of surface ^{125}I labeled (13) material which had been immunoprecipitated by anti-Lyt-2 antibodies. As shown in Fig. 3, a single broad band of approximately 40,000 MW was immunoprecipitated from both CTL clones. In contrast, control immunoprecipitation of surface labeled C57BL/6 thymocytes by anti-Lyt-2 antibodies resulted in 2 distinct bands of about 34,000 and 38,000 MW, in agreement with other recent studies (14, 15). Again, no obvious differences could be detected in the Lyt-2/3 molecules expressed by clones L3 and C10.

EFFECTS OF ANTI-LYT-2 ANTIBODIES ON SECRETION OF LYMPHOKINES BY CLONES C10 AND L3

Recent studies from our laboratory have demonstrated that CTL clones can secrete lymphokines when stimulated by antigenically

Table I. Effect of monoclonal anti-Lyt-2 antibodies on secretion of macrophage-activating factor (MAF) by CTL clones C10 and L3[a]

CTL clone supernatant		Relative MAF activity[b]	
Source	Concentration (%)	Control	Anti-Lyt-2
L3	50	87	6
	5	65	6
C10	50	83	80
	5	80	41

[a]CTL clones C10 or L3 (2.5×10^5/ml) were washed and exposed to 5×10^6 irradiated (2000 rads) T-cell-depleted allogeneic (DBA/2) spleen cells in the presence or absence of monoclonal anti-Lyt-2 antibodies (1:200 dilution of ascitic fluid). After 24 hours, supernatants were harvested and tested for MAF activity.

[b]Cultured bone marrow macrophages (5×10^4) were incubated for 24 hours with the indicated concentration of CTL clone supernatant plus lipopolysaccharide (100 ng/ml). ^{51}Cr-labeled P-815 tumor target cells (10^4) were then added for an additional 20 hours. Relative MAF activity is equivalent to percent specific ^{51}Cr release (corrected for release in the absence of added supernatant). Addition of anti-Lyt-2 antibodies to control supernatant preparations had no effect on MAF activity.

appropriate stimulating cells (5). It was, therefore, of interest to compare the effect of anti-Lyt-2 antibodies on such antigen-induced lymphokine secretion by clones C10 and L3. As shown in Table I, both CTL clones secreted macrophage-activating factor (MAF) when stimulated with irradiated T-cell-depleted DBA/2 spleen cells; however, in the presence of anti-Lyt-2 antibodies, secretion of MAF by L3 was totally abolished, whereas secretion by C10 was only slightly reduced. Thus, the differential inhibitory effects of anti-Lyt-2 antibodies on MAF production by the two clones paralleled the effects on cytolysis noted above.

Table II. Effect of monoclonal anti-Lyt-2 antibodies on proliferation and cytolytic activity of IL-2-independent CTL clones

CTL clone	Lyt phenotype[a]	Addition of anti-Lyt-2[b]	^{3}H-TdR incorporation (dpm)[c]		Percent specific lysis[d]
			C57BL/6	DBA/2	
AG 21.20	1^+2^+	-	450	21,372	43
		+	nt[e]	14,195	35
AG 39.2	1^-2^+	-	531	11,475	48
		+	nt	530	1

[a]Determined by flow microfluorometry (cf. Fig. 2).

[b]Cloned cells were pre-incubated with or without 1 μg of monoclonal anti-Lyt-2 antibodies for 30 minutes at 20°C.

[c]Cloned CTL (2×10^4) were incubated with 7.5×10^5 irradiated T cell-depleted syngeneic (C57BL/6) or allogeneic (DBA/2) spleen cells in a total volume of 0.2 ml. After 3 days, microcultures were pulsed with 1 μCi ^{3}H-TdR for 5 hours. Results are expressed as mean dpm of triplicate cultures.

[d] Measured in a 3.5 hour assay using lipopolysaccharide (LPS)-induced DBA/2 spleen cells as targets (effector:target cell ratio = 20:1).

[e]n.t., not tested.

EFFECTS OF ANTI-LYT-2/3 ANTIBODIES ON PROLIFERATION OF CTL CLONES

Most CTL clones, including L3 (8) and C10 (data not shown), are entirely dependent upon IL-2 for growth. However, it has recently been observed by Widmer and Bach (4) and by ourselves (1) that a small proportion of such clones are capable of proliferating to specific alloantigens in the absence of exogenously added IL-2. For example, Table II summarizes proliferation data for C57BL/6 anti-DBA/2 clones AG21.20 and AG39.2. These CTL clones were obtained by micromanipulating single cells from primary C57BL/6 anti-DBA/2 MLC cultures and growing up these cells in the presence of irradiated DBA/2 spleen cells and a source of IL-2. When restimulated by irradiated DBA/2 spleen cells in the absence of growth factor, most CTL clones (approximately 95%) failed to proliferate; however, as seen in Table II, AG21.20 and AG39.2 had stimulation indices of 47 and 22, respectively, as compared to stimulation with irradiated syngeneic (C57BL/6) spleen cells. Cytolytic activity of these 2 clones, when measured on LPS blast target cells, was comparable (43% and 48% specific lysis at a 20:1 effector:target cell ratio for Ag21.20 and AG39.2, respectively) (Table II). It should be noted, however, that testing of cytolytic activity on other blast and tumor target cells indicated differing immunological specificities of these 2 clones, with AG39.2 being directed against H-2D^d and AG21.20 being directed against a non K- or D- (perhaps I-) region encoded specificity of the H-2^d haplotype (data not shown).

When tested for proliferation and cytolytic activity in the presence of monoclonal anti-Lyt-2 antibodies, an interesting dissociation between clones AG21.20 and AG39.2 was observed. Whereas both functional activities were reduced to background levels by 1 μg of anti-Lyt-2 antibodies in the case of clone AG29.2, only a modest inhibition (approximately 20% in killing and 30% in ^{3}H-TdR incorporation) was observed for clone AG21.20 at this antibody concentration (Table II). This dissociation was confirmed in antibody titration experiments which showed that both antigen-dependent proliferation and cytolytic activity of clone AG39.2 were significantly inhibited by as little as 10 ng of anti-Lyt-2 antibodies while doses below 1 μg had no effect on either activity expressed by clone AG21.20. In specificity experiments using a variety of monoclonal antibodies directed against surface determinants present on CTL clone AG39.2, only antibodies directed against Lyt-2 or Lyt-3 inhibited proliferation; anti-Lyt-1, anti-Thy-1.2 and anti-H-2D^b antibodies had no effect (data not shown). Thus, inhibition of proliferation of AG39.2 appeared to be specific for antibodies directed against products of the Lyt-2/3 genetic locus.

In other experiments (data not shown), alloantigen-induced MAF release by clone AG39.2 was strongly inhibited by monoclonal anti-Lyt-2 antibodies, while no inhibition was observed with clone AG21.20. Thus, inhibition of lymphokine secretion went in parallel with proliferation and cytolytic activity for these IL-2-independent CTL clones.

DISCUSSION

It has been known for some time that antibodies directed against the Lyt-2/3 molecular complex on the surface of CTL are able to inhibit cytolytic activity (1, 2). More recently, we have demonstrated that this inhibitory effect is extremely heterogeneous when examined at the level of individual CTL clones (6). In the present study, we have therefore selected CTL clones of similar antigenic specificity but with dramatically different susceptibility to inhibition by monoclonal anti-Lyt-2 or anti-Lyt-3 antibodies in order to investigate this puzzling phenomenon in greater detail. Our results indicate that the expression of Lyt-2/3 antigenic determinants (as assessed by flow microfluormetry and by immunoprecipitation analysis) is both quantitatively and qualitatively similar in CTL clones of the "inhibited" (L3) and "uninhibited" (C10) phenotype. Furthermore, other antigen-dependent functional activities of these and other cloned CTL, such as proliferation and lymphokine secretion, exhibit a similar susceptibility (or lack thereof) to inhibition by anti-Lyt-2 antibodies as does cytolytic activity.

Recent analysis of the Lyt-2/3 molecular complex in thymocyte preparations by polyacrylamide gel electrophoresis under reducing conditions has demonstrated predominant peptides of 34,000 and 38,000 MW (14, 15). The present data confirm these observations and further demonstrate that a single molecular species of approximately 40,000 MW is immunoprecipitated from CTL clones C10 or L3 by these reagents (Fig. 3). This apparent difference in the expression of Lyt-2/3 by CTL clones and thymocytes may be related to the observation that peripheral T cells express only the higher (38,000) MW species (15). In any case, a more detailed comparison of the peptides immunoprecipitated from the thymocytes and the CTL clones (such as 2-dimensional gel electrophoresis) will be required before any conclusions as to structural differences can be made.

Although the inhibitory effects of anti-Lyt-2/3 antibodies on cytolytic function have been amply demonstrated at both the population (1, 2) and clonal (6, 9) level, little information is currently available concerning the effects of these reagents on other T cell functions. Recently, both Nakayama et al (16) and Hollander et al (17) reported that cellular proliferation and CTL generation in MLC could be partially inhibited by conventional and monoclonal antibodies directed against Lyt-2/3 antigens; however, since these studies were carried out with heterogeneous populations in which activation of CTL may depend on amplifier cells and/or soluble factors, it is difficult to interpret the cellular basis of this inhibition. With the recent demonstration that certain CTL clones

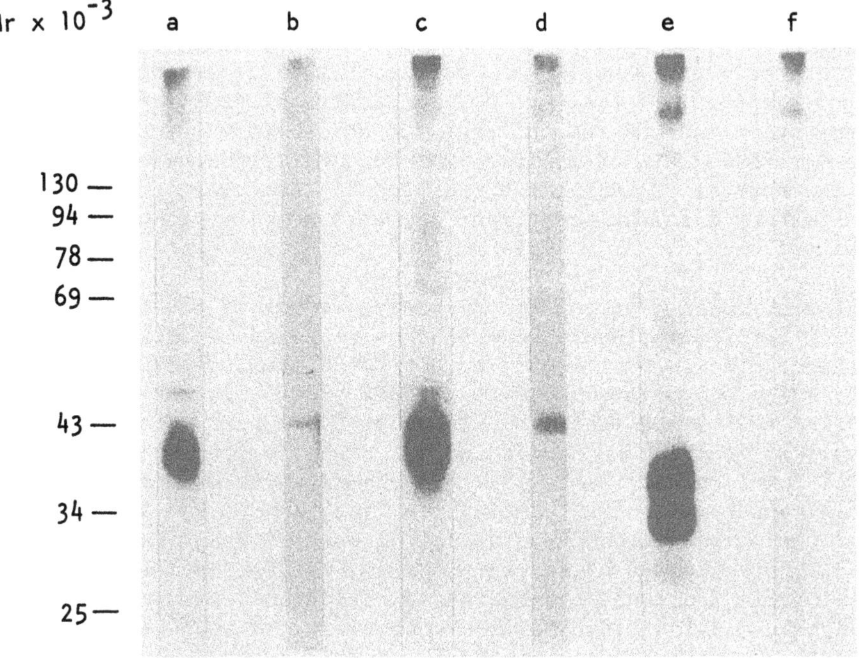

Fig. 3 Immunoprecipitation analysis of Lyt-2 antigens on surface ^{125}I-labeled CTL clones C10 and L3. Cells from C57BL/6 anti-DBA/2 clones C10 (a) or L3 (c), in addition to control C57BL/6 thymocytes (e) were surface ^{125}I-labeled according to the glucose oxydase/lactoperoxidase method (13) and lysed with 0.5% NP40. Cell lysates ($2x10^6$ cpm, corresponding to approximately $1-2x10^6$ cells) were incubated with monoclonal anti-Lyt-2 antibodies (53.6.7; reference 10) coupled to CNBr-activated sepharose. After 2 hours at 4°C beads were washed and proteins extracted in 2% SDS. Samples were electrophoresed on a 10% acrylamide SDS gel. Control lysates of C10 (b), L3 (d) and thymocytes (f) were reacted with an unrelated monoclonal antibody directed against β-galactosidase (kindly provided by Dr. R. Acolla).

can proliferate to alloantigens in the absence of exogenously added IL-2 (reference 4 and this report), it is now possible to investigate the inhibitory effects of anti-Lyt-2/3 antibodies on CTL proliferation in a defined system. In the present report, we demonstrate that the alloantigen-induced proliferation of some (but not all) CTL clones can be completely abrogated by monoclonal anti-Lyt-2 or anti-Lyt-3 antibodies. That this inhibiton of proliferation is specific for Lyt-2/3 molecules on the CTL clones is further supported by the finding that comparable concentrations of monoclonal antibodies directed against Thy-1, Lyt-1 or H-2D have no significant inhibitory effect. Thus it is possible that at least part of the inhibitory effects of anti-Lyt-2/3 antibodies on proliferation and CTL generation in bulk MLC cultures may be due to a blocking effect on the activation CTL of precursors. More direct experiments in which the effects of such antibodies on CTL precursors are assessed under limiting dilution conditions may shed some light on this complex problem.

Of particular interest in the present study is the observation that anti-Lyt-2/3 antibodies can block several (presumably independent) functional activities in certain CTL clones. For example, proliferation, cytolytic activity and MAF production were inhibited when clone AG39.2 was incubated with anti-Lyt-2 antibodies (Table II), while lymphokine secretion and cytotoxicity were inhibited in parallel for clone L3 (Table I). For clones which were insensitive to inhibition by anti-Lyt-2 antibodies (such as C10 and AG21.20), none of the aforementioned functional parameters was affected. The fact that a number of mechanistically distinct phenomena including cytolytic function, lymphokine secretion and cellular proliferation should all exhibit similar sensitivity to inhibition by monoclonal anti-Lyt-2/3 antibodies in certain cloned CTL lines suggests a common pathway for the initiation of these apparently unrelated events. In this context, it seems reasonable to assume that the initial event leading to triggering of these various functional activities would be specific recognition of alloantigenic determinants by the cloned CTL. If so, the results obtained would imply that anti-Lyt-2/3 antibodies can, in fact, block antigen recognition by CTL rather than merely interfere with a secondary process which is, in some way, required for the expression of cytolytic function.

How then can these findings be reconciled with the fact that other cloned CTL lines are not inhibited in any of the aforementioned functions by monoclonal anti-Lyt-2/3 antibodies? Since these "uninhibited" CTL clones apparently express Lyt-2 and Lyt-3 at a similar density (Fig. 2) and in a comparable molecular form (Fig. 3) as "inhibited" clones, it is possible to exclude trivial explanations such as a failure of the antibodies to react with the uninhibited cells. Why, then, should the reaction of these antibodies with Lyt-2/3 determinants on certain clones not lead to inhibition of antigen recognition functions? One attractive hypothesis to explain these discrepant experimental findings would be to postulate that the role of the Lyt-2/3 molecular complex is to stabilize the binding between the CTL antigen receptor and the appropriate antigenic determinant(s) on the target (or stimulating) cell (Fig. 4). Irrespective of how this stabilization process might occur at the molecular level, one important corollary to this postulate would be that, as the number and/or affinity of CTL antigen

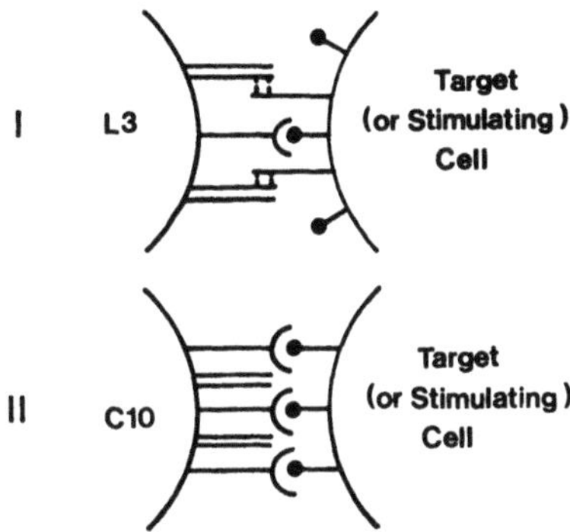

Fig. 4. Model to explain differential inhibitory effects of monoclonal anti-Lyt-2/3 antibodies on CTL clones.

I. Effector cell (prototype L3) has few and/or low affinity antigen receptors (—C). Binding to target (or stimulating) cells is stabilized by the Lyt-2/3 molecular complex (==).

II. Effector cell (prototype C10) has many and/or high affinity antigen receptors. Stable binding does not require Lyt-2/3.

receptors increased, the requirement for Lyt-2/3 molecules in order to stabilize the binding would decrease. Thus, in an operational sense, the ability of a particular CTL clone to be inhibited by monoclonal anti-Lyt-2 antibodies would be inversely proportional to the number and/or affinity of its antigen receptors.

Although such an hypothesis cannot be experimentally tested in the absence of any molecular definition of CTL antigen receptors, it is, nevertheless, interesting to compare some aspects of anti-Lyt-2/3 inhibition at the clonal level with what might be predicted by such an "affinity maturation" model. Firstly, the observed inhibition of lytic activity of CTL clones by monoclonal anti-Lyt-2 antibodies is very heterogeneous. In contradistinction to the extreme situations represented by clones such as L3 and C10 (this report), data obtained with a larger number of CTL clones (reference 6 and unpublished results) suggest that the degree of inhibition of lytic activity of individual clones is distributed in a continuous (rather than "all or none") fashion. Such a continuous distribution would be consistent with the concept of a wide range of receptor affinities. Secondly, the degree of inhibition of CTL by anti-Lyt-2 antibodies, measured either at the population or clonal level, is dramatically reduced when the CTL have been derived from precursors selected by _in vivo_ priming with the appropriate alloantigens. Thus, CTL populations or clones obtained either from alloimmune peritoneal exudate cells (6) or from restimulated populations of alloimmune spleen (this report) are much more difficult to inhibit with anti-Lyt-2 antibodies than CTL obtained in primary MLC. If CTL responses like antibody responses (18), select in vivo for precursors of high affinity, it is reasonable to assume that such differences in affinity might be reflected in the clonal progeny of such cells maintained in vitro. In such a case, quantitative inhibition experiments of CTL clones with monoclonal anti-Lyt-2/3 antibodies such as those described in this report, may prove to be a useful tool for making operational estimates of the relative affinity of CTL antigen receptors. Such inhibition experiments, using CTL clones derived from in vivo primed precursors in other antigenic systems (e.g., minor histocompatibility antigens, virus-associated antigens), are currently in progress in an attempt to test the general validity of this hypothesis.

ACKNOWLEDGEMENTS

We are grateful to the following for providing monoclonal antibodies used in this study: Dr. J. Ledbetter (Lyt-1, Lyt-2, Lyt-3), Dr. F. Fitch (Thy-1.2, Lyt-2), Dr. G. Hammerling (H-2D^b) and Dr. R. Accolla (β-galactosidase).

REFERENCES

(1) Nakayama, E., Shiku, H., Stockert, E., Oettgen, H.F., and L.J. Old. 1979. Cytotoxic T cells: Lyt phenotype and blocking of killing activity by Lyt antisera. Proc. Natl. Acad. Sci. 76:1977.

(2) Shinohara, N., and D.H. Sachs. 1979. Mouse alloantibodies capable of blocking cytotoxic T-cell function. I. Relationship between the antigen reactive with blocking antibodies and the Lyt-2 locus. J. Exp. Med., 150:432.

(3) Davignon, D., Martz, E., Reynolds, T., Kurzinger, K., and T.A. Springer. 1981. Monoclonal antibody to a novel lymphocyte function-associated antigen (LFA-1): mechanism of blockade of T lymphocyte-mediated killing and effects on other T and B lymphocyte functions. J. Immunol. 127:590.

(4) Widmer M.B., and F.H. Bach. 1981. Antigen driven helper cell-independent cloned cytolytic T lymphocytes. Nature. In press.

(5) MacDonald, H.R., Sekaly, R.P., Kanagawa, O., Thiernesse, N., Taswell, C., Cerottini, J.-C., Weiss, A., Glasebrook, A.L., Engers, H.D., Kelso, A., Brunner, K.T., and C. Bron. 1981. Cytolytic T lymphocyte clones. Immunobiology. In press.

(6) MacDonald, H.R., Thiernesse N., and J.-C. Cerottini. 1981. Inhibition of T cell-mediated cytolysis by monoclonal antibodies directed against Lyt-2: Heterogeneity of inhibition

at the clonal level. J. Immunol. 126:1671.

(7) MacDonald, H.R., Cerottini, J.-C., Ryser J.-E., Maryanski, J.-L., Taswell, C., Widmer, M.B., and K.T. Brunner. 1980. Quantitation and cloning of cytolytic T lymphocytes and their precursors. Immunol. Rev. 51:93.

(8) Glasebrook, A.L., and F.W. Fitch. 1979. T-cell lines which cooperate in the generation of specific cytolytic activity. Nature 278:171.

(9) Sarmiento, M., Glasebrook, A.L., and F.W. Fitch. 1980. IgG or IgM monoclonal antibodies reactive with different determinants on the molecular complex bearing Lyt-2 antigen block T cell-mediated cytolysis in the absence of complement. J. Immunol. 125:2665.

(10) Ledbetter, J.-A., and L.A. Herzenberg. 1979. Xenogeneic monoclonal antibodies to mouse lymphoid differentiation antigens. Immunol. Rev. 47:63.

(11) Boyse, E.A., Itakura, K., Stockert, E., Iritani, C.A., and M. Miura. 1971. Ly-C : a third locus specifying alloantigens expressed only on thymocytes and lymphocytes. Transplantation 11:351.

(12) Glasebrook A.L., Sarmiento, M., Locken, M.R., Dialynas, D.P., Quintans, J., Eisenberg, L., Lutz, C.T., Wilde, D., and F.W. Fitch. 1981. Murine T lymphocyte clones with distinct immunological functions. Immunol. Rev. 54:225.

(13) Hubbard, A.L., and Z.A. Cohn. 1975. Externally disposed plasma membrane proteins. I. Enzymatic iodination of mouse L-cells. J. Cell. Biol. 64:458.

(14) Reilly, E.B., Auditore-Hargreaves, K., Hammerling, U., and P.D. Gottlieb. 1980. Lyt-2 and Lyt-3 alloantigens: Precipitation with monoclonal and conventional antibodies and analysis on one- and two-dimensional polyacrylamide gels. J. Immunol. 125:2245.

(15) Ledbetter, J.A., Seaman, W.E., Tsu, T.T., and L.A. Herzenberg. 1981. Lyt-2 and Lyt-3 antigens are on two different polypeptide subunits linked by disulfide bonds. Relationship of subunits to T cell cytolytic activity. J. Exp. Med. 153:1503.

(16) Nakayama, E., Dippold, W., Shiku, H., Oettgen, H.F., and L.J. Old. 1980. Alloantigen-induced T-cell prolifeation: Lyt phenotype of responding cells and blocking of proliferation by Lyt antisera. Proc. Natl. Acad. Sci. 77:2890.

(17) Hollander, N., Pillemer, E., and I.L. Weissman. 1980. Blocking effect of Lyt-2 antibodies on T cell functions. J. Exp. Med. 152:674.

(18) Celada, F. 1971. The cellular basis of immunologic memory. Prog. Allergy 15:223.

IDENTIFICATION OF LYSIS-RELEVANT MOLECULES ON THE SURFACE OF CTL: PRIMARY SCREENING OF MONOCLONAL ANTIBODIES FOR THE CAPACITY TO BLOCK CYTOLYSIS BY CLONED CTL LINES

Deno Dialynas, Michael Loken, Marion Sarmiento, and Frank W. Fitch

Department of Pathology
University of Chicago
Chicago, Illinois 60637

Cytolytic T lymphocytes (CTL) couple antigen recognition with cytolysis of the target cell. The recognition (conjugate formation) and lethal hit components can be distinguished operationally. Both the antigen recognition structure and the lethal hit activity are unidentified. It is possible that the antigen recognition structure on CTL is modified so as to possess this lethal hit activity (1). Implicit in the work described here is the not unreasonable assumption that the molecule(s) responsible for recognition and for the lethal hit exist on the surface of the cytolytic T lymphocyte.

As neither antigen binding nor lethal hit activity has been demonstrated once the cell membrane is solubilized with detergents or mechanical methods, the intact cell so far constitutes the endpoint in the purification/identification of these activities. Given that cytolysis involves components on the cell surface, cytolysis should be generally amenable to blocking by antibodies. One can, therefore, use the resolution of monoclonal antibodies, in conjunction with an intact cell as part of a blocking assay, to bypass the aforementioned endpoint. At the same time, one then also has the probes with which to manipulate, genetically map and biochemically analyze the relevant molecule(s), and determine the extent of expression on different tissues/cell types/clones, etc.

It is not unreasonable to assume that the antigen recognition structure expressed on the surface of the cytolytic T lymphocyte is clonally unique. It is also not unreasonable to assume that a cytolytic cell expresses, on its surface, lysis-relevant molecule(s) which are not expressed on the surface of a non-cytolytic cell. Such assumed restricted expression can serve as the basis of a hybridoma screening assay. Eventually, though, the antibody must be shown to block cytolysis.

We have adapted the blocking assay to the sceening of hybridomas. The primary screen consists of analyzing hybridoma well supernatant fluid (SF) for the capacity to block the receptor-mediated cytolysis of a relevant tumor target by the immunizing cloned CTL line. Secondary screens of the hybridoma SF analyze either the blocking of receptor-mediated cytolysis by a cloned CTL line reactive with a different alloantigen or the blocking of lectin-mediated cytolysis of an irrelevant tumor target by one of several cloned CTL lines.

We modified the standard blocking assay (2) so as both to optimize sensitivity to blocking while retaining specificity and to make more efficient use of cloned CTL and tumor target cells. The parameters of these modified assays, which were empirically determined, are given here for the cloned CTL lines B18 and L3. These cloned cells are specific for $H\text{-}2K^d$ and $H\text{-}2D^d$ murine alloantigens, respectively (3). The fact that one is working with a cloned CTL line, for which CTL activity per cell is constant (4), means that one can derive a very reproducible assay. The sensitivity of the assay is optimized using anti-Lyt-2 monoclonal antibodies (2) as prototype blocking antibodies. As Thy-1 is not required for cytolysis (5), specificity of the assay is monitored using an anti-Thy-1 monoclonal antibody (6) as a prototype non-blocking antibody. The parameters given here for B18 and L3 are based on the kinetics of lysis of the relevant $H\text{-}2^d$ tumor target P815 by these cloned CTL lines (Fig. 1).

Fig. 1A. Parameters of the blocking assay. Effector cells are pretreated either with monoclonal antibody or with 20% agamma horse serum (AGH) in Dulbecco's modified Eagle's medium (DMEM) for $\underline{A}$ minutes at 5°C. The cells are then assayed in a short-term ^{51}Cr-release assay for cytotoxicity against a given target cell. EDTA (10mM final concentration) is added after $\underline{B}$ minutes of incubation at 37°C. The amount of ^{51}Cr released into the supernatant is determined at $\underline{C}$ hours total incubation.

Fig. 1B, C. Kinetics of lysis of the relevant $H\text{-}2^d$ tumor target P815 by the cloned CTL line B18. A, B, and C are defined as in Figure 1A. The analysis here is carried out at an effector to target ratio of 4 (10,000 B18 : 2500 P815).

Fig. 1D, E. Kinetics of lysis of the relevant $H\text{-}2^d$ tumor target P815 by the cloned CTL line L3. A, B, and C are defined as in Figure 1A. The analysis here is carried out at an effector to target ratio of 2 (5000 L3 : 2500 P815).

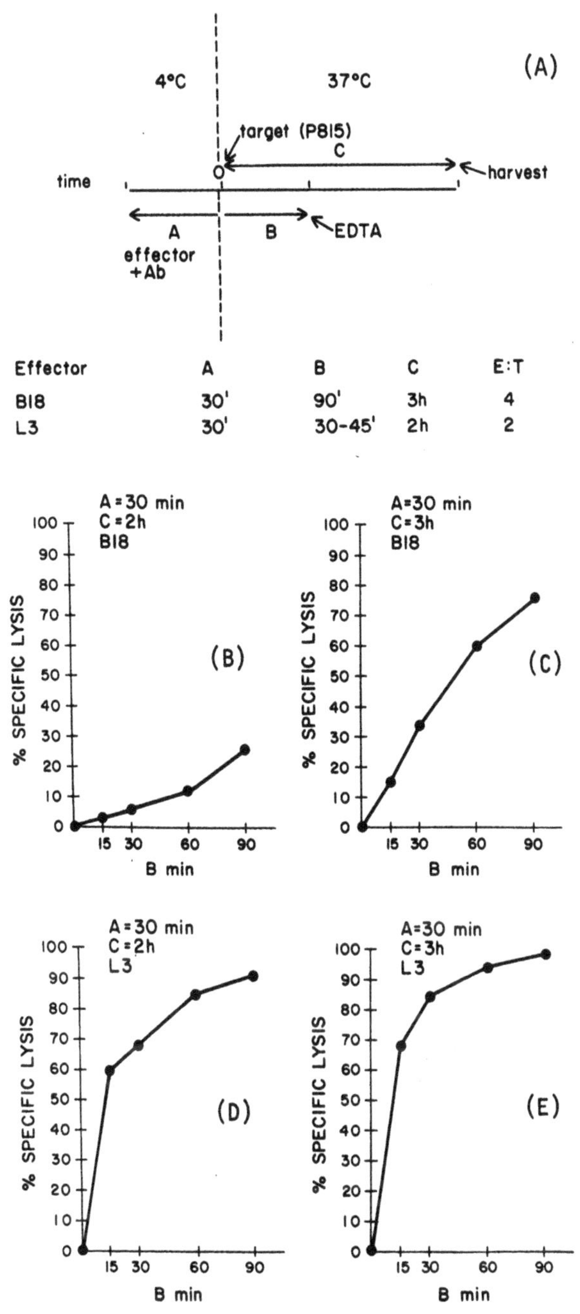
(A)
4°C
37°C
target (P815)
C
harvest
time
A
B
EDTA
effector
+Ab
Effector A B C E:T
B18 30' 90' 3h 4
L3 30' 30-45' 2h 2
A=30 min
C=2h
B18
(B)
% SPECIFIC LYSIS
B min
A=30 min
C=3h
B18
(C)
A=30 min
C=2h
L3
(D)
A=30 min
C=3h
L3
(E)

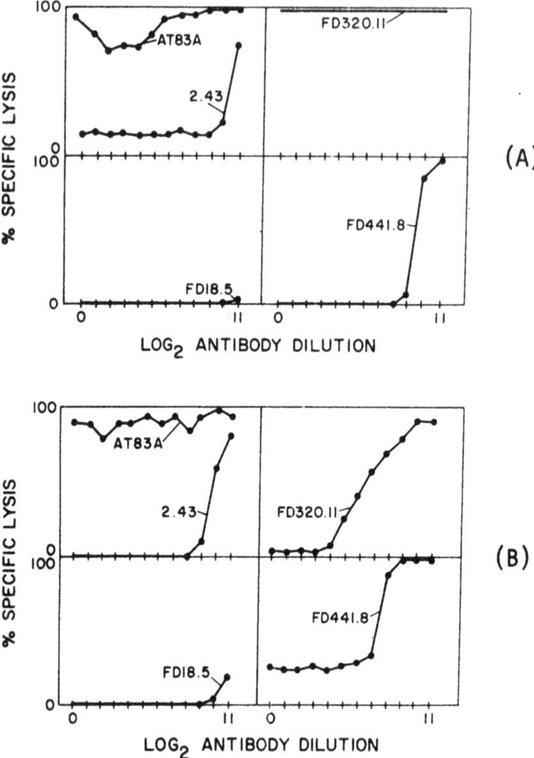

Fig. 2A. Titration of blocking activity of monoclonal antibodies on the cloned CTL line B18. The values of A, B, and C used here are those given for B18 in Figure 1A. This analysis was carried out at an effector to target cell ratio of 4 (10,000 B18 : 2,500 P815). Hybridoma culture SF was serially diluted as shown. Monoclonal antibody AT83A (IgM) is specific for Thy-1.2. Monoclonal antibody 2.43 (IgG2b) is specific for Lyt-2.2.

Fig. 2B. Titration of blocking activity of monoclonal antibodies on the cloned CTL line L3. The values of A and C used here are those given for L3 in Figure 1A; the value of B used here is 60 minutes. This analysis was carried out at an effector to target cell ratio of 2 (5,000 L3 : 2,500 P815). See the legend to Figure 2A for other details.

To obtain antibody-secreting hybridomas, we injected a Lewis rat intravenously three times, at two-week intervals, with B18 cells. Three days after the third injection, spleen cells from the rat were fused with drug-marked (HAT^s) SP2/0 myeloma cells (7). Seven days after culture under selective (HAT) conditions, SF from hybridoma wells were screened for the capacity to block receptor-mediated cytolysis of P815 by either B18 or L3. Hybridoma cells from those wells

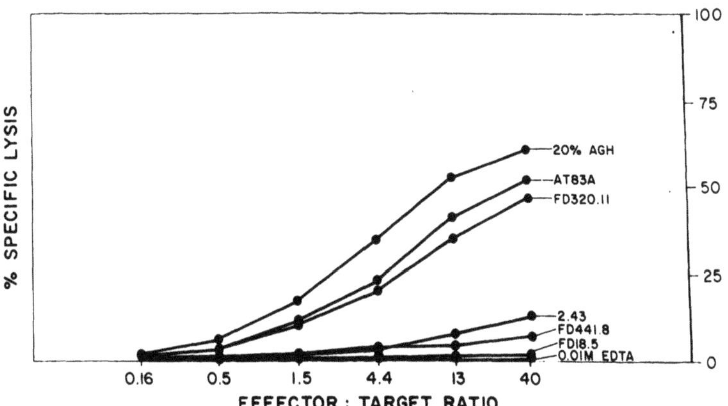

Fig. 3. Characterization of blocking activity of monoclonal antibodies of B10 anti-DBA/2 1° MLC Day 5 effector cells. The values of A, B, and C used here are 30 minutes, 30 minutes, and 2.5 hours respectively. Hybridoma culture SF was used undiluted. The effectors were serially diluted three-fold; 5000 P815 target cells were used. The negative control (unblocked curve) is defined by 20% AGH. The positive control (blocked curve) is defined by 0.01 M EDTA (EDTA was added immediately prior to the addition of target cells).

giving blocking were then cloned. Clones whose SF demonstrated blocking activity were expanded and the antibody they secreted characterized.

Seven such monoclonal antibodies currently being characterized fall into three groups as defined below. Group I (two antibodies) is represented by FD18.5. Group II (three antibodies) is represented by FD441.8. Group III (two antibodies) is represented by FD320.11. The antibodies in Groups I are IgG2a, and the antibodies in Groups II and III are IgG2b.

The grouping of these antibodies is based partly on the blocking profiles given in Figure 2. Antibodies in Group I can be distinguished from antibodies in Group II by analyzing blocking of receptor-mediated lysis of P815 by L3. Antibodies in Group III can be distinguished from antibodies in Groups I and II by analyzing blocking of receptor-mediated lysis of P815 by B18. For reference, the blocking activity of these antibodies directed against B10 anti-DBA/2 1° MLC day 5 effector cells is given in Figure 3. FD18.5, FD441.8, and FD320.11 also block receptor-mediated cytolysis by two TNP-reactive cloned CTL lines, one line restricted to H-$2D^{b,d,s}$ and the other line restricted to H-$2D^{b}$ (8).

SDS-PAGE analysis of immunoprecipitates under reducing conditions indicates that the antigen recognized by each of the antibodies

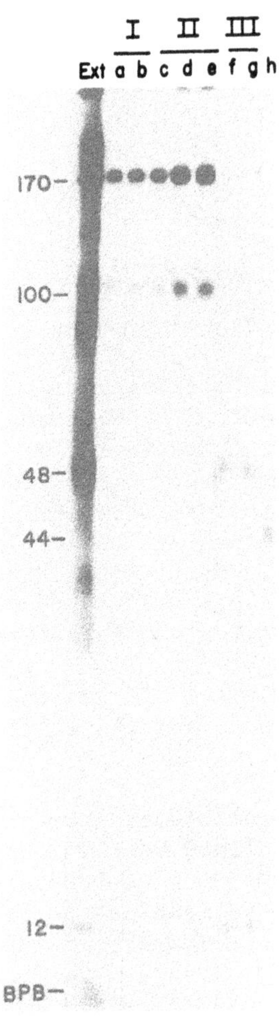

Fig. 4. Autoradiograph of proteins isolated from ^{125}I surface-labeled L3 cells by extraction with Nonidet P-40 and immune precipitation with monoclonal antibodies. Proteins were analyzed on a 12% SDS-(DATD)-polyacrylamide slab gel (14 X 24 X 0.075 cm). Ext: surface-labeled proteins extracted from L3 cells with Nonidet P-40. BPB: position of bromophenol blue. Group I: a, 18.5; b, 196.14. Group II: c, 251.10; d, 270.1; e, 441.8. Group III: f, 95.4; g, 320.11; h, 3.155 (anti-Lyt 2).

in Groups I and II consists of a 170,000 dalton molecular weight subunit and a 100,000 dalton molecular weight subunit (Figure 4). This, in conjunction with other data presented here, suggests that the antigen being recognized is analogous to the recently identified LFA-1 (9,10,11). The corresponding analysis for Group II antibodies, however, indicates that they recognize an antigen which consists of a 48,000 dalton molecular weight subunit and a 12,000 dalton molecular weight subunit. This, together with other data presented here, suggests that these antibodies recognize a framework H-2D/D determinant.

FACS analysis is consistent both with the interpretation of the SDS-PAGE data and with the distinction between Groups I and II based on the blocking data. Each of the antibodies in Group I, II and III stains essentially all cells from B10 spleen, lymph node, bone marrow, and thymus; they also stain the cloned CTL lines B18 and L3. Representative FACS curves are given in Figure 5. It is interesting that Group I antibodies, which appear to have the greater blocking activity based both on SF blocking titer and blocking activity on L3, characteristically appear to react with fewer sites on a given cell than do Group II antibodies. Each of these antibodies also stains B10 anti-DBA/2 1° MLC day 5 effector cells, B10 Con A blasts, B10 LPS blasts, and a cloned Mls^a-reactive amplifier T cell line, designated L2.

Several interesting questions remain to be resolved with respect to our anti-LFA-1 antibodies. Do Group I antibodies react with a subset of the molecules with which Group II antibodies react? Given that these antibodies were screened by a blocking assay, will they demonstrate restricted binding to only one of the subunits of the LFA-1 complex? Can these antibodies be used to generate an LFA-1$^-$ variant of the cloned CTL line L3, and what elements of the cytolytic pathway would be lost/retained (5)? Do any of these antibodies react with an allotypic marker of LFA-1, thus allowing preliminary genetic mapping of the structural gene? What necessary role, if any, does the LFA-1 complex play in cytolysis?

We have recently determined that these anti-LFA-1 monoclonal antibodies, which block receptor-mediated lysis by B18 and L3, also block Con A-mediated lysis of an irrelevant target cell by these cloned CTL. However, they do not block PHA-P-mediated lysis of an irrelevant target cell at least by the L3 CTL line. Therefore, these anti-LFA-1 monoclonal antibodies do not react with the active site responsible for the lethal hit. Whether or not this active site is elsewhere on the LFA-1 complex, or on an independent molecule, remains to be determined. The broad distribution of LFA-1 would argue for the latter case.

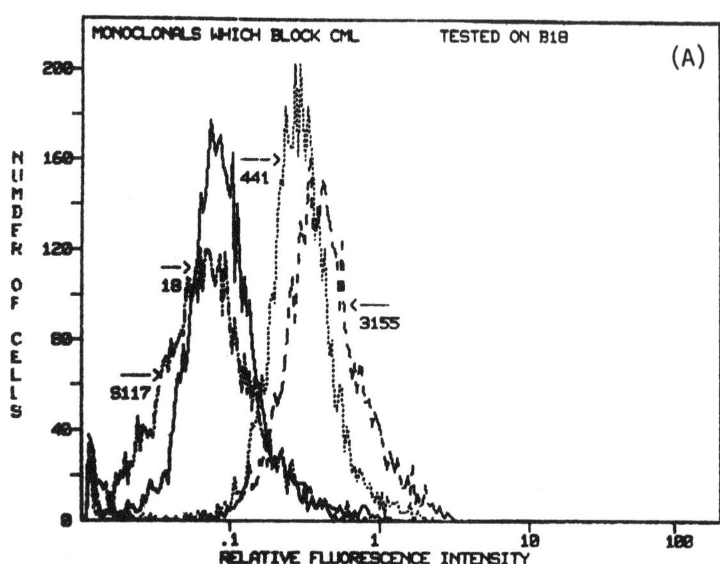

Fig. 5A. FACS analysis of binding of monoclonal antibodies by the cloned CTL line B18. The negative control is defined by S11.7, an inappropriate mouse monoclonal antibody (IgM) specific for H-2D^{d} (Sue Tonkonogy, Duke University); the second stage antibody in this instance was a fluorescein-conjugated rabbit anti-mouse Ig. The positive control is defined by biotin-conjugated 3.155, an IgM monoclonal antibody specific for Lyt-2; the second stage antibody in this instance was fluorescein-conjugated avidin. For FD18.5 and FD441.8, the second stage antibody was a fluorescein-conjugated mouse anti-rat Ig. Cells were analyzed by flow cytofluorometry using a modified FACS IV. In all experiments, 10^4 live cells as determined by exclusion of Propidium Iodide were analyzed. Results are expressed in histogram form with the ordinate representing cell number, and the abscissa representing the log of fluorescence intensity in arbitrary units where one decade is represented by each gradation along the x-axis.

Fig. 5B. FACS analysis of binding of monoclonal antibodies by the cloned CTL line L3. See the legend to Figure 5A for details.

Fig. 5C. FACS analysis of the binding of monoclonal antibodies by B10 spleen cells. The negative control is defined by using 20% AGH in the first stage. The positive control (not shown) is defined by using a monoclonal antibody specific for H-2K^{b}. The second stage antibody in these instances was a fluoresein-conjugated mouse anti-rat Ig. Cells were analyzed as described in Figure 5A.

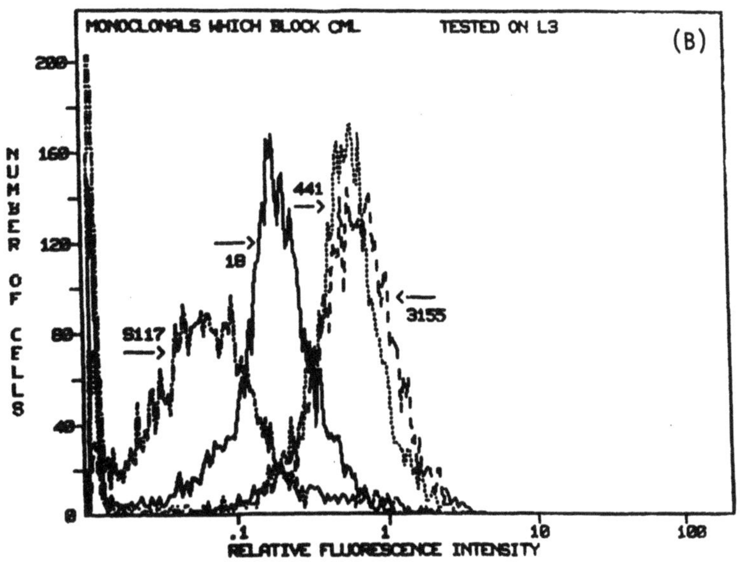
MONOCLONALS WHICH BLOCK CML
TESTED ON L3
(B)
NUMBER OF CELLS
200
160
120
80
40
0
S117
18
441
3155
.1
1
10
100
RELATIVE FLUORESCENCE INTENSITY

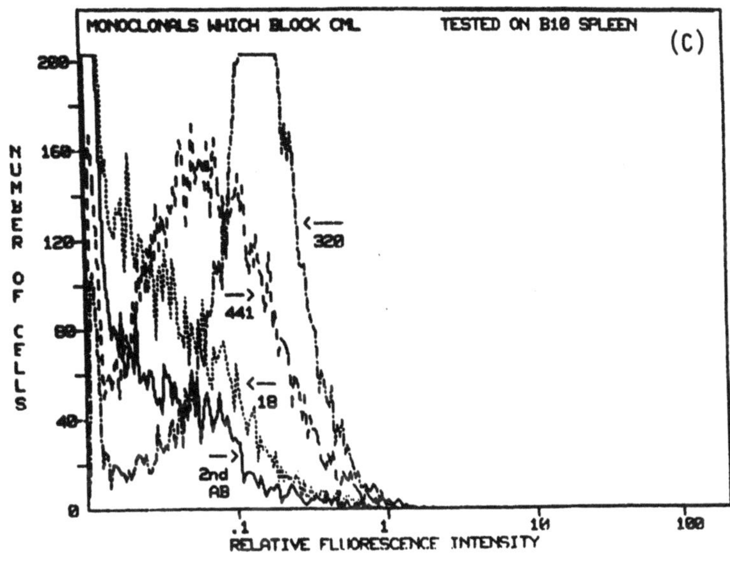
MONOCLONALS WHICH BLOCK CML
TESTED ON B10 SPLEEN
(C)
NUMBER OF CELLS
200
160
120
80
40
0
320
441
18
2nd AB
.1
1
10
100
RELATIVE FLUORESCENCE INTENSITY

ACKNOWLEDGMENTS

This research was supported by USPHS Grants AI-04197, AI-14872, and CA-19226. Deno Dialynas is supported by Training Grant 5T32-CA-09267. The authors gratefully acknowledge the technical assistance of Yukio Hamada, David Houck, LaVerne Decker, and Daisy Freeman. We also acknowledge the assistance of Frances Mills in the preparation of the manuscript.

REFERENCES

1. Geiger, B., K.L. Rosenthal, J. Klein, R.M. Zinkernagel, and S.J. Singer. Selective and unidirectional membrane redistribution of an H-2 antigen with an antibody-clustered viral antigen: Relationship to mechanisms of cytotoxic T-cell interactions. Proc. Natl. Acad. Sci. 76:4603. (1979)
2. Sarmiento, M., A.L. Glasebrook, and F.W. Fitch. IgG or IgM monoclonal antibodies reactive with different determinants on the molecular complex bearing Lyt2 antigen block T cell-mediated cytolysis in the absence of complement. J. Immunol. 125:2665. (1980)
3. Glasebrook, A.L., and F.W. Fitch. Alloreactive cloned T cell lines. I. Interactions between cloned amplifier and cytolytic T cell lines. J. Exp. Med. 151:876. (1980)
4. Glasebrook, A.L., and F.W. Fitch. T-cell lines which cooperate in the generation of specific cytolytic activity. Nature 278:171. (1979)
5. Dialynas, D.P., M.R. Loken, A.L. Glasebrook, and F.W. Fitch. Lyt-2^-/Lyt-3^- variants of a cloned cytolytic T cell line lack an antigen receptor functional in cytolysis. J. Exp. Med. 153:595. (1981)
6. Sarmiento, M., M.R. Loken, and F.W. Fitch. Structural differences in cell surface T25 polypeptide from thymocytes and cloned T cells. Hybridoma 1:13. (1981)
7. McKearn, T.J., F.W. Fitch, D.E. Smilek, M. Sarmiento, and F.P. Stuart. Properties of rat anti-MHC antibodies produced by cloned rat-mouse hybridomas. Immunol. Rev. 47:91. (1979)
8. Wall, K.A., and F.W. Fitch. Effects of concanavalin A pretreatment on cloned cytolytic cells. (This volume). (1982)
9. Kürzinger, K., T. Reynolds, R.N. Germain, D. DaVignon, E. Martz, and T.A. Springer. A novel lymphocyte function-associated antigen (LFA-1): Cellular distribution, quantitative expression, and structure. J. Immunol. 127:596. (1981)
10. Pierres, M., C. Goridis, and P. Golstein. Inhibition of murine T cell-mediated cytolysis and T cell prliferation by a rat monclonal antibody immunoprecipitating two lymphoid cell surface polypeptides of 94,000 and 180,000 molecular weight. Eur. J. Immunol. In press. (1981)
11. Trowbridge, I.S., and M.B. Omary. J. Exp. Med. In press. (1981)

A CLONE SPECIFIC MONOCLONAL ANTIBODY WHICH INHIBITS T CELL-MEDIATED CYTOLYSIS

David W. Lancki, Marc I. Lorber, Michael R. Loken,
and Frank W. Fitch

Department of Pathology
University of Chicago
Chicago, Illinois 60637

Functionally defined cloned T lymphocytes represent a homogeneous population of cells uniquely suited for the analysis of cell surface molecules involved in specific allorecognition. T cell clones expressing either cytolytic or amplifier functions have been derived in this laboratory from unidirectional secondary C57BL/6 anti-DBA/2 mixed lymphocyte culture (MLC) and have been maintained in long term culture (1). One cytolytic clone, designated L3, has been found to express cytolytic activity for the H-2D^d gene product (2). The L3 cell line has been used in the present study to derive and characterize a monoclonal antibody which reacts specifically with that cell line, and which is capable of inhibiting antigen specific cytolysis in the absence of complement.

Hybrid mouse-mouse cells were obtained by fusing spleen cells from a C57BL/6 x DBA/2 (BDF$_1$) mouse, which had been immunized with L3 cells, with the mouse SP2/0-Ag14 cell line (3). Supernatants from wells containing hybrid cells were screened for their ability to block the cytolytic activity of L3 against P815 mastocytes using a minor modification of the micro-blocking assay developed in this laboratory (by Dialynas, et al, this volume) for screening xenogeneic monoclonal antibodies against cloned cytolytic cell lines. One monoclonal antibody, FP384.5, strongly inhibited the cytolytic activity of L3 against P815 target cells. This antibody was further characterized for reactivity against L3, other cloned T lymphocytes and normal tissues.

Unlike other previously reported antibodies which inhibited T cell mediated cytolysis, the blocking activity observed with the monoclonal antibody FP384.5 is specific for the L3 cytolytic cell line. Figure 1 compares the effects of FP384.5 on the antigen

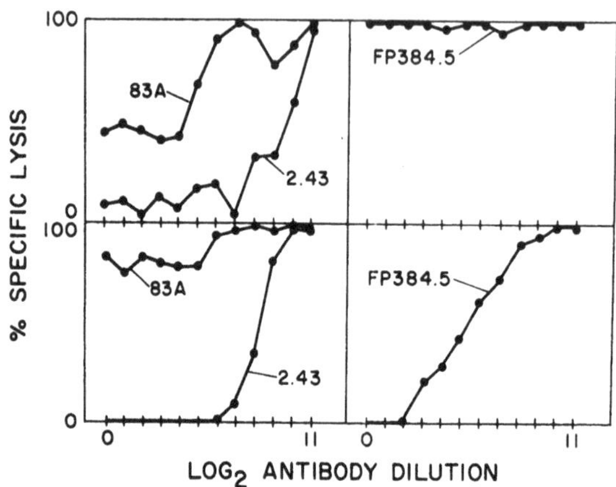

Fig. 1. Effects of FP384.5 monoclonal antibody and 2.43 (anti-Lyt-2.2) monoclonal antibody on the lytic activity of L3 and B18 cloned cytolytic cells. A fixed number of L3 (5×10^3) or B18 (1×10^4) cells were preincubated for 30 minutes at 4°C with various dilutions of 2.43 (anti-Lyt-2.2), 83A (anti-Thy-1.2), of FP384.5 supernatant fluids and tested for cytotoxicity against 2.5×10^3 ^{51}Cr-labeled P-815 target cells. After the addition of the target cells incubation at 37°C was continued for 90 minutes (18) or 60 minutes (L3) before the addition of EDTA to block further lytic activity. Incubations were continued at 37°C for a total of 180 minutes (B18) or 120 minutes (L3) before harvesting.

specific lytic activities of L3 and B18, a C57BL/6 cytolytic T cell clone specific for H-2K^d (2). L3 lytic activity was blocked over a range of FP384.5 antibody concentrations, while B18 lytic activity was unaffected over the same range of antibody concentrations. In contrast, a potent anti-Lyt-2.2 monoclonal antibody, 2.43, blocked both L3 and B18 cytolysis in a manner consistent with previous observations (4,5). The effects of an irrelevant (anti-Thyl.2) antigen specific antibody, 83A, are also shown for comparison in Figure 1. The specificity of the blocking activity of FP384.5 has been further tested using several other cloned cytolytic cell lines, including a cell line, 18.19, having specificity for TNP modified self (H-2^b) antigen, and a cell line, 38.5, reactive against TNP modified-alloantigen. The lytic activity of these clones was unaffected by FP384.5 antibody over a range of effector to target cell ratios (data not shown). The blocking activity of FP384.5 is further distinguished from the blocking observed with anti-Lyt-2 or anti-LFA antibodies in that FP384.5 does not strongly inhibit the cytolytic activity of five-day unidirectional C57BL/6 MLC cells responding to CBA, BA/2, B10.D2, or B10.A(5R) stimulating cells (Table I).

TABLE I. Failure of FP384.5 Monoclonal Antibody to Inhibit 5 Day MLC

			% Specific Lysis							
Target	Effector	E:T Ratio	20% AGH Exp.1	20% AGH Exp.2	AT83A Exp.1	AT83A Exp.2	2.43 Exp.1	2.43 Exp.2	FP384.5 Exp.1	FP384.5 Exp.2
P815	L3 Control	8		72.9		69.4		1.1		13.5
	0-1 B6αDBA/2	50	57.0		48.1		7.2		51.1	
		27		67.6		68.9		27.2		68.4
	0-1 B6αB10.D2	50	43.8		37.2		5.4		45.6	
		35		71.1		74.9		25.2		64.7
	0-1 B6αB10.A(5R)	50	37.7		31.7		8.2		38.5	
		33		65.4		67.5		19.5		53.5
AKR-A	0-1 B6αCBA	33		19.7		24.9		2.1		22.7

Effector cells obtained from the indicated MLC were preincubated with 20% AGH control or hybridoma culture supernatants (undiluted) for 30 minutes. The appropriate target cells (P815 or AKR-A) were added to the culture and the lytic reaction was allowed to proceed for 45 minutes. Lysis was stopped after 45 minutes by the addition of EDTA (5) and the incubation was continued for an additional 2 hours.

A recent investigation of anti-Lyt-2 blocking activity at the clonal level has indicated that the susceptibility of certain CTL clones to inhibition by anti-Lyt-2 antibodies does not correspond with the capacity of these clones to specifically bind the anti-Lyt-2 antibodies (6). We have investigated the correlation of blocking activity and the expression of the cell surface determinant detected by FP384.5. Cells were examined by indirect immunofluorescence using a fluorescence-activated cell sorter (FACS IV, BD FACS Systems, Mountain View, Calif.) equipped with a four decade logarithmic amplifier (Nozaki Assoc., Palo Alto, Calif.). Figure 2a shows the typical immunofluorescence profile observed with FP384.5 on the cloned L3 cells. The relative fluorescence intensity was 2.5 times greater than when L3 was reacted with an inappropriate third party antibody (data not shown) or with second antibody alone. The cytolytic clone B18 (Figure 2b) and other cytolytic or amplifier T cell clones (data not shown) did not stain with FP384.5. Blocking of L3 cytolysis of P815 mastocytes does not appear to be due to specific binding of FP384.5 to the target cell, since, FP384.5 does not stain P815 cells above the levels observed with inappropriate antibody controls.

The potential expression of FP384.5 determinants on nucleated normal tissues from C57BL/6 and BDF_1 mice was also investigated. The results shown in Figure 2c were obtained with C57BL/6 spleen cells; they indicate tht FP384.5 did not stain a detectable portion of the cell population. Similar results were obtained with the cells derived from C57BL/6 and BDF_1 lymph node, thymus and bone marrow preparations.

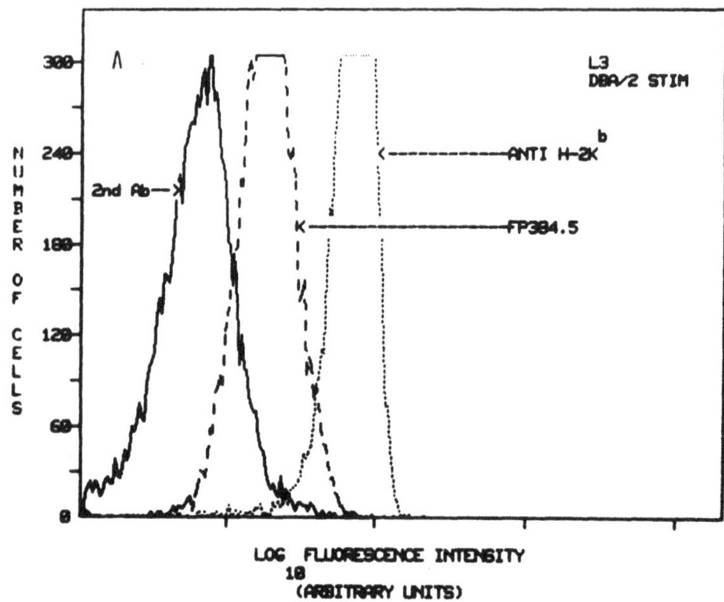

Fig. 2. Expression of cell surface FP384.5. Proliferating cultures of cloned cytolytic cells, L3 (panel A) or B18 (panel B), or normal lymph node cells of C57BL/6 origin (panel C) were harvested. Cells were centrifuged over a discontinuous Ficoll-Hypaque gradient (7), washed extensively, and distributed for fluorescence staining. A two stage technique was used with staining being accomplished at room temperature in the presence 0.2% sodium azide. The first stage antibody, FP384.5 or control monoclonal reagent as indicated, was incubated under saturating conditions with 10^6 cells for 15 minutes. The second stage antibody was a fluorescein-conjugated rabbit anti- mouse Ig in all experiments. Cells were analyzed by flow cytofluorometry using a modified FACS IV as described in the text. In all experiments, 10^4 live cells as determined by exclusion of Propidium Iodide were analyzed (8). Results are expressed in histogram form with the ordinate representing cell number, and the abscissa representing the log of fluorescence intensity in arbitrary units where one decade is represented by each gradation along the x-axis.

The results obtained using two analytical approaches, antibody blocking of cytolytic activity and antibody binding, suggest that the monoclonal antibody FP384.5 is clone specific. The specificity of reaction distinguishes FP384.5 from other classes of blocking antibodies, including anti-Lyt-2 and anti-LFA antibodies. Although the determinant detected by FP384.5 is distinct from those detected by other blocking antibodies, the nature of the molecule bearing

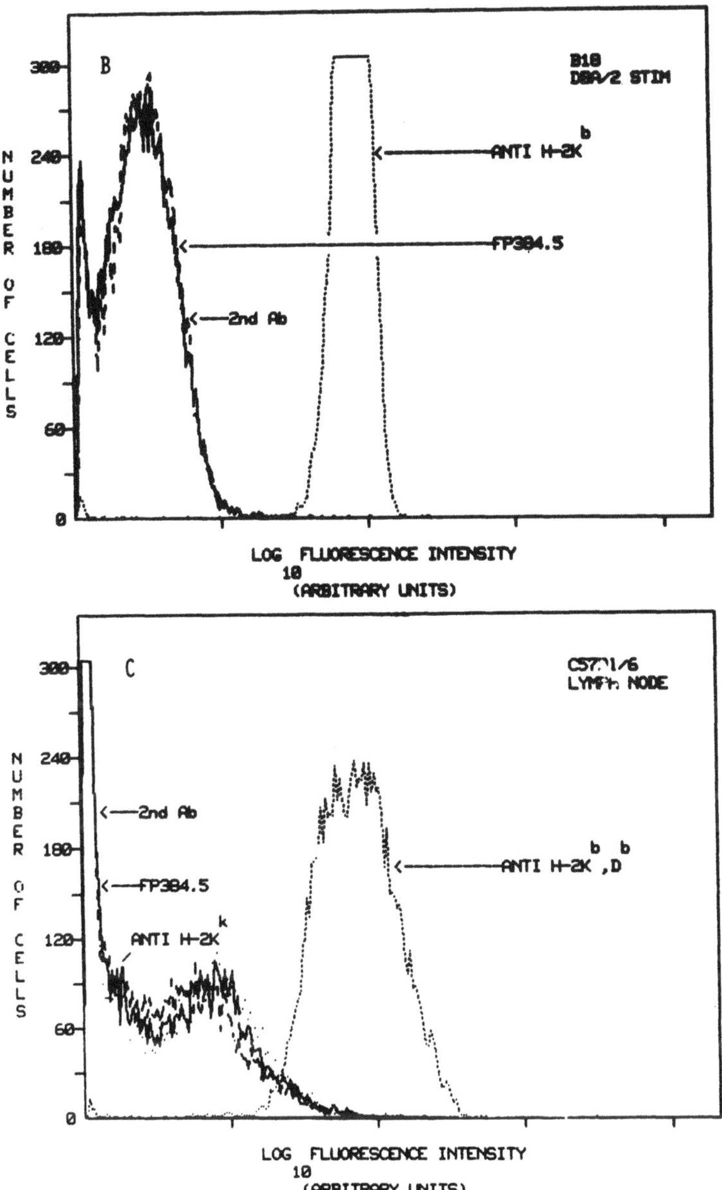

the determinant remains to be established. The ability of FP384.5 to block L3 cytolysis suggests that this antibody recognizes a clone specific determinant closely associated with the cytolytic response. The unique interpretation of these observations is at present premature, however, it is possible that the determinant detected by FP384.5 represents an idiotypic determinant on the molecule (T cell receptor) which imparts specificity in the L3 cytolytic response.

ACKNOWLEDGMENTS

This research was supported by USPHS Grants AI-04197, AI-14872, and CA-19226. David W. Lancki is supported by Training Grant 5T32-GM-07543. Marc I. Lorber is the recipient of American Cancer Society Postdoctoral Fellowship #PF-2049. The authors gratefully acknowledge the technical assistance of Yukio Hamada, David Houck, LaVerne Decker, and Daisy Freeman. We also acknowledge the assistance of Frances Mills in the preparation of the manuscript.

REFERENCES

1. Glasebrook, A.L., and F.W. Fitch. T cell lines which cooperate in the generation of specific cytolytic activity. Nature 278:171. (1979)
2. Glasebrook, A.L., and F.W. Fitch. Alloreactive cloned T cell lines. I. Interactions between cloned amplifier and cytolytic T cell lines. J. Exp. Med. 151:876. (1980)
3. McKearn, T.J., F.W. Fitch, D.E. Smilek, M. Sarmiento, and F.P. Stuart. Properties of rat anti-MHC antibodies produced by cloned rat-mouse hybridomas. Immunol. Rev. 47:91. (1979)
4. Nakayama, E., H. Shiku, E. Stockert, H.F. Oettgen, and L.J. Old. Cytotoxic T cells: Lyt phenotype and blocking of killing activity by Lyt antisera. Proc. Natl. Acad. Sci. 76:1977. (1979)
5. Sarmiento, M., A.L. Glasebrook, and F.W. Fitch. IgG or IgM monoclonal antibodies reactive with different determinants on the molecular complex bearing Lyt-2 antigen block T cell mediated cytolysis in the absence of complement. J. Immunol. 125:2665. (1980)
6. MacDonald, H.R., N. Thiernesse, and J.-C. Cerottini. Inhibition of T cell-mediated cytolysis by monoclonal antibodies directed against Lyt-2: heterogeneity of inhibition at the clonal level. J. Immunol. 126:1651. (1981)
7. Davidson, W.F., and C.R. Parish. A procedure for removing red cells and dead cells from lymphoid cell suspensions. J. Immunol. Methods 7:291. (1975)
8. Krishan, A. Rapid flow cytofluorometric analysis of mammalian cell cycle by propidium iodide staining. J. Cell Biol. 66:188. (1975)

INHIBITION OF HUMAN T CELL MEDIATED CYTOLYSIS BY MONOCLONAL ANTIBODIES TO EFFECTOR CELL SURFACE STRUCTURES

Bernard Malissen, Claude Mawas and Najet Rebai

Centre d'Immunologie INSERM-CNRS de Marseille-Luminy
Case 906
13288 Marseille Cedex 9 - France

Monoclonal antibody (mAb) technology has recently permitted the delineation of human functional T cell compartments involved in the generation of T and B cell responses (for review see 1,2,3). Most of these mAb were initially selected for their differential staining of lymphoid or T cell subpopulations. This approach relies on the assumption that the cellular distribution of some cell surface antigens matches the occurrence of given immunological functions. Nevertheless, when introduced in the absence of complement in functional assays such as T cell mediated cytolysis or specific proliferation to soluble or cellular antigens, only a small percentage of these functional subset-discriminating mAb was shown to modulate immunological functions and thus to define "Lymphocyte functionassociated antigens" (4).

In order to directly relate cell surface molecule(s) to given immunological functions we have recently developed a protocol in which mAb were selected for their ability to inhibit specific human T cell mediated cytolysis in the absence of complement, rather than for their restricted binding to cloned lines of human cytotoxic T lymphocytes.

After a brief review of the cytolysis-inhibitory mAb reported in the literature, a description will be given of some of our results obtained using the above-mentioned protocol. MAb inhibiting human T cell-mediated cytolysis by interfering with target structures (5) are outside the scope of this review.

mAb SELECTED FOR THEIR BINDING TO HUMAN T CELL STRUCTURES AND SUBSEQUENTLY SHOWN TO HAVE CYTOLYSIS-INHIBITING ACTIVITY

Several mAb recognizing T cell antigens were recently found to inhibit the effector phase of specific T cell mediated cytolysis. The characteristics of these blocking mAb are summarized in Table I. Effector cells were generally incubated at room temperature from 30 min. (6,7) to 2 hr (8) in the presence of various dilutions of mAb before addition of target cells. Target cells were usually PHA-stimulated lymphocytes.

Except for an early report (9) in which no cytolysis inhibiting effect was observed, OKT3 mAb (10,11) appeared as the most potent and constant inhibitor of specific T cell cytolysis. In addition, this mAb was previously shown (9) to block: (a) T cell specific proliferative responses to conventional and alloantigens, (b) generation of cytotoxic T cells when added at the initiation of mixed lymphocyte culture, and (c) ability of T cells to provide help for B cell Ig secretion in a pokeweed mitogen-driven system. On the other hand, OKT3 mAb was demonstrated to be a potent peripheral human T cell mitogen (12) when the cells were grown in xenogeneic serum but not in human plasma (6); it is not yet clear how to reconcile the above-mentioned data showing either inhibition or stimulation of human T cell proliferation by OKT3 mAb.

The other mAb described in Table I: OKT5 (13,14), OKT8 (15), Leu-2a and Leu-2b (8,16) were shown to define different epitopes of the same cell surface structure by competitive binding experiments (17). On ^{125}I-labeled peripheral T cells, this 76,000 dalton unreduced glycoprotein resolved under reducing conditions into a 32,000 dalton band occasionally appearing as a 30,000-32,000 dalton doublet (A. Van Aghtoven, personal communication). Comparative quantitative changes during T cell maturation, comparative tissue distribution and comparative biochemistry all have indicated (16) that this human cytotoxic/suppressor cell surface structure presented a strong homology with the murine Lyt-2 and Lyt-3 antigens. The fact that killing in CML was more effectively blocked by Leu-2a mAb than by Leu-2b mAb is compatible with the recognition by Leu-2a of a critical epitope of the antigen "closely associated with cytotoxic function" (8).

mAb SELECTED FOR THEIR ABILITY TO BLOCK THE CYTOTOXIC ACTIVITY OF CLONED LINES OF HUMAN CYTOTOXIC T LYMPHOCYTES (CTL)

From peripheral blood lymphocytes of volunteers hyperimmunized with cells from a selected donor, a collection of cloned CTL lines was established (18). Clones specific for HLA-A2, HLA-Cw3 and HLA-Bw60 were isolated. All have been stable as regards fine specificity and lytic activity for more than 16 months. They are E rosette pos-

TABLE I. Characteristics of monoclonal antibodies which block human T lymphocyte mediated cytolysis in the absence of complement

Reference	Monoclonal Antibody	Specificity	Cytotoxic combination and target used for blocking studies	Binding to target
Chang et al., 1981 (6)	OKT3	Detects a 19,000 mol. wt. glycoprotein expressed on all circulating peripheral T cells and on MLC responsive thymocytes.	Peripheral mononuclear cells stimulated against an Epstein-Barr virus transformed B cell line or against allogeneic mononuclear cells. Cytotoxicity tested after a 6 day MLC on EBV transformed cells. OKT3 caused more than 90% inhibition of cell lysis whereas OKT8 and OKT5 (see below) caused slight inhibition (20-30%).	No (see Ref. 10)
Platsoucas and Good 1981 (7)	OKT5 OKT8	Define approximately 80% of thymocytes and 25-35% of peripheral T cells (cytotoxic/suppressor subset). Precipitate from ^{35}S-labeled PHA-activated T lymphocytes a 76K glycoprotein under non-reducing conditions and a 30-32K doublet under reducing conditions.	Peripheral mononuclear cells stimulated with allogeneic mononuclear cells in primary or secondary MLC cytotoxicity tested on day 7 (1° MLC) or on day 3 (2° MLC) using PHA stimulated blasts. Significant but moderate inhibition of the specific cytotoxicity by the OKT5 and OKT8 mAb was only observed in some experiments.	n.d.
	OKT3	See above	Significant and consistent inhibition of the specific cytotoxicity by OKT mAb.	
Evans et al. 1981 (8)	αLeu-2A αLeu-2b	Cross-blocking experiments indicate that these 2 mAb define the same surface antigen expressed on 22-46% of peripheral T cells and 57-84% of thymocytes. They recognize on iodinated PBL a 32K molecule under reducing conditions. Analysis under non-reducing conditions revealed that the 32K subunit(s) are disulfide-bonded into a variety of multimeric forms.	Same cytotoxic combination and target as in Platsoucas and Good (1981). Specific cytolysis blocked by Leu-2a and to a lesser extent by Leu-2b.	n.d.
Malissen et al. (this paper and 20)	B9.1 B9.2 B9.3 B9.4 B9.7 B9.8 B9.11	These 7 mAb define at least 4 different epitopes of the same structure and precipitate from ^{125}I-labeled CTL clones a 30K molecule under reducing conditions and a major band of ca. 76K under non-ducing conditions.	Cloned CTL lines derived from an in vivo allosensitized individual and tested either on PHA activated cells or on EBV-transformed B cell lines. Heterogeneity of inhibition at the clonal level.	See text

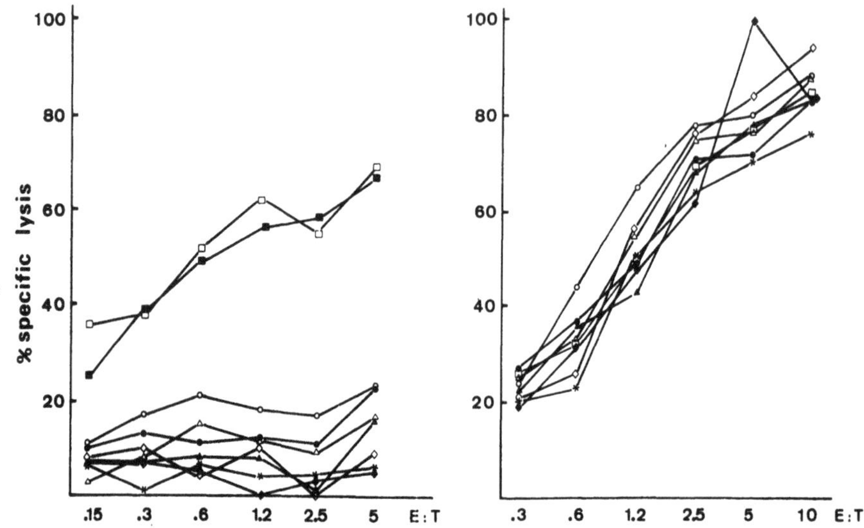

Fig. 1. Differential effect of various monoclonal antibodies on lytic activity of two CTL clones derived from the same individual and respectively directed to HLA-A2 (left panel) or to HLA-Cw3 (right panel). Various dilutions of effector cells were incubated for 30 min. at room temperature in the presence of 1/4 final dilution of supernatant fluid from cloned hybridomas B9.1 (○), B9.2 (●), B9.3 (▲), B9.4 (◆), B9.7 (◇), B9.8 (△), B9.11 (*) and B8.12.2 (anti-HLA-DR monomorphic, ■). Specific lysis in the presence of HAT selective medium alone is represented by open squares. Cytotoxicity was assayed on HLA-A2, Cw3 positive PHA blasts.

itive, surface immunoglobulin negative, Fc and C3b,d receptor negative, HLA-A, B, C and β2m positive. They were also found Ia-like-positive using either alloantibodies (19) or xeno-monoclonal antibodies for detection (18; and manuscript in preparation). In an attempt to raise mAb interacting with the specific cytolytic activity of CTL clones, BALB/c mice were immunized with cells from a human anti-HLA-A2 specific CTL clone; mAb derived from the immunized animals were initially screened for their ability to block the cytotoxic activity of the immunizing CTL clone. Effector cells (50 μl) were preincubated for 30 min. at room temperature with 50 μl of mAb supernatants; 100 μl of ^{51}Cr-labeled PHA activated target cells were then added. ^{51}Cr release was measured after 4 H of incubation at 37°C. An anti-HLA-DR mAb (B8.12.2) reacting with 100% of cloned cytotoxic T cells wa used to demonstrate that CTL performed lysis without measurable alteration even when large amounts of "irrelevant" mAb were bound to their surface. Seven mAb (B9.1,

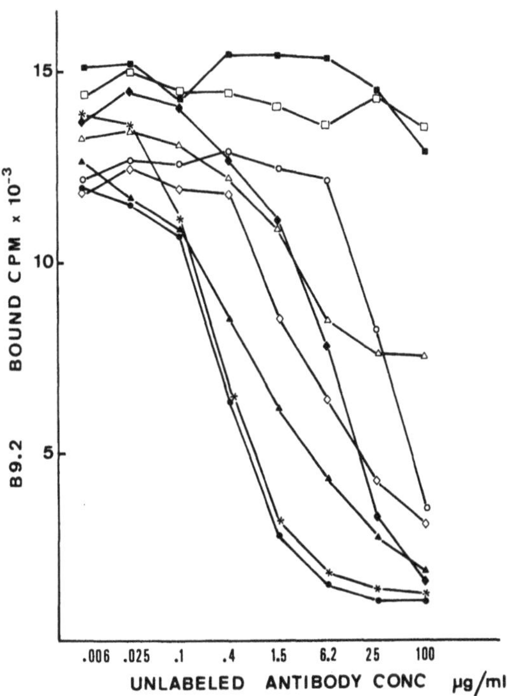

Fig. 2. Autoradiograph of SDS-PAGE analysis of surface-iodinated CTL clone proteins immunoprecipitated by mAb. An anti-HLA-A2 CTL clone was surface labeled with ^{125}I using the glucose oxidase modification of the lactoperoxidase technique, extracted with NP40 detergent and immunoprecipitated with mAb for analysis on 10% SDS-polyacrylamide gels run under reducing conditions. Immunoprecipitations were with the following mAb: A : B9.1; B : B9.2; C : B9.4; D : B9.7; E : B9.8; F : B9.12 (anti-HLA heavy chain); G : B9.3; H : B9.11; I : background (staph A coated with an anti-I-A^k mAb); J : B8.12.2 (anti HLA-DR monomorphic mAb); and K : B1.1.G6 (anti-β2m). The positions of molecular weight marker proteins are indicated at the right: (1) phosphorylase a, 94,000; (2) bovine serum albumin, 68,000; (3) actin, 42,000; (4) DNAse I, 31,000; (5) carbohydrase, 29,000; (6) trypsin inhibitor, 22,500; (7) cytochrome C, 12,500.

B9.2, B9.3, B9.4, B9.7, B9.8 and B9.11 shortened below to B9.1 to B9.11) were selected on the basis of their strong cytolysis inhibiting activity (Fig. 1, left panel); they pertained to various immunoglobulin isotypes (IgG1, IgG2a, IgG2b and IgG3). Results obtained with this panel of blocking mAb (20) may be summarized as follows.

Cytolysis-inhibiting Effects of B9.1 to B9.11 mAb Were Exerted at the Effector Cell Level.

B9.1 to B9.11 mAb stained about 20% of 5 day PHA-activated peripheral mononuclear cells used as target cells. Since mAb bound to target cell antigens such as HLA (5) were previously reported to block CTL mediated lysis it was important to use effector/target cell combinations in which mAb did not bind to the target cells. Epstein-Barr virus transformed B cell lines used in our laboratory did not bind mAb B9.1 to B9.11 as shown by cytofluorometric analysis; in addition, they were specifically lysed by our cloned CTL lines, in contrast to the results obtained using uncloned MLC combinations (unpublished observations). Their utilization as target cells did not impair the ability of the B9.1 to B.911 mAb to inhibit cytolysis. This strongly suggests that the cytolysis inhibiting effect of these mAb was exerted at the effector cell level.

Preliminary Biochemical Characterization Showed That B9.1 to B9.11 Precipitated the Same Macromolecule (Fig. 2)

The polypeptide immunoprecipitated from the ^{125}I-labeled immunizing CTL cloned line had an apparent molecular weight of 30,000 in SDS polyacrylamide gel run under reducing conditions. Analysis under non-reducing conditions revealed that the 30K reduced subunit was disulfide bonded into multimeric forms.

Topological Analysis of the Epitopes Detected by B9.1 to B9.11 mAb

Competitive binding studies (Fig. 3) were performed as previously described (21); they indicated together with comparative phylogenetic distribution of the recognized structure (M. Jonker et al., in preparation), that the seven mAb were defining at least four different epitopes on the same molecule.

Heterogeneity of Inhibition by B9.1 to B9.11

When analyzed on a large panel of CTL clones derived from an in vivo allosensitized donor (18), B9.1 to B9.11 mAb were only able to inhibit 10% of the CTL clones. This heterogeneity of inhibition could be demonstrated on a large range of effector-to-target ratios as well as on a wide range of mAb concentrations. This phenomenon did not change with time during clonal expansion, which argues against transient differences linked to growth phases of the cloned cells.

Flow cytofluorometric analysis indicated that both inhibited and uninhibited CTL clones expressed comparable amounts of the antigens recognized by these mAb. The inhibition was not related to the HLA-A, B or C specificity or to the lytic activity of the CTL clones.

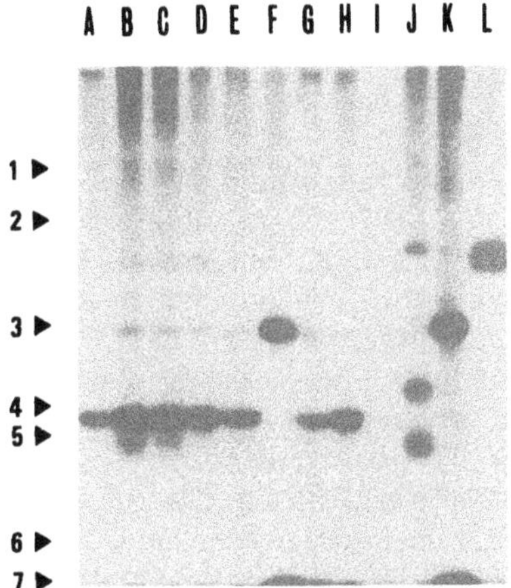

Fig. 3. Competitive inhibition of binding of ^{125}I labeled B9.2 mAb to PHA activated blasts by the following cold mAb: B9.1 (o); B9.2 (•); B9.3 (▲); B9.4 (♦); B9.7 (◇); B9.8 (△); B9.11 (*); B8.12.2 (anti-HLA-DR monomorphic mAb, ■) and B9.12 (anti-HLA-heavy chain, □).

DISCUSSION

Analysis of the B9.1 to B9.11 mAb on CTL clones revealed a heterogeneity in their cytolysis-inhibiting effect. Similar experiments done in mice (22) with anti-Lyt-2 mAb, have demonstrated that the majority of CTL clones derived from spleen primary MLC were inhibited by anti-Lyt-2 mAb, whereas only 15% of CTL clones derived from alloimmune peritoneal exudate lymphocytes were significantly inhibited at an equivalent mAb concentration. Our findings may explain the fact that inhibiton of the specific cytolysis of MLC populations by the OKT5/OKT8 mAb (7) was only observed in some experiments: this inconsistency may reflect fluctuating ratios of blocked to unblocked CTL from experiment to experiment in a given population.

Thus, interaction of B9.1 to B9.11 mAb with CTL surface structures is not sufficient for inhibition of cytotoxicity to occur; the corresponding structures may have different "functional connections" (23) from one CTL clone to another. Alternatively, CTL clones may differ otherwise than by the functional connections of these structures, and still be different as to their inhibitability by these mAb. The analysis of the OKT phenotype of human cytotoxic T cells from mixed lymphocyte cultures or from cloned cytotoxic T cell lines has also led to puzzling results. Functional studies on FACS separated lymphocytes showed that cytotoxic T effector cells sensitized in MLC were contained in the $OKT4^-$, 8^+ compartment, whereas inducer/helper T lymphocytes were phenotypically distinct and defined as $OKT4^+,8^-$ (13,24). On the other hand, study of the OKT phenotype of cytotoxic T cell clones (25) revealed that only 1 out of 8 CTL clones analyzed corresponded to the $OKT4^-,8^+$ phenotype; in addition, 3 out of the 6 $OKT8^-$ CTL clones were shown to express the OKT4 antigen. A similar $OKT4^+,8^-$ phenotype was found for an anti-HLA-A29 cloned cytotoxic T cell line (J.J. Van der Poel, personal communication). Analysis with mAb of Ia-like antigens on human cytotoxic T cells has led to the same type of discrepancy. Early work on Ia^+ and Ia^- MLC subpopulations indicated either that the Ia^+ subset included the cytotoxic effector cells (26) or that Ia^+ and Ia^- subsets exhibited similar levels of specific cytolytic activity (27). However, it was later found that all examined short-term (25) or long-term (18,19 and manuscript in preparation) in vitro maintained CTL clones were clearly Ia positive. It could be that the clonal growth promoters used (conditioned medium or mitogen stimulated PBL) favored the development of Ia^+ lymphocytes. However, as for the tissue distribution of the Lyt-1 antigen in mice (28,29), possible differences in the sensitivity of the various methods of detection and of separation used must also be considered.

In conclusion, mAb technology has now clearly permitted the definition of two human T cell surface structures associated with the inhibition of specific T cell-mediated cytolysis. OKT3 mAb interaction with a 19,000 dalton molecule may affect other immunological functions such as specific proliferation and T cell help, in addition to CML. A large panel of mAb (OKT5, OKT8, Leu-2a, Leu-2b and B9.1 to B9.11) defines another structure or a group of related structures (30,000-32,000 daltons under reduced form and ca. 76,000 daltons under non-reduced form), probably equivalent to the murine Lyt-2, Lyt-3 antigens. Analysis of B9.1 to B9.11 mAb cytolysis inhibiting effect at the level of CTL clones revealed an heterogeneity in the inhibition not simply linked to the presence or to the absence of these antigens on CTL clones. Similar findings were initially reported in mice using mAb directed against Lyt-2 (22). Selection of cytolysis-inhibiting mAb using "B9.1 to B9.11 unblocked CTL clones" will allow, by avoiding the selection of anti-Lyt-2/Lyt-3 like mAb, to probe for other T cell cytolysis associated structures.

ACKNOWLEDGEMENTS

This work was supported by INSERM (CRL 79.5.118.1) and DGRST (80.7.0218).

REFERENCES

1. Reinherz, E.L., and S.F. Schlossman. The differentiation and function of human T lymphocytes. Cell 19:821 (1980).
2. Haynes, B.F. Human T lymphocyte antigens as defined by monoclonal antibodies. Immunological Rev. 57:127 (1981).
3. Reinherz, E.L., and S.F. Schlossman. The characterization and function of human immunoregulatory T lymphocyte subsets. Immunology Today 69-75 (1981).
4. Davignon, D., Martz, E., Reynolds, T., Kürzinger, K., and T.A. Springer. Monoclonal antibody to a novel lymphocyte function-associated antigen (LFA-1): mechanism of blockade of T lymphocyte-mediated killing and effects on other T and B lymphocyte functions. J. Immunol. 127:590 (1981).
5. McMichael, A.J., Parham, P., Brodsky, F.M., and J.R. Pilch. Influenza virus-specific cytotoxic T lymphocytes recognize HLA molecules. Blocking by monoclonal anti-HLA antibodies. J. Exp. Med. 152:1955 (1980).
6. Chang, T.S., Kung, P.C., Gingras, S.P., and G. Goldstein. Does OKT3 monoclonal antibody react with a antigen-recognition structure on human T cells? Proc. Natl. Acad. Sci. USA 78: 1805 (1981).
7. Platsoucas, C.D., and R.A. Good. Inhibition of specific cell-mediated cytotoxicity by monoclonal antibodies to human T cell antigens. Proc. Natl. Acad. Sci. USA 78:4368 (1981).
8. Evans, R.L., Wall, D.W., Platsoucas, C.D., Siegal, F.P., Fifrig, S.M., Testa, C.M., and R.A. Good. Thymus-dependent membrane antigens in man: inhibition of cell-mediated lympholysis by monoclonal antibodies to TH2 antigen. (1981).
9. Reinherz, E.L., Hussey, R.E., and S.F. Schlossman. A monoclonal antibody blocking human T cell function. Eur. J. Immunol. 10:758 (1980).
10. Kung, P.C., Goldstein, G., Reinherz, E.L., and S.F. Schlossman. Monoclonal antibodies defining distinctive human T cell surface antigens. Science 206:347 (1979).
11. Van Agthoven, A., Terhorst, C., Reinherz, E., and S.F. Schlossman. Characterization of T cell surface glycoproteins T1 and T3 present on all human peripheral T lymphocytes and functionally mature thymocytes. Eur. J. Immunol. 11:18 (1981).
12. Reinherz, E.L., Kung, P.C., Goldstein, G., and S.F. Schlossman. A monoclonal antibody reactive with the human cytotoxic/suppressor T cell subset previously defined by a hetero antiserum termed TH2. J. Immunol. 124:1301 (1980).
13. Terhorst, C., Van Agthoven, A., Reinherz, E., and S.F. Schlossman. Biochemical analysis of human T lymphocyte differentiation antigens T4 and T5. Science 209:520 (1980).
14. Reinherz, E.L., Kung, P.C., Goldstein, G., Levey, R.H., and S.F. Schlossman. Discrete stages of human intrathymic differentiation: analysis of normal thymocytes and leukemic lymphoblasts of T-cell lineage. Proc. Natl. Acad. Sci. USA 77:1588 (1980).

15. Ledbetter, J.A., Evans, R.L., Lipinski, M., Cunningham-Rundles, C., Good, R.A., and L.A. Herzenberg. Evolutionary conservation of surface molecules that distinguish T lymphocyte helper/inducer and cytotoxic/suppressor subpopulations in mouse and man. J. Exp. Med. 153:310 (1981).
16. Van Wauwe, J.P., De Mey, J.R., and J.G. Goossens. OKT3: a monoclonal anti-human T lymphocyte antibody with potent mitogenic properties. J. Immunol. 124:2708 (1980).
17. Platsoucas, C.D., and R.A. Good. Inhibition of specific cell mediated cytotoxicity by monoclonal antibodies to human T cell antigens in the absence of complement. In "Mechanism of lymphocyte activation." Proceedings from the 14th Leucocyte Culture Conference. Elsevier-North/Holland, in press (1981).
18. Malissen, B., Kristensen, T., Goridis, C., Madsen, M., and C. Mawas. Clones of human cytotoxic T lympocytes derived from an allosensitized individual. HLA specificity and cell surface markers. Scand. J. Immunol., in press (1981).
19. Goulmy, E., Blokland, E., Van Rood, J.J., Charmot, D., Malissen, B., and C. Mawas. Production, expansion and clonal analysis of T cells with specific HLA restricted male lysis. J. Exp. Med. 152:182s (1980).
20. Malissen, B., Rebai, N., Mawas, C., and A. Liabeuf. Human cytotoxic T cell clone structures associated with expression of cytolysis. Analysis at the clonal cell level of the cytolysis inhibiting effect of 7 monoclonal antibodies. Submitted for publication.
21. Pierres, M., Rebouah, J.P., Kourilsky, F.M., Dosseto, M., Mercier, P., Mawas, C., and B. Malissen. Cross-reactions between mouse Ia^k and human DR antigens analyzed with monoclonal mouse alloantibodies. J. Immunol. 126:2424 (1981).
22. MacDonald, H.R., Thiernesse, N., and J.C. Cerottini. Inhibition of T cell-mediated cytolysis by monoclonal antibodies against Lyt-2: heterogeneity of inhibition at the clonal level. J. Immunol. 126:1671 (1981).
23. Golstein, P., Pierres, M., Schmitt-Verhulst, A.M., Luciani, M.F., Buferne, M., Eshhar, Z., and Y. Kaufmann. Functional relationships of lymphocyte membrane structures probed with cytolysis and/or proliferative inhibiting H35-27.9 and H35-89.9 monoclonal antibodies. Submitted for publication.
24. Reinherz, E.L., Kung, P.C., Goldstein, G., and S.F. Schlossman. Separation of functional subsets of human T cells by a monoclonal antibody. Proc. Natl. Acad. Sci. USA 76;4061 (1979).
25. Moretta, L., Mingari, M.C., Sekaly, P.R., Moretta, A., Chapuis, B., and J.C. Cerottini. Surface markers of cloned human T cells with various cytolytic activities. J. Exp. Med. 154: 569 (1981).
26. Reinherz, E.L., Hussey, R.E., and S.F. Schlossman. Absence of expression of Ia antigen on human cytotoxic T cells. Immunogenetics 11:421 (1980).

27. Moretta, A., Mingari, M.C., Haynes, B.F., Sekaly, R.P., Moretta, L., and A.S. Fauci. Phenotypic characterization of human cytolytic T lymphocytes generated in mixed lymphocyte culture. J. Exp. Med. 153:213 (1981).
28. Nakayama, E., Shiku, H., Stockert, E., Oettgen, H.F., and L.F. Old. Cytotoxic T cells: Lyt phenotype and blocking of killing activity by Lyt antisera. Proc. Natl. Acad. Sci. USA 76:1977 (1979).
29. Ledbetter, J.A., Rouse, R.V., Micklem, H. Spedding, and L.A. Herzenberg. T cell subsets defined by expression of Lyt-1, 2, 3 and Thy-1 antigens. Two-parameter immunofluorescence and cytotoxicity analysis with monoclonal antibodies modifies current views. J. Exp. Med. 152:280 (1980).

MOLECULAR INTERACTIONS IN T-CELL MEDIATED CYTOTOXICITY: DISCRIMINATION BETWEEN THE BINDING AND LETHAL HIT STAGES OF CYTOLYSIS

Benjamin Bonavida

Department of Microbiology and Immunology
UCLA School of Medicine
University of California
Los Angeles, California 90024

INTRODUCTION

The role of cytotoxic T lymphocytes (CTL) in immunity has been well documented. The exact mechanism, however, by which a CTL kills a corresponding target cell is not known. Several studies have investigated the mechanism of lysis using different probes and these have been reviewed extensively (1-4). These studies showed that T-cell-mediated cytotoxicity (CMC) can be resolved into at least three distinct steps, namely recognition or binding, programming for lysis or the lethal hit, and target cell disintegration in the so-called lymphocyte-independent phase. These studies have therefore suggested that multiple cell-cell interactions between effector cell (EC) and target cell (TC) may be involved in cytolysis.

Although our understanding of the physiological requirements and the cellular processes in CTL-mediated cytolysis has been greatly enlightened by recent studies, the molecular mechanism involved in target cell lysis remains to be resolved. Several different approaches have been adopted for the study of cell surface molecules of CTL involved in target cell lysis, such as the role of the T cell idiotype, the role of protease inhibitors, and the effect of blocking antibody directed against CTL (5).

Our laboratory has chosen the antibody blocking approach to delineate the biochemical nature of CTL-associated antigens involved in lysis. Our rationale is that if a particular antiserum inhibits the lysis of target cells by CTL, then it may be inferred that the cell surface determinants on CTL recognized by the antibodies may be involved in the cytolytic process. Consequently, we have analyzed functionally and biochemically two blocking antisera, namely anti-Lyt 2 antibodies and a xenogeneic rat anti-CTL serum (RAT*). In this manuscript, we will only summarize our findings to date and present the salient features of our systems.

MATERIALS AND METHODS

These have been described in detail elsewhere (6-9).

RESULTS AND DISCUSSION

Blocking by Lyt-2 Antibodies

Blocking of Recognition by Lyt-2 Antibodies. Several independent groups have recently reported that the addition of Lyt-2 antibodies to a CTL cytotoxic reaction resulted in inhibition of the CMC in the absence of exogeneous complement (10-11). The mechanism, however, of the α-Lyt-2 mediated inhibition was not known and was therefore extensively analyzed in our laboratory. Two main questions were investigated, namely (a) the stage(s) during the cytolytic process at which the inhibitory activity of the anti-Lyt 2 antibodies was manifested and (b) whether the expression and loss of Lyt-2 antigens on CTL correlated strongly with the functional expression of CTL-mediated cytotoxicity.

(a) The first question pertaining to the stage at which anti-Lyt-2 antibodies inhibit cytolysis was examined using different experimental designs and taking advantage of the single cell cytotoxicity assay (12). Several characteristics of the anti-Lyt-2 antibody mediated inhibiton of T-CMC were examined (7) and are summarized in Table I. The results of such experiments showed clearly that α-Lyt-2 antibodies inhibit the formation of conjugates but have no effect on lysis once binding takes place. Therefore, α-Lyt-2 inhibits the recognition step of CTL mediated target cell lysis. These results suggested that Lyt-2 antigens or closely associated molecules are important in the recognition phase of T-CMC.

(b) The above studies showed that α-Lyt-2 antibodies interfere with the initial recognition step in cytolysis, thus preventing a subsequent phase of the cytotoxic pathway to take place. Based on these findings, it was predicted that in cases whereby Lyt-2 antigens are removed, binding or lysis by CTL should not take place. This prediction was examined and verified (9). Thus, CTL treatment with trypsin was shown to selectively remove Lyt-2 antigens from CTL. The antigens Lyt-1, H-2, and Thy 1.2 were trypsin resistant under the conditions used. Furthermore, it was found that Lyt-2 antigens of CTL recover quickly following trypsin treatment and that the appearance of Lyt-2 antigens paralleled the recovery of

Table I

CHARACTERIZATION OF ANTI-LYT-2 ANTIBODY MEDIATED INHIBITION OF T-CMC

1. Anti-Lyt-2 antibodies from allogeneic or monoclonal sources inhibit T-CMC (derived from _in vivo_ or _in vitro_) in the absence of complement.

2. Inhibition by anti-Lyt-2 is directed against the Lyt-2^+ CTL.

3. Inhibition by Lyt-2 antibodies is not H-2 restricted and effective against all strains of mice tested.

4. Lyt-2 antibodies inhibit LDCC and ODCC by CTL.

5. Lyt-2 antibodies inhibit the initial formation of lymphocyte-target cell conjugates.

6. Addition of α-Lyt-2 antibodies to preformed conjugates do not inhibit lysis as tested in the single cell cytotoxicity assays and in assays preventing recycling.

7. There is a good correlation between Lyt-2 expression and cytotoxicity as follows:

   a. Trypsin treatment of CTL removes selectively Lyt-2 but not Lyt-1, H-2, or Thy 1.2 antigens and results in failure of CTL to form conjugates and mediate lysis.

   b. Kinetics of recovery of Lyt-2 antigens parallels the ability of CTL to form conjugates and mediate lysis.

conjugate formation and lysis (Table I). Clearly, these findings suggested that there exists a good correlation between the presence of Lyt-2 antigens and the ability to form conjugates and corroborate the above findings in section (a). The trypsin experiments suggest that since not all cell surface proteins are removed by trypsin digestion, the association between the expression of Lyt-2 antigens and the functional activities of PEL are not fortuitous. However, the findings do not eliminate the possibility that some additional membrane associated molecules susceptible to hydrolysis by trypsin may also be involved in lysis.

What is the Role of Lyt-2 Antigens of CTL? Clearly, Lyt-2^+ CTL seem to require Lyt-2 antigens or closely associated antigens to initiate cell-cell contact with target cells. Two questions arise, namely, the functional role of Lyt-2 antigens in Lyt-2^+ CTL and how Lyt-2^- CTL mediate their recognition and cytolysis.

It is possible that the observed inhibition of cytotoxicity by Lyt antisera may be attributed to the fact that Lyt-2 antigens are closely linked to or are integrated parts of a molecule such as the antigen receptor. Thus, Lyt-2 antibodies may block antigen receptor function by steric hindrance. The steric hindrance must be specific for Lyt-2 antigens since other antibodies directed against CTL associated antigens such as Lyt-1, H-2, and Thy 1.2 do not inhibit CTL function. Alternatively, Lyt-2 antigens may be involved in the binding, serving as an anchoring device in Lyt-2^+ CTL.

Cytotoxic CTL which are Lyt-1^+2^- have been directed primarily against the I-region determinants of the MHC. The fact that these cells or CTL clones are cytotoxic suggests that Lyt-2 antigens are not involved in lysis in this system. Therefore, if the anchoring hypothesis is correct, it may be that the nature of target antigens recognized by CTL dictates the requirement of CTL associated molecules in binding.

Blocking by RAT* Antibodies

Blocking of the Lethal Hit Stage of Lysis by RAT* Serum. We have recently reported that a xenoantiserum, RAT* serum, directed against CTL can inhibit CTL cytolysis at the lethal hit stage of cytolysis (6,8). Several studies have been performed to analyze the blocking phenomenon and to biochemically characterize the CTL-associated molecules recognized by RAT* serum.

The inhibition of T-CMC by RAT* revealed that it occurs at the post-recognition stage or the lethal hit stage of lysis. This conclusion was based on two main observations: (a) The antiserum did not alter CTL-target conjugates when added before and after interaction of CTL to target cells and (b) the antiserum was inhibitory when added after binding took place and at the Ca^{++}-dependent stage of lysis. Thus, RAT* serum, in contrast to α-Lyt-2 antibodies, inhibits the post-binding events. Several additional characteristics of the blocking activity by RAT* serum are summarized in Table II.

These results suggested that RAT* serum inhibition of CTL lysis may be due to interference in the mechanism of lysis. Therefore, biochemical analyses were performed to delineate the nature of CTL associated molecules recognized by RAT* and which be involved in lysis.

Biochemical Analysis of CTL Membrane Antigens Recognized by RAT* Antibody. We have initiated studies to characterize the molecular nature of antigens recognized by RAT* serum. Cell surface glycoproteins were radiolabeled by sodium periodate and tritiated borohydride or by lactoperoxidase ^{125}I iodination. Detergent solubilized radiolabeled cell surface proteins were immunoprecipitated

Table II

SUMMARY OF FINDINGS WITH RAT* SERUM AND MONOCLONAL ANTIBODIES

Blocking Activity

1. After extensive absorption on tumor cells (P815) and thymocytes, RAT* serum reacts with PEL-CTL > spleen T > B cells > thymocytes as analyzed by FACS.

2. RAT* serum blocks T-CMC (antigen specific and nonspecific) in the absence of C'.

3. Blocking is at the level of the effector T cells.

4. Blocking is seen by IgG and $(Fab')_2$ derived from CTL. Blocking is seen by monoclonal antibodies.

5. Blocking is not idiotype specific.

6. The blocking activity of RAT* serum is not removed by absorption with thymocytes but is removed by CTL.

7. Blocking is primarily at the post-binding phase during the lethal hit stage of lysis.

Biochemical Analyses

1. Cell free extract from CTL neutralizes the blocking activity of RAT* IgG. Selectivity in neutralization is observed.

2. Immunoprecipitation patterns on reduced SDS gels.

   a. ^{125}I-labeled CTL results in precipitating one band of 95K.

   b. Label with $^{3}HBH_4$ of low specific activity results in two bands of 95K & 180K.

   c. Label with $^{3}HBH_4$ of high specific activity results in three major bands of 95K, 140K, and 180K.

   d. Label with ^{125}I-lactoperoxidase results in three major bands of 95K, 140K, and 180K.

3. Major bands are glycoproteins as determined by trypsin treatment.

4. Absorption of RAT* IgG by CTL but not thymocytes removes all three bands.

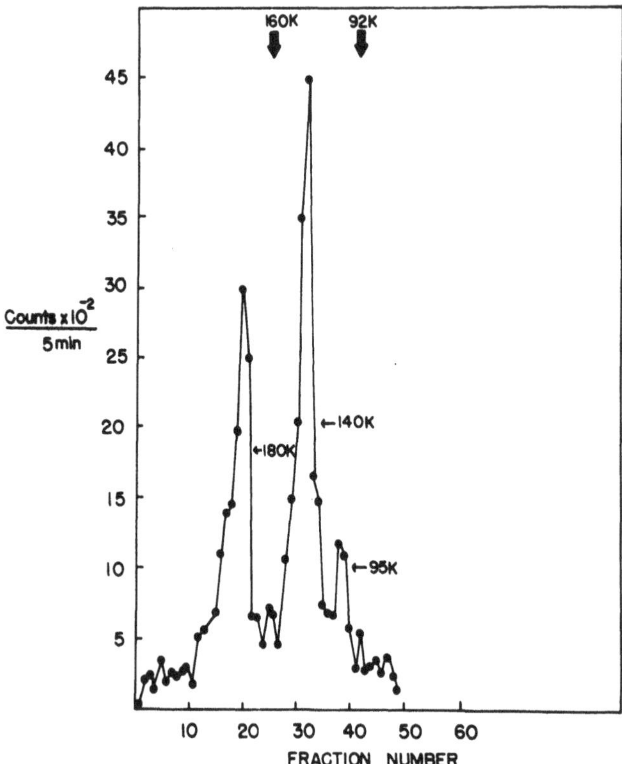

Fig. 1. Immunoprecipitation of periodate-oxidized CTL radiolabeled with $^3HBH_4$. The solubilized membranes are immunoprecipitated with staphylococcus A and analyzed on 7.5-15% gradient SDS gel.

with RAT* serum and analyzed on SDS-PAGE. The findings of Wexler et al (13) and Hiserodt et al (14) demonstrate that three major glycoproteins of CTL are reacting with the RAT* serum and/or its IgG fraction. Molecules of 95,000, 140,000, and 180,000 daltons are resolved by SDS-PAGE under reduced or non-reduced conditions (Figure 1). The inhibitory activity of RAT* serum as well as its abiity to immunoprecipitate the three glycoproteins is removed by absorption with CTL populations but not with thymocytes. These results suggest that these three glycoproteins may be involved in the mechanism of lysis. Of interest, independently Kurzinger et al (15) have produced a monoclonal antibody (M7/16) that inhibited CTL killing at the binding phase. It immunoprecipitated two glycoproteins of 95,000 and 180,000 daltons. Moreover, Pierres et al (16) have also reported similar findings except that the monoclonal antibody blocks CTL at the lethal hit stage. It is not clear at the present time the relationship between our findings and those of others. Further studies should delineate the role of CTL molecules in the mechanism of lysis.

Comparison Between Antigen Specific CMC (SCMC) and Antigen Non-specific LDCC and ODCC

The above studies done in the antigen specific system have also been compared to the antigen nonspecific cytotoxicity system (7-9). The results of these studies showed that both α-Lyt-2 and RAT* antibodies block LDCC and ODCC. The various parameters used for SCMC were also true for LDCC and ODCC. Thus, it appears that the mechanism of both SCMC and LDCC are similar and share similar molecular interactions leading to lysis.

How do our findings help in the elucidation of the mechanisms of LDCC and ODCC? The studies show that a common mechanism or molecular interaction is involved in the triggering of the cytolytic process. Thus, if CMC is viewed as a multi-stage process involving multiple interactions, LDCC and ODCC can also be viewed as being the result of bypassing antigen-receptor recognition by the lectin. A model exlaining this system has been proposed by several investigators who have suggested that the lectin serves to bridge or glue effector to target cell and to activate the effector cell (17-19). The model proposes a requirement for lectin to initiate contact between effector cell to target cell and to activate the CTL through a specific lectin receptor: the lectin may be part of the antige receptor or may be a different molecule. This bridging and and activation model is supported by a variety

Table III

EVIDENCE SUPPORTING THE BRIDGING-ACTIVATION MODEL IN LDCC AND ODCC

1. Requirement for T cell mitogens to mediate LDCC and ODCC suggesting activation.

2. Pretreatment of effector cells with most lectins or by modification with IO_4 leads to LDCC and ODCC.

3. Blocking of CMC by antibodies directed against binding or lethal hit stages of lysis suggesting interaction in addition to antigen/receptor recognition in lysis.

EVIDENCE SUPPORTING THE RECEPTOR-MHC MODEL

1. Blocking of LDCC and ODCC by anti-H-2 sera directed against target cells.

2. Poor LDCC with $H\text{-}2^-$ targets.

of experimental findings. On the other hand an alternate model has been proposed by Berke et al (20-21) that suggests LDCC is the result of interaction of the antigen receptor with lectin modified MHC antigens on the target cell. Clearly, the focus of the bridging-activation model has been at the level of the cytotoxic cell and the strength of the receptor-MHC model has been directed at the level of the target cell (22). Table III summarizes the evidence for both models.

Concluding Remarks

The approaches used in these studies with antibody blocking reagents have been adopted in an effort to unravel the molecular basis of CTL-mediated target cell lysis. The blocking of the lethal hit step by RAT* serum suggests that the "programming for lysis" step may be a molecular activation step in which the expression of the lytic component takes place. What is the nature of this lytic step? Several studies have suggested the involvement of enzymes such as proteases, phospholipases or lypmphotoxins (23-26). Such moieties may be triggered by the target or lectin and may directly or through a soluble mediator induce the lytic reaction. The notion of soluble mediators in CTL mediated cytotoxicity has been entertained but never proven. The closest that our laboratory has come to implicating a role of soluble cytotoxic mediators in cell-mediated cytotoxicity has been in the natural killer system (27-28). Such studies are described by us in a separate paper in this volume.

SUMMARY

The molecular characterization of cytotoxic T lymphocyte (CTL) associated membrane antigens that may be involved in the mechanism of lysis has been investigated. This was achieved by the generation and characterization of antibodies that block cell-mediated cytotoxicity (CMC) at either the recognition/binding or the lethal hit stages of the lytic event. Thus, Lyt-2 blocking antibodies were shown to inhibit CTL-target binding and RAT* (rat anti-mouse T cells) antibodies were shown to inhibit the lethal hit stage of lysis.

Blocking of CTL by anti-Lyt-2 antibodies was achieved with both allogeneic antiserum and monoclonal antibodies. Blocking was shown to affect the effector CTL and was specific such that other allo-antisera directed against CTL (e.g., anti-Lyt 1, anti-H-2, anti-Thy 1.2) were not inhibitory. The mechanism of inhibition by anti-Lyt 2 antibodies indicated that (1) the addition of Lyt 2 antibodies before the formation of lymphocyte-target cell conjugates resulted in reduction of the frequency of conjugates; (2) the addition of Lyt 2 antibodies after conjugate formation did not result in either dissociation of the conjugates or inhibition of lysis of bound targets; (3) trypsin treatment of CTL removed selectively Lyt 2 antigens (but not Lyt 1, H-2, Thy 1.2 antigens) and inhibited conjugate formation and lysis; (4) recovery of Lyt 2 antigens from trypsin treated CTL was directly correlated with recovery of CTL-mediated binding to target cell and cytolysis. These studies showed that Lyt 2 alloantigens or closely linked determinants of CTL appear to be involved in the binding or recognition step of the cytolytic process.

Blocking of CTL by RAT* serum absorbed with various tissues was shown to be directed at the CTL, and was devoid of any activity against target cells. The mechanism of blocking by RAT* serum revealed that (1) blocking is not idiotype specific; (2) it did not inhibit lymphocyte-target cell conjugates, and (3) it inhibits the lethal hit stage of cytolysis. Biochemical characterization showed that RAT* serum recognized three major glycoproteins on CTL of 90, 140, and 180,000 Mr. These studies showed that RAT* antibodies inhibit the lethal hit of cytolysis and that the three major glycoproteins recognized by RAT* may be involved, all or in part, in the lethal hit step of cytolysis.

We have also investigated the mechanism of antigen-nonspecific CMC in both lectin-dependent cellular cytotoxicity (LDCC) and oxidation-dependent cellular cytotoxicity (ODCC). The results obtained with Lyt 2 and RAT* blocking antibodies indicated that both antigen-specific and antigen-nonspecific cytotoxicity by T cells share similar pathways in the process of lysis.

In conclusion, we have shown that blockig antibodies may be used as probes in the delineation of the various stages involved in lysis and in the molecular determination of CTL associated molecules required for lysis. These studies should contribute to a better understanding of the mechanism of T-cell mediated cytotoxicity.

REFERENCES

1. Berke, G. Prog. Allergy 27:69 (1980).

2. Golstein, P., and E.T. Smith. Contemp. Top. Immunobiol. 7:273 (1977).

3. Henney, C.S. Contemp. Top. Immunobiol. 7:245 (1977).

4. Martz, E. Contemp. Top. Immunobiol. 7:301 (1977).

5. Bonavida, B., Fan, J., and J.C. Hiserodt. Membrane antigens of cytotoxic T lymphocytes associated with cytotoxic function. Immunology Today, in press (1982).

6. Effros, R.B., Hiserodt, J.C., and B. Bonavida. J. Immunol. 125:1879 (1980).

7. Fan, J., Ahmed, A., and B. Bonavida. J. Immunol. 125:2444 (1980).

8. Hiserodt, J.C., and B. Bonavida. J. Immunol. 125:256 (1981).

9. Fan, J., and B. Bonavida. J. Immuno. 127:1856 (1981).

10. Nakayama, E.H., Shiku, H., Stockert, E., Oettgen, H.F., and L.J. Old. Proc. Natl. Acad. Sci. 76:1977 (1979).

11. Shinohara, N., and D.H. Sachs. J. Exp. Med. 150:432 (1979).

12. Grimm, E.A., and B. Bonavida. J. Immunol. 123:2861 (1979).

13. Wexler, H., Fan, J., Hiserodt, J.C., and B. Bonavida. Submitted.

14. Hiserodt, J.C., Fan, J., Wexler, H., and B. Bonavida. Submitted.

15. Kurzinger, K., Teynold, T., Germain, R.N., Davignon, D., Martz, E., and T.A. Springer. J. Immunol. 127:596 (1981).

16. Pierres, M., Goridis, C., and P. Golstein. Eur. J. Immunol. In press (1981).

17. Bonavida, B., and T.P. Bradley. Transplantation 21:94 (1976).

18. Gately, M.K., and E. Martz. J. Immunol. 119:1711 (1977).

19. Green, W.R., Ballas, Z.K., and C.S. Henney. J. Immunol. 121:1566 (1978).

20. Berke, G., Hu, V., McVey, E., and W.R. Clark. J. Immunol. 127:776 (1981).

21. Berke, G., McVey, E., Hu, V., and W.R. Clark. J. Immunol. 127:782 (1981).

22. Bonavida, B. Letter to the Editor. J. Immunol. In Press.

23. Hudig, D., Haverty, T., Fulcher, C., Redelman, D., and J. Mendelsohn. J. Immunol. 126:1569 (1981).

24. Hatcher, V.B., Oberman, M.S., Lazarus, G.S., and A.I. Grayzel. J. Immunol. 120:665 (1978).

25. Frye, L.D., and G.J. Friou. Nature 258:833 (1975).

26. Granger, G.A., Hiserodt, J.C., and C.F. Ware. In "Biology of Lymphokines" Edited by S. Cohen, E. Pick, and J.J. Oppenheim. Academic Press, New York, p. 141 (1979).

27. Wright, S.C., and B. Bonavida. J. Immunol. 126:1516 (1981).

28. Wright, S.C., Hiserodt, J.C., and B. Bonavida. Transpl. Proceed. 13:770 (1981).

DISCUSSION

P. Golstein

This anti-serum that you are working with is a rat anti-mouse anti-serum, and it should contain some of the antibodies -- equivalent to the monoclonal antibodies -- that people have been working with. It should contain, for example, an H35-89.9 mAb equivalent, or one equivalent to Eric's. So it is not really a surprise that you should immunoprecipitate the two same bands with the antiserum. What is perhaps more surprising is the functional data, because your anti-serum has been reported to block not only at the post-recognition phase but actually at the post-lethal hit phase; i.e., after EDTA. This is something that we have never observed. For instance, H35-89.9 mAb or the other monoclonals never block at post-EDTA. So maybe you're dealing with other antibodies in addition to those that have been characterized in terms of immunoprecipitated products.

B. Bonavida

This is very true. We cannot go only by analysis of molecular weight of precipitated products. The activity we described on post-binding events may have absolutely nothing to do with what we define by immuno-precipitation. One is a molecular weight profile and one is a biological activity, which may or may not have anything to do with each other. Until we get monoclonal antibodies that would have an activity on the lethal hit, I think identity of the two would be at this point speculative.

R. Herberman

What about the effect of your antibody on NK functions?

B. Bonavida

We've noticed that the original serum we have generated does block NK both in the ^{51}Cr assay and also by neutralizing the NK cytotoxic factor. But we also notice that different batches of serum block NK activity variably.

APPENDIX

Prior to the Workshop, participants were asked to submit one or two questions that they felt should be discussed at some point in the proceedings. A list of these questions was distributed to each session chairman to use if discussion seemed to be lagging. As it turned out, there were never any gaps in the presentations or subsequent arguments that needed filling. However, as an indication to the community at large of what the participants felt were some of the crucial questions in cytotoxicity, an abbreviated list is presented below.

Complement and ADCC

Is there any indication of Ca^{++} flux in ADCC?

Can we be absolutely sure that ADCC does not involve complement? I.e., could complement components be produced by the effector cell and secreted locally?

NK

Are NK cells specific? Are NK cells part of the T cell lineage?

CTL

How is it possible to distinguish between recognition systems and effector mechanisms in cell-mediated cytolysis?

What are the post-recognition requirements to mediate lysis?

How can the role of calcium in cell-mediated cytolysis be further defined?

Is there a role for soluble mediators in cytotoxicity?

Are extracellular mediators of cytolysis secreted products or shed membrane fragments?

Does T kill involve a stimulus-secretion process?

Can cell surface associated and/or extracellular proteases mediate target lysis directly through limited proteolysis, or indirectly by regulation of superoxide formation or phospholipase activation?

Is lysis caused by a membrane enzyme fixed in the CTL surface, or by a releasable lymphotoxin-like substance?

How much is a mechanical process (related to CTL mobility in the area of TC contact) excluded as a mechanism for the lethal hit itself?

Is there any compelling evidence for a CTL lytic apparatus distinct from the T cell receptor?

Is there transfer of components between killer and target membrane?

Do cell surface recognition molecules, on either killer cells or targets, have a direct lytic potential, either prior to or as a consequence of, specific conjugate formation?

LDCC, Target Antigens, Role of the Target Cell

Is lectin induced kill identical to specific kill except for a bypass of specific recognition?

Do all cytolytic mechanisms involve target cell MHC proteins?

What makes a target a "good" target?

mAb, Clones and Hybridomas

How can CTL clones be reactivated in order to express their specific cytotoxic function.

Do Lyt 2 antigens play an important role in cytolysis?

What killer and/or target cell molecules are involved/required for lysis?

Do CTL express differentiation antigens involved in cytolysis?

What have we learnt about CTL mechanism from hybridomas and/or clones?

PARTICIPANTS

A.C. ALLISON[1]	Centre d'Immunologie INSERM-CNRS de Marseille-Luminy, Case 906, 13288 Marseille cedex 9, France.
G. BERKE	Department of Cell Biology, The Weizmann Institute of Science POB 26, Rehovot 76100, Israel.
B. BONAVIDA	Department of Microbiology and Immunology, UCLA Los Angeles, CA 90024, USA.
P. BONGRAND	Laboratoire d'Immunologie, Hopital Ste. Marguerite, B.P. 29, 13274 Marseille cedex 9, France.
B.D. BRONDZ[2]	Cancer Research Center, Karchirskoye Chaussee 6 Moscow 115 478, USSR.
M. CASTELLAZZI	Institut de Recherches en Biologie Moleculaire, Unite de Genetique Cellulaire, 2 Place Jussieu, 75221 Paris cedex 5, France.
W.R. CLARK	Molecular Biology Institute, UCLA Los Angeles, CA 90024, USA
F.W. FITCH	Department of Pathology University of Chicago 950 East 59th Street Chicago, IL 60637, USA.
R. FRADE	Institut de Cancerologie et d'Immunogenetique, 16 Av. P.-V. Couturier, 94804 Villejuif cedex, France.
B. GENETET	Centre Regional de Transfusion Sanguine, Rue Pierre Jean Gineste, 35000 Rennes, France.
A.L. GLASEBROOK	Swiss Institute for Experimental Cancer Research Chemin des Boveresses, CH-1066 Epalinges s/Lausanne, Switzerland

R. GOLDFARB	Immunology and Infectious Disease Central Research Pfizer, Inc., Groton, Connecticut 06340, USA.
P. GOLSTEIN	Centre d'Immunologie INSERM-CNRS de Marseille-Luminy, Case 906, 13288 Marseille cedex 9, France.
W.R. GREEN	Fred Hutchinson Cancer Research Center, 1124 Columbia Street, Seattle, WA 98104, USA.
M.G. HANNA	Frederick Cancer Research Center Frederick, MD 21701, USA.
M. HENKART	Immunology Branch, National Cancer Institute, NIH Bethesda, MD 20205 USA
P. HENKART	Immunology Branch, National Cancer Institute, NIH, Bethesda, MD 20205, USA.
C.S. HENNEY	Fred Hutchinson Cancer Research Center, 1124 Columbia Street, Seattle, WA 98104, USA.
R.B. HERBERMAN	Laboratory of Immunodiagnosis, National Cancer Institute, NIH, Bethesda, MD 20205, USA.
V. HU	Department of Biochemistry, School of Medicine, Uniformed Services, University of the Health Sciences, 4301 Jones Bridge Road, Bethesda, MD 20014, USA.
Y. KAUFMANN	Department of Cell Biology, The Weizmann Institute of Science, POB 26, Rehovot 76100, Israel.
R. KIESSLING	Department of Tumor Biology, Karolinska Institute, S 104 01 Stockholm, Sweden.
P.J. LACHMANN	MRC Centre, Hills Road, Cambridge CB2 2QN, England.
S. LADISCH[3]	Ludwig Institute for Cancer Research, Chemin des Bouveresses, CH-1066 Epalinges s/Lausanne, Switzerland.
S. LEVY	Institut d'Hematologie, Faculte de Medecine, 1 Place de l'Hopital, 67000 Strasbourg, France.
T.J. LINNA	Experimental Station, Central Research and Development Department, E.I. Du Pont Company, Wilmington, Delaware 19898, USA.

H.R. MAC DONALD	Ludwig Institute for Cancer Research, Chemin des Boveresses, CH-1066 Epalinges s/Lausanne, Switzerland.
I.C.M. MAC LENNAN	Department of Immunology, The Medical School, Vincent Drive, Birmingham B15 2TJ, England.
B. MALISSEN	Centre d'Immunologie INSERM-CNRS de Marseille-Luminy, Case 906, 13288 Marseille cedex 9, France.
E. MARTZ	Department of Microbiology, University of Massachusetts, Amhert, Massachusetts 01003, USA.
M.M. MAYER	Johns Hopkins School of Medicine, 725 N. Wolfe Street, Baltimore, MD 21205, USA.
M.M. MESCHER	Department of Pharmacology, Harvard Medical School, 25 Shattuck Street, Boston, MS 02115, USA.
M. NABHOLZ	Swiss Institute for Experimental Cancer Research, Chemin des Boveresses, CH-1066 Epalinges s/Lausanne, Switzerland.
C.F. NATHAN	Rockerfeller University, 1230 York Avenue, New York, NY 10021, USA.
P. PERLMANN	Department of Immunology, University of Stockholm, S-10691 Stockholm, Sweden.
M. PIERRES	Centre d'Immunologie INSERM-CNRS de Marseille-Luminy, Case 906, 13288 Marseille cedex 9, France.
J.E. RYSER	Department of Pathology, Faculte de Medecine, Universite de Geneve, 40 Bd. de la Cluse, 1211 Geneva 4, Switzerland.
C. SANDERSON	Division of Immunology, National Institute for Medical Research, Mill Hill, London NW7 1AA, England.
A.M. SCHMITT-VERHULST	Centre d'Immunologie INSERM-CNRS de Marseille-Luminy, Case 906, 13288 Marseille cedex 9, France.
A. SILVA	Swiss Institute for Experimental Cancer Research, Chemin des Boveresses, CH-1066 Epalinges s/Lausanne Switzerland.
E. SIMPSON	Clinical Research Centre, Watford Road, Harrow, Middlesex HA1 3UJ, England.

S.R. TARGAN Department of Microbiology and Immunology, UCLA, Los Angeles, CA 90024, USA.

D. ZAGURY Universite Pierre et Marie Curie, UER 61, 4, Place Jussieu - Tour 32, 75005 Paris, France.

[1]Present address: Syntex Research Corp., Palo Alto, California, USA.

[2]Dr. Brondz, who was planning to attend the Workshop, was not allowed to do so by the USSR Ministry of Health. He was, however, allowed to submit a written contribution to this volume.

[3]Present address: Dept. Pediatrics, UCLA School of Medicine, Los Angeles, CA 90024 USA.

INDEX

GPSR Compliance
The European Union's (EU) General Product Safety Regulation (GPSR) is a set of rules that requires consumer products to be safe and our obligations to ensure this.

If you have any concerns about our products, you can contact us on

ProductSafety@springernature.com

In case Publisher is established outside the EU, the EU authorized representative is:

Springer Nature Customer Service Center GmbH
Europaplatz 3
69115 Heidelberg, Germany

www.ingramcontent.com/pod-product-compliance
Ingram Content Group UK Ltd.
Pitfield, Milton Keynes, MK11 3LW, UK
UKHW051131260726
13967UKWH00010B/2990
* 9 7 8 1 4 6 8 4 8 9 6 0 6 *